DEPRESSION, STRESS, AND ADAPTATIONS IN THE ELDERLY

Psychological Assessment and Intervention

P.S. Fry, Ph.D.
Professor of Educational Psychology
Chairman of Developmental Studies
University of Calgary
Calgary, Alberta, Canada

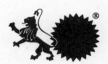

AN ASPEN PUBLICATION®
Aspen Publishers, Inc.
Rockville, Maryland
Royal Tunbridge Wells
1986

Library of Congress Cataloging in Publication Data

Fry, Prem S.
Depression, stress, and adaptation in the elderly.

"An Aspen publication."
Includes bibliographies and index.
1. Geriatric psychiatry. I. Title. [DNLM: 1. Adaptation, Psychological—in old age.
2. Aged—psychology. 3. Aging. 4. Depression—in old age. 5. Stress, Psychological—in
old age. WT 150 F947d]
RC451.4.A5F79   1986   618.97′689   85-30673
ISBN: 0-87189-255-3

Editorial Services: Jane Coyle

Library of Congress Catalog Card Number: 85-30673
ISBN: 0-87189-255-3

Printed in the United States of America

1 2 3 4 5

This book is warmly dedicated to

my mother *Kishni Dua*
my mother-in-law *Ann Fry*

and to

the loving memory of my father *Beharilal Dua*
and my father-in-law *Johann Justus Fry*

Table of Contents

Preface

The aging process is often conceptualized as a gradual, downward trajectory with ever-increasing levels of inadequacy, impairment, and physical and psychological decline. This has led to widespread myths and misconceptions concerning the utility and feasibility of assessing and treating the psychological problems and disorders of the elderly. The highly negative views of the functional disorders of the elderly and their depression and stresses tend to confound caregivers and trained mental health professionals and ultimately contribute to poor care of the aged. Bias against the elderly and the scant attention paid by behavioral scientists to their problems of depression and stress reaffirm in the elderly an all-too-common self-perception that they are not fully capable of independent living, problem solving, and decision making.

The elderly are especially endangered as a result of the medical view that the aged suffer from many untreatable and irreversible conditions. Because of this notion the distinctions between the treatable and nontreatable aspects of psychological disorders are often ignored in the clinical assessment of a majority of the elderly. Frequently insufficient time is spent in formulating the goals of assessment or in distinguishing the relatively mild and benign changes of normal aging from the severe disruptions of function. Because of the prejudiced nature of the health care system, the elderly are often overmedicated with drugs and pharmaceutical preparations that cause more damage than good. Although depression and stress reactions are widespread among the elderly, they go largely unrecognized, and if recognized, they are frequently susceptible to misdiagnosis and mistreatment.

Persons over the age of 65 constitute about 17 percent of the population, and approximately one-quarter of the 24 million older citizens are said to have medical and psychological problems severe enough to warrant professional attention. There is a critical shortage of mental health professionals with adequate training and skills of demonstrated value to offer the elderly. If applied systematically, the considerable knowledge of gerontology will lead to a substantially better understanding of the psychology of aging. There are, however, areas of clinical and behavioral assessment and therapeutic intervention where much has to be learned about goals, procedures, practices, and intervention strategies suitable for the elderly.

The need for increased involvement of researchers and mental health professionals with the aged is undeniable. In most communities there are few clinicians and practitioners with sufficient clinical training and expertise to qualify them for working with the elderly.

ix

Training programs in geropsychology or clinical psychology of aging exist at few universities, and continuing education opportunities in this area are rare. The large discrepancy between the mental health needs of the elderly and the degree to which these needs are being met by professional training institutes and mental health delivery systems has been amply documented by national councils and commissions on aging. The training needs for mental health professionals require that clinical knowledge and research evidence be transmitted to practitioners and those in training. Society does not by and large love and respect the elderly but tends to isolate them and place them in dependent roles. Thus what is urgently needed is an eclectic orientation to intervention and treatment of the elderly that will help them to maintain their independence in the community so that they may determine for themselves the level of care they desire. The major intention of this book is to integrate new developments in assessment and therapy that have specific applications to older persons living in community settings rather than long-term custodial and institutional settings.

This book represents an effort to present in one volume a discussion of the applied multidimensional aspects of the assessment and treatment of depression and stress in the elderly. The book is intended, first and foremost, for mental health practitioners providing care and treatment for depression, stress, and problems of adaptation in the elderly. It is assumed that practitioners have considerable knowledge about the concepts of aging. Hence a discussion of foundational materials, theoretical issues, and controversial research findings has been kept to a minimum. No attempt has been made to curtail the bibliographies, however. Practitioners also need to broaden their perspective on the goals of assessment and integrate their clinical practice with the growing body of up-to-date information on the aging process, late-life depression and stress. Hence, a number of chapters discussing aspects of assessment have been included in the book.

Although written primarily for clinical practitioners, it is hoped that the book will also serve as a useful resource to instructors in clinical psychology of aging, as a comprehensive text to graduate students, and as a reference in all educational programs for the training of mental health professionals in the geriatric field. Other practitioners training in nursing, social work, medical psychology and sociology of aging, and community health services will also find the volume useful.

PLAN OF THE BOOK

This book provides a comprehensive introduction to clinical practice and the psychology of aging. In clinical work with the elderly it is important to recognize that their problems are usually multiple and typically include biological, psychological, physical, and social-environmental components. Because of the widespread myths and apprehensions about what occurs with old age, it is important for professionals to have accurate foundational information about the aging process. In clarifying the multidimensional aspects of the aging process, it is important for mental health practitioners to recognize a biopsychosocial basis for assessment and evaluation. Chapter 1 provides such a theoretical framework for approaching the health care needs of the elderly. It reviews the basic psychobiological changes with normal aging (as distinguished from the more serious disruptions in functioning as a result of disease states) and examines some of the fears, anxieties, and uncertainties that most older persons may experience with aging.

It is reassuring for practitioners to know that clinical practice with older persons is growing in many diverse and exciting ways. New approaches to the assessment and treatment of psychological problems are emerging, and caregivers and clinicians are concerned with developing positive concepts for assessment and treatment that are uniquely relevant and important to problems of late life.

Chapters 2 through 6 present a comprehensive introduction to the goals and principles of assessment as well as the specific issues of assessment and evaluation that are uniquely relevant to clinical practice with the elderly. In clarifying the multidimensional aspects of assessment, Chapter 2 stresses the interaction of physical, social, and psychological problems that tend to characterize the functioning of the elderly and that present serious challenges and demands to professionals who must assess and plan intervention. Special considerations in terms of interviewing procedures, testing procedures, and the absence of age-appropriate norms for most psychological tests are discussed. Special cautions and precautions necessary to the evaluation of mental health status and mental status examinations of the elderly are discussed, and difficulties in neuropsychological and ecological assessment are examined. Because of the multiplicity of problems presented by the elderly clients, the need for multifunctional behavioral assessments is advocated.

Chapters 3 through 6 are organized around specific psychological problems and disorders of importance to the elderly. The specific types of problems (depression, stress reactions, cognitive impairment, functional disorders, and adjustment) are among the most prevalent problems witnessed in the elderly. Each chapter provides an in-depth examination of the psychodynamics of a specific clinical problem and discusses signs, symptoms, assessment procedures, and guidelines for the effective management of the clinical and functional disorder. Figures and tables highlight assessment procedures, therapeutic considerations, and management strategies.

Throughout these chapters the focus is on differentiating the relatively mild and benign disorders of normal aging from the more severe disruptions of functioning associated with organic conditions and disease states. Knowledge of the etiology and course of various disorders such as depression, stress reactions, and cognitive impairment is necessary and will assist the clinician in diagnosing and differentiating the large number of potentially treatable and reversible conditions from the few irreversible ones. Even when impairments are due to irreversible conditions, it is important for the professionals to recognize that it is possible to identify treatable aspects of the irreversible conditions and to train families and support systems to provide adequate care for their elderly members.

In Chapters 7 through 13, therapeutic interventions are discussed, including a review of the special considerations in psychotherapy and intervention with the elderly. Procedures of individual, group, and family therapy are described. Several case studies from the author's experience as a clinician and researcher have been included to illustrate important techniques for the practitioner in training. Since grief, death, and dying constitute the most common source of depression and stress among the elderly, a separate chapter (Chapter 9) is devoted to the understanding and care of the bereaved and dying.

In approaching issues of treatment, a combination of supportive, cognitive-behavioral, and pharmacal therapies are presented in Chapters 8, 10, 11, and 13 as the most effective way of working with the elderly. Although a detailed knowledge of psychopharmacology and pharmacotherapy is not considered the domain of the average mental health practitioner, a basic understanding of pharmacologic medication and its effects is a prerequisite for clinical practitioners working with the elderly. Chapter 12 presents an overview of psychotropic medication and pharmacotherapies. What is strongly emphasized are the broad considerations of the side effects of drugs and the cautions, precautions, and dietary concerns in the pharmacologic treatment of the elderly.

The final chapter of the book (Chapter 14) is devoted to a discussion of future directions in the care of the elderly. Since only 5 percent of the older adults are institutionalized and a majority of the elderly live out their entire life span in the communities, what is suggested is the development of a community-based system of care in which the elderly may determine for themselves the level of care they desire and the extent of control over their lives they wish to exercise. Because of current tendencies to see the aged as confused and helpless, or as needing to be taken care of, institutional treatment and custodial care have become the modal treatment for the elderly. There is a recent, strong trend toward deinstitutionalization of the elderly—a trend that reconfirms the ability of a majority of the elderly to function independently for many years of their later life. With increasing age and physical and cognitive decline, some elderly may need supportive and protective services. It is imperative therefore that issues of home care, social support networks, training of family members as caregivers, and preventive mental health factors be considered at the level of policy making. It is through a community-oriented health care system that the capacities of older persons to live as fully functioning lives as possible can be enhanced.

Acknowledgments

I would like to thank all those who made the completion of this book possible. The project was initially suggested to me by R. Curtis Whitesel, senior editor of Aspen Systems Corporation, who died shortly after helping me develop the plans for this book.

Most of the clinical examples that appear in this book have been drawn from the author's longitudinal research on psychotherapy for depression with the elderly funded by the Social Sciences and Humanities Research Council of Canada (Grant No. 492-83-0020) and the Department of National Health and Welfare, Canada (Grant No. 4558-26-10). I am indebted to these agencies for their financial support and also for the opportunity for clinical application of knowledge to the understanding and care of the elderly.

My experience in working on this book during the past two years has taught me to appreciate the substantial contributions of other people. I recognize how indebted I am to each of them.

I would like to express appreciation to Dr. Clifford M. Christensen and Dr. Nancy J. Osgood, who read much of the text and supplied many helpful, supportive, and useful comments. I wish to thank Lynne Hill, whose patience and skill in typing the manuscript was incomparable—she has labored through several manuscripts in the past three years with unequaled skills—and Margaret J. Samuelson, who always knew where everything was and who gave invaluable help in organizing library materials and references.

I am grateful for the support and consideration given by my family and especially want to thank my husband David, my son Shaun, my sisters Bhag, Sheila, and Shanta, and my brothers-in-law Julian Fry, Yudhishter Malik, and Om Kumar Khurana. I am indebted to my friends Dr. Barry Frost, chairman of the school, community and clinical psychology program, and Barbara J. Tooma, whose encouragement helped me through some rather difficult times.

My education and training have been strongly influenced by Dr. Dorothy L. Harris, who gave me the concepts and tools necessary to be a researcher and clinician.

Anne Gousha, associate editor, Margaret Quinlin, editorial director, and Jane Coyle, senior editor at Aspen Systems Corporation, have been vigilant and supportive throughout the process and have made my association with Aspen a pleasure.

PSF

A Biopsychosocial Approach to the Health Care of the Elderly: Implications for Assessment and Intervention

The geriatric practitioner understands well that the physical and mental health of elderly clients cannot be divorced from their environment and that individuals' physical well-being affects and is affected by their psychological and ecological well-being. The potent impact of psychological and environmental factors on health is particularly evident in the aged because they are often subject to much greater stresses than are younger persons and often have fewer physical, emotional, and material resources with which to withstand them (Coe, 1983).

Many biophysical and psychological sources of these stresses are clearly bound up with environmental factors that tend to increase the aged individuals' sense of isolation and depression. Social factors frequently associated with mental health risks are reduced income, bereavement, diminished mobility, and changes in the neighborhood. Mental health risks and disorders of the elderly are also frequently associated with a high rate of acute and chronic physical illnesses known to produce crippling disability and depression among an increasing percentage of elderly individuals in the seventh and eighth decade of life. An estimated 50 percent of elderly medical patients show mental health problems requiring psychological care just as importantly and urgently as medical care. The frequency with which these multifaceted problems are presented to the geriatric practitioners or geropsychologists will continue to increase to 18 percent to 20 percent of the total population by the year 2020 (Coe, 1983).

It is feared that unless mental health practitioners serving the elderly are prepared to work in close cooperation with medical practitioners and to understand how medical illness can influence the etiology, prognosis, and treatment of psychological problems, the mental health of our senior citizenry is likely to become worse instead of better. To support such an argument, one would only have to adduce data on depression, alcoholism, suicide, and social isolation in the elderly (Bigot & Munnichs, 1978). This trend is not surprising and is often attributed to lack of practitioner interest in gerontological psychosocial concerns and problems.

Elderly people are the victims of widespread prejudice and bias (Coe, 1983). Dealing with the elderly has not been popular with health professionals, who have tended to be nihilistic and have regarded the aged as hopeless, helpless, and unworthy of careful evaluation and treatment (Eisdorfer & Cohen, 1978). Neither the medical profession nor the

1

clinical psychology and mental health profession has been immune to this discrimination. Similar prejudices are found also in the lay public and volunteer workers. Unfortunately even when professionals are committed to the stance of the elderly, they are often unable to provide routine or long-term psychological care. The most glaring impediment to such care and intervention is the professionals' lack of knowledge about clinical gerontology or about biological processes in senescence that have immediate or long-term relevance to the psychological health of the elderly.

This is the problem to which the geriatric practitioners or clinical gerontologists must address themselves. The broader efforts of the profession of psychologists and practitioners as a whole to deal with the mental health needs of older adults require that biological, psychological, and sociological knowledge about the aged be transmitted to the practicing clinician. It is a problem that might best be tackled through the dissemination of a clinically useful biopsychosocial concept of psychological care. Such an approach, if it is to be effective, might be based on the premise of a holistic health care model involving an understanding of biological and psychological aging and the reciprocity of the effects on the health of the elderly.

Problems of assessment and treatment discussed in this book are predicated on the notion that the multifaceted problems of the elderly in the community require a multidisciplinary and multifunctional solution. Geropsychologists, geriatric physicians, and mental health professionals are challenged to coordinate their skills with the services of other health professionals in the community to provide more comprehensive and holistic care to the depressed and stressed elderly.

To meet the challenge, it is imperative that geropsychologists, clinicians, and mental health professionals be knowledgeable about both the psychology and psychobiology of the aged. It is important to understand prevalent late-life disorders and to determine at least generally which derive directly from intrinsic biologic aging and which derive from the interaction of environmental and psychosocial factors.

This chapter addresses some of these foundational questions and prepares the groundwork for a better understanding of the holistic concepts advocated for assessment and treatment of the elderly. This foundational chapter presents the major thesis of the book and emphasizes the need for practitioners to adopt a biopsychosocial approach to assessment and treatment. More specifically stated, this chapter has a threefold purpose: (1) to present a rationale for a biopsychosocial approach to health care of the elderly, (2) to direct the mental health practitioner's attention to some of the critical biological processes of aging and age-related changes having implications for psychological care, and (3) to discuss some well-identified fears and anxieties that frequently characterize the elderly and are thought to predispose them to physical disease and stress.

A detailed discussion of any single aspect is beyond the scope of this foundational chapter. Only those aspects that have immediate and critical relevance for the practitioner are reviewed here.

THE BIOPSYCHOSOCIAL APPROACH TO HEALTH CARE OF THE ELDERLY: THE HOLISTIC CONCEPT

The components of a biopsychosocial framework of psychological care for the elderly gain greater clarity when they are viewed within a specific frame of reference. Our discussion has relevance not only for the 5 percent chronically ill ambulatory elderly for whom comprehensive care must be provided over an extended time. It has even greater significance for the vast proportion of 90 percent to 95 percent of the elderly population who are functioning in the community at a socially acceptable level despite the diagnosis of some measure of mental problems and the presence of mental symptoms. Although many elderly can hold their psychological difficulties in check and balance their physical and psychological energies quite well, there is compelling evidence that many elderly need structured psychological care well beyond the routine expressions of reassurance, support, and sympathy.

Recent research findings attest to the validity of this contention. It has been established beyond doubt that in the elderly population, especially, there is a close relationship between the physical and psychological state—between soma and psyche—and to varying degrees between psyche and soma. A great majority of geriatric health and service professionals subscribe to this hypothesis in principle; yet they have ignored the mandate it carries to adopt a biopsychosocial approach to mental health care. Many primary care professionals believe that the overworked organization of their practice cannot afford a detailed consideration of both the psychological and biological components of the multiple disorders and diseases in the elderly. Others are strong proponents of the view that neither medical disease nor psychological states in the elderly can be treated effectively unless due attention is given to their physical illness, fears, anxieties, depression, emotional liability, and overall psychological status.

This thesis acquires clinical clarity when it is considered in specific relationship to some of the most commonly encountered diseases in old age: coronary heart disease and decline in cerebral blood flow hypertension. These illnesses may intervene only when additional exogenous stress is imposed on a somewhat compromised physiological system (Nowlin & Busse, 1977). The elderly coronary heart patient may often not present with chest pain but instead appear confused and disoriented, giving the impression of severe depression.

Admittedly the precise nature of the interrelationship between the physical risk factors and the psychological events is not fully understood. Nor has it been determined which combination of physical health variables and psychosocial stress phenomena is most pernicious in terms of the elderly person's predisposition to mental disorders or somatic illness.

Generally speaking, the concept of a biopsychosocial framework of health care for the elderly is consistent with Reiser's (1975) biopsychosocial field theory of disease, which emphasizes the interaction and interrelationship of the physical, mental, psychological, and environmental systems. The concept of a biopsychosocial orientation to the health care needs of the aged incorporates Lipowski's (1975) ecological viewpoint, which states that the "study of every disease must include the person, his body, and his human and nonhuman environments as essential components of the total system" (p. 6). The ecological approach is of particular significance in the assessment, evaluation, diagnosis, and management of psychological disorders and dysfunctioning of the elderly.

The determinants of a holistic model of health care relevant to the elderly follow. The specific life-cyle components of the model are adapted and summarized from Lipowski's (1975, pp. 7–11) ecological theory. Figure 1–1 portrays the various components of the biopsychosocial field of the elderly and depicts the multiplicity of the interactions among the biological, social, and psychological dimensions.

Intrapersonal Factors. These involve biological variables, such as age, sex, and constitution, and psychological variables, including personality dimensions, experiences,

Figure 1–1 The Biopsychosocial Field of the Elderly

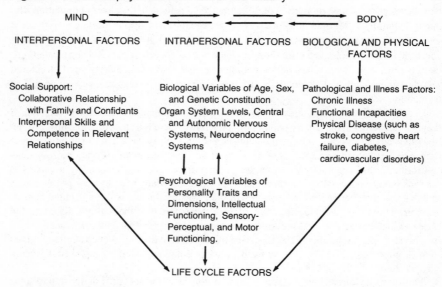

MIND ⟷ ⟷ ⟷ ⟷ BODY

INTERPERSONAL FACTORS   INTRAPERSONAL FACTORS   BIOLOGICAL AND PHYSICAL FACTORS

Social Support:
  Collaborative Relationship
    with Family and Confidants
  Interpersonal Skills and
    Competence in Relevant
    Relationships

Biological Variables of Age, Sex,
  and Genetic Constitution
Organ System Levels, Central
  and Autonomic Nervous
  Systems, Neuroendocrine
  Systems

Pathological and Illness Factors:
  Chronic Illness
  Functional Incapacities
  Physical Disease (such as
    stroke, congestive heart
    failure, diabetes,
    cardiovascular disorders)

Psychological Variables of
  Personality Traits and
  Dimensions, Intellectual
  Functioning, Sensory-
  Perceptual, and Motor
  Functioning.

LIFE CYCLE FACTORS

1. Past social experiences including
   accomplishments and adversities,
   bereavement, stressful events, losses,
   economic instability
2. Past physical experiences including acute
   illness, psychobiological predispositions to
   illness and psychological disorders

3. Current functioning with respect to behavioral
   and intellectual effectiveness; current hopes, and
   motivation; attitudes toward aging
4. Future perspectives including anxieties, fears,
   and depression with respect to future functioning

---

stressful events, losses, grief and bereavement, and prospects for health, safety, and the availability of health care delivery systems. Both these classes of variables inherent in the elderly person include psychobiological predispositions and states as well as those obtaining at the onset of old age and throughout its duration.

Old age frequently adds an important variable influencing the person's responses to illness. As Lipowski (1967, 1973, 1975) notes, some degree of reversible or irreversible brain damage and consequent proneness to cerebral decompensation often complicate physical illness and hospitalization in individuals over the age of 65. Lipowski (1975, p. 8) observes that cognitive disorganization impairs rational evaluation of the illness and the environment and adds a source of psychological stress and disorganizing anxiety. In old age especially, the individual is more likely to be affected by any chronic disability that enforces dependence on others and interferes with daily activity. In the opinion of most gerontologists such stress and anxiety must not be overlooked in the holistically oriented biopsychosocial approach to the health care of the elderly.

The patient's psychobiological state at the onset of old age must be taken into account and so must the stability of the person's life situations, economically, socially, and emotionally. It has been observed that the greater the magnitude of life changes, losses, related conflicts, and adaptive demands (Rahe, 1972), the more vulnerable is the elderly person to problems of mental and physical ill health. This suggests that psychosocial stress plays a dual role, first in enhancing the elderly person's susceptibility to illness and second in impairing the host's capacity to cope with it physiologically and psychologically.

Interpersonal Factors. These factors are concerned with examining the nature of the elderly person's relationship with other people, especially family members, social support agents, case workers, and other health care professionals (Busse, 1975).

In old age especially, loss of important relationships resulting in widowhood, grief, and bereavement is said to precipitate despair and the concomitant effects of hopelessness and helplessness (Maddison & Viola, 1968; Parkes, 1972; Rees & Lutkins, 1967). Beginning with Engel's (1962) work on a unified concept of health and disease, increasing attention has been given to the crucial importance of monitoring family relationships in order to influence the course of mental health. Other relevant relationships include those with employers, friends, and neighbors who are a vital part of the elderly person's social milieu.

Sociocultural and Economic Factors. These factors represent the values and attitudes that the elderly themselves and the relatives and health care professionals have toward aging and old age. The values include the attitudes toward the social role and social value of the elderly in the society in general and in the immediate social milieu. Knowledge about reversible and irreversible physical and emotional conditions of old age varies with socioeconomic groupings. Members of the lower socioeconomic groups especially have anticipitory fears of poverty, abandonment, and rejection by family and friends. Such fears intensify their anxiety. Attitudes toward old age in the elderly person's social milieu influence the person's determination to live life to its fullest or to withdraw socially and emotionally.

Pathology and Illness-Related Factors. These factors represent functional incapacities, physical handicaps, chronic illness, and physical disease and injury. The subjective meaning of these factors for the elderly person in relation to the past history of physical and emotional health and the present adaptive capacities to adjust to chronic illness are important determinants of psychological health. Any disease, injury, or disability that jeopardizes or destroys the person's positive image of physical or intellectual strength has intense personal and subjective meaning for the elderly and makes the person more vulnerable to frustration, agitation, and conflict. The attitudes of the elderly person's physician toward handicaps and the prospects for rehabilitation invariably influence the course and outcome of the rehabilitation process.

Nonhuman Environmental Factors. These factors represent physical aspects of the elderly's environment. Kornfield (1972) has discussed the psychosocial effects of hospital and institutional environments. Poor elderly from city slums or rural areas often live in environments characterized by extreme poverty and squalor. Relocation of the elderly to environments of unfamiliarity, monotony, or social isolation may arouse anxiety or precipitate disorientation and sometimes facilitate marked cognitive impairment or disorganization in the elderly. In view of the multiple and ever-continuing efforts of the elderly to retain physical and psychological equilibrium in the changed environment, some elderly continue to experience life-long changes in feeling tone, including anxiety, helplessness, and depression.

Most elderly are unable to visualize a solution to their problems of loneliness, isolation, and continuing physical decline in the foreseeable future. As a result many elderly fear that their usual patterns of activity must undergo change and that their social interaction with family, friends, and associates must be modified. Often these modifications are viewed as being disproportionately intrusive on their lives.

Last and most important, many elderly suffer from a manifest disturbance of one or more organ systems. Common chronic diseases in late life are strokes, congestive heart failure, diabetes, and cardiovascular disorders, all of which alter the spatiotemporal perceptions and subjective meaning of life for many elderly.

This biopsychosocial model of adaptation proceeds on the premise that the elderly client's behavior cannot always be fully understood or evaluated solely in terms of superficial manifestations. Bigot and Munnichs (1978) suggest a life-cycle strategy that would take account of the elderly's past, present, and future perspectives and needs. It would allow a deeper understanding of those aspects of the elderly person's current functioning (e.g., feelings, hopes, personal desires) that, while not directly related to clinical observations of anxieties, fears, and depression, are nevertheless likely to determine the elderly person's responses to the individuals, objects, and events in the social milieu and also to influence the care, treatment, and rehabilitation the elderly may receive from the physician, mental health professionals, and paraprofessionals.

THE LIFE-CYCLE STRATEGY IN HEALTH CARE OF THE ELDERLY

The practitioner must bear in mind that during the life course the elderly individual's behavior may have become affected by the impact of historical events (e.g., war, severe economic depression, or recession), environmental variables (e.g., race and social class), and societal expectations and value orientations. According to Bigot and Munnichs (1978), historical events and developmental variables are likely to have a differential impact on the behavior of individuals born at different points in historical time (intercohort differential effects) but may also have this kind of impact on the behavior of individuals born at roughly the same point in historical time (intracohort differential effects). Thus, several authors and researchers (e.g., Bengston & Cutler, 1976; Laufer & Bengston, 1974) contend that the behavioral aspects in human aging become progressively more difficult to understand unless this is achieved in relation to the individual's past, present, and future perspectives. What is advocated here is the significance of a life-cycle approach to the understanding of the health care needs and vulnerability of the elderly (see Figure 1–1). If properly managed, a life-cycle approach to health care of the elderly would require the following initiatives on the part of the health care practitioner.

Intimacy of Contact. If the mental health practitioner is to establish a therapeutic relationship with the elderly client, the practitioner needs contact with the elderly person at regular intervals and over time. It is important that prejudices and predetermined attitudes and patterns of relationships with the elderly be eliminated and their previous contributions and their present values and needs be recognized.

Mental health practitioners and clinicians need some familiarity not only with the elderly individuals' intrapsychic environment but also with their external environment. They need to consider in detail the matrix of the psychological caregiving relationship between themselves and the elderly person—its components, assessment, evaluation, and appropriate utilization—and to develop an approach that might most accurately be described as psychodynamic in orientation. This is not to imply that the mental health practitioner is expected to function in the capacity of psychoanalyst or psychotherapist. For the most part, however, the practitioner may be expected to function as a protagonist of the elderly, a friend, and a consultant to the physician in the treatment of the medically ill elderly or the emotionally upset and anxious elderly. The life-cycle approach proceeds on the premise that if properly managed, the relationship between the psychological caregiver and the elderly client is the most vital tool available in both assessment and treatment.

Alternating Need for Self-Sufficiency and Dependency. Families of the elderly often thwart the person's efforts to achieve even minimum adaptation by placing a high premium on the person's disabilities and the need to protect, thus fostering a dependency on the social environment and the custodial care system. Many elderly, by contrast, continue to place a high premium on independence and self-sufficiency. Despite the decline in biological functioning and socioeconomic constraints, many elderly for a variety of reasons do not wish to rely on others for their most basic needs. It is the mental health practitioner's overriding obligation to foster adaptation in the elderly clients by helping them to be as self-sufficient and independent as possible in their capacity for work, sex, and leisure and on the basis of these needs to develop or maintain a psychodynamic life style.

Adaptation. Chronic illnesses are prevalent in greater numbers among those elderly who are socially isolated, and their occurrence increases steadily with age. Thus it is important that the mental health practitioner be quite familiar with the broader concepts of both primary and secondary aging processes and be knowledgeable about adaptational processes of the aged and mechanisms of adaptation commonly used or acquired by the elderly.

One of the overriding psychological goals of the mental health practitioners in the geriatric setting is to foster the elderly client's adaptation to a life style compatible with the long-range social-emotional and environmental needs and preferences of the elderly person and with the identified affective or medical stress the client perceives. Thus the practitioner's assessment of the behavior of elderly individuals and interventions on their behalf must necessarily be geared toward the achievement of this goal.

Ego-Identity. As Erikson (1959) notes, at this stage of late adulthood the status of ego-integrity is of fundamental importance. The basic conflict is between the acceptance of one's life as useful and successful versus a sense of despair and fear of death. Two components of self-esteem often extremely important to elderly persons are their measure of the value of their life to themselves and to others and the more subtle but extremely important measure of their capacity to deal successfully with physical illness, socio-economic changes, and psychological trauma. Busse (1975, p. 72) observes that practitioners must assess the extent to which the elderly perceive that they have resources to survive a period of illness successfully or determine whether they lack the necessary reserve strength and must therefore be helped to accept reliance on others to meet their basic needs. In a life-cycle approach the mental health practitioner's task would also include helping disabled and chronically ill elderly to alter their ego ideal by contemplating their past contributions and to be proud of themselves for their ability to accept their current incapacitations.

To the degree that the relationship of past, present, and future physiological and psychological risk factors is acknowledged in the health status of the elderly, both the medical and the mental health practitioners must work in close cooperation. Working in unison, they are in an ideal position to provide for the psychological care of the vulnerable elderly and thereby reduce the impact of physiological and emotional stress factors. The interdependence of biological variables on the one hand and age-specific social and psychological variables on the other hand stands at the heart of the holistic and life-cycle concept of health care. Even under the most unpropitious conditions, effective management of the elderly individuals' health status begins with the understanding of both the psychological and the physiological states. In other words whether in settings of preventive, palliative, or emergency care, interventions should be guided by the elderly individuals' unique psychological and biological needs.

The provision of psychological care, however, cannot be limited to clinical psychologists or geropsychologists who engage in a particular type of psychological practice; nor can it be limited to a particular type of medical community or social setting that provides custodial care (see Kosberg, 1973; Vicker, 1974; Wolk & Wolk, 1971). There is a growing awareness among geriatric practitioners that in the 1970s only 5 percent of the aged in the United States and Canada lived in institutions (Botwinick, 1973). In 1985, two-thirds of the elderly are seen in ambulatory or outpatient settings. Within a biopsychosocial framework of health care for the elderly, protagonists must be the physicians, clinical psychologists, geriatric practitioners, geriatric social workers and nurses, trained volunteers, and adults in the family whose practice must be structured to facilitate the implementation of a psychosocial approach to the elderly. As Strain (1978, p. 4) notes, "the achievement of this psychosocial goal requires a model of care that addresses itself to the biological and psychological sources of the (elderly) individuals' strengths and their maladaptive behaviors, stresses, conflicts and regression" within a life-cycle framework.

The battle for improved health care of the elderly must therefore be fought on many fronts—in community health care settings, custodial institutions, day-care centers, group homes for the elderly, and the home. Reforms in each of these sectors are sorely needed. Even if reforms are implemented, care of the elderly will fall short of the ideal unless psychological care is administered by all members of the health care team working both in the specialties and tertiary care settings in the communities. Unless geriatric health practice is restructured within a biopsychosocial framework, it will remain unresponsive to the needs of the elderly.

Evidence regarding the significance of the biopsychosocial approach using a life-cycle strategy is still awaited and will depend on longitudinal and sequential design evaluations of elderly cohorts. This approach has stimulated thought on the subject of geriatric care among scores of social and behavioral scientists, psychologists, doctors, nurses, and social workers. Their cooperation in providing a holistic or whole-patient care is expected to be most meaningful in meeting the biopsychosocial needs of the elderly.

This book delineates such a framework of biopsychological health care assessment and treatment for the elderly and demonstrates its applicability to various segments of the elderly populations. There are segments of the elderly who can control the situation of physical and psychological care by economic resources, while there are other segments who are socially and economically depleted. All sectors must be considered sufficiently worthwhile by the communities and social institutions that they will be adequately cared for in old age.

PSYCHOBIOLOGICAL CHARACTERISTICS OF AGING

Lately there has been an intense renascence of interest in the biological and physical dimensions of psychological health care of the elderly. Part of the interest can be attributed to an emerging need to develop a specialty in psychogeriatric care.

Researchers (Moment, 1978) have approached the psychobiological processes and characteristics of aging from two general points of view: microscopic (or intrinsic) theories and macroscopic (or extrinsic) theories. Microscopic theories refer to events in the cells themselves or in the processes within and between cells. For instance, each time a cell reproduces, there is a tendency for errors to occur in the new cell. Finch (1978) notes, for example, that with time the number of highly specialized cells that do not divide decreases, and waste products build up in cells that are not lost. Taken together, changes in cell function might produce a progression of degenerative neural, endocrine, and metabolic events. These observations form the bases for a number of specific notions on the biological aging processes.

Several distinct but potentially overlapping theories have emerged to explain why aging occurs. It is imperative for the professional or paraprofessional to be familiar with the more commonly accepted genetic explanations, wear-and-tear theory, and autoimmune theory explaining senescence. The basic concepts are defined in Table 1–1. For a more detailed discussion of the biological theories of aging, the reader is referred to Behnke, Finch, and Moment (1978) and Finch and Hayflick (1977).

Genetic Theories

Genetic control of aging implies first that senescence is the result of some programmed, hence controlled, time-dependent degeneration of the organism and second that at least

---

Table 1–1 Biological Context of Aging

Genetic Theories
These theories propose that biological aging is controlled by a prewired genetic program that determines a predictable life span.

Autoimmune Theory
This theory of senescence proposes that as errors accumulate in the cells of the body, the autoimmune system begins to attack these mutant cells. Healthy tissues around the mutant are damaged, and in the end the body is in effect self-destructing (Beaubier, 1980).

Wear-and-Tear Theories
These theories of aging stress the effects of various physical and emotional insults on the life span. They link environmental events to increased probability of senescence and death. Organ systems may simply wear out, or some key parts may deteriorate. Disease might be responsible for organ wear and tear, and aging may be accelerated by atmospheric and climatic conditions.

Somatic Theory
This theory proposes that aging occurs as a function of the incapacity of the species to repair DNA (Deoxyribonucleic Acid). Every time a cell is replaced, mutation can occur. Mutations can accumulate with age, curtailing cellular functions (Curtis 1965). Eventually the cells become so inefficient that death ensues.

Free-Radical Theory
This theory proposes that free radicals are created during the normal process of cell metabolism and bond with other waste materials in the body to provoke the destruction of the immune system. Diets rich in vitamins E and C might help to fight the production of free-radicals by slowing cell metabolism, but gradually presence of free radicals provokes an accumulation of waste material in cells (Beaubier, 1980).

some of the aging processes are under the control of genetic mechanisms. In other words, according to genetic theory biological aging is controlled by a prewired genetic program. Rockstein (1958, 1975) has found the strong basis for a genetic theory of aging in species-specific differences in behavior and life span. Studies of the heritability of longevity among different races also suggest a genetic basis to aging. The observation by life insurance company actuaries that the offspring of long-lived parents tend to have a greater expectation of life than those of short-lived parents, implies inheritance of the factors controlling overall longevity (Lansing, 1959). Among humans there are sex differences in life expectancy, with women averaging two to seven years' greater longevity than men.

There is little dispute that an overall genetic control of life span exists in human and animal organisms studied, but there is much conflict as to what factors ultimately cause aging and death in humans as opposed to animals. Also not resolved is the question of whether the factors causing aging are purely genetic or purely stochastic or indeed, as commonly accepted, there is some contribution from both groups.

Role of Gene Redundancy

This theory has been proposed as fundamental to the expression of maximum life span (Medvedev, 1972; Cutler, 1974). It is argued that increased susceptibility to stress with age may result from mutation because cell redundancy is lost. A large (redundant) number of cells all perform the same task, enabling the body to cope easily with stressful situations. As errors accumulate and cells die, fewer cells perform more of the time, producing fatigue in the remaining healthy cells (Barrows, 1971; Brash & Hart, 1978). From a cellular and structural perspective, Hayflick (1977a, 1977b) has argued for the probability that the life span is, to some extent at least, determined by the role of types of protein synthesized by a cell, which in turn is determined by the genetic messages that the cell can utilize and the successive activations and repressions of which that cell line is capable.

These views all point to the consequences of differentiation in the cells of the species. It is suggested that all cells have a built-in genetically programmed life span, which varies with the genetically programmed life span of the species but may be modified within rather closely defined limits by extrinsic factors (Franks, 1974). The range of variation found in any biological system is sufficient to explain the observed variation in aging and death (Rowlatt & Franks, 1978). Gerontologists generally agree that to some extent genetic factors control aging, longevity, and death.

Immunologic Theory of Aging

Walford (1969, 1974) sees aging as due to an increasing immunogenetic diversification leading to a loss of tolerance toward self in the cells and resulting in "prolonged minor-grade histoincompatibility reactions" within and against the body's own tissues. He has labeled this the *autoimmune phenomena*. The exact reason for this diversification is not clear, but Walford suggests that somatic mutations in the cells of the immune system might account for cellular alterations. Alternatively, as a result of somatic mutation the lymphoid cells might become more, rather than less, tolerant with age and fail to destroy aberrant cells (e.g., cancer cells).

There is little doubt that the immunologic processes in the advanced years of life produce alterations in the immunoglobin concentration, as well as a marked increase in its variability, compared to immunologic processes found in the young and middle-aged adults (Buckley & Dorsey, 1971). Some immunoglobins produced in the young appear to be highly specific to an antigen. However, with aging, changes occur in the synthesis of these immunoglobins, resulting in a diminution in the tendency of the immunoglobins to react with only specific antigens. Weiner (1977) notes that the overall result is that broad spectrum antibodies are produced, and a range of cross-reactions with several chemically similar antigens may take place. From this perspective, then, aging may be due to alterations in the autoimmune systems. Those processes that repel infection and other foreign bodies may begin at some point to attack and weaken or destroy healthy cell structures.

A considerable amount of work, both clinical and experimental, has been carried out to determine how the functional capacity of the immune system declines with aging. For detailed reviews see Walford (1969, 1974). According to Walford (1969) other tissues that are part of the immune system (e.g., appendix, tonsils, lymph nodes) also show gross age-related changes. Basically the immune system produces antibodies that neutralize foreign agents that enter an organism, but as the immune system ages, there is some possibility that it loses its ability to distinguish between self and foreign elements. Thus healthy tissues may be self-destructed, and protection against infected or cancer cells may disappear markedly with old age (Adler, 1974; Beaubier, 1980).

In discussing the implications of cellular aging, Rockstein and Sussman (1979) note that because the important components of cells can be replaced only so many times, the basic material of the cell nucleus (i.e., the DNA, deoxyribonucleic acid) may be used up as we grow older. As a result there is an age-related reduction in enzyme activity and production, and this running out of the DNA without prompt replication produces further malfunctioning RNA (ribonucleic acid) and related enzymes (Shock, 1977).

Somatic Theory

Another plausible explanation for cellular deterioration and ultimate death is provided by somatic theory. It is argued that every time a cell is renewed, genetic error or mutation can occur. Mutations will then accumulate with age, curtailing cellular functions (Curtis, 1965) and ultimately causing cells to become so inefficient that death occurs.

Another source of change at the cellular level is an accumulation of waste products. The accumulation of pigmented, particulate material has been observed in the cells in most aging animals. This material is found typically in fixed postmitotic cell groups and is commonly referred to as *aging pigment* or *lipofuscin*. The origin and accumulation of this waste material pigment have been discussed at length (Bourne, 1973), but few agreements have been reached.

Perhaps one of the few points of agreement about the aging pigment lipofuscin is that it tends to accumulate with age. In human myocardium the amount of pigment is directly proportional to age (Strehler, 1964, 1977). After a certain threshold of this waste material is reached, the increasing level of lipofuscin leads to a loss of RNA. Mann and Yates (1974) suggest that when the lipofuscin concentration reaches a very high level in old age, it causes alterations in cellular metabolism leading to eventual atrophy and death of the cell.

Uncontrolled Free Radical Compound Reactions

These have been considered an important source of cellular damage especially during aging (Demopoulos, 1973). According to Marx (1974) escape of free radicals, produced either endogenously or exogenously (i.e., whether they are byproducts of metabolic processes of cells or come from environmental sources) seems a potential source of irreversible damage to cellular DNA. The damaged DNA would accumulate damage and so produce an ever-increasing number of faulty proteins.

The mechanisms by which free radicals might cause damage to cell constituents are now being elucidated, and this insight has given impetus to efforts to control the effects of free radicals in the biological systems of the elderly. For example, control of free radicals in cell structures through the use of vitamin E and vitamin C has been shown to increase the number of doubling of which those cells are capable before cell death. Also the inclusion of antioxidant compounds and fat-restricted and calorie-restricted diets as significant influences on life span is being tested in many cases to study free-radical damage effects in the process of aging (Beaubier, 1980). Hershey (1974) has proposed that we will soon learn how to break down the changes that occur with aging in the protein synthesis in the tissues and the ground substance around all tissues, thus allowing aging systems to be replaced and rejuvenated.

Each microscopic theory offers some cause for optimism in the battle against aging. Overall, it is concluded that aging results in a marked decline in the rate of protein synthesis or in a faulty programming of protein synthesis with the effects of this change being predominantly linked to various environmental stresses and various physical insults on the survival of the organism (Denny, 1975). These effects draw attention to the macroscopic wear-and-tear theories.

Wear-and-Tear Theories

These theories emphasize the notion of stress, environmental pressures, and the probability of senescence and ultimate death of the human organism. These theories of human life focus on forces that affect the organism as a whole and offer the most commonsense explanation for aging as a result of general wear and tear of the system. Some of the more specific wear-and-tear concepts follow.

Entrophy Theory

This theory discusses the relationship between the amount of organization in a system and the amount of energy available for work (Gould, 1978). Some basic life substance and energy are used up as the organism lives and endures. From a social evolutionary perspective it is reasonable to argue that the greater the cybernetic capacity of the organism (i.e., its ability to adapt to and cope with external events, both stressful and pleasurable), the more the organism is able to assimilate and synthesize new information and the more efficiently the organism is able to utilize the available reservoir of energy. It is in this context that the concept of entropy is fundamental to longevity.

The idea that each life is assigned a fixed, predetermined amount of energy that is genetically controlled in terms of both energy resources and energy consumption represents a notion important to life span and individual life history of the aging and aged organism.

Stress Theory

This theory attributes aging to a lifelong accumulation of insult to our bodies from stress, emotional tension, and physical trauma (Timiras, 1972). Disease and illness, especially chronic illness, might be responsible for wear and tear either because of specific effects (e.g., a heart attack) or interactions that are so defective (e.g., hypertension, high blood pressure) that the organism is no longer able to survive. Particularly with the elderly, stressful external events interact with the individual's cognitive and physiological response systems to produce wear and tear in the elderly's ability for coping with external events, such as socioeconomic losses or loss of loved individuals. Elderly people are especially vulnerable to death following relocation, retirement, loss of a significant other, or some personally significant events (Rowland, 1977). According to wear-and-tear theories of aging, stressful events are thought to have a cumulative, negative effect on the whole person. The entire psychobiology of the individual is affected adversely, which predisposes the person to disease and ultimately death.

Aging and the Brain

All persons have some changes in brain structure and functioning as they age, and it is widely thought that older persons suffer sufficient neuronal loss in some parts of the brain that significantly impairs their cognitive functioning, memory, and judgment. The interested reader is referred to Brody (1973) for a complete explanation of the structural changes in the brain associated with aging. Huyck and Hoyer (1982, p. 82) present a list of senescent changes (at the intracellular and intercellular level) commonly observed in the brain of elderly persons:

- accumulation of lipofuscin
- shrinking of the cell nucleus
- depletion of glycogen in the cell
- reduction of vasopressin
- neuronal loss
- increased neurofibrillary tangling
- decreased amounts of water and inorganic salts in the cell
- changes in the neurotransmitter substances (serotonin, norepinephrine)
- changes in rate of neural conduction
- decreased amount and distribution of Nissl substance

With advancing age, loss of neurons in the brain, increased neurofibrillary tangling, and increasing number of senile plaques are generally linked with senile dementia. Senile dementia is a disease associated with several marked pathological changes in the brain structure, especially the presence of senile plaques. Senile plaques are degenerated cell structures located at synapses between cells. They may affect the conductance of nerve impulses across cells. The neurofibrillary tangles are found within brain neurons, and these masses of tangled fibers interfere with cell metabolism or the transfer of substances from the neurons to the axons (Tomlinson & Henderson, 1976). Senile dementia is characterized by a progressive decline in memory, attention span, cognitive functioning, and physical self-care skills relative to previous levels (Hughes, 1978).

Although some of the abnormal changes associated with senile dementia (e.g., senile plaques, neurofibrillary tangles, and granulovacular changes) are also observed in normal aging, the degree of such changes is far greater in senile dementia patients. Mild mental impairment is associated with diffuse brain damage in about 5 percent of the elderly. Unlike gradual cognitive deterioration in normal aging, senile behavior is generally found when the presence of senile plaques in large numbers throughout the brain causes a rapid deterioration in the brain structure. According to Terry and Wisniewski (1975) senile dementia is the primary diagnosis of almost 1 million adults (i.e., about 5 percent) over the age of 65 years.

Diagnosis of dementias and brain diseases often requires extensive knowledge of neurophysiology and gerontology. The relationships between the normal and abnormal aging, and physical and psychological processes become more obscure (Levy, Derogatis, Gallagher, & Gatz, 1980). Our ignorance of the borderline between biology, chemical processes, and psychology is cogently illustrated by the facts of dementia and other organic brain syndromes. It is difficult to distinguish between the various types of dementias (e.g., the primary neuronal degeneration and cerebrovascular disease). The fact that the incidence of cognitive diseases resulting from senescent processes in the brain increases sharply with advancing age is a cause for much concern as more people are surviving into advanced old age (Pfeiffer, 1977; Eisdorfer & Cohen, 1978).

Aging and Intelligence

Practitioners need to be more fully informed of the changes in intellectual processes and intellectual functioning over time (see Baltes & Labouvie, 1973 for a discussion of age-related changes). Empirical evidence on the significance of longitudinal change is restricted to a few studies. Evidence has unequivocally indicated the stability of intelligence scores (based on tests of verbal ability) till 70 years or so. Stable scores are also reported on performance subtests till about age 70 (see Eisdorfer & Wilkie, 1973; Wilkie & Eisdorfer, 1973).

It would appear that little, if any, loss occurs in the normal elderly individual when intelligence is measured in terms of stored information (Botwinick, 1977). Indeed Botwinick (1978) has argued that verbal abilities are also maintained and may even increase in the later years of life. This is especially true for individuals of initially high or average ability. By and large stability rather than decline in scores has characterized the healthy noninstitutionalized groups examined in a number of studies (Granick & Birren, 1969; Granick & Patterson, 1971; Jarvik, 1975; Schaie, 1975), suggesting that in the healthy older persons cognitive decline may be a myth.

For example, older people perform best on the Information, Vocabulary, and Comprehension subtests of the *Wechsler Adult Intelligence Scale* (WAIS). These tests all involve verbal abilities and are influenced to a substantial extent by experience and education. Longitudinal studies since 1970 suggest that except for speeded performance tasks there may be no change in the elderly individuals' performance in cognitive tasks, at least up to the eighth decade (Jarvik & Cohen, 1973). Perceptual-integrative intelligence on the other hand appears to decrease with age, and poor performance by older adults is seen on the WAIS subtests of Digit Symbol, Picture Arrangement, and Block Design—measures that depend on the processing of novel information. This decline in the elderly persons' perceptual-integrative performance is attributed in part to their slower speed of performance in cognitive tasks.

Horn and Cattell (1967) have suggested that there are variations in the rate of change in the two components to intelligence: fluid and crystallized. Fluid intelligence is probably biologically based and is associated with the efficiency of the central nervous system. It is suggested that with aging, fluid intelligence may decline, reflecting perhaps decreased efficiency of the central nervous system. By contrast crystallized intelligence, which depends on the interaction of the organism with its environment, is maintained in old age, reflecting perhaps the continuance in late life of the acculturation factor in intellectual functioning.

The etiologies of intellectual decline may qualitatively differ with aging. For example, studies examining the relationships between health status and intelligence measures (e.g., Birren, Butler, Greenhouse, Sokoloff, & Yarrow, 1963; Reitan & Davison, 1974; Wilkie & Eisdorfer, 1973) have shown that certain physiological conditions and disease states prevalent with advancing age serve to magnify the decline in measured intelligence. High blood pressure and cardiovascular disease may be an important cause of deterioration in cognitive performance in later life.

One may assume numerous perspectives when attempting to interpret the disease- and age-related changes in intelligence. Overall, however, several studies report stability in intellectual functioning until advanced old age. Other studies report a decline in the intellectual performance of older persons associated with disease and illness states, principally cardiovascular disease, blood pressure, and arteriosclerosis. At the same time it is reasonable to conclude that some age-related declines occur even in the absence of pathology.

As suggested by biological theories of aging, individual variations in cognitive performance are genetically programmed at the cellular level. Many elderly of certain gene pools may not experience much decline while in the case of others the organism may run out of genetic program or accumulate too many errors in cell function to withstand further intrinsic or extrinsic strain. The evidence is not sufficient to make precise statements about the nature of ontogenetic changes in intellectual performance, but it is enough to challenge seriously the often-stated stereotype of a general performance decrement during old age (Baltes & Labouvie, 1973, p. 177).

Aging and Cognitive Functions

The research findings on age changes in cognitive functioning reflect a number of declines in attentional processes, including memory, perceptual, and cognitive process. Only broad patterns of change observed with aging are discussed here.

Attentional Processes

One of the earliest age-related changes is noted in the effectiveness of the attentional processes, which are responsible for translating and moving information in the sensory storage to the stages of short-term and long-term memory. These are summarized in Table 1–2. The reader is referred to Hoyer, Rebok, and Sved (1979) and Walsh (1975) for a detailed discussion of this topic.

Of the many changes in the attentional processes summarized in Table 1–2, age-related losses in reaction time can have serious consequences in several areas of the elderly's functionings. Reaction time may account to some degree for the higher rate of accidents among the old (Birren, 1974). Most of the psychomotor slowness observed in older persons is probably a product of decline in reaction time. A related issue is whether slowing reaction time is a normal development in aging or whether the principal causes of such changes are physical illness, other pathological brain syndrome conditions, and sensory decrements. Common illness in the seventh and eighth decade of life may have the most dramatic effects on psychomotor response and reaction time, but more gradual and subtle changes in performance may occur in healthy elderly individuals.

Table 1–2 Age-Related Changes in Attentional Processes

1. *Age-Related Reduction in Speed and Accuracy in Attentional Performance*
   This is attributed to
   - perceptual noise factor, resulting in a reduction in the ability of the aged person to suppress interfering or distracting stimuli
   - stimulus persistence factor, resulting in a reduction in the ability of the aged person to process information efficiently because of the reduced rate at which stimulus information travels in the nervous system

2. *Age-Related Slowing in Central Perceptual Processing*
   This is attributed to
   - slowness in localization of sound, that is, decline in the ability to locate sound sources using time cues and intensity of sound cues
   - increased response persistence time, that is, increased time needed to identify ambiguous figures and to make ambiguous decisions
   - decline in reaction time, that is, slowing down in the reaction time caused by a slowing in the conductance of electrical impulses in the CNS of the elderly person

---

Aging and Memory

Most of the popular literature on aging suggests that with aging is a rapid decline in memory-related performance. However, it is important not to generalize from these popular notions. Some kinds of memory definitely do show an age-related impairment, which traditionally has been regarded as a deficit in registration, retention, or retrieval, or a combination of these deficits. From the outlook of the elderly, however, it is more useful to regard memory as a time-related process that may be classified as proceeding from the time of registration onward: immediate, short-term, intermediate, and long-term memory storage.

Although this taxonomy does not explicate the exact mechanisms of retrieval or retention that are impaired with aging, it does provide some insight into the time relations in the continuum of stimulus acquisition and recall that become impaired. The following broad trends have been observed and help to localize where interference effects in the memory may become most manifest in the elderly:

- It is generally accepted that immediate memory is impaired with aging. Such impairment may represent a registration deficit due to receptor dysfunction or an interference effect from the pattern of nerve activity.
- Most investigators also agree that short-term or primary memory worsens with aging. Primary memory refers to the storage for information that is actively being processed at a given time, and its decline may also be an interference phenomenon.
- Overall comparisons of primary memory and secondary memory (Craik, 1977; Walsh, 1975) suggest that with advancing age, the capacity of the primary memory (i.e., the amount of information that can be held for active processing at any given time) appears to be stable, but secondary or long-term memory, which involves a later retrieval of that information, especially under conditions of recall (as opposed to recognition) declines with age.

It should be noted, however, that memory and learning are extremely difficult to differentiate, and there can be no memory if learning has not occurred first.

The major difficulty in memory that elderly individuals experience may be at the point of registration. Older adults do relatively well in remembering things they must retain for a little while only, but when information is to be remembered for longer periods, it must be processed more "deeply" when learned. It would appear that one of the greater difficulties in memory with older adults is that they do not process new information as thoroughly or effectively as do younger adults; therefore the information is less likely to be available later (Craik, 1977).

Aging and Motivation

Overall it is maintained that a general decline in the motivation of the elderly influences their learning. Frequently, however, old persons do perform better on tasks that are personally relevant to them in comparison to their performance on meaningless tasks. The difficulty of the task also limits the learning performance of older adults. Frequently the elderly refuse to attempt tasks that appear difficult because of the anxiety generated in doing difficult tasks and failing. Eisdorfer (1968) notes that beyond a certain level of difficulty of the task, the motivation may become anxiety provoking and act as a deterrent to task performance. Especially with the elderly, practitioners need to understand that some learning situations produce an extreme state of psychophysiologic arousal that detracts from their ability to perform when learning is required. The response of the elderly adult is inhibited and the task is discontinued.

In conclusion, it is suggested that the elderly are less interested and less motivated to stay involved in meaningless memory tasks (e.g., paired-associates or nonsense syllables learning tasks). They remember different aspects of experience than younger adults; usually the aspects remembered by older persons are not those measured in research. From a psychological perspective most older persons convince themselves that there is an inevitable pathological decline in memory in the later years. Consequently they do not devote sufficient attention to organizing recall materials effectively. For this reason Beck (1967) suggests that most complaints about a decline in memory and forgetfulness should be associated with stereotypic age expectations and the tendency for many depressed elderly with low self-esteem to underestimate their abilities.

Sensory Processes and Aging

Pastalan, Mautz, and Merrill (1973) have given considerable attention to the manner in which sensory systems change as we grow older. The practical value of their research is in terms of how it can affect the quality of life in the elderly. A number of specific developmental changes have been observed in several sensory systems. These are summarized in Table 1–3. The interested reader is referred to Rockstein and Sussman (1979), Rossman (1976), McKenzie (1980), and Timiras (1972) for a detailed discussion of sensory losses with aging.

Physical, cognitive, and experiential factors complicate the study of sensory loss in the elderly. However, there is little doubt that age-related sensory impairments contribute to a general reduction in the individual's adaptiveness and responsiveness to external events. Reduced sensory efficiency may often lead to social and physical withdrawal and, for many elderly with visual and hearing losses in particular, make daily functions (e.g., walking, talking) increasingly difficult. Oyer and Oyer (1978) observed increased fatigue, irritability, tension, depression, negativism, and vulnerability as consequences of age-related

Table 1–3 Age-Related Changes in the Sensory Systems

VISION	HEARING	OLFACTION
Illumination	Auditory acuity declines with	Smell sensitivity declines with
Decreased pupil size, loss of	age. This condition is called	age probably as a result of
transparency in the lens,	*presbycusis*. However, loss of	changes in the olfactory bulb
increased thickness of the lens,	auditory acuity is not constant	and tract. The ability of the
and thickening of the capsule	across all frequencies but is	elderly to discriminate food
allow less light to reach the	more severe for high tones with	odors may decrease with
retina. Hence elderly persons	increasing age. Since high	decrease in taste sensitivity.
need twice as much illumination	frequency sounds are more	SOMESTHETIC SENSES
as a younger person.	difficult for the elderly to hear,	Older adults appear to decline
Accommodation	problems may appear in word	somewhat in terms of sensitivity
With increasing age the elasticity	discrimination and in	to pain. Decreases in tactile
of the lens decreases, and	understanding normal	sensitivity often occur in some
elderly persons experience	conversation.	older adults and may be seen
increasing farsightedness or		primarily in areas of the palms of
presbyopia.	TASTE	the hands and soles of the feet.
Visual Acuity and Color Acuity	The number of taste buds	With aging there is reduced
Loss of visual acuity—the ability	declines with aging. Elderly	efficiency of thermoregulation or
to distinguish detail at a	persons often require more	loss of ability to respond to
distance—is quite marked	concentrated solutions of the	extreme temperatures.
around the age of 70. Ability to	salty, sweet, and sour	
discriminate colors—especially	ingredients to determine	
blues and violets, which get	particular tastes. The aged may	
filtered out—declines steadily	acquire preferences for foods	
with aging.	with more spices.	

DISTURBANCES RELATED TO LOSS OF SENSORY ABILITIES

-Sensory deprivation can produce hallucinations   -Increased olfactory thresholds may create a
 as well as deterioration in normal elderly.   problem of decline in smell sensitivity.
-Suspiciousness produced by loss of visual
 acuity may be increased to paranoid
 dimensions.

hearing losses. Not being able to see traffic signs, hear horns, or observe emergency signals can therefore produce serious physical and emotional hazards for the elderly.

While findings concerning old-age losses in the sense of touch and pain are unclear, many caregivers of the elderly need to be reminded that cuts, burns, irritations, and infections may go unnoticed and untreated. Similarly reduction in taste and smell might cause many elderly to choose foods that have strong taste and to ignore the need for nutritious and healthful food.

Age-Related Changes in the Organs

The structure and function of almost every organ in the human body are affected by the passage of time, and a progression of change is noticed in the heart, nervous system, respiratory and digestive system, kidneys, and pancreas. A few of the predominant changes with marked implications for the day-to-day functioning of the elderly are summarized in Table 1–4. The interested reader is referred to Rockstein (1975), Gutmann (1977), and Lindeman (1975) for an excellent discussion of age-related changes in the organ functions.

Table 1–4 Age-Related Changes in the Organs

1. MUSCULAR STRUCTURE CHANGES
   -Muscle weight decreases.
   -Number and diameter of muscle fibers decrease in late life and hypertrophy sets in.
   -Valves of the heart become thicker and less flexible.
   -Atrophy increases.
2. CARDIOVASCULAR SYSTEM
   -As individuals age, heart and blood vessels become more and more rigid due to changes of the physicochemical properties of collagen.
   -Maximal oxygen consumption, exercise stroke volume, heart rate, and cardiac output all decline with age. Peripheral vascular resistance increases. Capacity of the aging cardiovascular system to respond to stress declines significantly.

3. RESPIRATORY SYSTEM
   -Aging is accompanied by morphologic changes of the thorax and lungs.
   -The alveolar walls become thinner and the number of capillaries is reduced.
   -The number and thickness of the elastic fibers that form the supportive tissue of the lungs are reduced.
   -Pulmonary arterial walls thicken with age.
   -The costal cartilages become more rigid with advancing years and begin to calcify.
   -The intercostal muscles tend to become atrophic and weaker. Compliance of the chest wall diminishes with age interfering with the exhaling-inhaling function of the lungs. Shortness of breath (severe shortness called emphysema) is observed in very old age.

4. EXCRETORY SYSTEM
   Kidney Function Changes
   -Weight of kidney decreases by about 20 percent.
   -The ability of kidney to maximally dilute urine is diminished.
   -Inability of kidney to eliminate nonvolatile waste products increases and leads to disease states, which lower maximal urine osmolality and renal function.
   Digestive System Changes
   -Abilities of the intestinal system to secrete adequate volumes of gastric juice to assist digestion decline.
   -Atrophy in the mucosa that lines the gastrointestinal tract increases.
   -Digestion of food is inadequate and becomes the major cause of poor nutrition, diarrhea, or constipation in the elderly.
   Gall Bladder/Liver Changes
   -The prevalence of gallstones increases.
   -Liver size declines with age, and enzyme changes in liver may affect metabolism of drugs in the body.

Acute and Chronic Diseases in Later Life

According to Wilder (1971) the increased risk of circulatory, respiratory, and digestive system decline with aging is reflected in the high incidence of chronic health problems in the elderly. Of all individuals over the age of 65 an estimated 85 percent report at least one chronic illness and about one-half of the older population report some limitation in their daily physical and psychosocial functioning due to a chronic disorder (Hendricks & Hendricks, 1977).

Heart disease and cerebrovascular lesions account for about 70 percent of deaths after middle age. Surveys indicate that heart disease and hypertension are definitely indicated in at least one-half of all persons over the age of 65, while 25 percent to 30 percent have various abnormalities more remotely associated with heart disease.

Other common chronic problems associated with old age include cerebrovascular and arteriosclerotic diseases that ultimately affect the brain and constitute the fifth most frequent cause of death in the elderly populations (National Center for Health Statistics, 1971). This category of chronic illness factors may take the form of a stroke, which in effect is a cerebrovascular accident caused by an existing embolism that has traveled from one part of the body to one of the cerebral arteries, or by a thrombosis, a constriction that develops in the brain (Insel & Roth, 1976). Kimmel (1974) indicates a greater incidence of high blood pressure, cardiovascular diseases, gastrointestinal disorders, and lung diseases among persons from lower socioeconomic levels. Other chronic disorders that cause disruption in the normal functioning of many elderly are diabetes, high blood pressure, and hypokinetic diseases resulting from lack of physical conditioning. Thus the elderly's capacity to respond to stressors is further reduced as a result of blood pressure, diabetes (Shock, 1968; Upton, 1977), and poor physical conditioning. Since the risk of age-related illnesses increases with diabetes, there is a further slowing down in the rate at which many body functions return to normal following stress.

Of all the ills that bring about stressful physical and mental impairments in old age, the most distressing are those affecting the brain. These chronic conditions are associated with slow and long-term cognitive and personality changes that frighten patients and their families (Eisdorfer & Cohen, 1978; Pfeiffer, 1977). Some of these brain syndromes are the result of degenerative changes in the brain cells, while others are caused by chemical and metabolic disorders.

The trend toward decline in health as a result of chronic disease states is significant for old age in general. However, a majority of older persons are not rendered markedly unable to function in their daily lives. Bouvier, Atlee, and McVeigh (1975) have noted that approximately 60 percent to 65 percent of persons over the age of 65 encounter little change in their normal functioning and have no difficulties in carrying out major tasks. It is estimated that another 20 percent have minimal difficulty in major activities of daily life such as household work and outside tasks. Cole (1974) estimated that about 5 percent of the community elderly are restricted in their activities because of the effects of chronic diseases and related disabilities.

Thus the application of absolute standards of health is not useful in addressing the question of what it means for the aged to be healthy. If the definition of health implies complete mental, physical, and social well-being in functioning, then it must be conceded that few older persons can be considered healthy. However, despite the presence of potentially disabling conditions and the severity of some chronic impairments it is possible for many elderly to have adequate resources and to develop coping styles that help them to lead well-functioning lives (Lowenthal, 1981; Lowenthal & Chiriboga, 1972; Lowenthal & Robinson, 1976). The need for appropriate means of assessment and evaluation of disease-related psychological disorders is becoming increasingly significant in order that effective prevention, remediation, and rehabilitation of the elderly individuals' problems may be achieved. The practitioner's in-depth understanding and awareness of the psychobiological status of the elderly is becoming increasingly important to the task of clinical assessment and treatment of the elderly.

FEARS OF THE ELDERLY AND THEIR SOCIAL-EMOTIONAL CONSEQUENCES

A life-cycle orientation to the understanding of the biopsychosocial field of the elderly (see Table 1–1) reinforces the concept that age-related fears and anxieties play a key role in the long-term adaptations and adjustments of the elderly. No clinician or practitioner treating the elderly can afford, therefore, to neglect these fears or to overlook their social and emotional effects on the mental outlook of the elderly.

Although the contents of many of the elderly's fears and anxieties, and intervention and treatment programs for dealing with them, are detailed in later chapters, a brief overview is presented here of those fears attributed mainly to ageism and presumed to be the products of long-term social prejudices against elders. Brief comments are also made about their management. In each case the essential goal of management is to make both the elderly person and the practitioner more aware of the detrimental effects of ageism and society's stereotypic beliefs and myths about the aging process on the mental outlook and behavioral functioning of the elderly.

Gerontologists and suicidologists (e.g., Birren, 1964; Farberow & Moriwaki, 1975) contend that the primary fears and concerns of many elderly relate to the day-to-day problems of living and coping with physical hardship, loneliness, and personal suffering. These are not necessarily abstract issues but are linked to the elderly's concerns about everyday functioning, for example, shopping for groceries, dealing with everyday weather conditions, staying warm, having heat for the winter. There are also grave fears about the recurrence of nonnormative events. Many elderly who may have experienced two world wars, economic depression, and political dislocation and who may have sought political asylum and refugee status may have come face to face with impending catastrophe. For such elderly it would not be surprising if they constantly suffer nightmares, anxiety, and fear about exposure to similar hardships in old age.

Clinicians and geropsychologists attentive to uncovering the obstacles to successful aging and life satisfaction need to understand and evaluate many of the excessive concerns and fears of the elderly before a rewarding intervention network can be built. Such assessment cannot necessarily be made through an office interview with an elderly client. It can be done more adequately when the clinician has full knowledge about the client's background, life stresses and life style; the friendliness, hostility, safety, or danger of the client's environment, and the attitudes and interpersonal characteristics of the social network on which the elderly client is dependent. Knowledge of these factors and some tentative assessment of the client's loss reactions and the persistent themes of fear will lead the practitioner or clinician to a realistic appreciation of the depression and depressive disorders that the client may manifest. The opportunities for support as well as the psychological stressors (in the form of fears and anxiety) inherent in the environment may then be correctly appreciated from the perspective of the elderly subject.

The clinician's recognitions of other pervasive fears in the elderly such as psychological loss of self-image, loss of status, and loss of role play a part of utmost importance in establishing effective communications with the elderly (Pfeiffer, 1980). Persistent themes of fear and anxiety that pose considerable emotional hardship to the elderly need to be assessed systematically in any diagnostic workup plan or psychosocial evaluation of the elderly. Specific fears that may impinge on the daily functioning of the elderly follow.

Fear of Sensory Deprivation

Butler and Lewis (1973) believe that fear of anticipated loss of hearing is a widespread problem among the elderly. Indeed hearing impairment is the most difficult sensory loss for the elderly person. When the elderly first begin to experience small signs of hearing impairment, loss of visual acuity, or other sensory deficits, their fears may generalize to other aspects of their general functioning, for example, orientation and ability to process data, accurate interpretation of their environment as well as the ability to maintain daily activities such as driving a car, concentrating on tasks and conversing. Any significant diminution or threatened diminution in sensory acuity may cause many elderly to become sufficiently fearful, paranoid, and tense as to complicate communication in the physician's office (Cooper & Curry, 1976; Cooper & Porter, 1976).

Fear of Mental Decline

Another common fear is that decline in mental abilities is almost inevitable in late years. This pervasive belief is particularly vicious because, as Palmore (1980) notes, it can become a self-fulfilling prophecy. The invasive belief that mental decline is inevitable in old age may make serious inroads not only on practical coping abilities but also on the thinking abilities of many elderly. It may convey to the elderly person that the breach of the thinking center has occurred and the end cannot be far away. As noted by Palmore (1980), the fear of the inevitability of loss, whether it be slowing of response speed, loss of intellectual ability, learning ability, or integrative functions, can be just as stressful as the actual loss. Such fear, or perception of fear, can result in mental illness if it becomes severe enough.

The practitioner's assessment of such fears may help to facilitate communication so that more accurate evaluation of cognitive abilities is possible. Clinicians should be aware that such anxieties and fears may often cause depression and other psychiatric symptoms and may lead the client to behave as if there were an organic brain syndrome. The clinician must try to assess the actual mental competence of the elderly client and share reassuring information with the client.

Contrary to the fear-inducing beliefs held by many elderly concerning the inevitability of mental decline, the facts indicate that many aged continue to be quite creative in later life (Butler, 1967). Dennis (1966) found that creativity remained high in many elderly who were creative in their earlier years. Palmore (1974) also provided data, based on seven long-term investigations, that subjects with advanced education, working without time pressure, show little or no cognitive deterioration with age. It may be true that reaction time tends to slow somewhat with advanced age, but among healthy aged this slowing is only an average one-tenth of a second, and many older persons have faster reaction time than younger persons (Palmore, 1974).

Much of the cognitive disorientation and actual dysfunctioning that many elderly fear is at least partly attributable to the stereotypic and self-defeating beliefs that have been ingrained in their minds. Clinicians can help to alleviate the fears of mental impairment. Despite declines in perception and reaction time, studies of older workers under actual working conditions show that they perform as well as young workers, if not better on most measures. It may be true that older persons often require somewhat longer time to learn material, but given extra time, they can learn as well as younger persons (Botwinick & Thompson, 1966).

Thus, the elderly need to be told that the evidence does not justify the inevitability of serious mental decline in old age. The main detrimental effect often resulting from the elderly's deep-seated fears concerning mental incompetence may be disorientation and declining vigor because of mental inactivity.

Fear of Mental Illness

A related prejudice against the elderly is the belief that many or most are senile and that mental illness is common, inevitable, and untreatable among the aged (Palmore, 1980). This social prejudice is transformed into a fear in the minds of many elderly who become intensely worried about maintaining control over their lives and their environment. Palmore (1980, p. 229) observes that this belief is particularly vicious because it can become a self-fulfilling prophecy. The deep-seated anxiety or fear can lead many elderly to turn inward and withdraw and thus confirm the original belief that they are declining mentally.

Clinicians should be aware that fear of mental illness among the aged, as at any age, may cause severe depression and other psychiatric symptoms. Clinicians need to monitor the cues and signs of this fear and other related fears in any psychosocial evaluation. A number of researchers (Binstock & Shanas, 1976; Pasamanick, 1962; Harris, 1975; Leighton, 1965) are convinced that serious mental illness is not inevitable for a majority of older persons notwithstanding the high levels of psychosocial stresses that the elderly encounter in their day-to-day life. Lieberman's (1978) research evidence suggests that successful adaptation in old age is the rule rather than the exception. There seems to be no intrinsic connection between aging and social disintegration or mental ill health. Clinicians also need to be personally assured that the facts about the so-called inevitability of mental illness in the aged clearly contradict such beliefs and must communicate this assurance to the elderly clients.

Clinicians who are concerned with explaining the relationship between old age and mental health or illness have drawn attention to the complexity and diversity of the parameters involved in assessing mental illness. Although there is some evidence from clinical observations that age is associated with some mental decline and resulting disorientation, the relationships are neither clear-cut nor easily interpretable. As Pasamanick (1962) and Leighton (1965) have observed, the definitions of mild or severe forms of mental illness are obscure. Clinical assessment of mental illness in the elderly is therefore largely a function of arbitrary definition. Since it is relatively difficult to determine what proportion of mental illness among the aged is at least partly attributable to the elderly's psychological stresses, fears, and anxieties, it is important for clinicians to assess such emotional factors and attempt to reduce or ameliorate the elderly's fears concerning mental illness in advancing years.

Similarly it is relatively difficult to determine what proportion of mental illness among the aged is reversible or responsive to some form of treatment (Palmore, 1980). Thus, it is important for clinicians to ensure that when working with elderly clients, their fears concerning their mental or emotional health are objectively assessed and that the depressed elderly are not allowed, without substantial reason, to accept a defeatist attitude that little can be done to save them from even the milder forms of mental illness. It is important also to stress with elderly clients that mental illness is at least partly caused by social and psychological stress and that the elderly can help to enhance their well-being by reduction of stress and a proper regimen of relaxation, diet, and motivating activity.

Fear of Loneliness and Segregation

Among the most intense fears of old age are loneliness and fear of segregation. While there is considerable evidence (see Babchuk, 1978; Bates & Babchuk, 1961) to suggest that the idea of loneliness associated with old age is statistically false, nevertheless this fear is a frequent topic of conversation among the elderly. Good clinicians will do what they can to help their clients avoid becoming isolated, and therefore the objective assessment of fears related to loneliness and segregation may contribute most to the alleviation of these fears. In assessing these anxieties or in assessing their contribution to the mental well-being of the elderly, the clinician would need to assess the client's way of life. As Butler (1975) notes, a person who has developed a balanced portfolio—different skills, activities, and roles and engrossing activities—should in theory have less fear of loneliness. However, in practice the general abstraction that loneliness and segregation are inevitable in old age frequently contributes to considerable depression and cognitive disorientation in the elderly. Should even mild isolation and loneliness begin, it is likely to precipitate more fear, anxiety, and depression.

There is little evidence from social-psychiatric research to contradict this impression. Butler and Lewis (1973) and Bunch (1975) showed a significant relationship between actual or threatened loneliness and segregation and suicide in the elderly. Butler and Lewis (1973) identified isolation-induced helplessness, uselessness, and meaningless of life as diagnostic clues for depression and suicide in old age. They advise the clinicians and mental health workers to be alert to these cues of threatened isolation and depression. Myers, Murphey, and Riker (1981) regard the elderly's actual or potential fears of loneliness and isolation as an important area of diagnostic assessment in that many old people's internal resources become weak when the availability of external social resources is threatened. Without question older people living in circumstances of threatened or actual loneliness and isolation are a special at-risk group (Myers, Murphey & Riker, 1981), and suicide indicators are potentially established. Most preventable suicides are related to depressive reactions resulting from perceived loneliness and isolation (Butler & Lewis, 1973).

Thus several authors suggest that diagnostic assessment of the elderly's fear of loneliness should consider the role of their previous psychosocial functioning and the role of the old person in the social system and should take cognizance of special needs and values. Other factors to consider are the family and social supports available to the older person (Lawrence, 1981). Continual encouragement and reinforcement for maintaining social involvement should be given. Stimulating and enjoyable activity and interpersonal attachments constitute a cluster of social functions that may be partially incompatible with loneliness and help to alleviate some of the fears stemming from the prospects of segregation and isolation.

On a more realistic note a number of authors (e.g., Neugarten & Gutmann, 1958; Gutmann, 1969) view the elderly person's withdrawal from the world as a form of mastery of the external stimuli and as an attempt on the part of many elderly to adapt to rapid changes in their environment. Advanced age per se does not call for a differential assessment of the individual's isolation and withdrawal patterns. Some persons function on a high social active mastery level throughout their lives; by the same token there are isolated and withdrawn youngsters. The difference is that aged persons face rapid changes and frequently encounter external losses and risks that are real and continue unabated. In the face of many actual severe deprivations and risks the elderly person may decide to be practical and resort to a life of detachment, relative passivity, and withdrawal. Gutmann (1969), who studied the age-related withdrawal patterns in various cultures, noted that after the age of 65, cognitions of active mastery and instrumental and productive ways of mastering the external world were often replaced by cognitions and ideations of a more passive, detached, and less risk-taking nature. Such observations, if valid, call for assessment approaches or psychosocial evaluations that attempt to determine whether the so-called regressive symptomatology of withdrawal and isolation is a reflection of adaptive function in elderly persons or should be viewed as an indicator of regression or emotional disorders.

Fear of Crime and Violence

While older people commit little crime, they are frequent victims of crime, especially robbery. As Bild and Havighurst (1976) have noted, fear of crime is one of the most frequently mentioned problems in the elderly. Police reports often do not indicate the ages of the victims and are therefore not always good indicators of the amount of criminal activity directed exclusively against the elderly. Antunes, Cook, Cook, and Skogan (1977), who studied patterns of personal crime against the elderly, noted that the most frequent crimes committed against the elderly are robbery and personal larceny. Thus as Antunes et al. conclude, while the total amount of crime against the elderly may be equal to or lower than for other age groups, the special physical and emotional vulnerability of the aged to predatory crimes has the effect of making them much more fearful of becoming victims. Since most elderly, especially those living in depressed, unclassed neighborhoods, are cautioned not to go out alone and to place secure locks in their homes, these suggestions have the effect of increasing the isolation and fears of older persons. Also, the disabilities of old age—deafness, slowness, spotty memories, and partial blindness—not only increase the vulnerability of the elderly people to predatory crimes against them but also tend to make the elderly more paranoid, suspicious, and anxious and therefore more prone to social isolation and psychiatric disorders or syndromes.

On the one hand the elderly's association with poverty, physical impairment, disability, and illness makes for their higher need for support and aid from outsiders; yet on the other hand their fear of moving out alone and fear of violence pose even greater problems in their adaptive ways of living. Therefore, geriatric mental health workers need to assess the fears of the elderly in order to determine what proportion of these fears has some basis in fact, to discover and assess what social or health problems might be resulting from such actual victimization or fear of victimization, and how the elderly are dealing with them. In consultation with other human resources agencies, mental health practitioners need to explore methods and techniques for giving appropriate service to older persons who are victims of crime or have fears of being victimized. Zarit (1980, p. 95) suggests that a buddy system or escort service might be developed so that older persons are not out alone too much, particularly those elderly who could more easily become victims of crime because of limited mobility.

Fear of Physical Illness and Physical Disability

In examining the psychodynamics of aging and the aged, Berezin (1972a, 1977b) notes that old age is accompanied by many physical disorders and the presence of many physical illnesses. A number of researchers (e.g., Butler, 1978; Eisdorfer, 1977) observe that 45 percent of the elderly have some physical limitations and are more prone to disease than any other age group. These ailments are not only disabling to organs, limbs, and the brain, causing decreased function and pain; these medical processes have been seen to erode activity, appearances, finances, and self-esteem (Goodstein, 1981, p. 226).

The elderly have frequently heard it said that they represent one-third of the nation's health bill and one-third of the family physician's practice time (Palmore, 1974, 1980). It is not surprising, therefore, that the elderly are convinced about the inevitability of physical illness and physical disability in old age and begin to anticipate illness and fear the outcomes. While some physiologic aging occurs naturally in body organs, biochemical and metabolic pathways, musculoskeletal systems, and central nervous system, what is unappreciated is the fact that the health and physical ability of most aged do not decline precipitously (Palmore, 1980) nor are they quickly disabling. Nevertheless, as a result of misinformation and the common prejudices against them, elders tend to overestimate the prevalence of illness, organic impairment, and other problems in old age. More seriously, this bias has led or is leading many elderly to fear old age and its concomitants of chronic physical illness, disease, and disability.

It is particularly important for clinicians and health professionals to assess the facts of health in the individual elderly person and to avoid those prejudices that foster and maintain unnecessary fear and anxiety concerning the effects of physical illness on the functioning of the elderly. It is important also to stress with elderly clients that inadequate physical health is at least partly a function of declining activity and may be due also to lack of stimulation, exercise, and proper nutrition. The encouragement to care for health and advice and information on how to maintain good health within a biopsychosocial framework may help to counter some of the pervasive anxiety about the inevitability of failing health in old age.

Special attention, however, should be given to the psychosocial stresses of those elderly who are chronically ill and who fear long-term hospitalization. In many respects the psychological tasks imposed by chronic illness in the elderly replicate the psychological tasks imposed on the child at various stages of development. Even after the experience of many decades of autonomy and independence, chronic illness can induce severe forms of fear in the elderly, especially those who must be hospitalized from time to time.

Special Anxieties of the Chronically Ill

Strain and Grossman (1975) postulate that all acutely ill or chronically ill elderly are vulnerable to the following types of fears and anxieties.

Fear of Strangers. When the elderly enter the hospital anticipating a long stay they must put their lives in the care of a group of strangers with whom they have no close ties and who may not be judged particularly competent to assume responsibility for their survival (Strain, 1978). This feeling is reminiscent of the fear of strangers first experienced in childhood. It produces a similar type of body tension, fearfulness, and fright that was experienced in childhood despite the elderly person's cognitive understanding that professionals are not strangers.

Separation Anxiety. This anxiety reflects the state of separatedness that the elderly feel from the environment that has provided support and gratification for many years. This anxiety is also reminiscent of the anxiety that the child experiences. Strain (1978) postulates that all individuals are vulnerable in this regard, and separation anxiety may be dramatically reactivated in many elderly who have experienced other stern environmental losses.

Fear of Injury to Body Parts. As Strain (1978) conjectures, once the elderly client enters the hospital, the body becomes the property of the physician. Routine hospital procedures may require the elderly client to assume a passive-submissive stance, which may stir up many frustrating-aggressive feelings. Feelings of frustration may reactivate in the elderly client the fears of bodily damage similar to those the child experiences.

Fear of Pain. According to Strain (1978) and Strain and Grossman (1975) the fear of physical and emotional pain cuts across all of the stresses that humans experience. In the elderly client vulnerable to many other stresses and sensitivities, the fear of pain is a realistic one. While individuals cope with pain differently at different stages of development and different phases of discomfort, the fear of physical pain may come from the realization that the body is weak and deteriorated, and the threshold for pain is relatively low.

Fear of Loss of Control of Bodily Functions. Elderly patients may agonize over the transient loss of bodily functions and may convince themselves, despite assurances to the contrary, that bodily functions will never be regained. Concurrent with the fear of losing bodily functions, the elderly client may also fear loss of mental functions. Often fear of loss of physical functions may also be translated into the fear of loss of mental functions.

Guilt and Fear of Retaliation. Often feelings of guilt and shame may accompany physical illness. Feelings of guilt may emanate from the permanent sick role that the elderly client may desire with friends, family, and the physician. Shame may come from the disfiguration resulting from a mutilating surgical procedure, for example, in an elderly client who because of a debilitating illness may not be able to dress properly or be socially presentable.

Some elderly clients' subconscious fear that their present illness is a punishment for previous sins toward friends and family is a major source of stress and anxiety. Strain (1978) notes that many elderly characteristically believe that their illness is a punishment for their sins of selfishness, ego-centeredness, and self-indulgence. "Despite the acquisition of logic, intelligence and experience, the perception of illness and hospitalization as retaliation by a 'higher being' for one's transgressions" (Strain, 1978, p. 23) persists in many elderly.

Although these fears related to long-term hospitalization are present to varying degrees in the elderly and in varying frequency, they inevitably take on different forms in different elderly, depending on the limited nature of personal resources that the elderly perceive themselves as having. Conversely those elderly who view themselves as having many personal cognitive-intellectual resources and capacities may characteristically refuse to surrender to these fears, even when it is obvious that their hospitalization may place severe limitations on their activities.

SUMMARY

This chapter has presented a rationale for the development of a biopsychosocial approach to the health care of the elderly and attempted to show that the experience of aging cannot be understood without an appreciation of the ways in which biological, psychological, and social aspects interact over the course of the life cycle to contribute to the health of the elderly. It is imperative for the geriatric mental health practitioner and geropsychologist to work in close cooperation and collaboration with other health professionals, including geriatric physicians and clinicians, for the development of optimal methods of health care for the elderly and effective procedures for assessment, evaluation, and intervention.

Despite the well-recognized relationship between biological changes and psychological changes, most geriatric practitioners do not have sufficient knowledge about the interface between biology and psychology. We can identify a body of knowledge about biological processes of aging that should be made an essential requirement for the systematic training of geropsychologists, clinicians, and geriatric mental health professionals. A skeletal overview of normal biological processes that change with aging as well as the sensory, perceptual, and cognitive alterations has been presented. Moving from the outside in, we see evidence of many age-related changes and age alterations in the structure and functions of many organs and organ systems, both in physiological indicators such as glucose tolerance and in psychological measures involving learning, memory, reaction time, and intelligence.

The extent of decline in psychological functions such as memory, problem solving, and learning is accentuated by some of the chronic illnesses common in later life. Although there is considerable variability of humans as they age, certain old age diseases such as heart disease or central nervous system (CNS) disorders serve to magnify normal aging deficits in performance. However, variations in individual performance may be attributed to the individual's physical conditioning or the preventive health care style that will help some older individuals maintain or regain their health; a sedentary life style characteristic of many elderly may contribute to early decline in some individuals.

Psychological functions may often change without evidence of physical alteration, as is seen in the functional disorders of later years. At the same time, physiological changes and biological decline may not affect the functioning of the aged to a great extent until some threshold is passed, thereby moving the individual into a pathological range of biological damage. The rate of aging is different for different organs, tissues, and their constituent cells, and there is a variety of theories to explain the nature and pace of aging and senescence. Genetic theories of aging propose that biological aging is controlled by a prewired genetic program that serves as the basis for a fixed life span. Wear-and-tear theories of aging, by comparison, emphasize that as persons age, not only is there an increasing likelihood that biological and psychological decrements will occur but also that there may be a decreased resistance to various physical and emotional insults on the survival of the aged organism. Overall, however, predictions about any given individual's functioning are difficult to obtain because of the variations in performance observed in the elderly. Although biological decline is real, there is no point at which the psychological growth of the individual necessarily ceases. The idea that biological senescence does not restrict psychological growth in old age is importantly related to the development of various intervention strategies.

Aging is, fortunately or unfortunately, a dynamic process, and the aged change in ways that are interactive with society, as well as those mediated by their own psychology. Old people greatly fear the possibility of mental and cognitive decline and impairment. They also have a tremendous anxiety about becoming obsolete. Although society restricts new learning opportunities and obstructs their social participation, a significant number of elderly succeed in leading productive and worthwhile lives. Clinicians can continue to provide opportunities for growth and enhancement through systematic strategies of assessment and intervention.

Our slowly increasing scientific understanding of the processes of senescence and prolongation of life by biological and psychosocial interventions is ultimately related to the development of various individualized interventions and preventive and remedial treatment programs for the care of the elderly. This recent interest in the synthesis of accumulating biological and psychosocial knowledge about aging and applying it to assessment and intervention is clearly one of the most significant trends in contemporary gerontology likely to have important consequences for the effective health care of the elderly.

This foundational chapter has addressed some of the basic questions that pertain to the health care of the elderly and to systematic assessment and intervention. What has been advocated is a holistic multifunctional approach to assessment and treatment. The views expressed in this foundational chapter represent the major thesis of this book. A significant assumption underlying the integration of the biopsychosocial perspective as described in this chapter is that it will guide the practitioner in meeting the challenge of working with older clients and in better understanding and analyzing psychological methods of assessment and treatment described in Chapters 2 through 14.

REFERENCES

Adler, W. (1974). An autoimmune theory of aging. In A. Cherwin & C. Finch (Eds.), *Physiology and cell biology of aging* (Aging Series, Vol. 8) (pp. 212–267). New York: Raven Press.

Antunes, G.E., Cook, F.L., Cook, T.D., & Skogan, W.G. (1977). Patterns of personal crime against the elderly: Findings from a national survey. *Gerontologist, 17*, 321–327.

Babchuk, N. (1978). Aging and primary relations. *International Journal of Aging and Human Development, 9*(2), 137–151.

Baltes, P.B., & Labouvie, G.V. (1973). Adult development of intellectual performance. In C. Eisdorfer & M.P. Lawton (Eds.), *The psychology of adult development and aging* (pp. 157–219). Washington: American Psychological Association.

Barrows, C.H. (1971). The challenge—Mechanisms of biological aging. *Gerontologist, 11*, 5–11.

Bates, A.P., & Babchuk, N. (1961). The primary group: A reappraisal. *Sociological Quarterly, 2*, 181–191.

Beaubier, J. (1980). Biological factors in aging. In C.L. Fry (Ed.), *Aging in culture and society* (pp. 21–41). Brooklyn: J.F. Bergin.

Beck, A.T. (1967). *Depression: Clinical, experimental and theoretical aspects.* New York: Harper & Row.

Behnke, A., Finch, C.E., & Moment, G. (Eds.). (1978). *The biology of aging.* New York: Plenum Press.

Bengston, V.L., & Cutler, N.E. (1976). Generations and the intergenerational relations: Perspectives on the age groups and social change. In R.N. Binstock & E. Shanas (Eds.), *Handbook of aging and the social sciences* (pp. 130–159). New York: Van Nostrand Reinhold Co.

Berezin, M.A. (1972a). Psychotherapy for the aged. *Journal of Geriatric Psychiatry, 4*, 34–45.

Berezin, M.A. (1972b). Psychodynamic consideration of aging and the aged: An overview. *American Journal of Psychiatry, 128*, 1483–1491.

Bigot, A., & Munnichs, J.M.A. (1978). Psychology of aging, long term illness and care of the older person. In J.C. Brocklehurst (Ed.), *Textbook of geriatric medicine and gerontology* (pp. 791–806). New York: Churchill Livingstone.

Bild, B.R., & Havighurst, R.J. (1976). Senior citizens in great cities: The case of Chicago. *Gerontologist, 16* (1, pt. 2), whole issue.

Binstock, R., & Shanas, E. (1976). *Handbook of aging and the social sciences.* New York: Van Nostrand Reinhold Co.

Birren, J.E. (1964). *The psychology of aging.* Englewood Cliffs, NJ: Prentice-Hall, Inc.

Birren, J.E. (1974). Translations in gerontology—From lab to life: Psychophysiology and speed of response. *American Psychologist, 29*, 808–816.

Birren, J.E., Butler, R.N., Greenhouse, S.W., Sokoloff, L., & Yarrow, M. (Eds.). (1963). *Human aging: A biological and behavioral study.* Washington: Government Printing Office.

Botwinick, J. (1973). *Aging and behavior.* New York: Springer.

Botwinick, J. (1977). Intellectual abilities. In J.E. Birren & K.W. Schaie (Eds.), *Handbook of the psychology of aging* (pp. 580–605). New York: Van Nostrand Reinhold Co.

Botwinick, J. (1978). *Aging and behavior* (2nd ed.). New York: Springer.

Botwinick, J., & Thompson, L.W. (1966). Components of reaction time in relation to age and sex. *Journal of Genetic Psychology, 108*, 175.

Bourne, G.H. (1973). Lipofuscin. *Progress in Brain Research, 40*, 187–201.

Bouvier, L., Atlee, E., & McVeigh, F. (1975). The elderly in America. *Population Bulletin, 30*(3), 3–36.

Brash, D.E., & Hart, R.W. (1978). Molecular biology of aging. In A. Behnke, C.E. Finch, & G. Moment (Eds.), *The biology of aging* (pp. 57–81). New York: Plenum Press.

Brody, H. (1973). Aging of the vertebrate brain. In M. Rockstein (Ed.), *Development and aging in the nervous system* (pp. 121–133). New York: Academic Press.

Buckley, C.E., & Dorsey, F.C. (1971). Serum immunoglobulin levels throughout the life-span of healthy man. *Annals of Internal Medicine, 75*, 673–682.

Bunch, M. (1975). Relationship between the month of birth and the month of death in the elderly. *British Journal of Preventative Social Medicine, 29*, 151–156.

Busse, E.W. (1975). Aging and psychiatric diseases of late life. In S. Arieti (Ed.), *American handbook of psychiatry* (Vol. 4, 2nd ed., pp. 67–89). New York: Basic Books.

Butler, R.N. (1967). The destiny of creativity in later life. In B. Levin & R. Kahana (Eds.), *Psychodynamic studies on aging* (pp. 20–63). New York: International Universities Press.

Butler, R.N. (1975). Psychotherapy in old age. In S. Arieti (Ed.), *American handbook of psychiatry* (Vol. 5, 2nd ed., pp. 807–828). New York: Basic Books.

Butler, R.N. (1978). Myths and realities of clinical geriatrics. In S.S. Steury & M. Blank (Eds.), *Readings in psychotherapy with older people*. Rockville, MD: National Institute of Mental Health.

Butler, R.N., & Lewis, M.I. (1973). *Aging and mental health: Positive psychosocial approaches*. St. Louis: C.V. Mosby Co.

Coe, R. (1983). Aged in the community. In F.U. Steinberg (Ed.), *Care of the geriatric patient* (pp. 605–613). St. Louis: C.V. Mosby Co.

Cole, P. (1974). Morbidity in the United States. In C.L. Erhardt & J.E. Berlin (Eds.), *Mortality and morbidity in the United States* (pp. 65–104). Cambridge: Harvard University Press.

Cooper, A., & Curry, A. (1976). The pathology of deafness in the paranoid and affective psychoses of later life. *Journal of Psychosomatic Research, 20,* 97–105.

Cooper, A., & Porter, R. (1976). Visual acuity and ocular pathology in paranoid and affective psychoses of later life. *Journal of Psychosomatic Research, 20,* 107–114.

Craik, F.I.M. (1977). Age differences in human memory. In J.E. Birren & K.W. Schaie (Eds.), *Handbook of the psychology of aging* (pp. 384–420). New York: Van Nostrand Reinhold Co.

Curtis, H.J. (1965). The somatic mutation theory of aging. In R. Kastenbaum (Ed.), *Contributions to the psychobiology of aging* (pp. 69–80). New York: Springer.

Cutler, R.G. (1974). Redundancy of information content in the genome of mammalian species as a protective mechanism determining aging rate. *Mech. Ageing Development, 2,* 381–408.

Demopoulos, H.B. (1973). The basis of free radical pathology. *Federation Proceedings of the Federation of the American Societies of Experimental Biology, 32,* 1859–1861.

Dennis, W. (1966). Creative productivity between 20 and 80 years. *Journal of Gerontology, 21,* 1–16.

Denny, P. (1975). Cellular biology of aging. In D.S. Woodruff & J.E. Birren (Eds.), *Aging: Scientific perspectives and social issues* (pp. 201–228). New York: Van Nostrand Reinhold Co.

Eisdorfer, C. (1968). Arousal and performance: Verbal learning. In G.A. Talland (Ed.), *Human aging and behavior* (pp. 189–216). New York: Academic Press.

Eisdorfer, C. (1977). Stress, disease and cognitive change in the aged. In C. Eisdorfer & R.O. Friedel (Eds.), *Cognitive and emotional disturbance in the elderly* (pp. 27–44). Chicago: Year Book Medical Publishers.

Eisdorfer, C., & Cohen, D. (1978). The cognitively impaired elderly: Differential diagnosis. In M. Storandt, I.C. Siegler, & M.F. Elias (Eds.), *Clinical psychology of aging* (pp. 7–42). New York: Plenum Press.

Eisdorfer, C., & Wilkie, F. (1973). Intellectual changes with advancing age. In L. Jarvik, C. Eisdorfer, & J.E. Blum (Eds.), *Intellectual functioning in adults: Psychological and biological influences* (pp. 21–30). New York: Springer.

Engel, G.L. (1962). *Psychological development in health and disease*. Philadelphia: W.B. Saunders Co.

Erikson, E.H. (1959). *Identity and the life cycle* (Psychological Issues, Vol. 1, No. 1). New York: International Universities Press.

Farberow, N.L., & Moriwaki, S.Y. (1975). Self-destructive crises in the older person. *Gerontologist, 15,* 333–337.

Finch, C.E. (1978). The brain and aging. In J. Behnke, C.E. Finch, & G. Moment (Eds.), *Biology of aging* (pp. 301–310). New York: Plenum Press.

Finch, C.E., & Hayflick, L. (Eds.). (1977). *Handbook of the biology of aging*. New York: Van Nostrand Reinhold Co.

Franks, L.M. (1974). Ageing in differentiated cells. *Gerontologia, 20,* 51–62.

Goodstein, R.K. (1981). Inextricable interaction: Social, psychologic and biologic stresses facing the elderly. *American Journal of Orthopsychiatry, 51,* 219–229.

Gould, R.L. (1978). *Transformations: Growth and change in adult life*. New York: Simon & Schuster.

Granick, S., & Birren, J.E. (1969). *Cognitive functioning of survivors vs. non-survivors: 12 year follow-up of healthy aged*. Paper presented at the 8th International Congress of Gerontology, Washington.

Granick, S., & Patterson, R.D. (1971). *Human aging, II: An 11 year biomedical and behavioral study*. Washington: U.S. Government Printing Office.

Gutmann, D. (1969). *The country of old men: Cross-cultural studies in the psychology of later life* (Occasional Papers in Gerontology, No. 5). Ann Arbor: Institute of Gerontology, University of Michigan–Wayne State University.

Gutmann, D. (1977). The cross-cultural perspective. Notes towards a comparative psychology of aging. In J.E. Birren & K.W. Schaie (Eds.), *Handbook of the psychology of aging* (pp. 302–326). New York: Van Nostrand Reinhold Co.

Harris, L. (1975). *The myth and reality of aging in America*. Washington: National Council of Aging.

Hayflick, L. (1977a). The biology of aging. *Natural History*, September, 22–30.

Hayflick, L. (1977b). The cellular basis for biological aging. In C.E. Finch & L. Hayflick (Eds.), *Handbook of the biology of aging* (pp. 159–187). New York: Van Nostrand Reinhold Co.

Hendricks, J. & Hendricks, C.D. (1977). *Aging in mass society*. Cambridge: Winthrop.

Hershey, D. (1974). *Life span and factors affecting it*. Springfield, IL: Charles C Thomas Pub.

Horn, J.L., & Cattell, R.B. (1967). Age differences in fluid and crystallized intelligence. *Acta Psychologica, 26*, 107–121.

Hoyer, W.J., Rebok, G.W., & Sved, S.M. (1979). Effects of varying irrelevant information on adult age differences in problem solving. *Journal of Gerontology, 34*, 553–560.

Hughes, C.P. (1978). The differential diagnosis of dementia in the senium. In K. Nandy (Ed.), *Senile dementia: A biomedical approach* (pp. 201–208). New York: Elsevier/North-Holland Biomedical Press.

Huyck, M.H., & Hoyer, W.J. (1982). *Adult development and aging*. Belmont, CA: Wadsworth Publishing Co.

Insel, P.M., & Roth, W.T. (1976). *Health in a changing society*. Palo Alto, CA: Mayfield.

Jarvik, L.F. (1975). Thoughts on the psychobiology of aging. *American Psychologist, 30*, 567–583.

Jarvik, L.F., & Cohen, C. (1973). A biobehavioral approach to intellectual changes with aging. In C. Eisdorfer & M.P. Lawton (Eds.), *The psychology of adult development and aging* (pp. 220–280). Washington: American Psychological Association.

Kimmel, D.C. (1974). *Adulthood and aging: An interdisciplinary, developmental view*. New York: John Wiley & Sons, Inc.

Kornfield, D.S. (1972). The hospital environment: Its impact on the patient. In Z.J. Lipowski (Ed.), *Advances in psychosomatic medicine* (Vol. 8), (pp. 252–270). Basel: Karger.

Kosberg, J.I. (1973). Nursing homes: A social work paradox. *Social Work, 18*, 104–110.

Lansing, A.K. (1959). General biology of senescence. In J.E. Birren (Ed.), *Handbook of aging and the individual* (pp. 119–135). Chicago: University of Chicago Press.

Laufer, R., & Bengston, V.L. (1974). Generations, aging and social stratification: On the development of generational units. *Journal of Social Issues, 30*, 181–205.

Lawrence, P. (1981). Applying skills with special populations. In J.E. Myers (Ed.), *Counseling older persons: Volume 2, Basic helping skills for service providers*. Falls Church, VA: American Personnel and Guidance Association.

Leighton, A. (1965). Poverty and social change. *Scientific American, 212*, 21.

Levy, S.M., Derogatis, L.R., Gallagher, D., & Gatz, M. (1980). Intervention with older adults and the evaluation of outcome. In L.W. Poon (Ed.), *Aging in the 1980s* (pp. 41–64). Washington: American Psychological Association.

Lieberman, M.A. (1978). Social and psychological determinants of adaptation. *International Journal of Aging and Human Development, 9(2)*, 115–126.

Lindeman, R.D. (1975). Age changes in renal function. In R. Goldman & M. Rockstein (Eds.), *The physiology and pathology of human aging* (pp. 19–38). New York: Academic Press.

Lipowski, Z.J. (1967). Review of consultation psychiatry and psychosomatic medicine. 1. General principles. *Psychosomatic Medicine, 29*, 201–224.

Lipowski, Z.J. (1973). Psychosomatic medicine in a changing society: Some current trends in theory and research. *Comprehensive Psychiatry, 14*, 203–215.

Lipowski, Z.J. (1975). Physical illness, the patient and his environment: Psychosocial foundations of medicine. In M. Reiser (Ed.), *American handbook of psychiatry* (Vol. 4, pp. 1–42). New York: Basic Books.

Lowenthal, M.F. (1981). Intentionality: Toward a framework for the study of adaptation in adulthood. In J. Hendricks (Ed.), *Being and becoming old* (pp. 3–19). New York: Baywood.

Lowenthal, M.F., & Chiriboga, D. (1973). Social stress and adaptation: Toward a life course perspective. In C. Eisdorfer & M.P. Lawton (Eds.), *The psychology of adult development and aging* (pp. 281–310). Washington: American Psychological Association.

Lowenthal, M.F., & Robinson, B. (1976). Social networks and isolation. In R.H. Binstock & E. Shanas (Eds.), *Handbook of aging and the social sciences* (pp. 432–456). New York: Van Nostrand Reinhold Co.

Maddison, D., & Viola, A. (1968). The health of widows in the year following bereavement. *Journal of Psychosomatic Research, 12,* 297–306.

Mann, D.M.A., & Yates, P.O. (1974). Lipoprotein pigments; their relationship to aging in the human nervous system. I. The lipofuscin content of nerve cells. *Brain, 97,* 481–488.

Marx, J.L. (1974a). Aging research (I): Cellular theories of senescence. *Science, 186,* 1105–1107.

McKenzie, S.C. (1980). *Aging and old age.* Glenview, IL: Scott, Foresman & Co.

Medvedev, Zh.A. (1972). Repetition of molecular-genetic information as a possible factor in evolutionary changes of life-span. *Experimental Gerontology, 7,* 227–238.

Moment, G. (1978). The Ponce de Leon trail today. In J. Behnke, C.E. Finch, & G. Moment (Eds.), *The biology of aging* (pp. 1–18). New York: Plenum Press.

Myers, J.E., Murphey, M., & Riker, H.C. (1981). Mental health needs of older persons. Identifying at-risk populations. *American Mental Health Counselors Association Journal, 3,* 53–61.

National Center for Health Statistics (1971). *Health in the later years.* Department of Health, Education, and Welfare. Washington: Government Printing Office.

Neugarten, B.L., & Gutmann, D. (1958). Age-sex roles and personality in middle age: A thematic apperception study. *Psychological Monographs, 72.*

Nowlin, J.B., & Busse, E.W. (1977). Psychosomatic problems in the older person. In E. Wittkower & H. Warnes (Eds.), *Psychosomatic medicine: Its clinical applications* (pp. 326–347). New York: Harper & Row.

Oyer, H.J., & Oyer, E.J. (1978). Social consequences of hearing loss for the elderly. *Allied Health and Behavioral Sciences, 2,* 123–138.

Palmore, E. (1974). *Normal aging II.* Durham, NC: Duke University Press.

Palmore, E. (1980). The social factors in aging. In E.W. Busse & D.G. Blazer (Eds.), *Handbook of geriatric psychiatry* (pp. 222–248). New York: Van Nostrand Reinhold Co.

Parkes, C.M. (1972). *Bereavement.* New York: International Universities Press.

Pasamanick, B. (1962). A survey of mental disease in an urban population. *Mental Hygiene, 46,* 567.

Pastalan, L.A., Mautz, R.K., & Merrill, J. (1973). The simulation of age-related losses: A new approach to the study of environmental barriers. In W.F.E. Preiser (Ed.), *Environmental design research* (Vol. 1, pp. 383–391). Stroudsburg, PA: Dowden, Hutchinson & Ross.

Pfeiffer, E. (1977). Psychopathology and social pathology. In J.E. Birren & K.W. Schaie (Eds.), *Handbook of the psychology of aging* (pp. 650–671). New York: Van Nostrand Reinhold Co.

Pfeiffer, E. (1980). The psychosocial evaluation of the elderly patient. In E.W. Busse & D.G. Blazer (Eds.), *Handbook of geriatric psychiatry* (pp. 275–284). New York: Van Nostrand Reinhold Co.

Rahe, R.H. (1972). Subjects' recent life changes in their near-future illness susceptibility. In Z.J. Lipowski (Ed.), *Advances in psychosomatic medicine* (Vol. 8, pp. 2–19). Basel: Karger.

Rees, D.W., & Lutkins, S.G. (1967). Mortality of bereavement. *British Medical Journal, 4,* 13–16.

Reiser, M.F. (1975). Changing theoretical concepts in psychosomatic medicine. In M. Reiser (Ed.), *American handbook of psychiatry* (Vol. 4, 2nd ed., pp. 477–500). New York: Basic Books.

Reitan, R.M., & Davison, L.A. (1974). *Clinical neuropsychology: Current status and applications.* Washington: Winston.

Rockstein, M. (1958). Heredity and longevity in the animal kingdom. *Journal of Gerontology, 13,* 7–12.

Rockstein, M. (1975). The biology of aging in humans: An overview. In R. Goldman & M. Rockstein (Eds.), *The physiology and pathology of human aging* (pp. 1–7). New York: Academic Press.

Rockstein, M., & Sussman, M. (1979). *Biology of aging.* Belmont, CA: Wadsworth.

Rossman, I. (1976). Human aging changes. In I.M. Burnside (Ed.), *Nursing and the aged* (pp. 81–91). New York: McGraw-Hill Book Co.

Rowland, K.F. (1977). Environmental events predicting death for the elderly. *Psychological Bulletin, 84,* 349–372.

Rowlatt, C., & Franks, L.M. (1978). Aging in tissues and cells. In J.C. Brocklehurst (Ed.), *Textbook of geriatric medicine and gerontology* (pp. 3–17). London: Churchill Livingstone.

Schaie, K.W. (1975). Age changes in adult intelligence. In D.S. Woodruff & J.E. Birren (Eds.), *Aging: Scientific perspectives and social issues* (pp. 111–124). New York: Van Nostrand Reinhold Co.

Shock, N.W. (1968). Biologic concepts of aging. In A. Simon & L.J. Epstein (Eds.), *Aging in modern society* (Psychiatric Research Report No. 23). Washington: American Psychiatric Association.

Shock, N.W. (1977). System integration. In C.E. Finch & L. Hayflick (Eds.), *Handbook of the biology of aging* (pp. 639–665). New York: Van Nostrand Reinhold Co.

Strain, J.J. (1978). The psychological determinants of adaptation to chronic illness. In J.J. Strain (Ed.), *Psychological interventions in medical practice* (pp. 19–34). New York: Appleton-Century-Crofts.

Strain, J.J., & Grossman, S. (1975). Psychological reactions to medical illness and hospitalization. In J.J. Strain & S. Grossman (Eds.), *Psychological care of the medically ill: A primer in liaison psychiatry* (pp. 23–57). New York: Appleton-Century-Crofts.

Strehler, B.L. (1964). On the histochemistry and ultrastructure of age-pigment. *Advanced Gerontological Research, 1,* 343–384.

Strehler, B.L. (1977). *Time, cells and aging* (2nd ed.). New York: Academic Press.

Terry, R.D., & Wisniewski, H.M. (1975). Structural and chemical changes of the aged human brain. In S. Gershon & A. Raskin (Eds.), *Aging, Vol. 2. Genesis and the treatment of psychologic disorders in the elderly* (pp. 127–141). New York: Raven Press.

Timiras, P.S. (1972). *Developmental physiology and aging.* New York: Macmillan Publishing Co., Inc.

Tomlinson, B.E., & Henderson, G. (1976). Some quantitative findings in normal and demented old people. In R.D. Terry & S. Gershon (Eds.), *Neurobiology of aging* (pp. 183–204). New York: Raven Press.

Upton, A.C. (1977). Pathobiology. In C.E. Finch & L. Hayflick (Eds.), *Handbook of the biology of aging* (pp. 513–535). New York: Van Nostrand Reinhold Co.

Vicker, R.L. (1974). *Factors among nursing home personnel which relate to their attitudes towards aging, with implications for in-service training programs.* Paper presented at 27th Annual Meeting of the Gerontological Society, October, Portland, Oregon.

Walford, R.L. (1969). *Immunologic theory of aging.* Copenhagen: Munksgaard.

Walford, R.L. (1974). Immunologic theory of aging: Current status. *Federation Proceedings of the Federation of the American Societies of Experimental Biology, 33,* 2020–2027.

Walsh. D.A. (1975). Age differences in learning and memory. In D.S. Woodruff & J.E. Birren (Eds.), *Aging: Scientific perspectives and social issues* (pp. 125–200). New York: Van Nostrand Reinhold Co.

Weiner, H. (1977). *Psychobiology and human disease.* New York: Elsevier.

Wilder, C.S. (1971). *Chronic conditions and limitations of activity and mobility: United States, July 1965 to June 1967.* Vital and Health Statistics. Series No. 10(61). Department of Health, Education and Welfare. Washington: Government Printing Office.

Wilkie, F.L., & Eisdorfer, C. (1973). Systemic disease and behavioral correlates. In L.F. Jarvik, C. Eisdorfer, & J.E. Blum (Eds.), *Intellectual functioning in adults: Psychological and biological influences* (pp. 83–94). New York: Springer.

Wolk, R.L., & Wolk, R.B. (1971). Professional workers' attitudes toward the aged. *Journal of American Geriatrics Society, 19,* 624–639.

Zarit, S.H. (1980). *Aging and mental disorders: Psychological approaches to assessment and treatment.* New York: Free Press.

Chapter 2

Clinical Assessment and Aging: Special Considerations

Working with the elderly, psychologists and practitioners are overwhelmed by the complexity of the assessment issue. No other client population of this size presents more diverse causative possibilities, including those endogenous antecedents of disorders of which most psychologists and geriatric caregivers are less than familiar (Hussian, 1981). The challenge of unraveling the intricate process of assessment and evaluation of the aged comes from the complexity of variables including the high incidence of behavioral, cognitive, and organic process interactions. There is also the increased variability in behavioral responses of the elderly due to differences in the social background and in environment. Rarely does the older person (particularly the person with a frail physique) present a simple or single-entity problem that belongs neatly to one discipline or professional expertise. Rather the interaction of physical, social, and psychological problems tends to be the rule and presents serious challenges and demands to professionals (Schaie & Schaie, 1977).

A delineation of the single-entity factors in the behavioral disorders of the elderly may not be enough for systematic clinical assessment as many of the factors may be seen by the clinical assessor to fit several categories of geriatric disorders. This chapter is devoted to a discussion of five major aspects. First, the question of aims and objectives of accurate assessment of geriatric symptoms and responses is discussed. Second, specific assessment interview techniques applied to the functional assessment of geriatric capacities and deficits are examined. Third, there is a discussion of the special considerations necessary in the mental health, mental status, and neuropsychological assessment of the elderly clients and specific modifications that must be made in the assessment processes and procedures. Fourth, there is a discussion of the assessment criteria used to determine the elderly client's psychological capacity to maintain an independent role. Fifth, the question of assessing the elderly individual's social support networks is discussed.

Since depression, stress, and cognitive impairment are among the most prevalent and clinically most significant in the elderly, Chapters 3, 4, and 5 are devoted to their clinical manifestations, assessment, and management. Similarly, assessing a large number of the functional disorders prevalent in the elderly is an onerous but extremely significant task for the clinical geropsychologist. Chapter 6 is devoted to the assessment and management of a variety of functional disorders.

The general aims and contents of assessment become clear throughout this chapter. However, specific aspects of assessment as they pertain to cognitive impairment and the underlying factors such as diagnosis of the reversible and irreversible dementias, delirium, focal brain damage, and other cognitive disorders are discussed in Chapter 4.

AIMS OF ASSESSMENT

As Schaie and Schaie (1977) note, assessment is inevitably related to the intent to do something for or to the individual being assessed. The types of problems and cognitive and behavioral disorders most prevalent and frequently encountered in working with elderly patients are considered. A number of issues of diagnosis are considered, and a number of aims and objectives must be achieved. These are summarized in Table 2–1.

Differentiation of Normal from Pathological Aging

The first aim of geriatric assessment is the accurate differentiation of pathological symptoms from normal concomitants of aging. A major issue in the clinical assessment of the elderly seems to be the need to establish criteria for what level or range of functioning is normal for this age group and what further age decrements are considered to be pathology. The diagnosis of psychopathology or the differentiation of psychopathology from normal aging becomes one of the major functions of assessment.

It is all too easy for the clinician to believe that many of the problems of the elderly are pathological, irreversible, and progressive, and therefore a detailed assessment is futile. These myths and stereotypes of the clinician can easily interfere with the conduct of objective and adequate assessment. The process of pathologizing may also involve a struggle for power in which older persons are perceived as patients and inevitably as losers. Often pathology does become the statistical norm, thereby creating confusion about what is normal and what is pathologic so that everything becomes pathologic and therefore inevitable (Eisdorfer & Keckich, 1980).

To counter the tendency to be pessimistic, it is important for the clinician to begin with an assessment of some of the adaptive skills and competencies that the elderly individual may have possessed to function adequately in the younger years. Some of these capacities and skills may have become extinguished or inhibited in old age through disuse or paucity of reinforcement. Others may have become inhibited by stress in late life, when many of the psychological systems may be operating near the edge of their reserve capacity. In differentiating between normal and pathological aging, it would be desirable for the clinician to anticipate a period of physiological and psychosocial strain in which capacities, skills, and behaviors will be in a period of flux.

The work of Abramson, Seligman, and Teasdale (1978) on models of learned helplessness indicates that dysfunctional behavior may be a direct consequence of the loss of mastery that characterizes the life style of many older persons with diminished physical, economic, and psychosocial resources. From this perspective, therefore, many depressive disorders can be evaluated as being normal in old age. An abreaction to normalization leads to the opposite pattern of avoiding or ignoring a diagnosis of pathology. Hence neither extreme of orientation, pathologizing or normalizing, is appropriate to good clinical assessment and care.

Table 2–1 Major Aims and Major Aspects of Psychological Assessment of the Elderly

Aims	Major Aspects of Assessment

1. Distinguishing normal from pathological aging	1. Mental health assessment
	  • morale and well-being
	  • life satisfactions
	  • coping styles
	  • personality traits
	  • successful role adjustment

2. Assessment of client's psychosocial needs	
3. Assessment of morbidity and risk factors	

4. Competence of the elderly clients to handle their own affairs	2. Neuropsychological assessment
	  • cognitive functioning assets and deficits
	  • sensory functioning assets and deprivations
	  • distinguishing relatively mild cognitive changes from severe disruptions of cognitive impairment
	  • distinguishing reversible from irreversible problems

5. Assessment of remediation and treatment needs	

3. Intellectual functioning
   • determination of whether intellectual competence is being maintained or is declining; determination of whether decline is gradual or rapid

4. Mental status assessment
   • orientation to time, place, and persons
   • capacity for cognitive task performance

5. Assessment of psychological capacity to maintain an independent role
   • capacity for basic self-care tasks
   • assessment of client's functional resources and strengths/deficits
   • distinguishing between reversible dependencies, disabilities, and emotional disorders and others that are of longstanding duration and therefore irreversible
   • assessment of the extent to which the elderly client can function without supervision or alternatively the extent of custodial care needed

6. Ecological assessment
   • assessment of excess disability, if evident
   • assessment of client's interactions with family, friends, and various professionals and paraprofessionals
   • assessment of the frequency, intensity, and duration of stressors in the client's environment
   • assessment of the extent of social support needed by the client to maintain independent living

7. Assessment of treatment programs necessary to client's functioning
   • assessment of client's capability to benefit from treatment programs

Table 2–1 continued

Aims	Major Aspects of Assessment
	• selection of treatment programs compatible with client's goals for independent functioning or need for custodial care
	8. Assessment of client's social support networks
	• stability of networks, structural features of the networks, and client's subjective views of the support networks available
	• primary relatives, friends, and confidants
	• frequency of interactions with attachment figures
	• losses in social support and the extent to which these losses can be remediated

Note: The major aspects of assessment are not discrete and frequently overlap with one another to generate new categories of geriatric assessment.

Assessment of Client Needs

In order to ensure that the assessment process includes a consideration of the personal preoccupations, attitudes, sensitivities, and unique reactivity of the individual client, the clinician's aim should be to determine the client's need for seeking assessment and to instill in the client a sense of purposefulness. With an effective assessment procedure, oriented to the needs of the client, the latter may feel emotionally supported and reassured by a psychological interview even when no substantial therapeutic intervention or regimen is instituted. By contrast, a most detailed and elaborate assessment procedure may be rejected by a client as useless or redundant if the client felt that the interviewer had merely pursued professional curiosity instead of responding to the practical needs of the client in seeking mental health assessment (Gurland, 1980).

It is surprisingly easy in assessment to overlook the fact that the primary purpose of the assessment is guided by the needs of the client to be reassured of functioning cognitively, emotionally, and socially at an acceptable level. From the viewpoint of the elderly patient the crucial quality of a method of assessment is the degree to which it conveys to the person a sense that someone in the health profession is concerned and taking the trouble to understand the individual's anxieties, problems, or concerns (Gurland, 1980, p. 673).

Morbidity and Risk Factors

From a developmental and preventive mental health perspective the primary purpose of the assessment would be to determine whether the client is at risk for mental illness that calls for preventive intervention. The objective is to assess the indicators of vulnerability to mental illness. Before concluding that the elderly client is at risk, it is useful to assess the presence of other psychosocial problems that may coexist or be of greater importance than the observed depression or observed dysfunctioning. For example, grief and losses, anxiety disorders, family conflicts, and longstanding personality characteristics have been reported as examples of concomitant factors contributing to mental illness in the elderly. In the assessment of risk and morbidity factors priority of attention must be given to the client's depressive disorders.

The purpose of the assessment at this point is to judge whether the client's attitudes, expectancies, and cognitions are part of a normal spectrum of behavior, feeling, or thinking or whether the symptoms reflect morbidity, poor morale, and disturbance of mood outside the range of normal reactions. Some cautions and precautions are advised, principally the following:

- The subject must be clearly informed that the purpose of the queries in the interview is to confirm that the patient is functioning well (Gurland, 1980). The subject is frequently reassured on this score only when the mental health questions are presented in the context of a full health query. Sometimes verification of information by a family member or trusted friend may have to be obtained, and this should be done with the informed consent of the elderly client.

- On a practical level it is important for the practitioner to recognize that even in the most informal and nonthreatening environment, many elderly clients become anxious and confused and may underreport or overreport their symptoms and complaints. Other indicators of vulnerability to mental illness that should be assessed include an evaluation of specific personal and environmental factors that might be contributing to perceptual impairment, recent life-stress events, the quality of the social support network, the individual's coping style, daily pleasant and unpleasant behaviors and events, social role functioning, and morale.

- In settings where it is impractical to assess the client's mental health and mental illness indicators so extensively, the interviewer should at least explore most of these areas. This will provide a more in-depth understanding of the background factors influencing the development or maintenance of the client's sense of vulnerability.

- It is important to orient the elderly client fully to the purpose of the mental health examination and the various paper-and-pencil tools that may be used. It is essential that this be followed promptly by an understandable explanation of the findings. The elderly client should not be left too long in a state of uncertainty about the prognosis.

Competence of the Elderly to Handle Their Own Affairs

The issue of competence to handle one's own affairs will often predominate in geriatric assessment, and many elderly may seek assessment in self-defenses i.e., to establish remaining competence defined as the presence of skills requisite for adequate daily functioning. Such an assessment may require the clinical evaluation of questions such as level of reality contact, intactness of judgment and problem-solving ability, as well as the adaptability to deal successfully with new stimulus situations without distortion of effect.

In such circumstances the aim of assessment would be to assist the client with decisions concerning the severity of disabling symptoms (Gaitz, 1969) and to determine if the client could be reasonably expected to remediate disabling psychological symptoms or to seek intervention for changed physical and social circumstances and social role. Dispositional questions will therefore be addressed as to whether physical limitations or accumulated cerebral losses may be actively inhibiting the ability of the individual to maintain independent functioning. The objective of assessment in these cases is frequently to obtain evidence that will permit the institutionalization or guardianship for a troublesome older relative (Schaie & Schaie, 1977).

Assessment of Placement, Remediation, and Treatment Needs

If the elderly client is judged to be at risk for mental illness, the major task of the assessment is to seek other clinical, laboratory, or psychological methods to evaluate the specific vulnerabilities, deficits, and disorders. The clinical or laboratory procedures may focus on a limited number of mental functions or disorders. Features that will often be evaluated are the intensity of the client's depressive states and suicidal or other dangerous impulses. The neuropsychological assessment discussed later in this chapter must attend to all symptoms of restlessness, agitation, disorientation, and confusional states. When medical emergency is indicated, completion of the assessment will extend beyond the interview techniques and neuropsychological testing to include a comprehensive functional assessment of physical, cognitive-perceptual, and environmental resources.

In those cases where unadaptive behavior may complicate the self-maintenance of the older person in the home or with the family, the objective of assessment may be to seek remediation of the symptoms. As it may be discerned, the clinician's assessment approach very much depends on differentiating the various primary purposes of the assessment.

Lewinsohn and Teri (1983) have expressed concern about the frequent inadequacy of the assessment procedure to provide precise specifications for the remediation of the elderly client. Although the older patient may not clearly understand the purpose of the functional assessment and evaluation and may be understandably fearful about the process and outcome, the clinical geropsychologist must advise the older patient about the symptoms and problems that can be remediated with assistance from the therapist, medical practitioner, and social worker or by means of personal self-control and self-mastery. It is imperative that the assessment require a delineation of both the global characteristics of the individual that will be affected or altered by the recommended intervention procedure and also the precise behaviors that are to be modified in the treatment. Schaie and Schaie (1977) have argued that any less specific assessment procedure would of necessity be superficial and wasteful in addressing the special concerns of the elderly.

THE TASK OF FUNCTIONAL ASSESSMENT

A primary functional purpose may be the determination of baseline behaviors to permit comparison following intervention and treatment (Schaie & Schaie, 1977). Reports from others and a complete social and educational history should supply the necessary information to determine the elderly client's preintervention level of competency. Dispositional questions will therefore be addressed to the relative importance or estimated efficacy of using psychotherapy, conditioning methods, drug treatment, milieu therapy, medical treatment, institutionalization, or home care. In clinical work with the elderly it is important to recognize that these problems are usually multiple and may typically include a systematic combination of medical, psychological, and social-environmental components of intervention and treatment.

What is suggested here is the evaluation of each client in terms of functional capabilities and potentials and deficits. This involves an assessment of the individual client's stresses, depression, and anxieties—what maintains them, what their social, affective, and cognitive concomitants are; and how psychological well-being in general can be improved. Gallagher and Thompson (1983) describe several aspects of the older patient's life that warrant inclusion in a functional assessment battery (see Table 2–2).

From their perspective also, the focus of functional assessment is on the multidimensional aspects of the client's functioning in the community or institutional setting. It takes into account the elderly's physical health status, mental and cognitive functioning, coping styles, social support systems, and other factors such as stressful events, morale and well-being, daily living skills, and adaptive skills.

A MULTIDIMENSIONAL APPROACH TO MENTAL HEALTH ASSESSMENT OF THE ELDERLY

The multidimensional approach ensures that all important physical and psychosocial assets or liabilities in the functioning of the individual receive some attention. (See Table 2–3 for a summary of the major characteristics and major functions of the multidimensional approach to assessment.) The mental health status of the elderly is often influenced by many factors, and as Gaitz and Baer (1970) note, it is sometimes impossible to determine which factors of stress, anxiety, fear, etc., are most influential. These functions are often intricately interrelated (Dovenmuehle, 1968) and frequently complicated by social factors, experiential factors, past adaptations, and cultural attitudes. Consequently, when a multidimensional assessment of the elderly is undertaken, the rigid distinctions between stress, anxiety, fears, intellectual functioning, perceptual functioning, and their relationship with disease states or behavioral disorders are dropped. Social, psychological, and physical dimensions all receive concurrent attention (see Table 2–3).

Although the multidimensional orientation may suggest a medical and psychosocial evaluation solely directed toward the elderly client, the correct interpretation would be that it integrally involves an evaluation of the whole person, the person's environment, and the environmental resources and liabilities. According to Gaitz and Baer (1970) the best practical application of a psychosocial evaluation eventuates only when we determine whether an individual can perform the tasks required for adjustment and adaptation in the milieu in which the client lives. For example, an elderly person with no social supports, few psychological resources of initiative and assertiveness, and limited medical facilities faces different problems than those living with the family or those living in institutions.

The complex interplay of fears, anxieties, stresses, personality dimensions, and psychological factors becomes abundantly clear when the factors are assessed concurrently and when one can observe how the various patterns of factors and trends in interaction affect the adjustment and coping of the elderly person. The overall psychological state of the elderly client assessed in terms of the interaction of the stresses and physical disease adds a very significant dimension to the mental health status of the elderly. For example, mental confusion in the elderly can be attributed to social isolation, emotional stresses, or losses as well as a series of brain diseases or organic brain syndromes. Overcoming social isolation, or helping the elderly deal with their fears or stresses, then becomes as integral a part of the evaluation and treatment as does the assessment of dementia.

Although practitioners and clinicians restrict themselves to those psychosocial problems that they are trained to treat, collaboration from social agencies, community services, families, and other psychiatric and medical personnel may be important for the total care of the elderly person. Although this multidimensional evaluation approach has been used with

Table 2–2 Assessment Battery for the Diagnosis and Functional Assessment of Elderly Depressed Patients

Domain	Instrument	Focus	Format	Reference
1. Physical Health Status	Health History Form Current Medication Form & perceived health rating	Self-report of past & current health status.	Yes/no to presence of symptoms or medication use (from list) severity rating/health status.	Raskin & Crook, n.d.
2. Mental Status & Cognitive Function	Mini-Mental State Exam	Orientation: immediate & delayed recall; constructional dyspraxia.	Interview questions/correct or incorrect.	Folstein, Folstein & McHugh, 1975
3. Differential Diagnosis	History	Timeline for symptom presence.	Clinician's judgment.	—
	Schedule for Affective Disorders & Schizophrenia (SADS)	Duration, intensity of mood disturbance & related symptoms.	Interview/rating of items on scale 0–6.	Endicott & Spitzer, 1978
	Brief Symptom Inventory (BSI)	Other psychiatric problems (e.g., anxiety).	Indicate how distressing symptoms are; 5-pt. scale.	Derogatis, 1977
	Brief Psychiatric Rating Scale (BPRS)	Presence of other psychopathology.	Interviewer rating of symptom intensity.	Overall & Gorham, 1962
4. Level of Depression	Hamilton Rating Scale for Depression Beck Depression Inventory (BDI)	Associated features, particularly somatic. Mood disturbance and related symptoms.	Interview—17 to 19 items rated 0–3. Self-rating: select 1 of 4 choices for intensity of symptom.	Hamilton, 1960 Hamilton, 1967 Beck, Ward, Mendelson, Mock, & Erbaugh, 1961
	Zung Self-Rating Depression Scale (SDS) Geriatric Depression Scale (GDS)	Same as above. Mood disturbance primarily; designed especially for elders.	Indicate frequency of occurrence of each symptom, presence or absence of each symptom (yes/no format).	Zung, 1965 Yesavage, Brink, Rose, Lum, Huang, Adey, & Leirer, in press
5. Personality	Eysenck Personality Inventory	Introversion/ extraversion; neuroticism.	True/false to whether items apply.	Eysenck & Eysenck, 1968
	Sixteen Personality Factor Questionnaire (16PF)	Separate bipolar factors related to personality traits.	Yes/no/don't know.	Cattell, 1956

Table 2–2 continued

Domain	Instrument	Focus	Format	Reference
6. Occurrence of Stressful Life Events	Health & Daily Living Questionnaire	Frequency of common stresses (e.g., sickness).	Indicate which of a standard list has occurred, when, & how much control.	Moos, Cronkite, Finney & Billings, 1980
7. Coping Styles	Health & Daily Living Questionnaire	How does person cope with stressful event and with depression.	Indicate which of a list of common coping strategies are used and how often.	Moos et al., 1980
8. Social-Support System	Social Support Index and Questionnaire	Perceived support obtainable from others and number in network.	Indicate true/false and describe number in network.	Wilcox, 1981
	Social Network Questionnaire	Amount, frequency, and quality of contact with significant others.	Interview questions and rating scale.	Thompson, Gallagher, & Peterson, 1979
9. Cognitive Distortions	Automatic Thoughts Questionnaire (ATQ)	Occurrence of dysfunctional thoughts.	Frequency and degree of belief in standard list of distorted thoughts.	Hollon & Kendall, 1980
	Young Loneliness Inventory	Perception of social isolation/ loneliness.	Select one of four alternatives for each item to reflect intensity.	Young, 1981
10. Expectancies	Hopelessness Scale	Pessimism regarding future and present.	True/false whether items apply.	Beck, Weissman, Lester & Trexler, 1974
	Target Complaints	Current problems (in own words) and goals for therapy.	Interview to obtain number and severity of primary complaints.	Mintz, 1981
	Expected BDI	Expected symptom picture at end of therapy.	Use BDI form; change instructions.	Steinmetz, Lewinsohn, & Antonuccio, in press
11. Attributions	Attributional Style Questionnaire (original)	Degree of internality, globality, and stability re causes of events.	Select cause for vignettes, then rate cause on these three dimensions.	Peterson, Semmel, von Baeyer, Abramson, Metalsky, & Seligman, 1982
	Attribution Index (modified for elders)	Same dimensions.	Vignettes chosen for relevance to elders.	Bisno, Thompson, Breckenridge, & Gallagher, 1982

Table 2–2 continued

Domain	Instrument	Focus	Format	Reference
12. Daily Behaviors	Pleasant and Unpleasant Activities Schedules (PES & UES)	Frequency and impact of number of pleasant and unpleasant everyday activities.	Indicate each dimension on 3-point scales.	PES: MacPhillamy & Lewinsohn, 1982 UES: Lewinsohn & Talkington, 1979
	Older Person's PES and UES: modified versions of above	Events selected for appropriateness for variety of elders.	Same.	Hedlund & Gilewski, In Gallagher et al., 1981
13. Social Adjustment	Social Adjustment Scale self-report (SAS-SR)	Adjustment to work, leisure, and family life.	Respond to specific questions along intensity dimension.	Weissman, 1980 Weissman & Bothwell, 1976
	Katz Adjustment Scales (KAS)	Frequency and satisfaction with leisure activities and social-role performance.	Four-point self-rating scales; relatives' form also available.	Katz & Lyerly, 1963
14. Well-being	Morale Scale	Level of well-being and satisfaction.	Indicate agreement with positive and negative statements.	Lawton, 1975
	Life Satisfaction Index	Same.	Agree/disagree with items reflecting outlook on life.	Wood, Wylie, & Shaefor, 1969

Source: From *Clinical Geropsychology: New Directions in Assessment and Treatment* (pp. 19–20) by P.M. Lewinsohn and L. Teri (Eds.), 1983, Elmsford, N.Y.: Pergamon Press, Inc. Copyright 1983 by Pergamon Press, Inc. Reprinted by permission.

mentally ill aged who must be hospitalized or institutionalized, the general principles underlying this approach seem applicable to the evaluation of the elderly person in general, regardless of predominant presenting psychosocial or medical concerns (Lawton, 1971; Palmore, 1980).

RANGE OF THE MULTIDIMENSIONAL ASSESSMENT INTERVIEW

According to Clausen (1969) the emphasis of clinical assessment must shift from a detailed record of symptomatology to an assessment of the mental health assets and strengths on the one hand and the limitations and impairments of function on the other hand (Gurland et al., 1970; Kendell et al., 1971). Such a broad assessment is most appropriately done through the interview approach rather than the psychometric approach. Some impor-

Table 2–3 Characteristics and Functions of the Multidimensional Approach to Mental Health Assessment of the Elderly

Characteristics	*Functions and Specific Assessment Objectives*
The approach ensures that all important physical and psychosocial assets and liabilities of the client will be assessed and will receive concurrent attention.	Analysis of the elderly client's problem situation Analysis of the antecedents and consequences of the elderly client's behavioral responses
The approach requires that the rigid distinctions between intellectual functioning, perceptual functioning, behavioral disorders, and physical dimensions be dropped and a more holistic picture of the elderly client be formulated.	Analysis of the elderly client's assets and deficits in functioning Analysis of the elderly client's social relationships and social support networks Motivational analysis
The approach requires that mental health status of the client be assessed not merely in terms of the client's psychosocial characteristics but equally with respect to environmental and ecological resources and liabilities.	Analysis of the elderly client's social-cultural-physical environment Developmental analysis of the elderly client in terms of past and present adaptations and adjustments
The approach requires that a number of miniinterviews (structured or semistructured) and follow-up meetings structured over time are more appropriate to assessment of the elderly than is a comprehensive single interview.	Identification of specific targets for remediation and intervention
The approach relies on interview technologies such as CARE or OARS methodology in which structured or semistructured interviews are designed to assess the functional status of the respondents, their perceptions of needed services, and their strengths and assets in physical and emotional health and activities of daily living.	

tant components of the broad band interview and the major advantages and disadvantages of interviewing methods are considered here.

Structured Diagnostic Interview

As Schaie and Schaie (1977) observe, interviews vary from a brief screening-type encounter to extensive systematic questioning. They also vary in the degree of structuring from a general encouragement to the clients to tell the therapist more about themselves to quite specific questions and specific tasks to be performed. The purpose may be to assess the psychiatric status of the client with respect to mental functioning, or alternatively the objective may be to assess intrapsychic processes.

Several examples are available of structured interview schedules developed to elicit comprehensive views of life history or life style. Butler and Lewis (1973) and Schaie and Gribbin (1975) have developed structured interview schedules incorporating a life review form and a life complexity interview schedule for use with older persons. Data elicited include personal and family status, community involvements, friendship patterns, medical information and health items, and psychiatric information including attitudes toward death and self. Such an interview schedule is instituted with the additional goal of determining the complexity of the elderly person's environment and history.

At its best the structured interview approach to assessing the psychological functioning of the client is quick and flexible, takes a rich variety of clinical information into account including data not easily objectified, and weighs and sifts these data in a logical manner (Gurland, 1973). Fortunately for the elderly patient there is a strong movement for clinicians to apply the methods of psychology rather than psychiatric diagnosis. This trend emerged with a gathering of interest in the degree and nature of the unreliability of psychiatric diagnosis and the clinical interview in assessing the interactive physical, psychodynamic, biochemical, and medical history of the elderly (Krietman, Sainsbury, Morrissey, Towers, & Scrivener, 1961; Ward, Beck, Mendelson, Mock, & Erbaugh, 1962). Such unreliability is partly associated with the heterogeneity and overlap of somatic, psychological, and medical symptoms shown by the elderly in different diagnostic groups.

In an effort to make assessment and diagnosis more reliable, the World Health Organization has sponsored an international glossary of diagnostic categories mutually respected by psychologists and psychiatrists in the performance of the interviews. Of equal importance is the introduction of structured interview techniques that resort to the format of psychological tests. The procedure has several advantages, principally the following:

- By applying the structured interview to assess the mental state of elderly clients, small units of behavior (including expressed feelings, ramblings, distractions, motility, etc.) can be noted. Thus one of the major advantages of the structured interview with the elderly is that the clinician or psychologist can record symptoms in detail, and these symptoms may be used for classifying the elderly subjects in terms of psychosocial evaluation and cognitive functioning levels.

- Many of the psychometric tests developed by psychologists to determine the severity of depression, and the adaptational and adjustment capabilities of the elderly, can be incorporated bodily in the structured interview. For example, a psychological test such as the abbreviated Mental Status Test (Kahn, Goldfarb, Pollack, & Peck, 1960) described in Chapter 4 can be embedded in the structured interview. Other items can also be added to expand those areas of mental status assessment considered of particular importance in the elderly such as disorientation, memory lapses, hypochondriasis, and general physical functioning.

- Alternatively the same structured procedure is intended to identify characteristics of successful aging. Indexes can be developed to provide measures of health, activity, social relations, and cognitive alertness.

Using diagnostic criteria for the assessment of depressive disorders (see Diagnostic and Statistical Manual of Mental Disorders (DSM-III, 1980)) it is possible to include into a semistructured interview items that help the clinician obtain ratings of the elderly patient's depressive symptoms and depressive functioning along a number of dimensions. Thus, the clinician can make clinical observations of the elderly person's responses, reactions, and interactions based on a number of symptomatology ratings and behavioral ratings of depression, such as elation, sadness, acute and chronic anxiety, neurotic tendencies, and emotional states. Assessment of depression can therefore be made reliably in the course of one structured interview.

Clausen (1969) notes, however, that in view of the need to keep the interview brief and not too tiring for the elderly client, the practitioner must accept that assessment procedures must be spread over a number of interviews. Observations concerning the affective or social role functioning may not be valid unless they are stretched over time. Therefore multiple miniinterviews with the client and follow-up meetings with the elderly's family members and friends are finding a significant place in the assessment techniques of the practitioner (Clausen, 1969).

A number of advantages may also accrue from repeated miniinterviews with the elderly client. Acutely anxious elderly may become sufficiently relaxed to reveal their diagnostic features. Some confusional states associated with agitation resulting from situational-external events may clear up after the elderly individual has had a chance to relax and think about the clinician's communications in the miniinterview. Thus several structured miniinterviews are able to achieve the major objectives of a psychiatric status interview intended to evaluate orientation, memory, judgment, and cognitive abilities as well as a functional status assessment of the client in relation to social adjustment, well-being, and coping strategies.

A number of standardized assessment interview procedures have been used in the multidimensional approach. Some of the more well-known standardized procedures follow:

Comprehensive Assessment and Referral Evaluation (CARE). The CARE (Gurland et al., 1970) semistructured interview guide is designed specifically for the elderly living in the community and provides an inventory of defined and precoded items on discrete depressive symptoms and problems with a view to promoting consistency in recording of subjects' responses. There is a comprehensive coverage of psychological, medical, nutritional, economic, and social problems, and positive assets as well as deficits are covered. There are questions on somatic concerns, cognitive function, affective states, and behavioral symptoms ratable from the interview. Sources of information include self-report of the elderly client, observations of the interviewer, psychological testing of the client, and reports from informants. The information gathered does not rely on the subject's assuming the sick role, nor is it restricted to hearsay evidence of a medical label. Specific symptoms are recorded to allow independent recognition of important depressive syndromes. The information elicited permits distinctions to be made among psychiatric, medical, and social problems. A systematic narrative summary of symptoms, according to prescribed guidelines, is prepared for each of the problem domains. As noted by Gurland et al. (1970, 1976, 1978), CARE has three important functions.

First, it enables the practitioner to obtain differential diagnosis of depressed elderly patients by providing ratings for severity of depression along lines of limited depression, which refers to depression that is transient or can be self-suppressed so that a substantial part of life is free of depression; pervasive depression, which refers to depression that pervades most aspects of life (depression that occurs regularly each day for a large proportion of the day and at the same time of the day); and corresponding vegetative symptoms (not accounted for by physical disease), self-depreciation cognitions, and suicidal cognitions.

Second, it allows for a differential diagnosis of depression and dementia. Criteria for diagnosis and severity of dementia are provided along lines of limited cognitive disturbance, which refers to an impairment of memory but with substantial aspects of living adequately performed; pervasive dementia, which refers usually to an impairment of memory that renders the subject incapable of certain task performance and renders it necessary for the subject to be supervised; and other dementia-related features such as progressive deterioration (not accounted for by a physical disorder) and incidence of lucid intervals. Subclassifications of pervasive dementia are also described in terms of specific ratings. The interview is so designed that symptoms can be examined in order to determine the nature of the problem, the factors contributing to the symptoms being reported and whether the symptoms have clinical significance or medical-physical significance, and what pattern of disturbance is indicated within the social-psychological or medical-physical functioning of the elderly person.

Third, according to Gurland et al. (1970, 1976, 1978), the semistructured CARE interview is designed to make older persons feel comfortable and relaxed in the exploration of their problem. Notwithstanding the fact that the structured interview techniques require a substantial amount of self-disclosure, and the current form of the interview takes about one hour to administer, the clinician is instructed to make the client feel like the central figure in the interview by giving warmth, support, and acceptance (Gurland et al., 1970).

Older American's Resources Services Questionnaire (OARS). This semistructured interview technique (Pfeiffer, 1970) with forced choice responses permits ratings of social resources, economic resources, mental health, and physical health. Like the CARE battery, the OARS is a reliable assessment technique designed to elicit, rate, and classify information on the social-emotional and physical health of the older person. Parts of this technique are designed to be completed by a multidisciplinary team working independently (e.g., psychiatrist and psychologist). Like the CARE battery, the OARS provides a numerical score indicating extent of and severity of depressive symptomatology.

Essentially the OARS methodology is designed to assess the functional status of the respondents, their perceptions of needed services, and interviewers' ratings of respondents' physical health, mental health, and activities of daily living (Fillenbaum & Smyer, 1981). One noteworthy feature of the OARS methodology is that it is designed to be interwoven into the fabric of a semistructured counseling interview in which respondents are encouraged to reflect also on subjective perceptions of loneliness, social support, nurturance needs, and other psychological leanings. The use of these batteries at the initial interview stage may provide an economical and effective way to begin the assessment process and to set the stage for later in-depth assessment of specific areas appropriate for a more complete assessment of all of the resources available to the individual.

In the total process of condensing and integrating the data, information obtained from informants who know the elderly person is often vital in determining the individual's condition. The variety of disciplinary skills at play all point to the importance of inter-disciplinary teamwork in the clinical assessment of the elderly. The team approach to clinical assessment of the elderly is based on the assumption that the functional status of various social, physical, and psychological systems is typically interdependent; physical and psychological functions are often intricately interrelated, frequently complicated by social factors and cultural attitudes, and cannot be understood except in relation to one another. All the relevant spheres are, however, discussed separately in an attempt to illustrate the breadth of the approach required in assessing the elderly subject's mental health status. In this sense the structured interview procedure, such as the CARE or OARS, is often a channel of communication between interviewers from different disciplines (such as clinical psychology and psychiatry, social work, nursing, medicine) as well as between the interviewer and the patient.

Kanfer and Saslow (1965) have elaborated on seven major areas that might be appropriate for analyses in the interview (see Table 2–3).

1. Analysis of the problem situation. This analysis requires that the exact problem (whether social, medical, or somatic) be identified as specifically as possible. This helps to clear targets for intervention. The frequency, intensity, and duration of each problem should be considered in the specific context of the situation. Zarit (1980, p. 127) proposes that problems should be classified as *excesses* or *deficits* of behaviors. For example, nonassertive and nondemanding ways of subjects that the staff may label as good behavior may actually be deficits in behavior that may lead to the client's tension or frustration. Continuous activity, accompanied by signs of agitation and anxiety, may be an indication of excess behavior that is not goal directed or problem solving in outcome.

2. Analysis of antecedents and consequences. This analysis involves determining what happens before and after the problem and what are its main consequences or effects on the cognitions, feelings, and reactions of the elderly person interacting with the environment (Zarit, 1980, p. 127). For example, the symptoms that are shared by depression, physical illness, and old age include sleep disturbance, appetite disturbance, slowing of movement, social dysfunctions, and fatigue. Although these are important symptoms of depression, they can also originate in physical illness, stress, and crises. The important point to assess is the precise precipitating factors that led to the depression, disturbances, or social dysfunctions and to determine whether the depression led to the social dysfunction or the converse.

3. Analysis of other assets and deficits in functioning. Kanfer and Saslow (1965) suggest that in addition to focusing on the problem behavior, it might be useful to determine what other positive qualities and deficits in functioning the elderly client may have. For example, an elderly client may have the necessary mobility, transportation facilities, and finances for social activities but may have few social skills or resources for satisfying social activities. It is often useful to ask "what would be different if you were cured or did not have this problem" (Zarit, 1980, p. 129). It may become apparent that the individual would have other behavioral or cognitive deficits if the presenting problem were treated. Thus identifying both deficits and assets can give important information for devising a treatment plan.

4. Analysis of social relationship. Elderly subjects' ideas about social relationships that lead to passive or unassertive behaviors are often associated with feelings of depression and anomie. Therefore, an important focus of the assessment should be the client's ideas about social relationships. The person's social network should be considered, especially vis-à-vis individuals who are affected by the target problem or have an influence over it (e.g., the healthy spouse of a disabled elderly patient).

5. Motivational analysis. The elderly patient's motivations for treatment should be considered with a focus on those persons, events, objects, or activities that are reinforcing or aversive for the client. The underuse of mental health facilities by the elderly (Lawton & Gottesman, 1974) may well be related to the fears that the clinician may assess their psychological health as being inadequate for purposes of leading an independent life. Self-referral by the elderly person may therefore be subject to much more serious selection problems than among the young (Atchley, 1969). An important question to ask in an assessment is why a person decided to seek treatment at this time. For example, if a person has been depressed for a long time but seeks help because her children recently moved away, a goal of treatment may be to help her develop new social relationships. If an elderly client voluntarily seeks assessment, a factor to be considered is whether the family is exerting pressure on the elderly person

to move to a nursing home. In brief, a motivational analysis helps to determine the specific purpose for which assessment is being sought.

6. Analysis of the social-cultural-physical environment. This involves determining how well persons fit in with the expected norms for a given behavior and for being functional in their current environment. It may be important to obtain the client's ideas about the expected norms and personal norms and to help the client establish a better balance between personal needs and the demands of the environment. Quite commonly, aged people may feel that they are expected to be passive and hold back their views on family functioning (Zarit, 1980). Such an expectation of passivity or incompetence may lead to tension and frustration in an elderly person. It may be important to help such elderly to reestablish their own standards of competence, behavior, and self-care and to reinforce them for effort to restore their cognitive functioning.

Of equal concern is the tendency of the young clinician to attend to stereotypes about the old rather than to the characteristics of the elderly client (Ahammer & Baltes, 1972). Cognitive impairments, especially decrements of memory and intellect, are one of the most common expectations that clinicians and families appear to have about the aged. The aging process in most cultural contexts is viewed to be a gradual downward trajectory. Such stereotypes can be reduced if clinicians make it their major goal in assessment to become familiar with the family environment of the elderly client and to evaluate the client's functioning relative to the socioeconomic status of the client, the functional roles (e.g., helpless, or sick role, or autonomous and competent role) that the client plays within the family context. Also to be considered are the family members' expectancies of the elderly person.

7. Developmental analysis. This analysis provides information about the elderly person's typical functioning in the past, affective problems that the client experienced, and treatment strategies that were effective. More commonly behaviors that were adaptive in the earlier life of an aged person may no longer be adaptive, and maladaptive behaviors may be precipitated by sudden and dramatic losses and changes characteristic of old age. Changes in health status, self-concept, and cognitive-behavioral skills are often pertinent in aiding a differential diagnosis between depression, somatic complaints, and dementia.

Some difficulties peculiar to the structured interview procedure may present a problem in the multifunctional assessment. Practitioners often come with preconceived expectations that the aged have deficits in general adaptational and cognitive function, and they may make on-line judgments at the end of an interview. Thus on-line decisions may be made as to whether to assign symptoms such as fatigue, disorientation, and memory confusions to the realm of normal aging, depressive disorders, or cognitive impairment. After the initial structured interview, more detailed observations in subsequent assessment are necessary before final judgments are made as to mental status and related physical, medical, or social health status of the elderly client. Thus the assessment procedure may become a protracted process, which may be unrealistic in the case of many elderly.

Overall, however, the information and data gathered by means of the CARE or OARS interview technique can result in the identification of specific targets for intervention. It also facilitates evaluation of the personal and environmental factors that are related to an individual client's functioning, providing information on the personality, stressful life events, coping styles, social support systems, and social function roles.

In settings where it is impractical to conduct such an extensive diagnostic interview, it is recommended that the clinician at least explore some of the areas. These will provide a more in-depth understanding of the background factors contributing to the current mental health status of the geriatric client and will help to reconstruct the client's life style and also to elicit the respondent's feelings regarding the problems of aging. Thus the clinician may obtain a more clear diagnostic picture, which could provide the basis for a tailor-made treatment plan later (Gallagher & Thompson, 1983). For example, the clinician may conclude that an elderly person with a significant number of stresses, some cognitive impairment, few coping strategies, and poor social supports is likely to need more immediate and long-term help than another client who has a stronger social support network and a variety of coping strategies in the behavioral repertoire.

Special Considerations for Interviewing and Intake

Various clinicians (e.g., Gurland, 1973; Hussian, 1981; Schaie & Gribbin, 1975) have suggested a number of modifications in the interviewing process that are particularly relevant to elderly persons. These are summarized in Exhibit 2–1.

1. Generally the interview should be shorter than with most age groups as even healthy elderly clients tend to show the effects of fatigue after approximately 40 minutes

---

Exhibit 2–1 Special Considerations in Assessment Interviewing and Intake of Elderly Clients

1. Arrange for interview to be relatively shorter for elderly clients, and monitor closely for effects of fatigue on client's attention and communication.
2. Establish rapport with client before focusing on client's disabilities, impairments, and deficits. Several miniinterviews may be necessary to establish the necessary rapport.
3. Questions assessing client's disabilities should be spaced throughout the interview rather than massed at the beginning or end of the interview.
4. It is important to be sensitive to the elderly client's individual qualities and cultural difficulties and to the client's resistance and avoidance in reporting feelings and in admitting to disorders.
5. Appropriate support, empathy, and intermittent positive reinforcement should be given frequently in order to elicit more information from the elderly.
6. Allow the elderly client sufficient time to react to questions that are of a sensitive nature.
7. Interviewer must be prepared to be patient with elderly clients having speech and communication difficulties. Interviewers must train themselves to speak slowly and clearly and to monitor the client's level of attention.
8. Due allowance must be made for old-age losses in auditory and visual acuity and reaction time.
9. Interviewer must maintain positive attitudes, be aware of stress and anxieties that older clients experience in situations of evaluation, and take appropriate and prompt steps to alleviate the elderly client's anxiety.
10. Interviewer must invariably arrange to close the interview on a positive and reinforcing note.

(Gurland, 1973). Hussian (1981) notes that elderly clients with some brain impairment may not attend for longer than 5 to 10 minutes, thus making it necessary for the interviewer to see the client several times until sufficient information is gathered. The interview should not exceed the limits of the client's attention and tolerance since beyond this point the chances of errors in communication will increase rapidly. However, as Gurland (1980) notes, most elderly clients can accept and appreciate the same length of interview suitable for younger persons.

2. Because of the emotional vulnerability of many older persons, questions that might be distressing or may focus intensely on the respondent's disabilities should be spaced throughout the interview rather than massed (Gurland, 1973). Questions that focus on the client's disabilities and impairments should be raised after the client is somewhat more relaxed. Distressing issues should not be raised toward the end of the interview unless the patient volunteers such matters. It is crucial in the closing phase of the interview not to overstress the elderly client by raising emotionally laden topics or by testing cognitive functions (Gurland, 1980). The last few minutes of the interview should be left to the client to control, in any way desired. The interviewer must always attempt to close the interview on a reinforcing note conveying the message that the client has been most cooperative and helpful in that phase of the assessment.

3. There is a particular need to be sensitive to individual personality and cultural differences in an older person's willingness to report feelings and behaviors. Gergen and Back (1966) noted, for example, that their more highly educated respondents were less reactive in an opinion-eliciting situation regardless of the behavior of the interviewer.

   One cannot assume with the elderly clients that they are highly motivated to provide information that will be useful to themselves or to their clinician. Even with the self-referred elderly client there will be the tendency either to overreport or to underreport complaints relevant to important diagnosis of discomfort or disorders. The clinician must bear in mind the greater cautiousness of the elderly, their anxiety about receiving negative feedback, and the extension of risk-avoiding behavior when confronted with a situation of evaluation (Furry & Baltes, 1973). Much avoidance behavior, however, can be easily modified when appropriate support and empathy are introduced in the assessment situation. Positive incentive and reinforcement, therefore, in the form of verbal encouragement and praise should be frequently given by the interviewer in order to elicit more information from the elderly client. It is important, however, that the reinforcement be delivered randomly and not be made contingent on certain types of information that suit the clinician's orientation (Hussian, 1981). A good assessment is both searching and comprehensive. Sensitive topics such as family conflicts, physical abuse, suicide, etc., cannot be ignored. Several brief interviews may be required by the clinician to establish the necessary rapport with the client.

4. In spite of measurable differences in the rate of responding of elderly people, it is important to allow the elderly clients sufficient time to react either to questions involving historical information or to test items. Of greater concern is the tendency of the young clinician to emphasize speedy responses, which interferes with the elderly client's ability to provide useful information.

5. Communication and perceptual impairment (especially partial deafness) may create a strain in the interview. Interviewers can train themselves to speak slowly, clearly,

and firmly and with their lips plainly visible to the elderly client. The interviewer should be prepared to be patient with elderly clients whose speech impairments, such as dysphasias and dysarthrias, will make communications rather difficult. Gurland (1980) suggests that the communication can be greatly improved by a good match between the interviewer's style and the patient's attention. For example, the interviewer should be sure to signal the delivery of a question by use of body movements such as leaning forward and looking straight at the client. Another consideration is that the client's attention should be focused on the interviewer. It is possible for the interviewer to monitor the client's level of attention by watching face and eyes and to ask a question when there is reasonable evidence that the client is attentive and alert.

6. The clinician ought to be satisfied that visual acuity and auditory defects are corrected to the point that the client can handle test performance or interview responses without significant interference. If questionnaires are being used, alternate forms of the questionnaire, often available in larger typefaces, are readily accessible and may facilitate accurate responding by the client. Apparent decremental findings on task performance, suspected confusion, slowed reaction time, and errors may be a function of poor lighting and contrast, imposing a strain on the inefficient receptors of the elderly client. Apparent perceptual distortion of visual and motor tasks in the aged may be a function of deficit in peripheral sensory function rather than be indicative of organic and functional pathology. In order to safeguard against these adverse and atypical diagnoses, the interview and assessment tasks should be conducted when the client is most rested and comfortable (Hussian, 1981) and lighting is sufficient. In other words information should be gathered when stimulus conditions are optimal.

7. Another major factor discussed by several clinicians (e.g., Butler, 1969; Schaie & Geiwitz, 1982) is the need for maintaining appropriately positive attitudes toward elderly clients. It is important for clinicians to be aware of the nature and impact of their attitudes, especially the negative attitudes, on the emotional functioning of the elderly client. The tendency of many older people to attempt to please the professional examiner may make it likely that the client may consciously or unconsciously become pessimistic about the outcome of assessment. Thus negative attitudes of the clinician may interfere with the conduct of objective and adequate assessment.

8. The interviewer must from the outset be aware of the common anxieties that older persons experience in being assessed by a clinician. The more anxious the older person gets, the more likely that person is to make errors in responding, to be hesitant to complete tasks that assess cognitive functioning. Under these circumstances the interviewer's concern about the elderly client's poor performance may create further anxiety or sometimes even frank hostility in the client. If the interviewer does not take prompt account of the client's anxieties, the quality of the interview may quickly deteriorate.

9. Most clinical assessment of older clients is based on the interaction between the client and other members of the family whose reportings may be useful to the clinician. For example, Blessed, Tomlinson, and Roth (1968) noted that information on apparent senile changes reported by the elderly person's family members correlated highly with clinical findings. Supplemental information from other sources such as the family and social networks of the elderly client should always be sought. Hussian (1981) stresses the need for routine informal validation of the client's reportings from external sources. Since denial or overreportings of symptoms are a

common phenomenon in the elderly, clinical diagnosis made on the basis of limited contact with the client is often open to question. Family members, relatives, and friends may be able to fill in gaps in the historical information, especially for elderly clients experiencing confusional states or partial lapses of memory. Family members may, for example, be able to provide more accurate intake data concerning the number, type, and quality of the client's social contacts; recent residential relocations; and changes in physical, financial, and social conditions. Pertinent data may include type of housing, adequacy of meal services, and the type and quantity of social and cognitive stimulation that characterizes the elderly person's environment. Such data are essential also to the accurate financial functional assessment of the elderly described earlier.

10. The medical approach may be warranted in many cases because of the many obvious physical symptoms or disease correlates of the older person's depression, affective disorders, and confusional states. In any case the medical advice must always be sought and considered. A behavioral assessment is also advocated in many cases since a majority of medical disorders in old age have obvious behavioral correlates. In short, the intake report must routinely obtain data concerning the use of potentially problematic medications and physical illness. It must include the acquisition of laboratory tests particularly as they pertain to hearing and vision tests, glucose levels, electrolyte assays, and other vital capacities of the geriatric client.

11. Diagnosis of behavior disorders may be needed in some cases for counseling the older individual to achieve better adjustment. The major issue in the study of behavior disturbances in the elderly seems to be the need to establish criteria for what level or range of behavioral functioning is characteristic for an aged group or what might be termed pathology. For example, behaviors reflecting passivity or withdrawal may be optimal for some elderly who have always had a disengaging life style while maintenance of activity may reflect the normative behavior of other old people. In either case, the identification of behaviors reflecting disorders necessarily depends upon the individual's personal mode of adaptation in old age. The latter should be of special concern to the clinical psychologist's assessment of the elderly client.

The ultimate goal of complete data assessment, of course, is to identify the treatable aspects of the elderly clients' dysfunctioning and to develop more adequately a plan for remediation, treatment, or prevention that will enhance the clients' overall life adjustment.

ASSESSMENT AND MODELS OF PSYCHOPATHOLOGY

The clinician's framework or model of psychopathology is critical because it influences whether the professional perceives that a person has a problem, whether treatment is likely to be effective if a problem exists, and what type of treatment to use. The means of assessment is dictated by the clinician's own beliefs about the nature of psychopathology in the elderly.

Medical Model

This model implies that various mental and emotional disturbances are due to structural damage to body organs, especially the brain, or to altered physiological processes, as in disorders of metabolism or endocrine function. In terms of the elderly this model provides an appropriate framework for conceptualizing some common psychiatric problems. Principal among these are brain disorders.

Another emphasis of this model is that disordered behaviors emanate from within the individual. The consequence of looking for causes within the individual is that critical interpersonal and environmental events that have a profound influence on dysfunctional behaviors may be missed. An overreliance on the medical model can lead to problems in the aged. There is a tendency to see any problem of older persons as due to a vaguely defined internal disorder: the aging process (Zarit, 1980). Aging is incorrectly perceived by many practitioners as involving a gradual deterioration in functioning in all areas. The aging process is often conceptualized as a gradual downward trajectory, with ever-increasing levels of impairment, until the person is helpless and incompetent.

This model of aging, however, has not been supported by empirical studies (Zarit & Zarit, 1983). Furthermore, estimates of the effects of aging on the physical and cognitive health have been exaggerated by a number of factors, including generational differences and the medical practitioner's lack of knowledge of biological and physiological processes in aging. Behaviors of the old are sometimes inappropriately labeled *senile* or *senescent*. The extent to which the process of biological aging is implicated in the development of behavioral problems of the elderly is difficult to ascertain accurately. It is likely that the aging process will contribute in varying degrees to the onset of behavioral and affective symptoms. The role of the medical model in assessment of pathology is prominent when a differentiation is required among physical illness accompanied by neuropathology or cognitive impairment as a result of illness or brain syndrome. Results of such evaluation would have obvious implications for the role of the medical model in the treatment of the cognitively impaired elderly.

Psychodynamic Model

Psychodynamic models of treatment and diagnosis form an important variant of the medical model. Rather than viewing the causes of disorders as medical illness, however, psychodynamic theories stress the importance of early psychological experiences as the roots of pathology manifested in adulthood. As with the medical model, psychodynamic writers emphasize that the symptoms reflect an underlying illness and that one must treat the deep-seated conflict that lies at the core of the symptoms. Again looking for causes within the individual brings the risk of ignoring critical interpersonal and other environmental effects.

Although the psychodynamic model has its limitations, it is valuable in its conceptualizations of intraindividual variables. The elderly may mask their depression through a variety of ego-defensive mechanisms. They commonly are reluctant to admit depression and use denial, counterphobic defenses, or express depressive symptoms through somatic complaints and hypochondriasis. Faced with loss, diminished capacity for flexible gratification, and withdrawal of supports, a failing self-esteem and a sense of hopelessness may threaten to overwhelm the older person (Salzman & Shader, 1979). In order to cope, the ego of the older person may employ a variety of adaptive defense mechanisms that are attempts to reduce the conscious awareness of psychic pain (Salzman & Shader, 1979). Ego defenses used when they were younger may still be available and even become exaggerated with age.

If questions have been appropriately focused, it should be possible to specify some of the particular interpersonal behaviors or ego defenses of the client that may be interfering with optimal functioning. With the aged client attention could appropriately be focused on issues such as intergenerational conflict, the client's need to retain independent functioning and the need, therefore, to deny limitations and to cover up, through denial, the presence of inadequacies and deficits in functioning.

In its mild form denial can help the elderly person by providing a coping mechanism to deal with some of the tensions and diminishing capacities. However, the denial is maladaptive when it leads to worsening of physical illness or failure to develop realistic coping mechanisms to deal with changes in later life. According to Salzman and Shader (1979) severe denial can lead to some restriction of the ego so that anything that produces discomfort or painful effect is avoided by an ensuing restriction of awareness. In the majority of elderly people denial is not so severe and is usually incomplete. Certain memories, cognitive abilities, and sensory functions are variably retained while others are excluded from consciousness and expressed in the form of somatic symptoms and problems of somatization.

Somatization is an ego process by which psychic phenomena such as depressive effects are converted into bodily symptoms. When it is severe, somatization in the elderly can become hypochondriasis, an obsessive concern and fear of bodily ill health. True illness and bodily dysfunction may form the focus for the development of such a somatic preoccupation. Depression can thus be disguised so that the effects are not openly felt (Salzman & Shader, 1979). Instead the elderly person experiences physical suffering.

Thus, from a psychodynamic point of view the clinician is concerned with causes lying within the individual and with the mechanisms of defense. When the focus of assessment is on intrapsychic processes and internal guilts and conflicts, the psychodynamic model would be the appropriate method of evaluation.

Cognitive-Behavioral Model

The behavioral model proposes that problem or maladaptive behaviors are governed by similar principles of learning as are other actions. The behavioral approach focuses on the specific adaptive and maladaptive actions, thoughts, or emotions and the contexts in which they occur. From this point of view assessment involves clarifying the presenting problems, obtaining a social history that focuses on the origins of the problem behavior, and identifying relationships in the person's current environment that may be controlling or reinforcing the maladaptive behaviors.

Unlike the medical model, there is less difficulty in the cognitive-behavioral model in differentiating normal from abnormal thought and behavior. In the medical model the professional uses relatively unreliable criteria to determine if symptoms suggest an internal conflict or disorder. In contrast a behavioral approach is not concerned with whether an illness is present. The focus is placed instead on the perception of problems in functioning by the individual or by persons closely associated with the client. When the client is self-referred, the goals of assessment are to determine the client's ability to retain independent functioning despite the presence of physical-affective disorders. When a person is brought to treatment by others, the process of assessment involves determining how each of the involved persons contributes to the problem situation.

Another array of behaviors that helps signal the presence or absence of depression is the cognitive component. In the geriatric patient expressions of loneliness, worthlessness, and sadness often occur before the more obvious behaviors of avoidance and reduced participation. The assessor should be alert to statements incorporating references to no longer being in control or being under the control of others. These are often the initial signs in a chain that may terminate in passive acceptance and a low level of responsibility (Hussian, 1981).

A cognitive assessment may indicate functional links between the problems presented by a patient and other behaviors. Depressed persons generally report their low spirits as the principal problem, but research in the last two decades has shown that depression is related to certain dysfunctional thoughts that lead to overly negative evaluations of one's self (Beck, 1967) and to the failure to engage in pleasurable activities. This process of identifying functional associations among thoughts, behaviors, and mood represents a different process from inferring a disease from overt symptoms.

Three models have been discussed: the medical, the psychodynamic, and the cognitive-behavioral. Each of these models has its own theory of the etiology of psychopathology and its own method of assessment. For example, the cognitively oriented clinician may look for psychological explanations for cognitive impairment; the medically oriented clinician may look for disease states, dementia, or brain syndromes to explain cognitive impairment. No one method of assessment has been shown superior in the assessment of the elderly. However, using only one method of assessment will not suffice. Each orientation offers something valuable to a more comprehensive assessment of the aged.

NEUROPSYCHOLOGICAL ASSESSMENT

Assessment of neuropsychological functioning in the elderly is important for a number of reasons. Principal among these is the clinician's need to assess the cognitive losses in old age. The task for clinicians working with older adults is to distinguish the relatively mild cognitive changes and decrements in memory and intellect of normal aging from the more severe disruptions of function and to differentiate between treatable and untreatable causes of cognitive impairment. Early and proper identification of potentially reversible problems will reduce the numbers of older persons suffering from cognitive impairment.

Thus the first main reason for trying to assess neuropsychological function in the elderly is the identification of pathological function that might be reversed or slowed with appropriate and timely intervention. Assessment techniques and procedures that fulfill these demands must measure the decrements in the central nervous system and decline in intellectual functions.

Detailed description and critique of tests and procedures used to assess normal or pathological cognitive function among aged persons that show potentials for differentiating among normal age range groups are considered in Chapter 6. The presence of premorbid conditions at the time of neuropsychological testing may make it virtually impossible for the clinician to assess accurately the elderly person's true level of behavioral function and the severity and the extent of the neuropsychological impairment. However, some of the factors and issues of major concern in assessing neuropsychological function in older adults need specific mention here.

The first concern for clinicians is that psychological tests may not always correlate with functional levels. This is especially true in the assessment of the elderly compared to other age groups. For example, Granick (1971) notes that many brain-damaged elderly persons may continue to live their lives in a competent fashion into the seventh or eighth decade of life without any recognition of the brain damage condition until it may happen to show up in autopsy. Thus the presence of mild cognitive impairment and no obvious behavioral incompetence should not come as a surprise to clinicians who use psychological tests to study correlates of functional levels. Conversely there may be instances of serious behavioral incompetence without any obvious signs of cognitive impairment on the psychological tests. This lack of concordance between the test measures and behavioral functioning poses a number of problems for the clinician, who must then seek other interview-related diagnostic procedures to understand the wide discrepancy between test results and behavioral functioning.

Three factors discussed by Davison (1974) help to explain the discrepancy. The first factor is age. The literature reflects ignorance of the clinical indexes of age-related decrement in specific functions. Unfortunately little information is available regarding behavioral indications of brain damage in the elderly. Tests that differentiate between normal and pathological functions among young groups cannot be assumed to do so with older persons. Tests of neuropsychological and neurophysiological assessment are not sophisticated enough to differentiate between stages of normal aging and neuropathology. Individual differences among normal older persons are also considerable. Even on those abilities reported to have the most age-related decline, such as memory or reaction time, some older persons perform at or near levels typical of the young (Schonfield, 1974). Validation of existing psychometric techniques with older groups has not been done sufficiently to differentiate cognitive changes of normal aging from the more severe disruptions of function due to brain damage, dementia, and Alzheimer's disease.

The second factor involved in explaining the wide discrepancy between neuropsychological test results and behavioral functioning levels is the time between the onset of the brain lesion and the testing. Studies with young groups have suggested that processes of compensation are initiated as soon as the physical loss has occurred. The extent and nature of compensation possible or likely for elderly persons, however, are not clearly understood. Further, agents causing lesions in the brains of the elderly are not properly understood. Physical loss in old age is seldom a discrete and clearly discernible phenomenon. Both in normal aging and several forms of pathological development of lesions, physical loss and cognitive decrements are slow and gradual, and the corresponding compensatory processes are also likely to occur slowly, gradually, and continuously (Davison, 1974). Thus behavioral characteristics or changes likely from brain damage or physical loss are not easily discernible or easily assessed. Schaie and Schaie (1977, p. 696) note the complicating effects of sensory and motor problems in neuropsychological assessment of the aged. Apparent decremental findings on intelligence tests, suspected reality distortions on projective techniques, as well as apparent perceptual distortion on visual motor tasks in the aged may all be a function of a deficit in peripheral sensory and motor function rather than being indicative of organic or functional pathology.

The third critical factor contributing to the difficulty in assessing neuropathology in the elderly is the incidence of other conditions at testing. Davison (1974) observes the diverse effects of drugs and medication (commonly taken by the elderly for their medical problems or their behavioral functioning). Salzman and Shader (1979) warn that the elderly are more likely to be taking drugs for treatment of medical problems, and with increasing age the homeostatic mechanisms that ordinarily re-create balance may become impaired. As a result of minor increase in the drug level of standard amounts of the drug, there may be unwanted toxic effects because of the decrease in the efficacy of the kidney and liver in excreting and metabolizing (Fann, Wheless, & Richman, 1976; Goldman, 1974). Polypharmacology including usage of barbiturates and depression-inducing drugs may lead to other psychiatric states such as confusion and delirium and exaggerated bodily symptoms causing cognitive impairment symptoms virtually indistinguishable from dementia (Gibson

& O'Hare, 1968; Hale, Marks, & Stewart, 1979). Premorbid conditions of stress, anxiety, and sleep disturbance so commonly experienced in late life may present attentional deficits that resemble those of dementia.

The clinician is advised to use a number of measures to assess anxiety and anxiety-eliciting situations posing serious threats to an elderly person who has suffered some recent incapacitations. Many investigators have considered changes in autonomic measures such as cerebral blood flow and elevations in blood pressure as indicators of the presence of anxiety or defensiveness. Psychophysiological measures of diffuse slowing in the EEG or Alpha slowing might indicate organic deterioration or intellectual impairment. They indicate promise for the development of assessment techniques that can facilitate an early diagnosis of cognitive impairment associated with organic deterioration in the elderly (Marsh & Thompson, 1977). Busse and Pfeiffer (1969) caution that this is not always a reliable and valid procedure for assessing the presence of anxiety since anxiety reactions in the elderly are often delayed responses to earlier events or stimuli not immediately observable at a given moment or time of testing.

Furthermore, knowledge of the psychophysiological manifestations of anxiety in the elderly is scarce. Clinical indexes of stimuli that produce anxiety in the younger person may not be at all helpful in determining the anxiety reactions of the elderly. Since the psychophysiological manifestations of anxiety undoubtedly change with age (Busse & Pfeiffer, 1969), the best recourse for the clinician is to develop rules of thumb to help determine the anxiety level of the elderly clients. One technique for measuring the client's body awareness of the presence of the anxiety is Mandler's Autonomic Perception Questionnaire (Mandler, Mandler, & Uviller, 1958). Although it has questionable validity when used with elderly clients who are confused and unable to eliminate distracting stimuli, this technique for assessing the presence of anxiety can be useful with a majority of elderly clients.

ASSESSMENT OF INTELLECTUAL FUNCTIONING

One of the most important contributions in the clinical assessment of the aged may very well be the determination of whether intellectual competence is maintained or declines as compared to previous levels of functioning (Schaie & Schaie, 1977). It is not at all clear whether intellectual decrement is a normal and gradual accompaniment of the aging process or whether it is a pathological decline in some elderly.

Although a detailed discussion of the topic is outside the purview of this chapter the implications of this problem for clinical assessment and for clinicians deserve specific mention here. Some of the most important concerns in intellectual assessment of the elderly are as follows:

(1) Clinicians need to be concerned with both the validity of intelligence tests and the reliability of norms of tests. All current intelligence tests assess the intellectual competence of the aged with respect to constructs defined for the young (see Schaie, 1974). Few intelligence tests estimate criteria relevant to the lives of the elderly. For the clinician, then, the essential issue is whether to measure the behavior of the elderly client with instruments developed essentially for the young and whether changes or decrements in intellectual functioning of the elderly should be determined by comparing them to younger peers.

(2) A second major concern is that of intelligence norms for this age group. Most norms are age-corrected norms based on cross-sectional studies. Moreover, norms for the older age group have typically been derived from special populations of the elderly, for example,

those who have been hospitalized for a time or those who have been under considerable environmental stress or are deeply anxious. Such norms are therefore highly questionable since they cannot help the clinician to determine whether any part of the intellectual deterioration or changes noted are a function of normal aging, brain pathology, disease states, or depressive conditions. Thus clinicians who conduct intellectual assessment of elderly clients in order to develop intervention strategies for working with intellectually impaired elderly, or for those with slowing intellectual capacities, are unable to identify the root cause of the problem.

For example, it is difficult to determine whether the intellectual decline should be attributed to aging or whether it signifies the development of a pathological syndrome. Similarly clinicians may not be able to identify the specific areas of intellectual functioning that are expected to improve with time and treatment and other deteriorations (e.g., memory decline) that are irreversible.

Unfortunately, as noted by Matarazzo (1972), there are as yet no data bases from which to project changes in norms that would be useful to the clinician. Schaie and Labouvie-Vief (1974) call attention to the fact that in normal aging there are few individual changes until the sixties and a limited decline thereafter on tests of intelligence in which speed is not involved. In the absence of age-corrected norms it is minimally possible to get a general picture of the elderly individual's functioning by means of a measure such as Wechsler's efficiency quotient (Wechsler, 1939), which is recognized to have renewed utility in terms of assessing the individual's obsolescence as compared to younger contemporaries (Schaie & Schaie, 1977).

(3) In addition to obtaining information on intellectual efficiency or competence, another important area in clinical assessment is the estimation of intellectual deficits or deterioration observed in measures of intellectual functioning presumed to hold up with age. Matarazzo (1972) notes the absence of deterioration measures for looking at age changes in the elderly. The Wechsler-related deterioration measures are the only ones known to be used in clinical practice. It is suggested that comparison of the overall verbal versus performance scores on the WAIS is a reasonable estimation of intellectual deterioration. Researchers maintain that extensive norms on the aged are available for the WAIS. However, the clinical utility of using the WAIS as an estimation of intellectual efficiency or deterioration in the aged is limited (Savage, Britton, George, O'Connor & Hall, 1972). The extent to which verbal versus performance scores, or vocabulary versus speed and learning tests, can help the clinician to distinguish between previous functioning levels and current intellectual efficiency is unknown. The extent to which these comparisons will help to distinguish between normal aging patterns and pathological patterns will depend on the development of reliable norms for the aged.

(4) More recently there has been a shift toward diagnosing deterioration in terms of the individual's unique history of previous occupation, socioeconomic status, and social roles. Deficits associated with normal aging are not necessarily valid criteria when assessing the current performance of individuals who, for example, held high level professional and functional roles. Schaie and Gribbin (1975) hypothesize a relationship between individuals' previous level of intellectual functioning, their present performance, and their previous socioeconomic status. They propose a model within which the clinician's knowledge of the elderly client's demographic status may help to provide estimates of the client's previous level of intellectual functioning, which can then be contrasted with the level of present performance.

The advantages and drawbacks of neuropsychological approaches mirror those of all psychometric tests used with the elderly except that in using intelligence scales and verbal-performance measures there is more risk of confounding factors such as education, motivation, and fatigue (Kahn & Miller, 1978). The only major advantage of administering intelligence scales is to affirm that there is no evidence of severe deterioration in cognitive functioning.

MENTAL STATUS EXAMINATION

Mental status tests that are an integral part of the neuropsychological assessment in elderly clients are also essential for confirming or disconfirming the presence of deficits in cognitive functioning. The most widely used clinical procedures and psychometric measures to assess mental status in elderly clients are still quite inadequate for distinguishing the behavioral functioning of depressed clients from cognitively impaired clients and for differentiating elderly with normal age-related symptoms of cognitive decline and those with dementia and brain syndrome. Thus mental status assessment may confirm the presence of cognitive loss but provides the clinician with little help in determining whether the problem has any treatable aspects. Because of the uncomplicated nature of the questions in the mental status assessment enquiry, subtle differences in the extent or severity of the cognitive loss cannot be easily determined.

Clinical Issues

Geropsychologists and other geriatric health practitioners may frequently omit a formal mental status examination either because the presence of intellectual impairment is so very obvious or because they wish to save time or avoid irritating the elderly persons. Kahn, Zarit, Hilbert, and Niederehe (1975) and Gurland (1973, 1976) suggest that the mental status examination of the cognitive impaired elderly person is central to the diagnostic differentiation of diffuse brain syndrome, delirium, and depression. However, to be diagnostically accurate and reliable, such assessments must be based on some structured guidelines and standards rather than on casual observations or the complaints of the nurses, family members, or the elderly clients. Some of the general and specific cautions in the administration of mental status examination are summarized in Exhibit 2–2.

While depressed elderly often give the impression of intellectual impairment and complain about poor memory and inability to perform tasks, the clinician can generally determine the extent of the elderly's disturbance of memory and intelligence by attending to the three essential cognitive processes of registration, retention, and recall of information and experiences. Unless clients have sensory deficits (such as hearing and visual losses), most older depressed patients who do not have dementia rarely have difficulty registering environmental events, even though they may appear uninterested in their surroundings.

Some elderly with acute psychic distress may have difficulties in retention of experiences or events that had definitely registered. Most elderly may be too agitated or restless to attempt to retain or remember information frequently asked for on the mental status examination or perform a cognitive task. For example, depressed older patients who are severely agitated may have difficulty with digit span testing. Persistent questioning may reveal that a given patient is cognitively more or less intact but is too agitated to perform on

Exhibit 2–2 Precautions To Be Observed in Mental Status Examination of Elderly
Clients

1. Establish rapport with client and gain client's trust and acceptance before mental status examination.
2. Rule out possibility of sensory deficits (especially hearing and visual losses) before mental status examination.
3. Rule out possibility of toxic effects accruing from medication and drug dependencies before mental status examination.
4. Assess the presence, if any, of agitation, acute anxiety, and depression resulting from recent stressful events before mental status examination.
5. Assess client's retention and recall by using information, experiences, and events that have been known to have registered.
6. Test client's memory for events by selecting events that are of considerable interest and significance to the elderly client.
7. Memory of recent events should be tested by asking client to recall events that occurred in the past 8 to 24 hours (e.g., name of visitors; important event of the day).
8. Memory of more remote events may be evaluated by asking client to recall dates of important past events (birthday, anniversary date, age) and names of persons who had considerable significance for the client.
9. An independent assessment should be obtained from the client's family of the extent of the client's motivation and interest in the surroundings before the mental status examination.
10. Assessment of client's capacity for basic self-care tasks should be done before the mental status examination.
11. The nature of cognitive tasks expected of the client in the mental status examination must make allowance for the limited educational attainment of some clients and also for the impoverished nature of the client's current environment.
12. Questions of understanding, recall, and integration of materials in the mental status examination must definitely take into account the life style, cultural bias, and previous interests of the elderly client.
13. Elderly clients should not be expected to engage in psychological tests that involve prolonged capacity for memory and attention.
14. Mental status tests should be supplemented by the use of other psychologic tests involving observation of behavioral symptoms of the elderly client.
15. Careful assessment of mental status should be conducted over a longer time to preclude the possibility of off-days or client's distress on a given testing day.

request. In clinical practice with the elderly, retention in such persons should be tested indirectly through questioning or through conversation about events that the clinician is aware had registered. Memory for recent and remote events may be found intact if the events being discussed are of sufficient significance to the elderly client. Recall need not always be tested by asking the individual to repeat a series of digits in forward or reverse order. As Blazer (1982) suggests, recent memory can be better tested by asking the client to recall certain events during the past 12 to 24 hours, such as names of visitors or dishes at a meal. Memory for remote events can be evaluated by asking the patient about important dates such as birth, marriage, ages of children, retirement. The important point here is that the cognitive activity or discussion should be of interest and significance to the elderly person.

The most common test of recall on the cognitive functioning test and mental status examination involves questions relating to time, place, person, and situation. Errors on these questions have been found to correlate highly with scores on dimensions of anxiety and agitation. It is important to put the client at ease before commencing on the cognitive testing. An older person may miss answers on questions of orientation because information such as dates or names of contemporary leaders had not been recently available. For various reasons older persons may not be exposed to experiences involving the names of the presidents or other current changes in the environment. Similarly, elderly persons living alone or with sensory deficits (such as loss of eyesight or hearing) may be poorly oriented to time and current events not because of cognitive impairment or memory disturbance but because of social and sensory deprivation. Such factors as social isolation or sensory deficits need to be ruled out by the clinician before a diagnosis of cognitive impairment.

Clinical experience suggests that even poorly motivated individuals are able to answer items of time, place, and person orientation correctly unless they are demented. Some elderly may be off by a few days on the day of the month but are unlikely to identify the month or year incorrectly, notwithstanding the severity of their agitation or psychic distress. Persons with diffuse brain damage on the other hand show persistent deficits in orientation questions and questions involving both recent and remote memory. Persons with a limited educational background and intelligence may present special problems for making an accurate assessment. Their performance on any cognitive tests, including mental status, may reflect an impaired range without necessarily reflecting a diffuse degenerative process. When dealing with an elderly person who has had little or no formal education, any items testing for ability to understand, recall, or mobilize previous learning or integrate new situations may often have poor validity. Mild impairments are likely to reflect a lifelong pattern and may not necessarily be signs of progressive or increasing decrements in ability to perform self-care activities.

Zarit (1980) notes that any test of mental status should be introduced only after some rapport builds up between the interviewer and the elderly client. Once the necessary rapport has been established, persons with good mental functioning will seldom resent answering simple questions of orientation or memory, especially if these aspects are tested indirectly through questioning or through techniques mentioned.

Blazer (1982) stresses that questions of understanding, recall, and integration of materials must take into account the life style and previous interests of the client and as far as possible must take into account the client's cultural bias. For example, the elderly Jewish grandmother who cannot remember the day of the month or the name of the president may be able to recall other culturally relevant information or incidents surrounding her favorite grandchild.

There is too much of a tendency to use tests of recall or intelligence that involve cognitive activity of little or no significance to the elderly client. Marginally impaired clients may feel offended or irritated and will then stop performing on a task or stop concentrating on a required activity and may give the impression of being more severely impaired than they actually are. In examinations to assess ability to abstract or ability to perform simple arithmetic calculations, the general fund of knowledge or specific abilities should be determined by the clinician asking questions about items, concepts, or ideas that are closely related to the previous experiences of the client. It is also important to ensure that such events did register.

A classic test for capacity for abstract reasoning is usually to interpret a well-known proverb such as "people who live in glass houses should not throw stones." A classic test for calculation is to ask the patient to subtract 7 from 100 and to repeat this operation until 0 is reached. Unfortunately such tests often irritate the elderly clients because of the unimportance of the cognitive activity or the attention required. A better test of abstraction for an elderly person who has lived on the farm is, In what way are a cow and a horse similar? Even clients with little or no formal education would have no difficulty in performing such a test of abstraction or would not be threatened if asked to classify objects such as animals, vegetables, and household tools into a common category.

The cognitive assessment is generally based on the time and assistance needed by the elderly client to respond to basic questions. Significant attention, however, must be paid to the client's ability to concentrate on the task in hand. Elderly clients should not be expected to engage in tests that involve prolonged capacity for memory and attention. On the whole the clinician must be careful not to rush the patient or penalize the patient for lack of speed when scoring the test.

Because of the coexistence of depression and primary dementing processes in later life, some systematic observations about neuropsychologic impairment are usually warranted. Most tests administered in the routine mental status examination are not sensitive to mild neuropsychologic impairment. Blazer (1982) suggests that the clinician may wish to supplement the orientation examination by administering a psychologic test such as the trailmaking test in the Halstead battery. Such a test, especially when supplemented by careful observations of the symptoms and functioning of the elderly, may be valuable for estimating impairment. Subtest discrepancy on the Wechsler Adult Intelligence Scale and evidence of aphasia may also document the start of a dementing process.

Wang (1980) noted that the Rorschach test is the most frequently used individual psychologic test for personality assessment of the cognitively impaired elderly. According to several clinicians, depressed elderly taking the Rorschach show tendencies toward restriction of attention to detail, shading responses, inanimate movement responses, autonomic responses, and marked delay to cards where spontaneity is expected. Such a test result, while noting general trends of constriction and reduction in the responses of the elderly, is of no value in distinguishing depression and dementia.

Zarit (1980) stresses the danger in using common and loosely formulated criteria such as memory problems, poor judgment, emotional flatness, and confusion as diagnostic criteria for judging the mental status of the elderly. There is ample clinical evidence to support the position that memory problems and poor judgment in the elderly can often be symptomatic of acute psychic distress and can occur without the presence of brain impairment. Similarly *confusion* is a vague, imprecise term most misused in mental status examinations of the elderly's orientation of time, place, and surroundings. Confusion is often manifested by elderly persons with a variety of stress-related problems. Given sufficient psychic stress, confusion, amnesia, and forgetfulness could assume an acute form. Unless a careful assessment of mental status is conducted over time, many elderly may be diagnosed as having chronic conditions or an organic brain syndrome condition. Thus observations of the onset of depression and the extent, pattern, and duration of confusion, amnesia, and memory problems that follow are essential for a differential diagnosis of depression and dementia in the elderly. It is recommended that these be treated as critical progressive steps in the mental status examination (Zarit, 1980; Blazer, 1982).

ASSESSMENT OF PSYCHOLOGICAL CAPACITY TO MAINTAIN AN INDEPENDENT ROLE

This issue is of vital importance whenever assessment procedures are used to determine whether an individual remains competent to manage affairs or whether the individual should be assigned to receive permanent or temporary custodial care given by family members or institutions. Determination of the individual's capability to maintain independent role function will depend first on the family members' evaluation of the elderly client's ability for self-care. While such observations are never sufficient in and of themselves, a routine effort should be made to obtain such information whenever possible.

The first task of the clinician is to assess the elderly client's level of dependence, which means the need for personal intervention by another in order to sustain life and maintain living arrangements. According to Gurland (1980) the importance of assessing dependence is that it is a pivotal concept with respect to the elderly person's capacity to remain in the community. It is assumed that one of the major determinants of dependence, especially in the elderly, is sheer inability to carry out basic self-care tasks. Excessive dependence will often denote the existence of cognitive impairment, cognitive disorders in handling routine tasks, or physical ill health and chronic fatigue and weakness. The degree of dependence may also be an indicator of the severity and the cause of, or an underlying, disorder or depression.

Unfortunately there is no clear-cut or objective way to assess the degree to which dependence in a given elderly client is a result of cognitive impairment, psychomotor retardation, learned helplessness, or poor motivation on the part of the client. The elderly cohorts of today grew up believing that dependency and helplessness are expected traits and tendencies in old age and are a means of adaptation in family relationships (Goldfarb, 1977). As such, dependence should be assessed only to the extent that it confirms the presence of cognitive impairment but not for reasons beyond that.

The clinician's major tasks will be to determine the mental status of the elderly person, to evaluate the current behavioral capabilities of the client to function in the independent home environment, and finally to assess the degree of social support available to the elderly client. Assessment of social support available is especially important in the care of a client who is mildly to moderately impaired but who resists the idea of institutionalization, hospitalization, or alternative settings of custodial care.

Inferences will have to be drawn from the various neuropsychological and intellectual functioning assessment data as to the client's ability to engage in routine self-care tasks and to meet the demands of the role requirements. Relatively simple rating scales that assess disability or handicaps in performing self-care functions have been found quite useful. This type of assessment is reflected in the work of Kelman and Muller (Kelman, 1962; Kelman & Muller, 1962). The Index of Independence in Activities of Daily Living (ADL) developed by Katz and his associates (Katz, Downs, Cash, & Grotz, 1970; Katz, Ford, Moskowitz, Jackson, & Jaffe, 1963) is probably the most widely used and empirically tested of these instruments. The instrument is designed to test vital functions such as ability to bathe, dress, go to the toilet, be continent, and feed. The ADL instrument provides index scores ranging from A (i.e., independent functioning in all six areas) to G (i.e., dependency in all six areas) in a wide variety of settings such as private home, hospitals, nursing homes, and housing projects for the aged. Although the self-care and general physical-psychosocial indexes are useful tools in the psychologist's armamentarium, they are somewhat narrow in scope.

Information from them must be supplemented by the clinician's observations through interview, home visits, and consultation with the family members and social workers.

Lawton (1970) has observed that a single assessment device is not likely to discriminate functions throughout the entire range of complexity. He proposes that a full assessment should contain data on all important levels of behavior, the major ranges of complexities within each level, and the major range of normative competence. Clinicians should provide reassurance of independent living to elderly clients and their families only on the basis of functional assessment data showing substantially maintained levels of physical and psychological function.

Even if strong evidence is presented by the functional assessment data that the present functioning level is below the basic level necessary for the client to meet the demands of daily living, it may still be very important to determine to what extent the elderly client perceives the present functioning to be sufficient or disabling. This counseling aspect of the assessment procedures may be particularly important in obtaining the client's cooperation in doing a valid and reliable functional assessment.

Reliable and valid psychometric procedures for assessing the psychological and functional capabilities of the elderly persons are not available. One of the major tasks of clinicians, therefore, is to develop their own procedures to determine the minimal levels of function and/or disorders. Such an assessment will enable them to make appropriate recommendations for a change of the client's status from independent to supervised living. Schaie and Schaie (1977, p. 715) stress the need to determine whether enough intellectual competence remains so that the persons concerned can engage in a prudent management of their daily affairs and in problem-solving efforts required for this purpose. Additional questions to consider are whether these elderly individuals have the self-confidence to maintain themselves in an environment that presents subjective and objective hazards.

ECOLOGICAL ASSESSMENT

According to Goldman (1971) the clinician's task is not simply to define the change in the elderly client's functional and psychological status, but more important it is to identify possible alternate living arrangements for the client and suggest alternative remedial ways of upgrading the functional level and successful role adjustment.

Final determination of the individual's capability to maintain independent role function must be based on the assessment of various professionals and semiprofessionals (e.g., physician, psychologist, family members, and social workers) who have identified problems and resources in that particular case. Data must be closely scrutinized to determine whether custodial care is available and whether the custodial care can be manipulated or structured to include the following environmental components advocated by Pincus and Wood (1970):

- privacy: the degree to which the environment allows the individual to maintain a personal domain
- freedom: the degree to which the client is permitted to exercise choice, decision making, or initiative
- resources: the degree to which the environment provides the opportunity for social interaction and leisure

- integration: the degree to which the environment affords opportunity for communication and community

- personalization: the degree to which the environment affords opportunity for personal interaction with professionals and other staff

Clinicians also need to assess the extent to which a given deficit is a reversible, as opposed to an irreversible deterioration and the extent to which a given elderly client requires a supportive environment to compensate for deficits in functioning.

It would seem advisable to reevaluate the client for excess disability (i.e., the discrepancy when the person's functional incapacity is greater than warranted by the actual impairment) (Brody, Kleban, Lawton, & Silverman, 1971). As far as possible, the elderly client should not be transferred to an environment that fosters unnecessary dependence. In the final analysis the goal is to help the older person, or those who can help the individual, to plan and function in an environment congruent with actual capacities.

Alternative new roles suggested to the elderly client may require lesser levels of competence that are well within the reach of the elderly person, making it possible to maintain an independent role. More often than not, the inference should be drawn that while status change is not yet mandatory, conditions can be specified under which such status change may become unavoidable.

Another major function of the clinician is the assessment of the client's capability to benefit from treatment programs. Before such an assessment is possible, the clinician must be able to identify and delineate a number of behavioral dysfunctionings or responses that need to be modified. Although it is generally agreed that elderly clients can benefit considerably from psychotherapeutic intervention, intervention programs that expect aged clients to accomplish major reorganization of personality are not likely to be successful. Assessment efforts must focus on the detection of resources and strengths that are at least partially intact in the elderly client and suggest how previously learned skills and capabilities can be integrated into the new adjustments or adaptations that the elderly client must undertake. Several divergent types of treatment programs can be suggested. The assessment effort must focus on helping to select a treatment program compatible with the client's goals for independent functioning or need for custodial care.

ASSESSMENT OF SOCIAL SUPPORT NETWORKS

Importance of Assessing Social Support Networks

According to Blazer (1980) the role of social support factors in late-life psychiatric disorders is relatively unexplored. Frerichs, Aneshensel, and Clark (1980) point out that social network forces vie in importance with biological and psychological forces in maintaining the elderly individual's health status. Because of the elderly person's obvious emotional impoverishment and restricted use of contacts, clinicians and researchers are increasingly concerned with attempts to restructure, maximize, and improve the emotional valence of their social networks. While there is some evidence that the rate of depression in the elderly is clearly related to the level of perceived network support (Frerichs et al., 1980), not enough effort has been made to devise strategies for accurately assessing the support system. Frerichs et al. (1980) note that spouses and immediate family members provide support to the elderly in times of physical or mental crisis. Little clinical analysis and assessment have been done on the influence of social networks in noncrisis situations.

Two possible etiologic factors that deserve special attention in geriatric psychology and psychiatry are social stress and social support, which play a significant causative role in mental illness. By evaluating in detail the social support systems of the elderly and by actively increasing and remediating the social support network, we can realize a significant gain in the life adjustment processes of many elderly. Increased success in the promotion of mental well-being of the elderly and assisting them to retain independent living for as long as possible will result directly from our accurate assessment of the future and present social support needs. Custodial care or institutionalization of the elderly can be delayed to a fair measure if adequate social support is available.

Social Support and Integrated Health of the Elderly

Social support is usually defined as help that would be available to the elderly individual in difficult or stress-arousing situations. Thus, it is suggested that elderly who are low in social support lack the interpersonal resources that would enable them to rely on other institutional supports in times of need. A number of writers have hypothesized that social support acts as a buffer against the stresses and shocks of daily life (Bowlby, 1973; Hirsch, 1980; Pfeiffer, 1980). Social support is embedded in the elderly individuals' matrix of relationship with family members including spouse, children, and grandchildren. Research with the elderly has shown that social support can ameliorate the effects of certain stressful life experiences such as losses, bereavement, and environmental dislocation (Fulton & Gottesman, 1980; Myers, Murphey, & Riker, 1981).

Social support is of value to the elderly in that it provides nurturance and is operative through an integration at the emotional level. Closely associated with this emotional support is the provision of task-oriented assistance. Moss (1973) speculates that social support would protect a more vulnerable subset of individuals (e.g., the elderly) who become shielded against environmental stressors and information incongruities by membership in support groups.

Client Factors: Concomitants of Social Support

Palmore (1980) regards families as the single most important and frequent source of aid and support for elders, serving as the primary source of financial aid and nursing care and most important the primary source of affection, esteem, and emotional gratification.

As explained by Blazer (1980), in the case of an elderly individual a social stressor such as loss of a spouse may affect the social system at many points. If the spouse provided a service to the elderly subject such as transportation and financial assistance, the survivor may find the remainder of the social system less reachable, and the duration, intensity, and frequency of the subject's interactions within the social system may also become threatened. Thus the single life-event (loss of a spouse) may become a source of chronic stress for an elderly individual.

Although most older persons continue to receive attention from one or other source, for a sizable number of aged, social contacts diminish drastically through death of friends and relatives. Blazer (1982, p. 99) postulates that a long-range decline in perceived social support contributes directly to an increase in major depressive reactions. His work confirms the significance of assessing the depth and breadth of social support systems of each elderly client. Pfeiffer and Busse (1973) suggest that social and emotional losses in interpersonal resources are intimately associated with stern depressive reactions in old age and may be a prime determinant of pervasive depression and suicide in the elderly (Zarit, 1980). Blazer (1982, p. 96) contends that this variable is potentially of very great value to researchers and clinicians in a number of ways. The continuing interaction between the elderly, their physical environment (e.g., the provision of an adequate diet, warmth, etc.), and their social environment (i.e., the durability, frequency, and intensity of social interactions) may be more predictive of health outcomes than discrete stressful events.

Social Environment and Social Support

In assessing the degree of social support available to the elderly individual, the practitioner would need to be familiar with the individual's general experience with the environment over time so that the practitioner can, during crisis, rely on those individuals in the elderly's social system who are likely to provide meaningful, appropriate, and protective feedback (Cobb, 1976; Nuckolls, Cassel, & Kaplan, 1972). Thus, the practitioner's assessment of the elderly individual's social system would require knowledge of

- the individual and groups of individuals in the social system in which the elderly person relates;
- the reactability, that is, the extent to which individuals can contact and use other individuals of importance;
- the intensity, frequency, and flexibility of interactions among the members of the social system;
- the cognitive, affective, and directive value orientations that guide the social system;
- the available interpersonal attachments;
- the individual's subjective evaluations of the dependability, reliability, and stability of the social network resources; and
- the instrumental support or concrete and tangible services accorded to the individual by the support resources.

Assessment of the Social Network

Snow and Gordon (1980) suggest that it is useful to set out the elderly client's social network diagrammatically as a circle, with the elderly individual at the center and the members of the social network on the circumference. According to Snow and Gordon, the network can then be examined to study the following features:

- Structural features, which include the number of people in the network, their geographical location, the frequency of contacts, and the number of tasks and services they can perform.
- Dynamic features, which include the emotional bonds between the elderly client and the individual members of the network, the frequency of interactions between individual members of the network, and the effects of each interaction on the elderly client and vice versa, and the general expectations, motivations, and resistances of others with regard to the client.

- The elderly client's subjective view of the network. This factor is important enough to warrant a detailed assessment by the clinician. It is rare in psychogeriatric clients that all intervention is limited to service by the professional. Much planning, management, and actual service will be delegated to members of the social network. A realistic evaluation of the client's subjective perceptions of the social network is therefore imperative.

The perceptions assumed to influence health outcomes in crises situations may be conscious perceptions of the environment. However, the effects of the social environment may also be mediated by unconscious perceptions when certain stressful and supportive stimuli may influence the organs of the human body without the organism's sensory awareness. The implications of this perspective of the social system for the mental health practitioner are not always clear. However, the clients' subjective perceptions of the support systems and attitudes and values concerning social stress and social support may actually play a more significant causative role in mental health or mental impairment than might the clinician's objective assessment (Dohrenwend & Dohrenwend, 1974).

According to Hemsi (1982) such an analysis is particularly important in the case of old people who are disoriented or confused. The emphasis of assessment of the social network should be twofold: (1) concentrating on the needs and demands of the elderly person and (2) concentrating on the needs of the members of the social network who may have some intense feelings about the client. The assessment itself should summarize the following:

- relevant points of history and relevant points of examination with respect to the client and to others in the social network of the client
- the nature of the problem as perceived by the elderly client and as perceived by the assessor and others in the social network of the elderly client
- the factors leading to the problem: mental illness, physical disease, social nuisance, and abandonment by family group
- services available—physical, psychological, and social services possible in terms of client self-care or in terms of what others in the social network can offer the client, for example, bathing, shopping for the client, and telephoning the client

PSYCHOMETRIC MEASURES FOR EVALUATING INDIVIDUAL SUPPORT NEEDS

The more commonly known psychometric measures or procedures that can facilitate the practitioner's task include the following.

The Social Support Questionnaire (SSQ). This measure (Sarason, Levine, Basham, & Sarason, 1983) consists of 27 items. Each item asks clients to list the people to whom they can turn and on whom they can rely in given circumstances and to indicate how satisfied they are with their level of social support. Specimen items include the following:

- Whom you can count on to console you when you are very upset?
- Whom can you really count on to help you in a crisis situation?
- Whom can you really count on to listen to you when you need to talk?

- With whom can you be totally yourself?
- Who do you feel really appreciates you as a person?

The test-retest reliability of the SSQ is quite acceptable; both components of the SSQ correlate significantly and negatively with measures of anxiety and depression (Sarason et al., 1983). On this scale, people high in social support report higher emotional well-being than those low in social support. While not standardized on a population of elderly, this scale shows good potential for such use. As a further extension of the SSQ scale, for each presenting problem the respondent is asked to rank-order three preferred choices for the question, "If you need advice very urgently would you seek the help of a family member (be specific about the family member), physician, clinic, clergyman, psychiatrist, friend, neighbor, any other person?"

Many of the items on the SSQ overlap with questions included in the OARS methodology for the semistructured interview. The SSQ has the advantage of being short (27 items), documented, and consisting of items that check on the perceptual and subjective impressions of the elderly subjects. It is designed to be a quick check on the general availability and degree of social support and interpersonal resources of each elderly client. It may form a part of the initial evaluation interview of the client presenting symptoms of psychological and social dysfunctioning.

Social Surround Measure. This (Lieberman, 1978) is a measure to assess social surroundings of a sample of middle-aged to elderly individuals across three ethnic groups. In this measure the focus is on three aspects: (1) the structural relationship with regard to social class status, marital status, and social mobility status; (2) the individual's relationship to the social network, including perceived amount and type of social resource (i.e., friends and family) and actual social context (e.g., the size of the social network including family network and the number of actual contacts with them) (this component assesses the degree to which the social contacts provide gratifications and the degree to which intimacy with spouse is an important source of satisfaction and well-being); and (3) characteristics of the person's neighborhood with regard to its quality and the degree of the individual's embeddedness. This scale has been validated on a crosscultural sample of elderly subjects and has yielded satisfactory reliability and validity.

Home and Family Networks Measure (HFNM). Pfeiffer (1980, p. 282) recommends this assessment procedure for looking at specific aspects of home and family personal networks of the elderly. According to Pfeiffer the objective of the inquiry is to assess the long-term social resources available to the elderly rather than the moment-to-moment social contacts. The assessment procedure is designed to take stock of marital status (with the presence of an intact marriage or spouse constituting a positive social support resource); living arrangements (with the availability of living quarters with the relatives constituting a positive social resource); availability of transportation during an emergency; availability of someone to provide continual care in the event of a serious or prolonged physical illness or depressive disorder; the personal social resources useful in the understanding and management of psychological distress of the elderly; and informal social support structures such as neighborhood groups, group homes for the elderly, extended day care, and church affiliation.

In advocating this measure, Pfeiffer (1980) contends that the availability of caregivers in the social environment is critically important in determining whether a depressed elderly can be cared for at home or should be hospitalized immediately. While these aspects of social support functioning must be routinely assessed with all elderly, a more desirable approach is to take a specific count of the available social networks that can monitor closely the moment-to-moment functioning of severely depressed elderly or those at risk for suicide (Blazer, 1982).

Burke and Weir (1981) believe that the encouragement of informal helping relationships would make a significant contribution to the emotional well-being of the client. These authors' commentary on the moderating effects of informal social support and helping relationships on life stress has a number of direct applications and implications for the elderly:

Although incidents of informal social support are prevalent in our society, they are far more accessible to individuals who are actively engaged in a variety of coping activities and who actively seek informal supports to maintain and reestablish their emotional equilibrium. Given the fact that many elders live lives of relative isolation and loneliness, even informal support systems and informal helping relationships are not as readily available or accessible to many elderly.

The personal and social stigma associated with the use of the social support services has also created a certain amount of resistance on the part of the elderly. In response to the elderly's obvious need for special assistance in coping with such stresses as mental confusion and disorientation, family breakdown, bereavement and social losses, financial losses, etc., several traditional professional services are considered too formal and should be made considerably more informal for meeting the needs of the elderly.

Since information about the assessment of the informal social resources cannot be assessed in an office interview, Pfeiffer (1980) recommends home visitation by the practitioner's assistant, associated nurse, or social worker. Through home visitation further knowledge can be acquired about the elderly client's integration into the community and the potentiality for adaptation into the community after the elderly client returns from the hospital following treatment. As Pfeiffer notes, assessment and evaluation of these factors will lead to a realistic appreciation of how the client functions 24 hours a day in the natural setting and to what extent the client needs environmental and social supports.

SUMMARY

This chapter has dealt with the adaptability of our present assessment and evaluation procedures to provide a detailed functional assessment of the elderly clients. The value of a functional approach to assessment lies both in identifying the abilities and resources of the elderly person and in pinpointing problems related to independent living.

The older individual brings, in addition to the usual problems encountered by the young, problems unique to this age group. There may be problems of neuropsychological decrements and intellectual functioning impairment. There may be problems of poor health, depression, and biochemical alterations. There may be considerable decrements in self-esteem, self-confidence, and autonomy. All these factors must be considered and used in order to evaluate the older individual's performance. Structured clinical interviews using the OARS and CARE methodology developed for geriatric use have been described as an example of the merging of techniques from different disciplines such as psychology, psychiatry, and medicine. However, these are lengthy instruments and may not be suitable for all clinical settings. The abundance of data gathered must be reduced to manageable proportions and presented in a form that can be assimilated by the geriatrician, the family members of the elderly client, and often the clients themselves.

This approach need not be implemented automatically on contact with every elderly client but is most often available in the geriatric facilities and opens up the possibilities of a team approach. The team approach is most advantageous in that the functional analysis of each client is considered and evaluated for treatment and remediation by shared perceptions rather than by one practitioner attempting to assimilate several consultants' reports.

However, despite its obvious necessity in some clinical settings, the multifunctional assessment procedure may be unrealistic for many others. It is vulnerable to inconsistency and bias on the part of the various members of the assessment team, to inefficient summarization of data, and to selective listening on the part of the clinician who translates the data into a decision on the management of the patient.

Current psychodiagnostic procedures for assessing cognitive impairment, intellectual functioning deficits, and sensorimotor and organic brain losses seem to be lacking in adequate norms for the elderly. As individuals grow older, their physical, psychological, and anxiety factors increase in complexity, their autonomic responses become less under their own control, and tests become more threatening. All of these factors must be considered in making inferences or decisions based on test results.

The new trend exemplified by the ecological assessment approach directs itself to the task of determining the older person's neuropsychological status, mental status, social status, physical health, and social support status. A study of these components of the person-environment interaction will help the clinician determine what an elderly client can do in particular situations and a given choice of situations. The ecological assessment will provide the basis for therapy, rehabilitation, screening, or placement of the older individual.

REFERENCES

Abramson, L.Y., Seligman, M.E.P., & Teasdale, J.D. (1978). Learned helplessness in humans: Critique and reformulation. *Journal of Abnormal Psychology, 87*, 49–74.

Ahammer, I.M., & Baltes, P.B. (1972). Objective versus perceived age differences in personality: How do adolescents, adults, and older people view themselves and each other. *Journal of Gerontology, 27*, 46–51.

Atchley, R.C. (1969). Respondents vs. refusers in an interview study of retired women: An analysis of selected characteristics. *Journal of Gerontology, 24*, 27–42.

Beck, A.T. (1967). *The diagnosis and management of depression.* Philadelphia: University of Pennsylvania Press.

Blazer, D.G. (1980). The epidemiology of mental illness in late life. In E.W. Busse & D.G. Blazer (Eds.), *Handbook of geriatric psychiatry* (pp. 249–271). New York: Van Nostrand Reinhold Co.

Blazer, D.G. (1982). *Depression in late life.* St. Louis: C.V. Mosby Co.

Blessed, G., Tomlinson, B.E., & Roth, M. (1968). The association between quantitative measures of dementia and of senile change in the cerebral gray matter of elderly subjects. *British Journal of Psychiatry, 114*, 797–811.

Bowlby, J. (1973). *Attachment and loss: Separation, anxiety and anger* (Vol. 2). New York: Basic Books.

Brody, E.M., Kleban, M.H., Lawton, M.P., & Silverman, H.A. (1971). Excess disabilities of mentally impaired aged: Impact of individualized treatment. *Gerontologist, 11*, 124–133.

Burke, R.J., & Weir, T. (1981). Moderating effects of social support on life stress: The case of depression. In J.P. Soubrier & J. Vedrinne (Eds.), *Depression and suicide* (pp. 155–159). New York: Pergamon.

Busse, E.W., & Pfeiffer, E. (1969). Functional psychiatric disorders in old age. In E.W. Busse & E. Pfeiffer (Eds.), *Behavior and adaptation in late life* (pp. 183–236). Boston: Little, Brown & Co.

Butler, R.N. (1969). Age-ism: Another form of bigotry. *Gerontologist, 9*, 243–246.

Butler, R.N., & Lewis, M.I. (1973). *Aging and mental health: Positive psychosocial approaches.* St. Louis: C.V. Mosby Co.

Clausen, J.A. (1969). Methodological issues in the measurement of mental health of the aged. In M.F. Lowenthal & A. Zilli (Eds.), *Interdisciplinary topics in gerontology: Colloquium on health and aging of the population* (pp. 111–127). New York: Karger.

Cobb, S. (1976). Social support as a moderator of life stress. *Psychosomatic Medicine, 38,* 300–314.

Davison, L.A. (1974). Introduction. In R.M. Reitan & L.A. Davison (Eds.), *Clinical neuropsychology: Current status and application* (pp. 1–18). Washington: Winston.

Diagnostic and Statistical Manual of Mental Disorders (DSM-III) (1980). Washington: American Psychiatric Association.

Dohrenwend, B.P., & Dohrenwend, B.S. (1974). *Stressful life events: Their nature and effects.* New York: John Wiley & Sons.

Dovenmuehle, R.H. (1968). The relationship between physical and psychiatric disorders in the elderly. *Psychiatric Research Reports, 23,* 81–87.

Eisdorfer, C., & Keckich, W. (1980). The normal psychopathology of aging. In J.O. Cole & J.E. Barrett (Eds.), *Psychopathology in the aged* (pp. 1–16). New York: Raven Press.

Fann, W.E., Wheless, J.C., & Richman, B.W. (1976). Treating the aged with psychotropic drugs. *Gerontologist, 16,* 322–328.

Fillenbaum, G., & Smyer, M. (1981). The development, validity, and reliability of the OARS multidimensional functional assessment questionnaire. *Journal of Gerontology, 16,* 428–432.

Frerichs, R.R., Aneshensel, C.A., & Clark, V.A. (1980). *Prevalence of depression in Los Angeles County.* Paper presented at the Society of Epidemiological Research, Minneapolis, June.

Fulton, R., & Gottesman, D.J. (1980). A psychosocial concept reconsidered. *British Journal of Psychiatry, 137,* 45–54.

Furry, C.A., & Baltes, P.B. (1973). The effect of age differences in ability on extraneous variables on the assessment of intelligence in children, adults, and the elderly. *Journal of Gerontology, 28,* 73–80.

Gaitz, C.M. (1969). Functional assessment of the suspected mentally ill aged. *Journal of the American Geriatrics Society, 17,* 541–548.

Gaitz, C.M., & Baer, P.E. (1970). Diagnostic assessment of the elderly: A multifunctional model. *Gerontologist, 10,* 47–52.

Gallagher, D., & Thompson, L.W. (1983). Depression. In P.M. Lewinsohn & L. Teri (Eds.), *Clinical geropsychology: New directions in assessment and treatment* (pp. 1–37). New York: Pergamon.

Gergen, J., & Back, W. (1966). Communication in the interview and the disengaged respondent. *Public Opinion Quarterly, 30,* 385–398.

Gibson, I.I.J.M., & O'Hare, M.M. (1968). Prescription of drugs for old people at home. *Gerontologia Clinica, 10,* 271–280.

Goldfarb, A.I. (1977). Psychotherapy in the aged. In S. Steury & M. Blank (Eds.), *Readings in psychotherapy with older people* (DHEW Publication No. ADM 77–409, pp. 182–191). Washington: Government Printing Office.

Goldman, R. (1974). Speculations on vascular changes with age. *Journal of American Geriatrics Society, 22,* 296–303.

Goldman, S. (1971). Social aging, disorganization and loss of choice. *Gerontologist, 11,* 158–162.

Granick, S. (1971). Psychological test functioning. In S. Granick & R.D. Patterson (Eds.), *Human aging II* (DHEW Publication No. HSM 71–91037, pp. 49–62). Washington: Government Printing Office.

Gurland, B.J. (1973). A broad clinical assessment of psychopathology in the aged. In C. Eisdorfer & M.P. Lawton (Eds.), *The psychology of adult development and aging* (pp. 343–377). Washington: American Psychological Association.

Gurland, B.J. (1976). The comparative frequency of depression in various adult age groups. *Journal of Gerontology, 31,* 283–292.

Gurland, B.J. (1980). The assessment of the mental health status of older adults. In J.E. Birren & R.B. Sloane (Eds.), *Handbook of mental health and aging* (pp. 671–700). Englewood Cliffs, NJ: Prentice-Hall, Inc.

Gurland, B.J., Fleiss, J.L., Cooper, J., Sharpe, L., Kendall, R., & Roberts, P. (1970). Cross-national study of the diagnosis of mental disorders: Hospital diagnoses and hospital patients in New York and London. *Comprehensive Psychiatry, 11,* 18–25.

Gurland, B.J., Fleiss, J.L., Goldberg, K., Sharpe, L., Copeland, J.R.M., Kelleher, M.J., & Kellet, J.M. (1976). A semi-structured clinical interview for the assessment of diagnosis and mental state in elderly: The Geriatric Mental State Schedule II: A factor analysis. *Psychological Medicine, 6*, 451–460.

Gurland, B.J., Kuriansky, J., Sharpe, L., Simon, R., Stiller, P., & Birkett, P. (1977–78). The Comprehensive Assessment and Referral Evaluation (CARE)—Rationale development and reliability. *International Journal of Aging and Human Development, 8*, 9–42.

Hale, W.E., Marks, R.G., & Stewart, R.B. (1979). Drug use in a geriatric population. *Journal of American Geriatrics Society, 27*, 374–377.

Hemsi, L. (1982). Psychogeriatric care in the community. In R. Levy & F. Post (Eds.), *The psychiatry of late life* (pp. 252–287). Oxford: Blackwell Scientific Publications.

Hirsch, B.J. (1980). Natural support systems and coping with major life changes. *American Journal of Community Psychology, 8*, 159–172.

Hussian, R.A. (1981). *Geriatric psychology: A behavioral perspective.* New York: Van Nostrand Reinhold Co.

Kahn, R.L., Goldfarb, A.I., Pollack, M., & Peck, A. (1960). Brief objective measures for the determination of mental status in the aged. *American Journal of Psychiatry, 117*, 326–328.

Kahn, R.L., & Miller, N.E. (1978). Assessment of altered brain function in the aged. In M. Storandt, I.C. Siegler, & M. Elias (Eds.), *Clinical psychology of aging* (pp. 42–70). New York: Plenum Press.

Kahn, R.L., Zarit, S.H., Hilbert, N.M., & Niederehe, G. (1975). Memory complaint and impairment in the aged. *Archives of General Psychiatry, 32*, 1569–1573.

Kanfer, F.H., & Saslow, G. (1965). An alternative to diagnostic classification. *Archives of General Psychiatry, 12*, 529–538.

Katz, S., Downs, T.D., Cash, H.R., & Gratz, R.C. (1970). Progress in the development of the index of ADL. *Gerontologist, 10*, 20–30.

Katz, S., Ford, A.B., Moskowitz, R.W., Jackson, B.A., & Jaffe, N.W. (1963). Studies on illness in the aged: The index of ADL, a standardized measure of biological and psychosocial function. *Journal of the American Medical Association, 185*, 914–919.

Kelman, H.R. (1962). An experiment in rehabilitation using nursing home patients. *Public Health Reports, 77*, 356–366.

Kelman, H.R., & Muller, J.N. (1962). Rehabilitation of nursing home residents. *Geriatrics, 17*, 402–411.

Kendell, R.E., Cooper, J.E., Gourlay, J., Copeland, J.R.M., Sharpe, L., & Gurland, B.J. (1971). Diagnostic criteria of American and British psychiatrists. *Archives of General Psychiatry, 25*, 123–130.

Kreitman, N., Sainsbury, P., Morrissey, J., Towers, J., & Scrivener, J. (1961). The reliability of psychiatric assessment: An analysis. *Journal of Mental Science, 107*, 887–908.

Lawton, M.P. (1970). Assessment, integration and environments for older people. *Gerontologist, 10*, 38–46.

Lawton, M.P. (1971). The functional assessment of elderly people. *Journal of the American Geriatrics Society, 19*, 465–481.

Lawton, M.P., & Gottesman, L.E. (1974). Psychological services to the elderly. *American Psychologist, 29*, 689–693.

Lewinsohn, P.M., & Teri, L. (Eds.). (1983). *Clinical geropsychology: New directions in assessment and treatment.* New York: Pergamon.

Lieberman, M.A. (1978). Social and psychological determinants of adaptation. *International Journal of Aging and Human Development, 9*(2), 115–126.

Mandler, G., Mandler, O., & Uviller, O. (1958). Autonomic feedback: The perception of autonomic activity. *Journal of Abnormal Social Psychology, 56*, 367–373.

Marsh, G.R., & Thompson, L.W. (1977). Psychophysiology of aging. In J.E. Birren & K.W. Schaie (Eds.), *Handbook of the psychology of aging* (pp. 219–248). New York: Van Nostrand Reinhold Co.

Matarazzo, J.D. (1972). *Wechsler's measurement and appraisal of adult intelligence.* Baltimore: Williams & Wilkins.

Moss, G.E. (1973). *Illness, immunity and social interaction.* New York: John Wiley & Sons.

Myers, J.E., Murphey, M., & Riker, H.C. (1981). Mental health needs of older persons. Identifying at-risk populations. *American Mental Health Counselors Association Journal, 3*, 53–61.

Nuckolls, K.B., Cassel, J., & Kaplan, B.H. (1972). Psychosocial assets, life events and psychiatric symptomatology: Change as undesirable. *Journal of Health & Social Behavior, 95*, 431–441.

Palmore, E. (1980). The social factors in aging. In E.W. Busse & D.G. Blazer (Eds.), *Handbook of geriatric psychiatry* (pp. 222–248). New York: Van Nostrand Reinhold Co.

Pfeiffer, E. (1970). *Multidimensional functional assessment: The OARS Methodology.* Durham, NC: Duke University, Center of the Study of Aging and Human Development.

Pfeiffer, E. (1980). The psychosocial evaluation of the elderly patient. In E.W. Busse & D.G. Blazer (Eds.), *Handbook of geriatric psychiatry* (pp. 275–284). New York: Van Nostrand Reinhold Co.

Pfeiffer, E., & Busse, E.W. (1973). Mental disorders in late life-affective disorders: Paranoid, neurotic and situational reactions. In E. Busse & E. Pfeiffer (Eds.), *Mental illness in later life* (pp. 107–144). Washington: American Psychiatric Association.

Pincus, A., & Wood, V. (1970). Methodological issues in measuring the environment in institutions for the aged and its impact on residents. *Aging and Human Development, 1*, 117–126.

Salzman, C., & Shader, R.I. (1979). Clinical evaluation of depression in the elderly. In A. Raskin & L.F. Jarvik (Eds.), *Psychiatric symptoms and cognitive loss in the elderly* (pp. 39–72). Washington: Hemisphere.

Sarason, I.G., Levine, H.M., Basham, R.B., & Sarason, B.R. (1983). Assessing social support: The social support questionnaire. *Journal of Personality and Social Psychology, 44*, 127–139.

Savage, R.D., Britton, P.G., George, S., O'Connor, D., & Hall, E.H. (1972). A developmental investigation of intellectual functioning in the community aged. *Journal of Genetic Psychology, 121*, 163–167.

Schaie, K.W. (1974). Translations in gerontology—from lab to life: Intellectual functioning. *American Psychologist, 29*, 802–807.

Schaie, K.W., & Geiwitz, J. (1982). *Adult development and aging.* Boston: Little, Brown & Co.

Schaie, K.W., & Gribbin, K. (1975). The impact of environmental complexity upon adult cognitive development. *Proceedings of the Third Biennial Meeting of the International Society for the Study of Behavioral Development*, Guildford, England.

Schaie, K.W., & Labouvie-Vief, G.V. (1974). Generational versus ontogenetic components of change in adult cognitive behavior: A 14 year cross-sectional study. *Developmental Psychology, 10*, 305–320.

Schaie, K.W., & Schaie, J.P. (1977). Clinical assessment and aging: General considerations. In J.E. Birren & K.W. Schaie (Eds.), *Handbook of the psychology of aging* (pp. 692–723). New York: Van Nostrand Reinhold Co.

Schonfield, D. (1974). Translations in gerontology—from lab to life: Utilizing information. *American Psychologist, 29*, 796–801.

Snow, D.L., & Gordon, J.B. (1980). Social network analysis and intervention with the elderly. *Gerontologist, 20*, 463–467.

Wang, H.S. (1980). Diagnostic procedures. In E.W. Busse & D.G. Blazer (Eds.), *Handbook of geriatric psychiatry* (pp. 285–304). New York: Van Nostrand Reinhold Co.

Ward, C.H., Beck, A.T., Mendelson, M., Mock, J.E., & Erbaugh, J.K. (1962). The psychiatric nomenclature: Reasons for diagnostic disagreement. *Archives of General Psychiatry, 7*, 198–205.

Wechsler, D. (1939). *The measurement of adult intelligence.* Baltimore: Williams & Wilkins.

Zarit, S.H. (1980). *Aging and mental disorders: Psychological approaches to assessment and treatment.* New York: Free Press.

Zarit, S.H., & Zarit, J.M. (1983). Cognitive impairment. In P.M. Lewinsohn & L. Teri (Eds.), *Clinical geropsychology* (pp. 38–80). New York: Pergamon.

Chapter 3

Assessment of Clinical Depression

Only recently have clinicians and researchers turned their attention to a number of critical issues concerning the problems of assessing depression and depression-related functional disorders in the elderly. After a delayed start there has been a substantial growth of interest in the area (Rehm, 1980). In this chapter some of the special problems of assessing depression in the elderly are considered. These problems emphasize the need to assess many different kinds of aspects of the biopsychosocial functioning of the elderly and to make more precise distinctions in symptomatology and etiologies of depression as present in the aged, in order to develop a complete picture of the causes and consequences of depression. Since depression in the elderly may resemble the familiar clinical syndrome seen in younger adults, it is important to consider the psychological and physical aspects of depression that are particularly relevant and unique to the elderly. A section of this chapter draws attention to certain physical and organic diseases of the aged that include depression as part of the clinical picture and present a differential diagnosis for the practitioner. The last section examines methods and scales used in measuring depression and critical evaluations of these instruments.

NEED FOR ASSESSING DEPRESSION IN THE ELDERLY

Most practitioners and researchers in aging would agree conclusively that depression is the most prevalent psychological disorder of the later years and that both in hospitalized and community samples depression is found more often than any other psychological disorders or problems. There is a growing recognition that older persons (65 years and over) represent the age group most vulnerable to episodic or chronic states of depression. While prevalence studies indicate that as many as 15 percent to 20 percent of all persons above 65 years of age living in the community show significant depressive symptomatology, the frequency of depressive states may be as high as 25 percent for those elderly living in institutional care settings.

Given the high prevalence of depression in later life, the questions most relevant to the assessment of depression in the elderly are linked first to the social, psychological, and physiological changes of the later years and second to a further clarification of the psychosocial, biological, and medical correlates found in many cases of depression in the elderly.

Since many elderly have somatic and organic complaints and often also show sadness, their symptoms should not automatically be dismissed merely as signs of depression or merely as part of the normal aging process. Most elderly have at least one chronic illness or health problem and have numerous somatic complaints that might present symptoms of depression. Hence the task of differentiating normal from pathological symptomatology becomes a difficult but important one for the clinician or practitioner.

Viewed from the perspective of the elderly, assessment of depression should take into account the following diagnostic considerations:

- As a first step, the assessment process must focus on distinguishing pathological disordered functioning from what might be normative disordered functioning for aging individuals.

- As a second step, the assessment process must be concerned with the identification of intrapsychic and situational factors that may be contributing to the affective disorders. Such knowledge of the internal and external factors contributing to depressive symptomatology provides valuable information for deciding on an appropriate course of therapeutic intervention.

- As a third step, the evaluative component of assessment must attempt to reassess outcomes or effects of various interventions on the interpersonal functioning of the elderly.

Looked at from an age-specific perspective, the clinical picture of depression, although similar for the elderly and younger persons, may be quite different in terms of causes, and different therefore in terms of goals of diagnosis and assessment. Perceptive gerontologists have known for a long time that both endogenous and reactive depressions in the elderly are frequently associated with unknown factors of biological or psychosocial stresses, neurotic preexisting conditions, or a predisposing personality structure. All the subgroupings described by Lehmann (1981) (see Figure 3–1) are recognized to be responsible for depression in the elderly.

Lehmann's classification stresses genetic and biochemical changes and the relation of depression to personality and psychosocial life changes. When applied to the elderly, the model suggests that physiological changes, such as decreased neurobiological responsiveness to stress, may also make older persons more vulnerable to recurrent feelings of depression. Similarly, psychosocial changes in aging are linked to assumed etiologies suggested in Lehmann's schematic representation, but none of them can unfortunately be defined with great precision. Nevertheless, a classification into endogenous depression, neurotic depression, reactive depression, and depressive personality is accepted by most gerontologists, geropsychologists, and clinicians.

That depression is the most prevalent psychiatric disorder in the aged is not surprising given the many unique changes in life circumstances that the elderly experience. Soldo (1980) stresses the increasing likelihood that the elderly individuals experience significant losses and other stresses as they age. Soldo (1980), for example, notes that 10 percent of the men 65 and older are widowed; in the 75 and older group the figure rises to one of four. Among women more than 50 percent of those aged 65 and over are widowed; at age 75 and older as many as 70 percent have lost their spouses.

According to Raskin and Sathananthan (1979) over 80 percent of the elderly, the equivalent of 18 million people, have chronic health problems that are multiple in nature.

Figure 3–1 Schematic Representation of Etiological Factors in Depressive Disorders

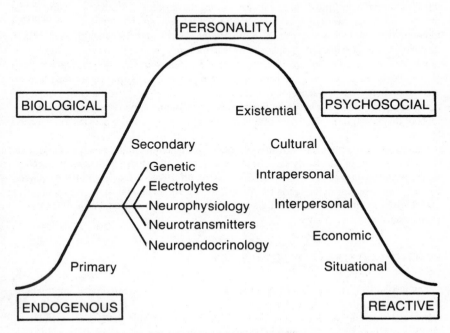

Source: From *Prevention and Treatment of Depression* (p. 5) by T.A. Ban et al. (Eds.), 1981, Baltimore, Md.: University Park Press. Copyright 1981 by University Park Press. Reprinted by permission.

Many of these older people (who are often also socially isolated) experience significant psychological reactions from stress caused by loss of health and social isolation. In summary, social isolation, together with chronic illness and loss of financial resources, is the most common factor leading to depression and stress in the elderly (Friedman & Sjogren, 1981).

A given clinical picture in an aged person may therefore result from one of several unrelated causes, some of which reflect past and present psychosocial and biological stresses and experiences and others that are age-specific and related to the later stage of life. All this argues that some of the depressive reactions of the aged are related to the developments of the aging period. Assessment of depression in the elderly must therefore be conceptualized from an age-specific perspective that takes into account the elderly's unique intrapersonal and interpersonal frailties, cultural sensitivities, and situational reactions to social and economic losses and temporary confusional states.

In the overall profile of the elderly there is increasing uncertainty as to whether depression in old age represents phenomena similar to or different from depressive disorders in earlier life. Although the feelings of hopelessness, despair, and confusion that the depressed elderly experience have much in common with the psychological experiences of youth and middle-aged persons, most practitioners and researchers (Zung & Green, 1973; Butler &

Lewis, 1977; Gurland, 1976; Pfeiffer & Busse, 1973) agree that depression in the elderly may be difficult to differentiate from symptoms of normal aging. In severe cases the clinician should have little difficulty in recognizing the depressive disorders because of the pronounced symptoms of dysphoric moods, loss of interest, suicide attempts, and psycho-motor retardation. In less severe cases, however, the elderly often deny being depressed and do not complain of sadness or dysphoria. Instead they may present the physician with signs of memory or concentration disturbances, lack of drive, or somatic problems that are present in other diseases such as organic brain syndromes. Careless or uninformed diagnosis of depression may lead to inappropriate treatment of various physical and mental symptoms that accompany old age. Thus there is a considerable risk in applying theories of etiology, tools of diagnosis, or evaluation procedures developed with younger persons to the problems of the elderly.

Other problems associated with an incomplete understanding of the age-specific depression phenomenon in the elderly stem from the fact that different disciplines are engaged in the study and evaluation of affective disorders, a situation that has led gerontological practitioners from different fields (geriatric physicians and clinicians, physiologists, and pharmacologists) to emphasize different classes of symptoms as important in the diagnosis of depression.

SYMPTOM CONTENTS OF DEPRESSION

Lewinsohn, Biglan, and Zeiss (1976) propose five classes of symptoms as important in the diagnoses of depression and depressive disorders across age groups and populations (presented in detailed diagrammatic form in Table 3–1): (1) dysphoria (feelings of sadness, apathy, and boredom); (2) behavioral deficits (inability for active social participation; psychomotor retardation and decreased verbal and physical activity); (3) behavioral excesses (excessive complaints about one's life situations, feelings of guilt, feelings of self-doubt and uncertainty); (4) somatic symptoms (headaches, sleep problems, fatigue, poor appetite); and (5) "cognitive" manifestations that reflect recurrent and persistent feelings of poor self-esteem, negative expectancies, and ideations of inadequacy, dependency, and self-criticism.

Lehmann (1981) schematically presents the modes and dimensions of the most characteristic depressive phenomena (Figure 3–2) and advocates the distinction between observable and nonobservable phenomenon. He groups the dimensions of behavioral, autonomic, and psychological reactions in the observable realm; in contrast, data on cerebral metabolism and psychodynamics are nonobservable and must be deduced or hypothesized. Until the 1960s many of the biogenic factors now known to contribute greatly to depression in the elderly have been strictly unobservable, and therefore depression in the elderly has been frequently misdiagnosed and inappropriately treated. Positron emission tomography is making it increasingly possible to observe directly metabolic processes in the brain and organic brain syndromes and dementias (Lehmann, 1981). Thus the semipermeable barrier between the observable and nonobservable phenomena of depression as indicated in Lehmann's schematic representation (Figure 3–2) will make it increasingly possible to differentiate in the elderly the treatment-resistant depressions (resulting from dementia, organic brain syndromes) from other more treatment-responsive depressions linked with psychosocial stresses. At the same time the rate of recovery from depression is becoming higher, both when active treatment is given for physical and biogenic imbalances known to

Table 3-1 Symptoms of Depression

Dysphoria	Behavioral Deficits	Behavioral Excesses	Somatic Symptoms	"Cognitive" Manifestations
Feelings dominated by sadness and blueness.	Minimal social participation—"I do not like being with people."	Complaints about: material problems—money, job, housing; material loss—	Headaches.	Low self-evaluation: Feelings of failure, inadequacy, helplessness, and powerlessness.
Loss of gratification—"I no longer enjoy the things I used to."	Sits alone quietly, stays in bed much of time, does not communicate with others, does not enter into activities with others.	money, property; the demands of others; noise; memory, inability to concentrate, confusion; lack of affection	Sleep disturbances: Restless sleep, waking during night, complete wakefulness, early morning awakening.	Negative expectation—"Things will always be bad for me."
Professes to have little or no feeling.		from others—"No one cares about me"; being lonely.	Fatigue—"I get tired for no reason."	Self-blame and self-criticism—"People would despise me if they knew me."
Feels constantly fatigued—"Everything is an effort."	Inability to do ordinary work.	Expresses feelings of guilt and concern about: making up wrongs to others; suffering	Gastrointestinal—indigestion, constipation, weight loss.	
Loss of interest in food, drink, sex, etc.	Decreased sexual activity. Psychomotor retardation.	caused to others; not assuming responsibilities;	Dizzy spells.	
Feeling of apathy and boredom.	Speech slow, volume of speech decreased, monotone speech, whispering.	welfare of family and friends; indecisiveness—"I can't make up my mind anymore;" crying,	Loss of libido. Tachycardia.	
	Gait and general behavior retarded.	weepy, screaming; suicidal behavior—"I wish I were	Chest sensations. Generalized pain.	
	Does not attend to grooming; neglect of personal appearance.	dead"; "I want to kill myself."	Urinary disturbances.	
	Lack of mirth response.			

Source: From *The Behavioral Management of Anxiety, Depression and Pain* (p. 94) edited by P.O. Davidson, 1976, Larchmont, NY: Brunner/Mazel. Copyright 1976 by Brunner/Mazel. Reprinted by permission.

Figure 3–2 Schematic Tabulation of Depressive Phenomena

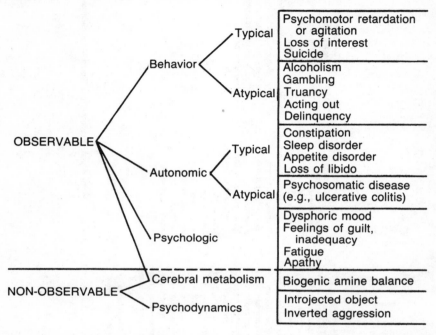

Source: From *Prevention and Treatment of Depression* (p. 10) by T.A. Ban et al. (Eds.), 1981, Baltimore, Md.: University Park Press. Copyright 1981 by University Park Press. Reprinted by permission.

be occurring with aging and when psychotherapy is offered for the observable psychosocial phenomena of depression in old age.

Until recently few studies have objectively considered the criteria for depressive disorders in the elderly. It is also not clear how the phenomena of depressive illness in the elderly can be distinguished from the normal variations of emotional, cognitive, physical, and volitional symptoms throughout the life cycle and whether depressions in later life represent the same or different phenomena from those in earlier years.

Clusters of Cognitive-Behavioral and Psychological Symptoms

Some observers have noted consistent clusters and groupings of verbal-cognitive and overt-motor symptoms of depression and depressive behaviors that distinguish late-life depression from depression of the earlier life.

Verbal-Cognitive and Overt-Motor Symptoms

This label has been used in the behavioral literature (e.g., Lang, 1968) to note those symptoms expressed primarily through verbalizations of dependency and helplessness. Paranoia may be a part of severe late-life depression.

Epstein (1976) noted that older depressed patients are more frequently described as manifesting an atypical pattern with symptoms of apathy, subdued self-deprecation, and psychomotor retardation emphasized more than in the young. Behavioral deficits include decreases in work and recreational activities and disturbances in sleep and mental functioning.

Pessimism, hopelessness, and guilt are often prominent symptoms of early depression before severe retardation becomes evident. Elderly subjects withdraw, may become mute, take to bed, and are unable to care for bodily functions. If able to speak, such patients sometimes say that any treatment efforts will be futile as they are hopeless and beyond assistance (Salzman & Shader, 1979). Fry (1984), who developed a geriatric scale of hopelessness, noted a number of major themes of hopelessness in the verbalizations of 138 elderly subjects between the ages of 65 and 80 years. This factor analytic study showed that the elderly expressed a keen sense of hopelessness about recovering lost physical and cognitive abilities, lost personal and interpersonal worth and attractiveness, lost spiritual faith and grace, and lost nurturance, respect, and remembrance from friends and family. Fry's findings also showed that hopelessness in the elderly subjects correlated significantly with subjects' self-ratings of depression and self-esteem and observer ratings of depressive disorders.

According to Caird and Judge (1974) depressed elderly may appear apathetic and expressionless, with poor attention or concentration. There may be frequent statements of self-deprecation such as "I am a real nuisance," "I'm sorry to be wasting your time," "I'm not good at anything." Suicidal ideations have also been noted as a frequent component of depression and must be taken seriously. Although some thoughts of suicide are associated with serious illness, depressive suicide ideation is often associated with decreased self-esteem and guilt (Salzman & Shader, 1979).

Agitation is more frequently seen in depressed older persons (Winokur, Morrison, Clancy, & Crowe, 1973). Chronicity is more frequently seen in elderly females, and recurrent depressive episodes accompanied by frustration and irritability are more frequently seen in older males (Winokur, 1973).

However, the preceding studies (Epstein, 1976; Winokur, 1973) were often concerned with distinguishing patients below and above the median age of 50 years, and it is therefore questionable as to whether these kinds of differences would hold true for the general population of elderly.

Somatic Symptoms

A number of authors (Raskin, 1979; Gurland, 1976; Zung, 1967) note the presence of transient depressive disorders accompanied by somatic complaints such as insomnia, loss of appetite, diffuse pain, troubled breathing, and headaches, which are more predominant in the elderly than in the young. Kahn, Zarit, Hilbert, and Niederehe (1975) observed frequent complaints about recent memory loss unrelated to cognitive impairment. Also in this category were typical complaints such as excessive fatigue, weight loss, hearing loss, and reduced vision (Pfeiffer & Busse, 1973).

The recognition that the elderly present a variety of somatic symptoms manifest in depression is an important consideration in the assessment of the elderly. However, a number of cautions and precautions are suggested in the assessment of somatic symptoms accompanied by verbal, cognitive, and overt-motor symptoms. Since somatic illnesses increase with age, it is not clear whether complaints about hearing loss, decreased visual acuity, arthritis, and other somatic symptoms in clinical or nonclinical samples represent correlates of depression or of actual health and physical health problems.

According to Epstein (1976) behavioral observations of older persons may help to make this differentiation between health and affective disturbance. Epstein recommends that this distinction is critically useful since somatic symptoms that are signs of depression are likely to respond to treatment of depression even in elderly persons with other physical illnesses such as cardiovascular disease. Although Steuer (1980) found fewer somatic symptoms in the elderly, a psychosocial evaluation of these elderly showed that lack of hope, decreased activity, difficulty in doing things, feelings of uselessness, and problems in decision making, combined with the somatic symptoms, contributed more greatly to depression in the elderly than in younger or middle-aged adults. Overall, Salzman and Shader (1979) caution that energy difficulties and fatigue (which often mimic depression) may be particularly difficult to evaluate in the elderly, as lassitude and apathy could also be signs of physical disease or drug toxicity in the elderly.

Hypochondriacal Symptoms

A number of researchers have commented on the frequency of hypochondriacal symptoms in the elderly (DeAlarcon, 1964; Brink, 1977; Goldfarb, 1974). DeAlarcon found hypochondriacal symptoms in 66 percent of the men and 62 percent of the women in elderly depressed samples. Of these clients with serious hypochondriacal symptoms, only 19 percent showed a lifelong concern for health, whereas for the majority of depressed elderly the concern for health was related to the onset of depressive symptoms in old age. Based on clinical behavioral observations, therefore, it can be suggested that hypochondriacal symptoms that first appear in old age (even in persons having concomitant physical illnesses) are likely to be related to depression.

Interpersonal Symptoms of Depression

Although this category has not been a part of the traditional symptomatology of depression, theory and research evidence are increasingly pointing to depressed elderly becoming withdrawn, excessively dependent, demanding, complaining, or manipulative. These deficits in the behavioral functioning of depressed individuals often lead to other psychiatric functional disorders in old age and are therefore not classified as depressive disorders in later life.

Selective Issues in the Assessment of Depression

Two significant issues emerge in most investigations and assessments of depression in elderly patients. The first issue is whether the depressive episode has occurred for the first time or whether there have been repeated depressive episodes beginning in early or middle life. From the standpoint of assessment it would be important for clinicians and geropsychologists to bear in mind the fact that the precipitants, symptoms, and response to treatment of depressive episodes would be evaluated differently in terms of how these episodes vary over time. A number of clinicians (e.g., Pfeiffer, 1977; Salzman & Shader, 1979; Zarit, 1980; Zung, 1980) suggest that elderly persons with repeated episodes are likely to respond to those treatments that worked best in the past. Hence a careful history should suggest an appropriate treatment plan of medication, psychotherapy, electroconvulsive therapy, or some combination of these interventions.

A second issue considered significant in the assessment of depression and the concomitant recovery is the client's age at first onset of a serious depressive episode. In the case of those elderly manifesting depressive symptoms for the first time, the lack of clear criteria for assessing the precipitants, symptoms, and methods of treatment poses a number of problems. First, it would not be clear how the transient mood states that the elderly subject reports on various symptom checklists are related to potentially more severe and persistent affective disorders (Gurland, 1976). Second, there is an increased prevalence of somatic symptoms in the mood states that may reflect health problems in some elderly persons and depressive disorders in others. The suggestion is that symptoms of depression take different patterns depending on the person's age at first onset of depression. As proposed by Zung (1980), assessment of first-time depression in the elderly (i.e., with onset of severe depressive symptoms after the age of 60) for purposes of planning intervention would necessitate a more thorough evaluation of the following basic life functions:

- behavior: withdrawal, disinterest
- growth: decrease in weight, sleep, and energy; impaired function of all body systems
- metabolic changes
- movement: decreased motor and joint mobility
- responsiveness: decreased tolerance for stress; diminution of impulse control; increased dissatisfaction and dependency
- adaptation: loss of coping and adaptive mechanisms; personal devaluation

Overall it is suggested that late onset of depression has a better recovery rate than does an early onset of depression and a history of treatment (Roth, 1955; Post, 1962).

NOSOLOGY AND CLASSIFICATIONS OF DEPRESSIVE DISORDERS

Recognizing the wide heterogeneity of disorders subsumed under the canopy of depression, a number of researchers and practitioners (e.g., Burrows, Foenander, Davies, & Scoggins, 1976; Coleman, 1976; Kolb & Brodie, 1982) have attempted to operationalize depression by examining in detail the various classification systems and diagnostic distinctions employed by researchers. Zung (1980) emphasizes the need for the establishment of a classification of depression that is jointly inclusive and mutually exclusive and brings order where order is lacking (Zung, 1980, p. 343) in the description of depressive disorders. Starting with nosology, a number of classifications of depressive disorders have been suggested. Each of these classifications presents one or more avenues toward an understanding of the etiology and treatment of depressive disorders but at the same time poses diagnostic dilemmas. A summary of the usual classifications attributed to depression and depressive disorders follows. However, it is uncertain whether all these distinctions apply strictly to the elderly, particularly since studies using rigorous diagnostic classifications are virtually nonexistent in the gerontological research.

Primary versus Secondary Depression

This classification of depressive disorders has been proposed by Woodruff, Murphy, and Herjanic (1967), who in the interest of simplicity attempted to avoid etiologic or symptomatic implications. According to Woodruff et al. a *primary depression* is defined as a depressive episode in a patient whose previous history does not include any psychiatric illness. A *secondary depression* by contrast is defined as a depressive episode in a patient who has had a preexisting diagnosable psychiatric illness. When this diagnostic classification (Figure 3–1) is applied to the elderly, a number of problems become obvious, which may limit the extent to which accurate diagnosis is possible.

First, the elderly exhibit a number of medical problems that obscure the primary or secondary nature of the depressive disorders. Older depressed patients tend to have more physical complaints and therefore report feelings of depression to a lesser extent than their younger counterparts (Blazer, 1982). Therefore, it is rather difficult to ascertain whether the depressive episode is primary or secondary in the diagnostic system.

Second, apathy and listlessness are characteristic of many aged who have been hospitalized for a long period, and these symptoms appear to be much more prominent in the aged than in the younger groups (Salzman & Shader, 1979). Increased irritability and delusions are observed more often in hospitalized elderly patients, and these symptoms do not necessarily suggest a clinical disorder but an acceptable response to the listless environment.

Finally, depression in the elderly can often be associated with cerebral dysfunction (cf., Post, 1975).

Unipolar versus Bipolar Depression

Perris (1966) and Leonhard (1959) propose a classification in which affective disturbances are categorized in terms of the occurrence of the disorders, the age of the patient, the family history, premorbid personality characteristics, and the presence or absence of precipitating factors.

In summarizing some characteristic distinctions between unipolar and bipolar disorders, Zung (1980, p. 346) describes unipolar depression disorders as involving only mania or only depression but not both, as contrasted with bipolar depressive disorders, which are characterized by both depressive and manic phases. Concerning median age at onset, unipolar disorders start at about age 45 as contrasted to bipolar disorders, which commence at an earlier average age of 30 years. As Zung (1980) observes, an examination of family history implies that specific heredity factors are more dominant in bipolar than unipolar disturbances. There are no differences noted in the reporting of precipitating factors or in the clinical ratings of anxiety or depressive symptoms in the two opposed classifications of unipolar and bipolar affective disorders.

A number of differences in signs and symptoms, clinical course, familial and genetic characteristics, and pharmacologic response have also been noted. Blazer (1982) notes a predominance of activity and agitation in the depressive episodes of the unipolar patients who show a propensity to hyposomnia and present somatic complaints more frequently. Unlike unipolar patients, bipolar patients exhibit more psychomotor retardation in the depressive phase. These patients are more passive and have a propensity to hypersomnia.

In examining the clinical course, it is observed that unipolar patients are less likely to suffer a recurrence and have a mean number of four to six depressive episodes as compared to bipolar patients, who show a greater likelihood of suffering recurrence and have a mean number of seven to nine depressive episodes. Comparatively speaking, bipolar patients are more likely to show symptoms of alcoholism and have higher rates of both attempted and completed suicides.

Observations of familial and genetic characteristics of the two groups of patients suggest a lower frequency of affective disorders among the relatives of the unipolar patients and a higher frequency of genetically based affective disorders in the relatives of the bipolar patients. In evaluating management procedures, Blazer (1982, p. 154) notes that unipolar depressives are responsive to tricyclic antidepressants whereas bipolar depressives are responsive to lithium carbonate.

In summary, then, genetic research and longitudinal follow-up have produced new and provocative findings in recent years. Studies of recurrent affective disorders have confirmed the distinction between unipolar and bipolar depressions and concluded that many first-time depressive disorders in the elderly are of a unipolar nature. Bipolar depressions tend to have an earlier onset, shorter episodes and cycles, more recurrences, and more frequent history of affective disorders in the clients' families (Lehmann, 1981).

Although new research developments are exciting and provide invaluable heuristic leads, in practice, however, the assessment of the biological, genetic, and psychosocial parameters of unipolar and bipolar depression continues to be a major problem. The major difficulty lies in the fact that many elderly patients may exhibit a number of medical problems that extend the duration of the depressive symptoms (Salzman & Shader, 1979). In both the unipolar or bipolar depressive and manic patients the presence of physical illness may contribute to the frequency of somatic complaints and apathy, and listlessness and psychomotor retardation may be evident across unipolar and bipolar patients. Salzman and Shader (1979) note that irritability and delusions generally characteristic of bipolar patients only are seen with a majority of depressed elderly who have been hospitalized for a long time.

Thus Blazer (1982) recommends that the traditional classification of unipolar and bipolar disorders, when applied to the elderly, needs to be supplemented by a detailed diagnostic workup by the practitioner. In his opinion a key to an accurate diagnosis is a history of the patient's past and present symptoms and a family history of affective disorders. When depressive symptoms occur or recur in late life, family members from at least two generations should be interviewed to determine whether the affective disorder might be predominantly bipolar and, in suspected cases of unipolar or bipolar affective disorders, whether the family history might assist in distinguishing manic episodes from other diagnostic entities.

Agitated versus Retarded Depression

Although all unipolar depressed patients cannot be categorized into this dichotomy, some authors (e.g., Gerner, 1979) suggest that the distinction has some value for both research and clinical practice with the elderly. One possible use of this distinction is that psychotropic medications can be differentially applied in treatment for patients diagnosed in terms of agitated versus retarded depression. Agitation typically refers to the presence of anxiety and activation across a number of domains. Many elderly persons may function continually at a high level of anxiety. The increased pressure of a new situation may lead to intense arousal, impairing the elderly person's ability to communicate rationally. Weight loss, loss of sleep, and psychomotor restlessness are also believed to be characteristic of the agitated subtype. By contrast, psychomotor fatigue; slowing, increased sleep often manifested by difficulty in getting up in the morning; and weight gain tend to suggest the retarded subtype. However, in describing the functioning of many elderly, Pfeiffer (1980) notes that patients are often characterized by both agitated states and fatigue, withdrawal and apathy, thus suggesting that agitation and psychomotor retardation features may coexist in the depressed aged.

For ease in conceptualizing the agitated-retarded distinction in the elderly, it has been suggested by a number of investigators (e.g., Kolb & Brodie, 1982; Jamison, 1979) that agitation-retardation be seen as a continuum of depression-related behaviors that vary in terms of both anxiety and the severity of the disorder. Kolb (1977) suggests that agitation be seen as simply the expression of anxiety, which under varying conditions may represent the persistent expression of the apprehension, tension, and feeling of prospective self-harm. In the elderly these feelings may arise from increasing constraints and threatening situations encountered in the changing environment. The internal uneasiness in response to threat may produce various behavioral and cognitive forms of psychomotor agitation in the aged. High levels of arousal, perhaps in response to lack of control in one's environment, would also explain some of the agitation in the depressed elderly.

Agitated features in the aged could also be viewed as occurring relatively early in the development of depression in later life. The agitation component in the elderly might best be conceptualized as a form of helpless anxiety. Excessive helplessness and agitation may also be found among those elderly individuals who respond rigidly in the face of threatened loss of attachments and hitherto stable sources of security.

By contrast, retardation features might best explain the behavior of those depressed elderly who have succumbed to the conflicts and tensions associated with perceived or real environmental losses. As noted by Beck (1972), psychomotor retardation is more frequently found in more severely depressed patients, and such retardation is associated with regressive behavior, withdrawal, and dependency states. Features of psychomotor retardation in the continuum might best correspond to states of hopelessness in the elderly, which emerge when anxiety and arousal diminish and yield to states of inhibited functioning. This conceptualization of psychomotor retardation is also congruent with Engel's (1966) discussion of patients who give up and give in and turn increasingly helpless in the face of changing life events.

Seligman (1975) has perhaps been much more explicit in proposing that helplessness is a characteristic feature of the depressive disorders, and his model of learned helplessness has many implications for depression in later life. He has argued that the initial anxiety and arousal in the elderly may yield to states of permanent dependency, regression, and loss of reactivity to the environment. The initial agitation would reflect the elderly's struggles to maintain control and to resist the loss of personal effectance. The psychomotor retardation would appear after the elderly person has succumbed to the external forces, and depression sets in.

Endogenous versus Reactive Depression

Kraepelin (1921) suggests that unipolar depression could be divided into endogenous and exogenous or reactive entities on the basis of emotional reactivity during the illness. In the view of Lehmann (1981; see Figure 3–1) endogenous disorders are alleged to be nonreactive to external events and are believed to be caused primarily by some biological disorder, such as hormonal endocrine dysfunction, or perhaps even transmitted through genetics. Endogenous depressions are also viewed as the more severe form of depression and as psychotic in nature. Lehmann (1981), following Lange (1928), has used the term *endogenous* to describe those depressive disorders preceded by genetic and constitutional stress factors and therefore predominantly related to internal factors such as degenerative or metabolic internal processes of nature. He has used the term *reactive* for those endogenous depressions preceded by environmental stress. In more general terms, however, *reactive* or *exogenous* depression is believed to be caused by external predisposing factors and external events rather than internal biological and metabolic processes and is not psychotic in nature.

Thus depression in the elderly may be seen essentially as the result of life experiences—a type of reaction to these experiences that protected the individual (Blazer, 1982, p. 8). Older depressed persons may be responding to social, psychologic, and biologic stress, and therefore reactive depression may be a method of adaptation (Willmuth, 1979). Antecedent or precipitating factors, such as stressful life experiences involving loss of self-esteem, financial failure, or loss of a spouse, could be seen as the primary circumstances leading to reactive depression. In drawing up distinguishing diagnostic criteria, Zung (1980, p. 344) notes the following distinctions that would have implications for assessment of the elderly.

Endogenously depressed patients characteristically are older; have a family history of depression; have a normal premorbid personality; report no identified precipitating events or factors; show diverse physiological symptoms such as decreased appetite, decreased weight, increased fatigue, sleep disorders that are reported to be worse in the morning, and diurnal variations that are at their worst in the morning; show pervasive depression; manifest psychomotor retardation and agitation; and show a variety of negative psychological symptoms such as loss of interest in life, self-reproach, guilt, and remorse.

By contrast, the reactively depressed patients characteristically are younger; have no family history of depression; manifest neurotic symptoms of inadequacy, hysteria, obsessiveness, etc.; report specific precipitating events leading to the depression; show fewer pervasive and less severe symptoms of depression; show fewer and less severe physiological symptoms of sleep disturbance, weight loss, etc.; and show less severe symptoms of apathy, self-pity, and guilt (Zung, 1980).

How clear-cut is the endogenous-exogenous dichotomy in the aged? A majority of researchers agree that the endogenous-reactive dichotomy cannot be applied to depressed elderly patients in any systematic and consistent way. The major problem is due to the wide variation and heterogeneity of symptoms in any single elderly individual. Post (1975) found that 78 percent of a depressed elderly sample disclosed precipitating factors before the onset of an affective disorder, implying a preeminence of reactive depression in the elderly. However, Post also found that there was no difference in the frequency of precipitating factors, the severity of depression or guilt feelings reported by endogenous or exogenous depressives in the elderly population. Moreover, Kolb (1977) reviewed data indicating that depressed patients showed a continuous distribution of somatic, organic, and psychogenic concerns. These findings argue against a model of depression (Figure 3–1) that rigidly stresses organic etiology on the one side and psychogenic factors on the other side.

It is not uncommon to find various features of both endogenous and exogenous depression in elderly patients with multiple physical illnesses and a long-term experience of institutionalization (Salzman & Shader, 1979). Thus, the severe depressive syndrome seen so frequently in later life might best be conceptualized as a secondary reaction to loss of functional ability, the effects of hospitalization and confinement, or both.

Elderly patients can have a reactive depression with severe psychomotor retardation and agitation and show severe fatigue, sleep disorders, and loss of interest in life resembling the psychological and physiological symptoms characteristic of endogenous depression (Post, 1975; Salzman & Shader, 1979). It is not clear at this time whether reactive depressions in the elderly differ qualitatively or only in degree from endogenous depressions. Thus Klerman (1971) suggests that these distinctions should be viewed as hypothetical constructs (having perhaps some limited value for treatment) rather than categories of illness. The general assumption is that reactive depressions are more like psychogenic disorders and therefore respond better to psychotherapy and intervention measures directed toward altering the external environment of the depressed elderly such as family group or social milieu. Endogenous depressions, by comparison, are assumed to be organic in etiology and therefore respond best to medical treatments that are somatic and alter the internal physical milieu of the elderly patient.

Situational versus Chronic Depression

In the last ten years there has been an increasing trend toward employing the terms *transient* and *situational* as opposed to *chronic* as descriptors of depression. From a pragmatic and management standpoint Akiskal (1978) prefers the use of terms such as *situational* as opposed to *reactive* in classifying depressed patients. This terminology has the effect of reducing some of the negative impact of psychiatric labels. In suggesting that the client is situationally depressed (as opposed to being reactively or endogenously depressed), the therapist may indicate to the depressed individual that there is more hope for recovery. Elderly clients who are told that they have situational depression could be persuaded to believe that more personal control may be acquired over the depression by focusing on the problem situations in the environment and gradually eliminating externally imposed restraints. As such, the notion of situational depression may give the depressed client some reason for exercising self-assertion and gaining control over situational events.

However, there are some difficulties in applying Akiskal's (1979) concept of situational depression to the elderly. Akiskal originally advocated the situational versus chronic distinction to draw attention to the fact that certain subtypes of depression are actually unrelated to predisposing life events. He viewed situational depression as a relatively transient dysphoric mood, which most individuals may experience as a reaction to negative life events and adverse environmental conditions. The implication is that full recovery is expected only when the depressive life situation is resolved, reversed, or changed for the better. Such reversal may not always be possible with those elderly whose life circumstances have changed drastically. Perhaps Akiskal's notion of situational depression has greater applicability to those elderly who have recently encountered a significant and difficult transient life situation. As emphasized by Post (1975), a majority of depressed elderly patients are successfully able to associate the onset of depressive states with a significant predisposing life event.

Winegardner (1981), who examined the cognitive, affective, and stress-related features of depression in three age groups of elderly persons living in nursing homes and living in the community, provided empirical data to support the notion that depressions in the elderly are associated with specific distressing situations. Situational life event problems were strong predisposing factors in the case of two groups of elderly. Winegardner (1981) also noted that in describing their depressions the younger subjects endorsed more items involving self-criticism and self-blame, while older subjects focused more on problem situations and external situations that contributed to their depression. Although further research is needed, these findings suggest that many elderly depressed patients will attempt to concentrate on external sources of situational stress and life problems for a longer time than younger individuals, who resort to negative self-attributions relatively early in the development of the depressive state.

However, over a prolonged period of episodic stress, chronic depression sets in with more severe and negative behavioral consequences. Chronic depression among the elderly may involve episodic but severe dysphoria or even significant recurrent unipolar depressive illness. Chronic states of depression may also involve greater degrees of psychopathology, including states of withdrawal, delusional thinking, and regressive features that closely resemble psychoticlike behaviors in which the elderly individual has increasing difficulties in maintaining adequate levels of adaptive functioning. Epstein (1976) is of the opinion that the elderly as a group are psychologically predisposed to chronic states of depression, and a significant proportion of the elderly may actually resign themselves to a state of chronic depression in later life. Some authors (e.g., Carp & Carp, 1981; Epstein, 1976) note that many elderly are convinced of the inevitability of certain losses in old age: loss of status, change in residential living status, loss of satisfying levels of income and other gratifications. Therefore, it may be that those elderly who view problem situations as the inevitable fact of later life are actually more vulnerable to serious chronic depression. Thus a significant loss in later life, such as loss of a spouse or loss of health, could serve as a major predisposing factor that might abruptly change a situational state of depression into a more severe and chronic disorder (Epstein, 1976).

Despite the difficulty involved in the definitions and diagnostic criteria, the distinctions between situational and chronic states of depression among the aged have clear implications for the outcome of depression. A more favorable prognosis has been suggested for those depressed elderly who are situationally depressed for the first time in later life, as opposed to persons who have experienced a number of intermittent dysphoric episodes. From the standpoint of prevention practitioners must be sensitive to the features that may predispose elderly individuals to more serious and chronic states of depression. Sensitivity to the elderly person's existing cognitive beliefs and expectations, behavioral and social interaction styles, and coping strategies could be significant areas to focus on and develop effective means of dealing with future problems and events.

Neurotic versus Psychotic Distinction

According to Zung (1980) the distinction between neurotic and psychotic depression is an important one, which needs to be upheld because of its usefulness to geriatric practitioners. The roots of the distinction between endogenous and reactive, and psychotic and neurotic depression date to the theoretical formulations of Kraepelin (1921). However, more recent theories have coalesced into the more recent distinction of endogenous versus neurotic depression, which many investigators (e.g., Klerman, 1975) treat as the equivalent of endogenous versus reactive, or of psychotic versus neurotic depression. In practice such classifications can be used broadly and interchangeably in the diagnosis of depression in the elderly, especially since the categorical or dimensional distinction used by clinicians is primarily in terms of clinical symptoms. From a management viewpoint a majority of elderly are diagnosed as being reactive or neurotic along multidimensional criteria. In Zung's judgment these sets of terms are not synonymous nor are they mutually exclusive in the elderly. It may well be that depressives can have a reactive depression of psychotic proportion or have an endogenous depression of neurotic severity.

For purposes of a simple distinction it is generally accepted that neurotic depression typically involves minimal to moderate mood disturbance while the psychotic classification usually requires more intense and pervasive dysphoria. Not only is there a pervasive alteration of mood in psychotic depression, but there is also decreased cognitive functioning, decreased reality testing, and greater distortion. By contrast a *neurotic depression* is defined as having mild impairment in mental functioning. The neurotic patient is aware of the declining ability and is able for the most part to function adequately. Gerner (1979) emphasized that neurotic forms have fewer and less severe disruption in physiological functions (such as sleep, appetite, and energy), only mild-to-moderate psychomotor agitation or retardation, fewer and less severe disturbance in psychological functions, usually intact reality testing, and an absence of delusion or other thought disturbance.

Zung (1980) believes that the critical distinction between neurotic and psychotic depression lies in the notion that psychotic depression implies the severe loss of capacity to meet ordinary demands of life. Therefore, care of such elderly individuals would require closer clinical assessment of their ability to function on a daily basis. Even moderate levels of dejected mood, physiological problems, and loss of interest could lead to impairment in adaptive capacity of some elderly persons. The Research Diagnostic Criteria (RDC) and various depression scales would have some value in rating the severity of depression in the elderly.

RELATIONSHIP BETWEEN DEPRESSIVE SYMPTOMS AND MEDICAL ILLNESS

In understanding diagnostic and etiologic classifications of depression in late life, another major difficulty is the distinction between depression due to medical diseases and illness, and the impact of depression on the medical and physical health of the elderly person. Thus the complex interplay of depression and illness needs to be understood in detail.

Garretz (1976) has noted that a dangerous cycle of depression and medical illness is common among the elderly. Symptoms of depression are often among the initial presenting symptoms of serious medical disease in elderly patients. This observation is confirmed by Wigdon and Morris (1977), who found that in a comparison group of medical histories covering a 20- to 24-year period for groups of moderately to severely depressed males the severely depressed suffered a significantly greater number of medical disorders per individual. A related and equally significant finding of these authors was that many of the medical disorders experienced by the depressed (i.e., cardiovascular disorders, diabetes, and arthritis) are especially associated with the aging process. Salzman and Shader (1979) postulated that the differential diagnosis of medically related depression versus the depression of psychogenic origin may be difficult to establish because in their view many manifestations of depression in the elderly (such as lassitude, anorexia, insomnia, diminishing energy, pain, protean somatic symptoms, and hypochondriasis) may be of psychogenic origin as well as parts of a medical disease.

The relationship between depressive symptoms and medical disease is even harder to establish when anxiety and depression are found together. McCrae, Bartone, and Costa (1976) found that anxious and depressed elderly males were far less concerned about their health than normal subjects, suggesting thereby that certain groups of depressed and anxious elderly may be overly concerned about their medical health while other depressed and anxious persons may be too little concerned. Thus, the clinician or physician should look for and evaluate both anxiety and depression in the elderly, and when these problems are found to coexist, appropriate psychotherapeutic, pharmacologic, or medical assessment modes should be used in responding to the anxiety, depression, and medical disease components. Careless or uninformed diagnosis and assessment of either the psychogenic depression as a predisposing factor to medical illness or medical disease factors as contributing to depression and anxiety can lead to inadequate treatment of various problems.

It has also been suggested that older persons may be diagnosed as clinically depressed more often in circumstances where in fact nutritional deficiencies may be present and leading to worsening physical and medical problems. The picture is further complicated by a tendency to equate processes of normal aging with depression, the effects of disease, and nutritional deficiencies.

With respect to assessment strategies the presence of anxiety, depression, and suboptimal nutrition should remind the clinician that medical illness might be present. All too often the emphasis in the assessment of the depressed elderly has been on psychopathology with a resulting neglect in assessing the strengths and weaknesses of the elderly person's general physical or psychological organization or medical status. Thus, emphasis should be placed on the need for integrative multidimensional (i.e., psychotherapeutic, biological, pharmacologic, dietary, psychiatric) approaches to diagnosis and assessment, in order to minimize the high probability of misdiagnosis when the perspective and tools of only one discipline are used (Gaitz & Baer, 1970). Whenever a relationship between depressive symptoms and medical disease is hypothesized or suspected by the practitioner or clinician, some of the following factors and potentialities need further consideration.

Depression as a Response to Physical Illness

Depression in the elderly may often be precipitated by physical illness. Verwoerdt (1980, 1981) contends that the severity, duration, and rate of progression of the physical illness are closely associated with the magnitude of depressive responses and reactions of the elderly to their illness. Verwoerdt noted that 60 percent to 85 percent of the elderly subjects have been able to identify the specific physical stimulus or bodily activity that precipitated feelings of depression (Busse, 1975).

Kavanagh, Shepherd, and Tuk (1975) and White (1971) observed that one of the most common illnesses of old age is cardiovascular disease, which can produce severe depressive illness in the patient in the early stage of the disease. This depression may be manifested in physical symptoms of fatigue, exhaustion, breathing difficulty, insomnia, etc., which may sometimes be falsely attributed to the failing heart and increase the danger of inaccurate diagnosis and therapeutic neglect. Schwab (1966) also noted that a vast majority of medical patients express some of the usual symptoms of depression, many of which may be a concomitant of their physical illness. Depressive symptoms such as guilt, crying, irritability, anxiety, and dependency, in addition to the generalized somatic problems encountered by the physically ill, are particular characteristics of physically ill elderly. With prolonged physical illness there may be a further increase in dependency, regression, and helplessness, and the social isolation that ensues (Payne, 1975) may contribute to further depression. Payne presented the clinical depressive symptoms of a 62-year-old woman who following a myocardial infarction was forced to rely increasingly on her husband for whom she had ambivalent feelings. The presence of physical illness and the concomitant helplessness led to an agitated depression with suicidal preoccupation.

Butler and Lewis (1977) found that 86 percent of the depressed elderly had physical health problems of one kind or another. In addition, sensory losses, especially losses of hearing and visual impairment, may exacerbate depressive symptoms by contributing to loss of control and independence and to further social isolation and related depression reactions. Thus Schwab (1966) suggests that geropsychologists and geriatricians should question the patients about object losses incurred in surgery or physical illness and the chronicity of the depressive symptoms and carefully evaluate the patient's reactions to the most recent illness. Based on the depressed elderly person's history the practitioner should determine if there has been a pattern of repeated episodes of depression with repeated incidents of physical illness. Both the severity of the depressive symptoms and the extent to which these depressive reactions are associated with precipitating physical illness factors should be determined and carefully evaluated before determining whether depression or physical and somatic concerns are the primary problem.

Medical Diseases Present with Depression

It is suggested that a medical examination, including a careful evaluation of neurologic deficits, endocrine system, and cardiac dysfunction, may provide further evidence of whether the depression may be a result of organic brain damage, thyroid glandular dysfunction, or the like.

Neurological Illnesses

Despite the difficulties that may be encountered in accurately assessing the mental status of patients with Parkinson's disease, there is some clinical evidence to suggest that as the duration of the disease increases, a proportion of the patients become demented (Celesia & Wanamaker, 1972). The decreased motility produced by this neurologic disorder (the peak incidence of which occurs in the sixth and seventh decades) may resemble the physical signs of retarded depression: fatigue, psychomotor retardation, and lassitude.

Pathological evidence has been presented to suggest that while dementia is not seen in all cases of idiopathic Parkinson's disease, neuronal loss is inevitably evident (Pearse, 1974; Martilla & Rinne, 1976) and Alzheimer-type dementia develops more frequently in Parkinson's disease. Boller, Mizutani, and Roessmann (1979) reported 55 percent of the Parkinson's disease subjects they studied had the neurologic deficits characteristic of Alzheimer-type dementia, and the occurrence of true depressive effect with Parkinson's disease was reported in 40 percent to 90 percent of the cases (Brown & Wilson, 1972).

Considerable debate has therefore ensued over the question of whether depressive symptoms are part of the neurologic etiology of the disease or are a secondary reaction to the chronic and progressive disability of the illness (Celesia & Wanamaker, 1972). It has been suggested, however, that the depressive symptoms of Parkinson's disease have responded well to electroconvulsive therapy.

Brain tumors are another common neurologic disease that may be a cause of depression. Of the various CNS tumors that may occur in the elderly, the commonest is the meningioma. The larger cranial capacity : brain volume ratio allows meningiomas to reach a larger size in the elderly (compared to younger patients) before brain compression and raised intracranial pressure develops. Gliomas are the most frequent type of primary cerebral tumor that may present as depression and may produce other general deficits in psychological functioning resembling clinical signs and symptoms of retarded depression: lability of emotions, lassitude, apathy, and withdrawal (Wilson & Bruce, 1955). Tumors of the frontal lobe, temporal lobe, and corpus callosum are likely to produce more emotional impairment (Rossman, 1969) with many of the clinical signs and symptoms of dementia and dementia-related depression.

Other neurologic disturbances that present with depression in old age may be vascular in nature: small silent strokes, intracranial aneurisms, mild or moderate head injuries occurring at an age when the walls of the arteries become thinner, and bacterial infections such as meningitis, cerebral syphilis, or simplex encephalitis. All these disorders may produce depressive symptoms (Strassman, 1957) and dementing syndromes characterized by mental symptoms (especially inattention, lack of initiative, fatigue, and irascibility) that are also characteristic of retarded depression.

Massey and Bullock (1979) note that depression in the elderly may lead to physical problems such as peroneal palsy that can be diagnosed only on medical examination, and inactive and depressed elderly with weight loss may be particularly prone to this condition. Often depression in the elderly may be linked to the sensory loss experienced in the area supplied by the peroneal nerve.

Endocrine Abnormalities

These are often associated with alterations in the affective states. In general, both hypo- and hyperfunctioning of the various endocrine systems are implicated in depression. The physical health assessment of the elderly should definitely evaluate hypothyroidism, a disease associated with 80 percent incidence of depressive symptoms. Addison's disease and Cushing's disease, although less common, may present as depression.

Cardiac Abnormalities

Cerebral anoxia resulting from cardiac insufficiency, emphysema, or both often precipitates severe depression or affective disorders. Anoxic confusion may follow after surgery, and family members of the elderly, unless cautioned by the physician, may express grave concern over the serious depression in the elderly relative. The severity, duration, and rate of progression of the illness (e.g., cancer) are factors in determining the magnitude of the depressive response of the elderly to sickness (Verwoerdt, 1976).

Additional factors that may determine the severity of a depression following medical disorders are the organ system involved and its role in the ego-maintenance of the elderly individual, for example, severe arthritis in the case of an elderly pianist; the degree of narcissistic attachment to the lost functioning (for example, the removal of a cancerous breast for a women may produce a sense of diminished womanhood that may lead to chronic depression); and the inability to maintain a positive body image subsequent to an organ loss or loss of parts or function (Verwoerdt, 1973).

Thus it is evident that in any diagnostic or assessment workup procedures with the elderly, depression may be inextricably linked with a physical disease or may in turn be the symptom of a medical illness. A clinician or physician may concentrate either on the depression or the physical illness and miss or fail to examine depression complaints that have a true physical origin, or conversely physical and somatic complaints that originate in clinical depression.

Nature of Depressive Equivalents or Masked Depression

Just as the relationship between depression and physical illness presents problems in routine psychological or mental health examination of the elderly, the presence of depressive equivalents or the translation of depression into physical terms can make the routine physical health status examination difficult. Pfeiffer and Busse (1973) note that many elderly patients with depression also present with an aggravation of preexisting physical illness. The use of somatic complaints to communicate sad affective states represents the use of an active ego-coping and adaptive mechanism. Thus some clinicians may decide not to take the somatic complaints or depressive equivalents seriously. Beyond a certain point, however, many manifestations of physical symptoms (e.g., weakness, anorexia, abdominal pain, gastrointestinal symptoms) are too dangerous to treat lightly (Blazer, 1982). A variety of these symptoms may be unconsciously used by elderly patients to disguise their depression as well as to communicate and ask for help (Ancherson, 1961; Lundquist, 1961). Thus treatment of depressive equivalents or forms of masked depression need to be considered in greater detail.

Gerner (1979) warns that many somatic symptoms may serve to "mask" depression and that "masked" depression may be found in as many as one-third of elderly individuals. The notion of masked depression assumes that an individual is depressed to an unknown extent but attempts to hide, disguise, or otherwise cover up the primary symptoms of dysphoria and dejection arising from loss of self-esteem or loss of productivity. Synonyms for the term *masked depression* include *depression sine depression, depressive equivalent,* and *occult depression.*

Based on clinical observations and interview data, a number of clinicians (Busse, 1975; Lesse, 1974; Salzman & Shader, 1979) note that somatic symptoms or somatic preoccupations, including gastrointestinal symptoms and abdominal pain, burning tongue, and other oral discomforts, are the most frequent expressions of masked depression in the elderly. Lassitude, easy fatigability, and loss of strength, if not associated with any clear physical illness, may be the early symptoms of masked depression. However, as Salzman and Shader (1979) warn, these somatic symptoms in elderly patients suspected of being depressed should not be taken lightly. From a psychodynamic perspective masked depressive symptoms are often unresolved feelings, involving ambivalence toward family members, anger, and guilt, which are turned inward in self-punitive ways if they are ignored by the gerotherapist, physician, or members of the family. This may explain why a relatively high number of elderly patients with hypochondriacal symptoms attempt suicide (Stenback, 1980).

Both Lesse (1974) and Gerner (1979) conclude that many elderly individuals with masked depression did not respond favorably to physical symptomatic treatments, often leading practitioners to employ more drastic treatment measures such as surgery or a more complicated medical regimen. Krietman's (1972; 1976) retrospective data also confirm that more than one-third of patients with masked depression symptoms had unnecessary surgery, which alone appeared to relieve their somatic symptoms.

In summarizing the psychodynamic picture of masked depression, Smith (1978) identified several personality, social, and demographic factors related to masked depression in the elderly. These factors include lack of creativity, sense of uselessness, isolation and segregation, bereavement, social stress resulting from loss of income, loss of status, and loss of family networks.

In summary, the assessment perspective advocated here stresses that the clinician should take serious note of the development of those somatic concerns or symptoms that do not correspond to known disease. The vagueness of the symptom descriptions in the elderly may have a signal value (Salzman & Shader, 1979) indicating that the elderly person is in need of emotional help.

INITIAL ASSESSMENT OF CLINICAL DEPRESSION: PRELIMINARY STEPS AND PROCEDURES

In most instances the primary feature of depression is dysphoria, a feeling of pessimism and sadness. Clinical depression, however, should be viewed as a cluster of behavioral, somatic, and cognitive symptoms. Depression in addition to being a negative mood state involves observable changes in behaviors, thoughts, and perceptions. The DSM-III (the Diagnostic and Statistical Manual of Mental Disorders, 1980) has identified several recognizable features of an episode of clinical depression, almost all of which are applicable to the elderly.

Necessary and Sufficient Symptoms of Clinical Depression

Three categories of depressive symptoms and features of depression that have special significance for the assessment of depression in the elderly can be distinguished from the schematic representations of Lehmann (1981) (Figures 3–1 and 3–2), and from Table 3–1 (Lewinsohn, Biglan, & Zeiss, 1976). These are as follows:

1. Behavioral and somatic symptoms such as headaches; sleep disturbances, especially restless sleep and insomnia; loss of libido; suicidal attempts; bodily preoccupation and hypochondriasis; memory impairment; and inability to concentrate. Some of these symptoms are common in old age and many are common in the depressed elderly, but not all of them are necessary or sufficient for establishing the presence of clinical depression in the elderly. Some of these symptoms may reflect the presence of organic and physical disease.
2. Psychological symptoms, depressed mood, and hopelessness. These are sufficient but not necessary for the diagnosis of depression in the elderly, many of whom may disguise their dysphoric moods and present more pronounced somatic complaint symptoms.
3. Organismic, negative symptoms, that is, reduction of interest (apathy), loss of capacity to experience pleasure (anhedonia), loss of energy, and fatigue states. These are necessary but not sufficient features of depression in the elderly. Many elderly may show organismic and negative symptoms arising from disorders other than depression, for example, chronic illness, diabetes, physical disability.

According to Lehmann (1981) the last category of necessary symptoms is postulated to be present in all depressions and is probably invariant across different cultures and ages. In the elderly the presence of two or three of these symptoms may be helpful in the uncovering of masked depression.

Methods for Evaluating Depression

Gallagher and Thompson (1983) have compared the operational definitions suggested by the Research Diagnostic Criteria (RDC) and the Diagnostic Statistical Manual of Mental Disorders (DSM-III) (Table 3–2). They note that the RDC criteria are more stringent but provide opportunity for more fine-grained distinctions between the symptoms of major depressive disorders and major depressive episodes and between episodic and chronic conditions.

RDC criteria have the advantage that they provide more evidence of daily functioning disorders, whether the depressed individual sought or was referred for help during the episode and whether the person took medication for relief of stress. Some of the additional qualifying information provided by RDC is especially useful to the clinician in the diagnostic evaluation of elderly clients. One of the disadvantages of using RDC with elderly

Table 3–2 Comparison of the Research Diagnostic Criteria (RDC) and DSM-III Criteria for Major Depression

RDC Criteria for Major Depressive Disorder (MDD)	DSM-III Criteria for Major Depressive Episode (MDE)
A. Mood Disturbance One or more distinct periods with dysphoric mood or pervasive loss of interest or pleasure.	Dysphoric mood or loss of interest or pleasure in all or almost all usual activities and pastimes.
In both systems, mood disturbance is characterized by descriptors such as: depressed, sad, downhearted and blue, hopeless, down in the dumps, don't care anymore, or irritable. While this disturbance does not need to be dominant, it must be prominent and persistent. Momentary shifts from dysphoric mood to another serious emotional state such as anxiety or anger would preclude a diagnosis of major depression.	
B. Related Symptoms At least five of the following are required as part of the episode and four for probable MDD:	At least four of the following must be present regularly:
1. Poor appetite or weight loss, or increased appetite or weight gain. 2. Sleep difficulty (insomnia) or sleeping too much (hypersomnia). 3. Psychomotor agitation or retardation (but not merely subjective feelings of restlessness or being slowed down). 4. Loss of energy, fatigability, or tiredness. 5. Loss of interest or pleasure in usual activities, or decrease in sexual drive not limited to a period of delusion or hallucinating. 6. Feelings of worthlessness, self-reproach, or excessive or inappropriate guilt. 7. Complaints or evidence of diminished ability to think or concentrate (e.g., slowed thinking or indecisiveness). 8. Recurrent thoughts of death or suicide, or any suicidal behavior.	
C. Duration Dysphoric features: 2 weeks for definite; 1–2 weeks for probable. Related symptoms: Not specified but presumed at least 2 weeks.	Dysphoric features: Not specified but presumed at least 2 weeks. Related symptoms: Must be present nearly every day for at least 2 weeks.
D. Exclusionary Criteria 1. None of the following which suggests schizophrenia is present: —Delusions of being controlled, or of thought broadcasting, insertions, or withdrawal. —Nonaffective hallucinations. —Auditory hallucinations. —More than one month of *no* depressive symptoms but delusions or hallucinations. —Preoccupation with a delusion or hallucination to relative exclusion of other symptoms or concerns. —Definite marked, formal thought disorder. 2. Does not meet criteria for schizophrenia, residual type.	1. Preoccupation with a mood-incongruent delusion or hallucination or bizarre behavior cannot be dominant in the clinical picture before or after the occurrence of an affective syndrome. 2. Mood disturbance cannot be superimposed on schizophrenia, schizophreniform disorder, or a paranoid disorder. 3. Organic mental disorder or uncomplicated bereavement is ruled out as a cause of mood disturbance.
E. Impairment of functioning. Sought or was referred for help during the dysphoric period, took medication, or had impairments in functioning with family, at home, at school, at work, or socially.	Not specified.

Source: From *Clinical Geropsychology: New Directions in Assessment and Treatment* (pp. 14–15) by P.M. Lewinsohn and L. Teri (Eds.), 1983, Elmsford, N.Y.: Pergamon Press, Inc. Copyright 1983 by Pergamon Press. Reprinted by permission.

clients is that most of the symptoms used to describe unipolar depression are also normal concomitants of the aging process (Gallagher & Thompson, 1983). It is suggested that by using the Schedule for Affective Disorders and Schizophrenia (SADS) (Endicott & Spitzer, 1978) along with RDC a more careful delineation can be made of major depressive disorders involving dimensions of physical health, aging, and cognitive functioning (Gallagher & Thompson, 1983). This comprehensive test battery is recommended when there is a real question as to the effects of aging on cognitive and affective functioning.

In each case of clinical depression specific criteria indicated by DSM-III and RDC are suggested for the identification and procedural steps in the initial diagnostic assessment of depression in the elderly. First, duration of two or more weeks must be established. The individual would need to be experiencing several symptoms of depression on a consistent basis for at least two weeks. If some of the dysphoric feelings, behavioral deficits or behavioral excesses, or somatic or cognitive symptoms described in Table 3–1 are not experienced over a stretch of time, then it can be assumed that the elderly person is not clinically depressed but is more likely showing transitory symptoms common in the older age group.

Second, the primary affective state or feelings during the initial interval should be established. Feelings of sadness and dysphoria are typical and prominent symptoms in the early depression before severe retardation becomes evident. However, as Raskin (1979) and Gurland (1976) have noted, many elderly depressed individuals may show little mood disturbance (Post, 1965) but may present a variety of somatic concerns (e.g., anorexia, abdominal pain, fatigue, and weakness) or a number of other psychological symptoms (e.g., aggravation of preexisting dependency, helplessness, or pessimism). In the latter instance these symptoms of dependency or pessimism may be seen as the elderly's attempts to cover up the primary symptoms of dysphoria and dejection (masked depression). Every depressive syndrome includes somatic symptoms, but in the depressed elderly persons the somatic symptoms become so predominant that their depressive basis remains completely hidden. Detailed inquiry about the nature of the somatic symptoms and complaints may lead to more positive information about the presence of clinical depression.

Third, if symptoms of helplessness, dependency, and pessimism are noted, it would be important to identify significant precipitating factors that may have led to the resurgence of helpless fatigue. Shinfuku (1981) suggests that an inquiry about significant events and experiences would help in the identification of precipitating factors in the many depressions of the elderly. These queries could be about

- death and disease of close relatives,
- physical accidents,
- family problems and conflicts,
- changes in living conditions,
- retirement,
- recent medications and drug ingestions, and
- diagnosis of terminal illness for self or close relatives.

Fourth, specific observations, monitoring, and inquiry should be made to ascertain the duration, intensity, and frequency of depressive symptoms pertaining to sleep irregularities; increased or decreased appetite; loss of appetite with accompanying weight loss; changes in psychomotor activity including signs of agitation, loss of energy, easy fatigability, bodily aches, loss of interest, and inability to experience pleasure; and difficulty in concentrating. Questions about suicide ideation should be asked directly. The syndrome of clinical depression is distinguished from symptoms of depression by the severity and duration of the depressed mood and by the continuity and sustained presence of four or more of the accompanying symptoms. In other words not all elderly with symptoms of depression suffer from a primary clinical depressive disorder. However, beyond the symptom level the sustained presence of a syndrome or a cluster of symptoms, behaviors, and functional disturbances more clearly suggests clinical depression.

Symptoms described in step 4 are very specific. There are essentially eight somatic, psychogenic, and cognitive areas related to the onset of depression according to DSM-III (1980) criteria. Other symptoms such as worry and anxiety, stress, loss of self-esteem, and inadequacy are not included as criteria for classification. The eight symptom areas are the most efficient indicators of true clinical depression as distinguished from lower levels of distress or from other psychological disorders (Spitzer, Endicott, & Robins, 1978).

Fifth, in order to diagnose normal mood changes in old age from clinical depression, it is useful to inquire about the effect of the mood changes, loss of appetite, insomnia, etc., on the day-to-day functioning of the elderly person. Just as depression has no single cause, there are no simple categories of effects and consequences that depression has on the functioning of individual elderly. However, there appears to be a general consensus that clinical depression leads to a greater degree of impairment in social and cognitive functioning. Thus a clinical level of depression is more likely if day-to-day functioning is diminished and everyday chores and responsibilities and essential self-care functions are being ignored. Increasing signs of helplessness and dependency in the performance of routine tasks are also smaller indications of the presence of clinical depression.

If significant problems are noted in the day-to-day functioning of the elderly person but no physiological causes account for the difficulty, and no accompanying symptoms of dysphoric mood, blues or agitation, and anxiety are present, then these are indications of masked depression. Kielholz (1981, p. 242) suggests that asking an elderly person the following questions may assist in the diagnosis of the devitalizing or vegetative symptoms that underlie masked depression:

- Can you enjoy things as usual?
- Do you find it difficult to make decisions?
- Are you interested in things as usual?
- Are you brooding more than usual?
- Do you feel that life has become pointless?
- Do you feel more tired and have less energy than usual?
- Do you have any trouble with your sleep?
- Do you get up in the morning earlier than usual?
- Have you lost your usual appetite and weight?
- Do you have any interest in sex?

The more affirmative answers obtained, the greater is the probability that depression is present.

Sixth, differential diagnoses of clinical depression, as distinguished from a dementia, organic brain syndrome, and neurological disturbances, is particularly important in evaluating the elderly. However, the differential diagnosis is a complicated process. It is important to rule out the impact of other significant endogenous and secondary health problems, neurological disturbances, etc., by means of an extensive diagnostic workup for the elderly depressed person. The latter comprehensive assessment is recommended for a major depressive condition. Initially, however, before the need or usefulness of a detailed diagnostic workup can be determined, it is important that information be obtained from the elderly person with respect to the six areas described. If specific inquiry in each of these areas yields positive findings and the frequency, intensity, and duration of several physical and psychological symptoms are maintained over a sustained period, then the primary problem is more likely to have assumed clinical proportions, and extensive diagnostic workup procedures will be warranted in order to establish whether the depressive disorder is mainly somatogenic, endogenous, or psychogenic (Figure 3–1) or a combination of one or more classifications.

COMPREHENSIVE DIAGNOSTIC WORKUP OF THE ELDERLY DEPRESSED CLIENTS

Overall, Lehmann (1981) suggests that most cases of depression can be easily diagnosed by observation of symptoms and behaviors and by general inspection. Some other cases will have to be diagnosed on the basis of a semistructured interview (Pfeiffer, 1980). In some cases of major depressive disorders, however, a comprehensive diagnostic workup will be imperative. As part of the comprehensive diagnostic workup evaluation procedure, it is recommended that several intricate psychosocial and environmental factors, physical loneliness, and mental status factors be examined.

The comprehensive diagnostic workup of elderly depressed individuals using the CARE or OARS methodology and procedures (Chapter 2) should be designed with the following goals in mind:

- Elicit a history of the patient's symptoms, medication data, and family history of depression.
- Evaluate the physical status with special attention paid to the evaluation of possible endocrine disorders, neurophysiological deficits, and other genetic conditions.
- Assess the mental status with special attention being paid to disturbances of mood, effect, motor behavior, perception, and memory.
- Test biological conditions of blood count, urinalysis, thyroxine levels, etc.
- Assess psychological status by means of psychological tests of depression, control, self-care, and social adjustment.

It is essential for the clinician to understand the complex interplay of family history, medical illness, cognitive functioning, and psychophysiological capacities and to be aware of the major implications.

Family History

For the geropsychologist and geriatrician it may suggest careful history taking of the affective status of the elderly patient. In addition to the history of physical health, it is instructive to obtain full knowledge of the patient's background factors such as heredity, childhood, work record, and sexual and marital experiences. A supplementary history obtained from members of the family, or friends, either before or after the interview is almost an imperative when dealing with those elderly who show many "depressive equivalent" symptoms in the form of somatic complaints (Weinberg, 1975) or who have a serious illness. The clinician should assess the client's most likely reason for mastering the depression and should guide the family of the elderly in understanding the nature of the somatic concerns of the elderly patient. Obtaining a family history from the elderly of affective stress and distress may be germane to understanding the responses of the individual.

Mental Health Examination

A mental health examination along the lines suggested next is central to a diagnostic workup of the elderly client:

- Overt behavior. It is suggested that the clinician can generally determine the patient's motor activity of restlessness, aimless walking, seclusion, inactivity, or the reverse such as agitated or repetitive activity. Facial expressions should not be missed. Does the patient portray perplexity, anxiety, or sadness? Does the patient speak so softly and quietly that the speech is barely audible or is the speech ebullient, distractible, and loud as to reflect agitation (Blazer, 1982)? Psychomotor retardation or underactivity is characteristic of masked depression in the elderly although older depressed patients may also commonly exhibit hyperactivity or agitation. Linn (1975) notes that there is an inability to sit still, and increased activity may take the form of repetitive behavior such as hand washing, washing the dishes many times, and adjusting pillows. The severely depressed elderly often has a grimaced face with eyes closed and indicates inability to move the extremities or do anything requiring activity.
- Mood status. This evaluation must be inferred from the presence of sadness, despair, anxiety, tension, loss of feeling, and paucity of ideation. Effect may vary considerably during the interview; however, effect in the depressed elderly is less susceptible to wide fluctuations and is sustained over time. Suicidal ideas may surface through a sense of self-reproach, depersonalization, or guilt (Weinberg, 1975). There may be passivity or projective experiences and thoughts. The elderly client may complain of somatic sensations that may in a sense be substitutes for an expression of emotional state.
- Process of thinking. This evaluation must be inferred from disturbances in thinking that may present as problems with the structure of associations, the speed of associations, and the content of thought. Agitated depressed elderly persons may pathologically repeat the same word or idea in response to a variety of probes. Upon questioning, depressed patients generally respond with statements such as, "I just can't do anything"; "I'm tired and can't think straight"; "I don't remember anything." Except in cases of severe depression and agitation, most depressed elderly demonstrate no disturbance of the structure of associations. Severely depressed persons may have

difficulty in maintaining logical connections in their thoughts but only rarely are depressed elderly incoherent and disoriented. The latter symptoms, if detected, may suggest delirium or early indications of dementia. Some depressed older persons demonstrate circumstantiality or the introduction into conversation of many details only distantly related to the main subject and may sound cheerful for a few seconds in response to an association.

- Distorted perceptions. Linn (1975) defines perception as the awareness of objects in relations that follow stimulation of peripheral sense organs. Typical disturbance of perceptions that is noted in elderly depressives is false sensory perceptions not associated with real external or internal stimuli (e.g., false perceptions of movement or body sensations and sounds, false perceptions of smell, touch, and taste). The depressed elderly are more likely than nondepressed elderly to reflect psychic distress in the form of body function symptoms.

- Cognitive impairment and dementia. It is estimated that 15 percent of all elderly persons diagnosed as being depressed show signs of cognitive impairment and other indications of dementia (Salzman & Shader, 1979) and that dementia occurs in up to 20 percent of persons over the age of 65 years and is the leading cause of geriatric patients admitted to psychiatric institutions for the first time (Sloane, 1980).

Because of the overlap of symptoms found in dementia and clinical depression in later life, misdiagnosis often occurs. McAllister and Price (1982) note that as many as 15 percent of the elderly patients diagnosed as demented by their physicians were later evaluated as suffering from depressive illness. However, misdiagnosis in the early stage of the dementia patients may be unavoidable since such patients may show emotional lability and typical symptoms of clinical depression rather than severe cognitive impairment.

The failure on the part of the practitioner to identify clinical depression as the primary disorder implies that there would be potential delay in providing the appropriate psychosocial attention and proper medication. The negative side effects of inappropriate medication may often contribute to making the patient's depressive condition worse. By contrast the practitioner's failure to identify dementia as the primary disorder in those patients who also show serious clinical depression is a diagnostic error that may lead to obvious delay in intervention for patients, especially for those patients who may have a form of dementia that responds favorably to treatment.

Medical Factors

Contribution of Drugs to Depression

Drugs, either prescribed by a physician or taken independently, are often responsible for the development of depression, especially in the elderly. Larson, Whanger, and Busse (1982) note that as age increases, the individual's responses to drugs also change. The changes in the elderly's mood may be due to alterations in metabolism, decreased capacity of the liver to detoxify, reduced renal capacity to excrete, decreased cerebral blood flow, and decreased overall body metabolism (Friedel, 1978; Beattie & Sellers, 1979). The body's capacity to maintain biochemical homeostasis is reduced (Larson, Whanger, & Busse, 1982). Thus, with respect to the elderly the addition of drugs to the body's system would increase the probability of side effects, particularly in response to benzodiazepines

(Greenblatt, Allen, & Shader, 1977) and such antidepressants as tricyclics (Nies, Robinson, & Friedman, 1977). A detailed discussion of the impact of drugs on the affective functioning of the elderly is presented in Chapter 12.

There is a disproportionately high use of psychotropic drugs—tranquilizers, sedatives, and antidepressants—by the elderly. Gibson and O'Hare (1968) felt that one-third of depressed elderly self-medicate in ways that are potentially dangerous. These self-medications may rapidly increase the susceptibility of the elderly to strange physiological responses produced as a result of interaction between the drugs, the naturally occurring morphologic changes, and the present medical status. Lamy and Kitler (1971) recommend, therefore, that a careful history be obtained of the elderly individual's medication, drugs, and alcohol consumption.

Depression and Nutrition

Schwab (1976) emphasizes that the elderly are at high risk of depression arising from suboptimal nutrition. Although the direct effect of various nutritional deficiencies is still not well understood (Todhunter, 1976), it is reasonable to assume that they contribute adversely to the medical and mental health and subsequently generate confusional states and depression. Although nutritional status is not often a common part of the clinician's therapeutic regimen, it is vital that evaluation of nutritional status be made central to any diagnostic workup of the depressed elderly (Whanger & Wang, 1974; Todhunter, 1976). Depression in the aged is often a concomitant of physical illness restricting nutritional intake and decreasing protein binding and absorption.

Such an interlaced process makes the task of assessing depression in the elderly extremely complex and challenging. Zung (1980) concludes that the greater the number of physical disorders, the more rigid and insecure will be the behavior patterns of the elderly, and the greater will be the perceptual distortion of the external stimuli. The resultant depression will tend to compromise further the rather tenuous physiological and psychological functioning of the aged and lead to more related feelings of sadness and depression.

Personal Psychosocial Factors

Assessment of psychosocial factors as interlaced with mental status factors is useful in the diagnostic evaluation of depressive disorders in the psychogenic classification. Assessment of the following factors are germane to an understanding of various functional disorders in the elderly:

- Grief reactions. These are common in late life and are frequently indistinguishable from a depressive disorder when only the symptoms are assessed; a history of significant loss and remission over time, without an increased risk for recurrence, partially distinguishes grief reactions from depression.
- Stress. Zung (1980) speculates that rarely are the elderly suffering from depressive disorders unaffected by the social and physical stress factors. Stress, according to Zung, refers to all psychic events or processes whether they originate from within the person or from without in the environment. Stress can and does occur at any age, but with aging, stress can become a greater risk factor for depression and mood disorders since the elderly's vulnerability to the vicissitudes of life are increased (p. 340). Stress in the elderly, classified as object losses of various kinds, includes various environmental

losses such as loss of status as a result of retirement, loss of physical health with physical disabilities, social isolation, and loss of role—all these losses of one kind or another contribute to the decrease in the elderly's self-esteem and the growth of pessimism. Clinicians therefore need to note that while a certain degree of pessimism may be considered normal neurosis of the aged, the gloomy outlook of the elderly may be magnified and distorted to such a degree that the individual develops despondent tendencies leading to severe depression and suicide (Zung, 1980).

Thus clinicians and physicians need to monitor the social-environmental factors that may be producing stress either in the form of real losses, threatened losses, or imaginary losses. Several factors that precipitate and exacerbate stress in the elderly and need to be monitored are discussed in Chapter 5.

RATING SCALES FOR DEPRESSION

The clinical assessment of depression in the elderly has traditionally employed a variety of self-report ratings and observer-ratings to assess the severity and intensity of depression. Self-report and observer-report measures of depression have traditionally been employed in research and clinical practice with adults, and this tradition has been extended to practice with older clients. These rating scales for measuring the severity of depression are of particular interest to the geropsychologist and practitioner because of their potential for cost-effectiveness. They can in a large number of situations be effectively used by semi-trained personnel, including nurses and adult members of the elderly's family. Their use is recommended during the initial screening and intake interview.

Rating scales have been designed for administration by a trained observer who may make observations and complete the scale during an interview or in the setting of daily contact with the client, or scales may be designed to be completed by the client. Procedures for repeated administration of the rating scales for depression with the client over time and consultation with the elderly person's family members about the severity of depression, are finding an increasingly important place in the assessment techniques of the practitioner. One important recommendation is that the interviewer be responsible for explaining and, wherever necessary, repeating self-reporting items and recording the responses.

Kochansky (1979) argues that to be effective, scales for assessing depressive symptomatology in the elderly should consist of items that focus on the physical and affective symptoms that are characteristic of the elderly, as well as those symptoms that are not age-specific. In other words these scales in order to be of optimal value should be sensitive to the wide spectrum of depressive symptomatology in the elderly, for example, ranging from apathy and physical complaint to severely depressed mood and major impairment of psychological functions (p. 132). Kochansky proposes that an optimal scale should have some capacity to differentiate the neurotic from the endogenous depression and depressive symptomatology from dementia.

The geropsychologist needs to be informed of both the research criteria and diagnostic statistical criteria of the depression measures. Hence details of specific items and comparisons of symptoms assessed by various depression rating scales are described to inform the clinician and the practitioner of those scales that are useful as research tools and others that have practical value for screening purposes.

Self-Rating Scales

Zung Self-Rating Depression Scale (SDS)

The Self-Rating Depression Scale (Zung, 1965) is a brief, 22-item screening inventory of the client's current depressive symptomatology. Zung (1965) designed the scale in order to measure three basic dimensions of depression: (1) physiological equivalents, (2) psychological factors, and (3) effect. Respondents are asked to indicate, on a four-point scale, how much of the time during the past week a specific statement was true. The SDS includes eight physiological statements, eight psychological statements, four emotional and affective statements, and two psychomotor statements.

The SDS has had more trials with the elderly than any other depression measure; see McNair (1979) for a review. However, the SDS has also been criticized because of its preponderance of somatic items (relative to those tapping psychological distress). See Blazer's (1982) comparison of symptoms assessed by various depression rating scales (Table 3–3).

Zung (1970) had 69 Methodist Retirement Home residents and Golden Age Club members complete the scale. He found no significant differences between these two groups, but he observed that they reported significantly higher depression scores than the younger normative group. Zung offered no explanation for these differences, but Blumenthal's (1975) interpretation is that the somatic items on the SDS such as constipation, weight loss, fatigue, and heart racing may have resulted in spuriously high total scores for those over 65. It is Blumenthal's contention that somatic complaints in persons 65 and older often reflect true physical problems rather than depression. In other words these items have different meaning for older than for younger adults.

An analysis of the rank ordering of the 20 SDS items for those aged 65 and older revealed that the normal aged individuals tended to rate the somatic items high and the depression items low. Specifically items reflecting decreased libido, psychomotor retardation, anorexia, diurnal variation, constipation, and confusion were ranked high, whereas depression and crying spells were ranked low (Zung, 1967). The suggestion is that the inclusion of somatic complaint items on a depression scale designed for use with elderly subjects with significant health problems may result in spuriously high depression ratings. However, one must be cautious not to label all somatic concerns, complaints of body slowness, and expressions of fatigue and apathy as normal for elderly subjects. One must be careful to disengage behaviors that can legitimately be ascribed to the aging process from those associated with depression.

Plutchik (1979) has critiqued the SDS in terms of reliability, validity, and administration procedures. In terms of reliability Plutchik (1979) points out that the format for altering items positively and negatively for symptoms requires frequent shifts in response sets. This procedure may confuse many older patients. He cites evidence to suggest that the best assessment items are written in a way that people use to express themselves spontaneously and naturally. McGarvey, Gallagher, Thompson, and Zelinski (1982) reported that the measure's internal consistency was below usual standards when used with the old-old and suggested that deletion of somatic items would improve the reliability of the scale for use with samples over the age of 70 years.

Plutchik (1979) has also raised a number of concerns regarding the validity of several SDS items. The primary concern is that several items appear inappropriate and may not be measuring depression. For example, the statement "I have trouble sleeping at night" may

Table 3–3 Comparison of Symptoms Assessed by Various Depression-Rating Scales

Symptoms	Beck (1967)	Hamilton (1960)	Zung (1965)	CES-D (Weissman et al., 1977)	ODS (Blazer, 1980)
Emotional					
Dejected mood	X	X	X	X	X
Negative feelings toward self	X			X	
Decreased life satisfaction	X		X	X	X
Loss of interest		X			X
Crying spells	X	X	X	X	
Irritability	X	X	X	X	X
Emptiness			X		
Fearfulness		X		X	
Cognitive					
Slowed thinking					X
Low self-evaluation			X		X
Negative expectations, hopelessness	X	X	X	X	X
Self-blame and self-criticism	X				
Worry		X			X
Indecisiveness	X	X	X		
Guilt feelings	X	X			X
Distorted self-image	X				
Loneliness				X	
Confusion		X	X	X	X
Preoccupation with health	X	X			
Helplessness					
Uselessness, sense of failure	X				X
Delusional					
Somatic					
Poverty					
Hallucinations					
Worthlessness		X		X	X
Sense of punishment	X	X			
Nihilistic					
Physical					
Fatigability	X	X	X	X	X
Sleep disturbance	X	X	X	X	X
Loss of appetite	X	X	X	X	X
Constipation		X	X		
Loss of libido	X		X		
Diurnal variation		X	X		
Weight loss	X	X	X		
Agitation		X	X		X
Retardation	X	X	X		X
Volitional					
Paralysis of will					X
Desire to withdraw socially	X	X			
Suicidal impulses	X	X	X		
Desire to receive help					
Work inhibition		X			

Source: From *Depression in Late Life* (p. 25) by D.G. Blazer, 1982, St. Louis: C.V. Mosby Company. Copyright 1982 by C.V. Mosby Company. Reprinted by permission.

be unclear for purposes of evaluating a patient who routinely takes sleeping medication. In addition, Plutchik (1979) raises questions of interpretation concerning SDS items related to loss of weight, trouble with constipation, clarity of mind, ease in doing the things one used to do, and so forth. There is little reliable evidence that these items are indicative of clinical levels of depression among the elderly as many of these symptoms frequently occur as a result of changes associated with aging and the effects of medication. Finally Plutchik (1979) suggests that it is often necessary to have an examiner present in order to weigh diagnostic decisions and clarify concerns raised by the patient.

Despite these limitations the SDS has had more trials with the elderly than any other scale because of its brevity and attempts to sample apparently core depressive symptoms in the emotional, cognitive, and physical domain.

Beck Depression Inventory (BDI)

The Beck Depression Inventory (Beck, Ward, Mendelsohn, Mock, & Erbaugh, 1961) is a 21-item, easily administered, self-report instrument that measures the nature and intensity of depressive symptomatology. Each item reflects a specific sign of depression, which is weighted in severity from 0 to 3. The construct of depression as used in this scale is an abnormal state of the organism reflected in signs and symptoms such as low subjective mood, pessimistic and nihilistic attitudes, loss of spontaneity, and specific vegetative signs (Table 3–3). This construct has been identified in many diverse types of patients who differ vastly in terms of other characteristics, such as degree of conceptual disorganization, presence of anxiety, and prognosis (Beck, 1972, p. 201). The BDI was designed for research purposes and was originally conceived as appropriate for discriminating levels of depression only in psychiatric populations.

Scoring procedures yield a total score that is obtained simply by adding the weighted values for each response endorsed by the patient. In the general adult population, scores of 0–9 are considered normal, the 10–15 range represents mild depression, 16–19 indicates mild to moderate severity of depression, 20–29 is judged as moderate to severe, and 30–63 represents severe depression. Scoring formats that separately evaluate cognitive, affective, physiological, and performance dimensions of depression can also be utilized. While the BDI is often presented as a self-administered inventory, the recommendation of observers and clinicians is that among a geriatric population its use be limited to administration by a trained interviewer who reads each statement and asks the elderly client to select the statement that fits best.

Beck (1972) sought to develop explicit rather than inferred behavioral criteria for evaluating depression. Toward this end, items were selected from the general literature on depressive symptomatology and clinical experience. Each subcategory describes a particular behavioral manifestation of depression and consists of a graded series of self-evaluative statements. The items were chosen on the basis of their relationship to overt manifestations of depression and do not reflect any particular etiology or viewpoint concerning the dichotomies (e.g., endogenous-reactive, neurotic-psychotic). The authors of this scale report that it is capable of discriminating between anxiety and depression, correlating 0.59 with clinical ratings of depression and only 0.14 with similar anxiety ratings.

Gallagher, Nies, and Thompson (1982) reported results of a reliability study using the BDI with persons over 60 years of age. They reported that the test-retest reliability of the BDI for depressed elderly outpatients was 0.79, and 0.86 for the nondepressed normal elderly persons. A further study (Gallagher, Breckenridge, Steinmetz, & Thompson, 1983) showed that the use of traditional cutoff scores for diagnostic classification had good agreement with diagnoses established using the Schedule for Affective Disorders and Schizophrenia (SADS) (Endicott & Spitzer, 1978). These results combined with those of Fry (1983; & Grover, 1982) suggest that the BDI appears to be relatively adequate as a clinical screening instrument for use with the elderly. Fry recommends that items should be read to elderly patients in order to avoid any misunderstanding of the meaning of a particular statement. Gallagher, Nies, and Thompson (1982) recommend caution in assessing the significance of physiological and somatic items as seen in the BDI, since many elderly patients experience bodily symptoms as a normal part of the aging process.

Caution is suggested also in the interpretation of extremely high or low total scores. Experience indicates that very high scores on the BDI (e.g., greater than 35) are found only in severely depressed inpatients. High scores among elderly outpatients may often indicate a need for immediate clinical evaluation, a cry for help from elderly clients who feel they are losing control or overwhelmed by their life circumstance. In these instances the client's outpatient psychosocial status should be carefully evaluated for feelings of loneliness, rejection, and social isolation. Similarly, very high scores, particularly among outpatients who indicate no depressive concerns, may be an indication of masked depression.

Gallagher and Thompson (1983) observe that the BDI is sensitive to change and is therefore a useful tool for assessing treatment progress. Change can be assessed by comparing total BDI scores across time or by examining changing patterns of item endorsement (see Table 3–3 for types of symptoms). For example, if a person has had intense weight loss, constipation, or fatigability but has been treated through medical attention, these items should be rated differently as treatment progresses, or if a patient has indicated a serious intensity of cognitive symptoms (loneliness, confusion, and helplessness) and these problems have been addressed through supportive therapy and social support intervention, these items should be rated differently in the course of treatment.

MMPI—Depression Scale (MMPI)

The depression scale of the Minnesota Multiphasic Personality Inventory (Hathaway & McKinley, 1951) is a 60-item scale developed originally to assess symptomatic depression. The primary characteristics of symptomatic depression underlying the development of this depression scale are poor morale, lack of hope, and a general dissatisfaction with one's own life situation. Many of the 60 items of the scale deal with various aspects of clinical depression such as denial of happiness, devaluation of personal worth, psychomotor retardation, lassitude and withdrawal, and decreasing interest in one's surroundings. Other items in the scale cover a diversity of behaviors that overlap with physical complaints, inability to control one's ideational processes, and generalized sadness.

In terms of the specific items included in the scale, it is reasonable to assess the MMPI—Depression Scale (D Scale) as being an excellent index of elderly persons' depressive symptoms, their discomfort and dissatisfaction with their current life situation, and their poor morale and lack of involvement in their environment. Despite its wide use, however, the MMPI poses a number of problems for use with a geriatric sample. The MMPI—D Scale is usually encased and interpreted within the context of the 566 items of the full scale. While the full MMPI scale would be far too lengthy a questionnaire to administer to the elderly, the use of the MMPI—D Scale in isolation has questionable validity, especially when used with an elderly population. Its most serious shortcomings when used with the elderly are its heterogeneity of symptoms and item contents and its lack of discrimination from anxiety.

On the positive side the MMPI scale has considerable support from geriatricians who have used it in their interviews with elderly subjects to determine the scope of severe and moderate levels of clinical depression (Harmatz & Shader, 1975; Schwab, Holzer, & Warheit, 1973; Taylor, Carithers, & Coyne, 1976; Wiggins, 1966). It has also accumulated a fair deal of statistical and normative background data among samples of the elderly (Harmatz & Shader, 1975; Schwab, Holzer, & Warheit, 1973). Taylor, Carithers, and Coyne (1976) have developed valid visual-analogue scales to measure MMPI substantive contents of depression, poor morale, social maladjustment, manifest hostility, psychoticism, family problems, poor health, organic symptoms, religious fundamentalism, and feminine interests. This set of 11 scales is based on a procedure employed in Wiggins' (1966) MMPI Content Scale and uses a 0 to 100 anchored self-rating scale. This abbreviated version of the MMPI scale may be appropriate for verbal administration to the elderly to determine not merely the scope of depression but also overall physical complaints, social adjustment, affective status, and psychosocial status.

Geriatric Depression Scale (GDS)

This (Brink, Yesavage, Lum, Heersema, Adey, & Rose, 1982) is a newly developed scale that has been standardized on an elderly population. It includes 30 items that refer to affective, cognitive, and behavioral symptoms of depression. The respondent confirms the presence or absence of the symptoms described in each statement (Do you often feel down-hearted and blue? Do you have trouble concentrating? Do you prefer to avoid social gatherings?). Using distribution scores on the GDS for community samples and hospitalized samples of elderly over the age of 55, Brink et al. (1982) provide natural cutoff points for three distinct levels of geriatric depression: (1) scores 0 to 10 for normal elderly with few complaints of depression, (2) scores 11 to 20 for mild depression, and (3) scores 21 to 30 for moderate to severe depression.

The scale with essentially a self-rating format can be administered in oral or written form. If administered in oral format, the subject must be instructed to give a clear yes or no response. A detailed examination of the items shows that the authors have attempted to avoid undue focus on somatic complaints, which although clearly a part of depressive disorders, do not characterize the milder forms of depression. Compared to most existing scales of depression, which are heavily loaded toward measuring somatic symptoms of depression, the GDS as a screening instrument focuses more on psychological and cognitive symptoms. These are assumed by the authors as having greater discriminative power. Items used in this self-rating scale were selected for their relevance to an elderly population from a larger pool of 100 items. Brink et al. (1982) and Yesavage et al. (1983) report satisfactory estimates of construct validity as well as sufficiently high test-retest reliability with their geriatric depression measure to consider its use in clinical settings. The GDS has been compared with the Hamilton Rating Scale for Depression (HAMD) and the Zung Self-Rating Depression Scale (SDS). Yesavage et al. note that the GDS, HAMD, and SDS were found to be internally consistent measures and that the GDS correlated significantly with the Research Diagnostic Criteria (RDC) symptoms.

Fry (1984) administered the GDS to 138 nonpatient elderly subjects between the ages of 65 and 80 years. Fry's findings showed that the elderly subjects' GDS scores correlated significantly with their scores on Fry's measure of geriatric hopelessness and also with the ratings of behavioral depression provided by observers and informants.

Clinicians whose practice includes a significant number of elderly patients and who need a short, portable, reliable, and valid instrument to screen depression are encouraged to use the GDS for further validity and reliability studies. Compared to other existing scales of depression, the GDS has the advantage of being validated within an elderly population. It has a simple, easily understood format and discriminates between nondepressed and mildly to severely depressed subjects.

In summary, a review of the studies that have used self-report measures indicates that the elderly persons' pattern of response to such self-report measures is distorted by the overlap between typical depressive symptomatology and changes associated with the aging process itself. It has also been suggested that age produces a differential pattern of response to depression questionnaires, with somatic physiological symptoms being more frequently selected by the aged and emotional psychological symptoms underreported (Zemore & Eames, 1979).

None of the available self-rating scales is ideal. Typically these scales (with one or two exceptions such as the Brink et al. [1982] scale) have been constructed and validated with younger subjects and have not been systematically applied to older patients. Thus symptoms, easily identified as depressive in nature in the young, may become difficult to distinguish from events of normal aging or from symptoms of coexisting medical conditions (Okimoto et al. 1982, p. 801). Despite these problems the results of the self-rating scales examined in this section often agree with diagnoses made by geriatricians in psychiatric interview.

The deficiencies of self-assessment scales for use with the elderly are obvious. They can be used only by cooperative patients who are literate and not too ill. In other words the elderly client must not suffer from a condition where noncomprehension or falsification of the scale's responses would be likely (Snaith, 1981). Establishing and maintaining rapport is important with all subjects. However, researchers have pointed out that the depressed elderly, more than other populations, often have limited attention span and decreased tolerance for ambiguity (Salzman & Shader, 1979). Sometimes they become angry with items they view as irrelevant to their stage of the life cycle (Salzman & Shader, 1979).

Observer Rating Scales of Depression

Kochansky (1979) notes that no observer-rating scales of depression have been developed specifically for the elderly. Three scales have been used in a number of studies involving older people. They are the Hamilton Psychiatric Rating Scale for Depression (HAMD) (Hamilton, 1960), the Zung Depression Status' Inventory (DSI) (Zung, 1972; Zung et al., 1974), and the Montgomery and Asberg Depression Scale (MADS) (Montgomery & Asberg, 1979).

Hamilton Psychiatric Rating Scale for Depression (HAMD)

The HAMD (Hamilton, 1960) is the most widely used observer-rating scale. It is a 17-item list of symptoms rated for the level of severity (0–4 or 0–2) by a clinician. Although the scale is designed to be used in conjunction with a clinical interview, ratings can also be made on the basis of other available data. The scale, developed on the basis of clinical observations of depressive symptoms, was designed to identify and diagnose symptoms of clinical depression as separated from the broad range of psychiatric symptomatology generally included in other measures of depression. Although no diagnostic breakdowns are provided, the scale covers the major symptomatology of both reactive and endogenous depressions frequently observed in hospitalized and institutional settings (Hamilton, 1967).

The scale items assess affective disorders and somatic symptoms: depressed mood, guilt, suicide, insomnia-initial, insomnia-middle, insomnia-delayed, work and interests, retardation, agitation, anxiety-psychic, anxiety-somatic, somatic symptoms and gastrointestinal symptoms, somatic symptoms general, genital symptoms, hypochondriasis, loss of insight, and loss of weight (Table 3–3).

These items are to be rated on a 0- to 2-point scale (0 = absent; 1 = slightly; 2 = clearly present) or on a 0- to 4-point scale (0 = absent; 1 = mild; 2–3 = moderate; 4 = severe). The ratings obtained on each of the symptoms are then added to give an overall depression score. Interrater reliability of the total score is high as various investigators have found it to range between 0.8 and 0.9 (Hamilton, 1960). The sensitivity to changes in the patients' condition appears also to be satisfactory (Hamilton, 1974, p. 136).

Unfortunately the HAMD has not been subjected to a geriatric normative study of the kind carried out by Zung and Green (1973) with regard to the Zung self-rating scale. Kochansky (1979) believes, however, that the HAMD is capable of assessing virtually all of the major dimensions of depressive symptomatology as it appears in the elderly and has the potential for assessing their severity, although it may be less sensitive at the low or mild end. It has been used in a few geriatric psychopharmacological studies (e.g., Sakalis, Gershon, & Shopsin, 1974) and appears to be quite sensitive to changes in depressive symptomatology (Kochansky, 1979).

Unfortunately the use of this scale is not strongly recommended because of its sensitivity to somatic concerns (which may reflect normal age-related changes and bona fide complaints associated with physical illnesses as well as depression). Unless the interviewer skillfully inquires about the health status and uses the information obtained to qualify Hamilton ratings, the scores can be falsely elevated (Gallagher, Slife, & Rose, 1982; Gallagher & Thompson, 1983; Waskow, 1981).

Zung Depression Status Inventory (DSI)

Like the HAMD scale this scale (Zung, 1972) has been used several times in geriatric psychopharmacological studies (Zung et al., 1974). The Zung DSI has items in common with the HAMD, but there are some important differences: the Zung DSI contains items that consider crying spells, confusion, emptiness, hopelessness, irritability, and personal devaluation. The Zung DSI seems to focus more than the HAMD on affective nuances of depression. However, in contrast to the HAMD the Zung DSI omits items that in their manifest-content assess guilt feelings, hypochondriasis, insight, paranoid symptoms, and obsessive-compulsive symptoms. The Zung DSI also assesses only sleep disturbances occurring in the late phase of sleep and only two items directly pertaining to somatic complaints. The Zung DSI, while stressing the affective dimensions of depression, fails to focus extensively on somatic dysfunctioning and complaints—a most important aspect of depression in the elderly.

Montgomery and Asberg Depression Scale (MADS)

The MADS (Montgomery & Asberg, 1979) was designed to assess the severity of depression and consists of 10 items scored by the clinician from 0 to 6. However, "the rater must decide whether the rating lies on the defined scale steps (0,2,4,6) or between them (1,3,5)"

(Montgomery & Asberg, 1979, p. 387). The items covered are apparent sadness, reported sadness, inner tension, reduced sleep, reduced appetite, concentration difficulties, lassitude, inability to feel, pessimistic thoughts, and suicidal thoughts. The MADS is relatively short in comparison to the HAMD and can be utilized by trained nurses and psychologists as well as by psychiatrists. Because of its brevity it has excellent potential for use with elderly patients, although unfortunately the MADS has not been subjected to a geriatric normative study. The interrater reliability of this scale was reported between 0.93 and 0.97, while the interrater correlation between "simultaneously performed" HAMD ratings during various stages of therapy is reported to range between 0.89 and 0.95 (Montgomery & Asberg, 1979, p. 396).

In summary, none of the observer-rated depression scales available for assessing depressive symptomatology in the elderly is ideal. None was designed to differentiate dementia or organic impairment symptoms from depressive symptoms in the elderly (Kochansky, 1979). None assesses memory, a function that may be impaired as a result of depression in the elderly, and none distinguishes between depression and motor retardation as a medical symptom. However, the prevalence of depression as identified by these instruments is similar to the estimated prevalence as tested by detailed diagnostic interviews. Blazer (1982) (see Table 3–3) and Kearns et al. (1982) compared a number of depression scales, one against the other, and concluded that in a comparison of assessment methods of severity of depressive symptomatology, most scales of depression, including scales of observer-ratings or self-ratings, had more or less equal performance. Burrows (1977) concludes, however, that no single rating is capable of distinguishing depressive symptomatology from other overlapping symptomatology that is inherently related to cognitive impairment or the effects of somatic, biochemical, and organic changes.

A main drawback of observer scales is that of rater bias. The rater may be influenced in scoring by a general expectation of how ill the elderly patient ought to be. Raters are influenced in their scoring of severity by their general experience of patients suffering from the disorder. Some see only clients from the community while those in hospitals deal with a different population of severely depressed elderly.

Abrupt changes in depressive symptomatology scores will need special consideration, particularly among older patients in whom there is a risk of suicidal attempt. More often than not, elderly patients with suicidal plans will attempt to mask the presence of symptoms in order to leave the hospital.

Conclusions

Among the self-rating scales the Beck Depression Inventory and the relatively new scale, the Geriatric Depression Scale, report reliabilities and validity indexes sufficiently high to consider their use in clinical and community settings. Both these scales are recommended for their brevity and their focus on core emotional, cognitive, and somatic depressive symptoms frequently observed in the elderly. The Geriatric Depression Scale has been validated strictly on samples of the elderly and has the advantage of not being heavily loaded on the measurement of somatic symptoms, which are not always indicative of depression in late life. The use of both these scales as initial screening instruments is greatly encouraged.

In settings where it is impractical to administer a comprehensive observer assessment battery but where preliminary observer-ratings of depressive disorders are considered important in the clinical interview, the use of the Hamilton Rating Scale for Depression as an interviewer-administered measure is recommended. The scale has had more trials with the elderly than any other interviewer-administered measure. Gallagher, Slife, and Rose (1982) suggest that because of the preponderance of somatic items its use be limited to those clinical interviews in which there are additional means to determine the true physical health status of the elderly client.

SUMMARY

This chapter has discussed etiologies and diagnostic classifications of depression in the elderly. It has also addressed several important issues in the assessment of depression and has described assessment steps and diagnostic procedures for assessing the nature of depressive disorders, the primary and secondary causes of the depressive disorders, and how assessment procedures used with the elderly may differ from those used with younger populations.

In summarizing the clinical picture it is obvious that depression is the most prevalent psychological disorder of the later years. However, it is also one of the disorders most vaguely defined in terms of specificity as to cause, origin, and methods of assessment. One of the problems has been the difficulty in defining clinical depression in terms of severity of symptoms (limited, latent, or pervasive depression), etiology (neurotic, psychotic, or agitated), and other functional features (stress, anxiety, sleep disorders, and self-depreciation).

Although the literature dealing with the diagnosis of elderly persons with depression is quite extensive, few studies concerned primarily with diagnosis have had success in differentiating depression and depressive disorders from normal aging processes. Gaitz (1977), for example, notes that one of the difficulties in assessing depression in the elderly lies in the definition of *normal aging* and in the selection of assessment measures that can be used to determine mood and affect changes normally experienced by a large proportion of elderly persons, as contrasted with other affect changes that are syndromes in later life and must be viewed as disorders. Busse (1975, p. 4) notes that depressive episodes in the elderly increase in frequency and depth in the advanced years. Feelings of apathy and inferiority, loss of self-esteem, and a wide array of physical symptoms distinguish the elderly depressed persons from the younger depressed persons, who experience greater guilt and hostility.

In the elderly the causes of depression are multiple and complex and often complicated by the frequent presence of physical illness, fatigue, psychomotor retardation, and also organic brain involvement. The types of depressive disorders presented by an elderly population are varied ranging from a symptom to a psychotic syndrome, an occasional episode to recurrent depressive episodes. In many cases of depression the depressive symptoms may not be independent of senile brain diseases. Perhaps the most difficult task in the differential diagnosis of depression in old age is the distinction from senile dementia. Indeed in many such cases depressive symptoms and general apathy and lassitude may be inextricably related to dementia or chronic mental confusion. In such cases it is not unusual for the elderly person to be unable to report precipitating events or give a personal history. Thus, depression in the elderly could be one of several disorders requiring a further clarification of the relative roles of brain disease and organic and biological correlates.

Some clinicians advance genetic explanations for the prevalence of depressive reactions in later life. While the genetic difficulties or faults do not interfere with reproduction, the manifestations of the genes, or genes of manic-depressive psychosis, may be increasingly postponed in successive generations—thus the appearance of greater depressive reactions in later life (Weinberg, 1975, p. 2417). It is not unreasonable to suggest that the types of depressive disorders manifested by elderly persons are probably more varied than at any other period in the life cycle. For example, depression in the elderly may be intricately linked with stress or anxiety. However, to regard depression as the direct consequence of stress, illness, or anxiety reaction to life events is a serious oversimplification. Genetics, early life experience, environmental stress, and personality all combine in various complex ways in the etiology of depression. Thus depression in the elderly may often emerge as a cluster of symptoms and syndromes rather than as single entities and may also involve different combinations of causes and precipitating factors.

Reactive depressions may need further clarification of the relative roles of psychosocial stress factors, anxiety-precipitating factors, and personal factors such as loneliness, lack of social support, and various kinds of losses such as bereavement and loss of status. There is also little evidence of how various other affective illnesses in old age such as chronic or acute anxiety can be distinguished from depressive disorders.

In summary, depression can present as a reaction to physical illness, as physical illness per se, as an accompaniment to physical illness, as an accompaniment to stress and anxiety, or as a result of chemotherapy. Having recognized that depression in the elderly is a frequent concomitant of physical disorders or functional disorders, one must place increased attention on the correct diagnosis of depression in the medically ill or the functioning impaired elderly.

At this point our understanding of many of these problems is limited in terms of methods of assessment, evaluation, and diagnosis. In part this lack of information and understanding reflects the imprecision in the current diagnostic categories and the assessment tools. Considerable progress has been made in developing new subclasses, as reflected in the Diagnostic and Statistical Manual of Mental Disorders (DSM-III). However, there is little agreement on how these categories of disorders help to classify the various depressions of the elderly. The development of more reliable assessment tools and procedures will in general lead to better descriptions of the types of depressive disorders occurring in old age and the related genetic, organic, or psychosocial factors contributing to these disorders.

A detailed comprehensive diagnostic workup may not be necessary in the case of all depressed elderly, and a few preliminary steps for assessing the duration, intensity, and frequency of depressive episodes may be sufficient for a diagnostic evaluation. In the case of severely depressed elderly the presence of many other somatic concomitants and psychosocial factors may require that the assessment be based on a comprehensive diagnostic evaluation of family history, medical history, cognitive functioning status, and psychosocial history. A multidimensional, multifunctional approach to assessment is therefore advocated (Gaitz & Baer, 1970).

REFERENCES

Akiskal, H.S. (1978). The nosological status of neurotic depression. *Archives of General Psychiatry, 32,* 756.

Akiskal, H.S. (1979). A biobehavioral approach to depression. In R.A. Depue (Ed.), *The psychobiology of the depressive disorders: Implications for the effects of stress* (pp. 409–437). New York: Academic Press.

Ancherson, P. (1961–62). Atypical endogenous depression. *Acta Psychiatrica Scandinavica,* supple., 160–163, 267–271.

Beattie, B.L., & Sellers, E.M. (1979). Psychoactive drug use in the elderly. *Psychosomatics, 20,* 474–479.

Beck, A.T. (1972). *Depression: Causes and treatment.* Philadelphia: University of Pennsylvania Press.

Beck, A.T., Ward, C., Mendelsohn, M., Mock, J., & Erbaugh, J. (1961). An inventory for measuring depression. *Archives of General Psychiatry, 4*, 53–63.

Blazer, D.G. (1982). *Depression in late life.* St. Louis: C.V. Mosby Co.

Blumenthal, M.D. (1975). Measuring depressive symptomatology in a general population. *Archives of General Psychiatry, 32*, 971–978.

Boller, F., Mizutani, T., & Roessmann, U. (1979). Parkinson's disease, dementia and Alzheimer's disease: Clinicopathological correlations. *Annals of Neurology, 7*, 329–335.

Brink, T.L. (1977). Depression in the aged: Dynamics and treatment. *Journal of the National Medical Association, 69*, 891–893.

Brink, T.L., Yesavage, J.A., Lum, O., Heersema, P., Adey, M., & Rose, T.L. (1982). Screening test for geriatric depression. *Clinical Gerontologist, 1*, 37–43.

Brown, G.L., & Wilson, W.P. (1972). Parkinsonism and depression. *Southern Medical Journal, 65*, 540–545.

Burrows, G.D. (1977). *Handbook of studies on depression.* Amsterdam: Excerpta Medica.

Burrows, G.D., Foenander, G., Davies, B., & Scoggins, B.A. (1976). Rating scales as predictors of response to tricyclic antidepressants. *Australian and New Zealand Journal of Psychiatry*, 53–56.

Busse, E.W. (1975). Aging and psychiatric diseases of late life. In M.F. Reiser (Ed.), *American handbook of psychiatry* (Vol. 4, pp. 67–89). New York: Basic Books.

Butler, R.N., & Lewis, M.I. (1977). *Aging and mental health: positive psychosocial approaches* (2nd ed.). St. Louis: C.V. Mosby Co.

Caird, F.I., & Judge, T.C. (1974). *Assessment of the elderly patient.* London: Pitman Medical.

Carp, F.M., & Carp, A. (1981). Mental health characteristics and acceptance-rejection of old age. *American Journal of Orthopsychiatry, 51*, 230–241.

Celesia, G.G., & Wanamaker, W.M. (1972). Psychiatric disturbances in Parkinson's disease. *Diseases of the Nervous System, 33*, 193–200.

Coleman, J.C. (1976). *Abnormal psychology and modern life.* Glenview, IL: Scott, Foresman & Co.

DeAlarcon, R. (1964). Hypochondriasis and depression in the aged. *Gerontologica Clinica, 6*, 266–277.

Diagnostic and Statistical Manual of Mental Disorders (DSM-III) (1980). Washington: American Psychiatric Association.

Endicott, J., & Spitzer, R.L. (1978). A diagnostic interview for affective disorders and schizophrenia. *Archives of General Psychiatry, 35*, 837–844.

Engel, G.L. (1966). A life setting conducive to illness: The giving up—given up complex. *Bulletin of the Menninger Clinic, 6*, 41–52.

Epstein, L.J. (1976). Depression in the elderly. *Journal of Gerontology, 31*, 278–282.

Friedel, R.O. (1978). Pharmacokinetics in the geropsychiatric patient. In M.A. Lipton, A. DiMascio, & K.F. Killam (Eds.), *Psychopharmacology: A generation of progress* (pp. 1499–1505). New York: Raven Press.

Friedman, J., & Sjogren, T. (1981). Assets of the elderly as they retire. *Social Security Bulletin, 44*(1), 16–31.

Fry, P.S. (1983). Structured and unstructured reminiscence training and depression in the elderly. *Clinical Gerontologist, 1*, 15–37.

Fry, P.S. (1984). Development of a geriatric scale of hopelessness: Implications for counseling and intervention with the depressed elderly. *Journal of Counseling Psychology, 31*, 322–331.

Fry, P.S., & Grover, S. (1982). Cognitive appraisals of life stress and depression in the elderly: A cross-cultural comparison of Asians and Caucasians. *International Journal of Psychology, 17*, 437–454.

Gaitz, C.M. (1977). Depression in the elderly. In W.E. Fann (Ed.), *Phenomenology and the treatment of depression* (pp. 447–449). New York: Spectrum.

Gaitz, C.M., & Baer, P.E. (1970). Diagnostic assessment of the elderly: A multifunctional model. *Gerontologist, 10*, 47–52.

Gallagher, D., Breckenridge, J., Steinmetz, J., & Thompson, L.W. (1983). The Beck Depression Inventory and Research Diagnostic Criteria: Congruence in an older population. *Journal of Consulting and Clinical Psychology, 51*, 945–946.

Gallagher, D., Nies, G., & Thompson, L.W. (1982). Reliability of the Beck Depression Inventory with older adults. *Journal of Consulting and Clinical Psychology, 50*, 152–153.

Gallagher, D., Slife, B., & Rose, T. (1982, April). *Psychological correlates of immunologic disease in older adults.* Paper presented at Western Psychological Association annual meeting, Sacramento.

Gallagher, D., & Thompson, L.W. (1983). Depression. In P.M. Lewinsohn & L. Teri (Eds.), *Clinical geropsychology: New directions in assessment and treatment* (pp. 1–37). New York: Pergamon.

Garretz, F.K. (1976). Breaking the dangerous cycle of depression and faulty nutrition. *Geriatrics, 31,* 73–75.

Gerner, R.H. (1979). Depression in the elderly. In O.J. Kaplan (Ed.), *Psychopathology of aging* (pp. 97–148). New York: Academic Press.

Gibson, I.I.J.M., & O'Hare, M.M. (1968). Prescription of drugs for old people at home. *Gerontologia Clinica, 10,* 271–280.

Goldfarb, A.I. (1974). Masked depression in the elderly. In S. Lesse (Ed.), *Masked depression* (pp. 236–249). New York: Jason Aronson.

Greenblatt, D.J., Allen, M.D., & Shader, R.I. (1977). Toxicity of high dose flurazepam in the elderly. *Clinical Pharmacology and Therapeutics, 21,* 355–361.

Gurland, B.J. (1976). The comparative frequency of depression in various adult age groups. *Journal of Gerontology, 31,* 283–292.

Hamilton, M. (1960). A rating scale for depression. *Journal of Neurology, Neurosurgery and Psychiatry, 23,* 56–62.

Hamilton, M. (1967). Development of a rating scale for primary depressive illness. *British Journal of Social and Clinical Psychology, 6,* 278–296.

Hamilton, M. (1974). General problems of psychiatric rating scales especially for depression: Psychological measurements in psychoplasmacology modification problems. In P. Pichot and R. Olivier-Martin (Eds.), *Modern problems of pharmacopsychiatry* (Vol. 7, pp. 125–138). Basel: Karger.

Harmatz, J.S., & Shader, R.I. (1975). Psychopharmacologic investigations in healthy, elderly volunteers: MMPI Depression Scale. *Journal of the American Geriatrics Society, 23,* 350–354.

Hathaway, S.R., & McKinley, J.C. (1951). *MMPI Manual* (rev. ed.). New York: Psychological Corp.

Jamison, K.R. (1979). Manic depressive illness in the elderly. In O.J. Kaplan (Ed.), *Psychopathology of aging* (pp. 79–95). New York: Academic Press.

Kahn, R.L., Zarit, S.H., Hilbert, N.M., & Niederehe, G. (1975). Memory complaint and impairment in the aged. *Archives of General Psychiatry, 32,* 1569–1573.

Kavanagh, T., Shepherd, R.J., & Tuk, J.A. (1975). Depression after myocardial infarction. *Canadian Medical Association Journal, 113,* 23–27.

Kearns, N.P., Cruickshank, C.A., McGuigan, K.J., Riley, S.A., Shaw, S.P., & Snaith, R.P. (1982). A comparison of depression rating scales. *British Journal of Psychiatry, 141,* 45–49.

Kielholz, P. (1981). Training general practitioners to treat depression. In T.A. Ban, R. Gonzalez, A.S. Jablensky, N.A. Sartorius, & F.E. Vartanian (Eds.), *Prevention and treatment of depression* (pp. 241–249). Baltimore: University Park Press.

Klerman, G.L. (1971). Clinical research in depression. *Archives of General Psychiatry, 24,* 305–319.

Klerman, G.L. (1975). Overview of depression. In A. Freedman, H. Kaplan, & B.J. Sadock (Eds.), *Comprehensive textbook of psychiatry/II* (pp. 1003–1011). Baltimore: Williams & Wilkins.

Kochansky, G.F. (1979). Psychiatric rating scales. In A. Raskin & L.F. Jarvik (Eds.), *Psychiatric symptoms and cognitive loss in the elderly* (pp. 125–156). New York: John Wiley & Sons.

Kolb, L.C. (1977). *Modern clinical psychiatry.* Philadelphia: W.B. Saunders Co.

Kolb, L.C., & Brodie, H.K.H. (1982). *Modern clinical psychiatry.* Philadelphia: W.B. Saunders Co.

Kraepelin, E. (1921). *Manic depressive insanity and paranoia* (translated by R.M. Barclay). Edinburgh: E.A. Livingstone.

Kreitman, N. (1972). Aspects of the epidemiology of suicide and "attempted suicide" (parasuicide). In J. Waldestrom, T. Larsson, & N. Ljungstedt (Eds.), *Suicide and attempted suicide* (pp. 45–52). Stockholm: Nordiska Boklandelms Forlag.

Kreitman, N. (1976). Age and parasuicide ("attempted suicide"). *Psychological Medicine, 6,* 113–121.

Lamy, P.P., & Kitler, M.E. (1971). Drugs and the geriatric patient. *Journal of American Geriatrics Society, 19,* 23–33.

Lang, P.J. (1968). Fear reduction and fear behavior: Problems in treating a construct. In J.M. Shlien (Ed.), *Research in psychotherapy III* (pp. 49–57). Washington: American Psychological Association.

Lange, J. (1928). The endogenous and reactive affective disorders and the manic-depressive constitution. In A.J. Bumke (Ed.), *Handbook of mental diseases* (Vol. 6, pp. 282–322). Berlin: Springer.

Larson, D.B., Whanger, A.D., & Busse, E.W. (1982). Geriatrics. In B.B. Wolman (Ed.), *The therapist's handbook* (pp. 343–388). New York: Van Nostrand Reinhold Co.

Lehmann, H.E. (1981). Classification of depressive disorders. In T.A. Ban, R. Gonzalez, A.S. Jablensky, N.A. Sartorius, & F.E. Vartanian (Eds.), *Prevention and treatment of depression* (pp. 3–17). Baltimore: University Park Press.

Leonhard, K. (1959). *Aufteilung der endogenen Psychosen*. Berlin: Akademie Verlag.

Lesse, S. (1974). *Masked depression*. New York: Jason Aronson.

Lewinsohn, P.M., Biglan, A., & Zeiss, A.M. (1976). Behavioral treatment of depression. In P.O. Davidson (Ed.), *The behavioral management of anxiety, depression and pain* (pp. 91–146). New York: Brunner/Mazel.

Linn, L. (1975). Clinical manifestations of psychiatric disorders. In A.M. Freedman, H.I. Kaplan, & B.J. Sadock (Eds.), *Comprehensive textbook of psychiatry* (pp. 783–825). Baltimore: Williams & Wilkins.

Lundquist, G. (1961–62). Somatic and mental stress as causative factors in depression. *Acta Psychiatrica Scandinavica* supple., 160–163; 267–271.

Martilla, R.J., & Rinne, U.K. (1976). Dementia in Parkinson's disease. *Acta Neurologica Scandinavica, 54*, 431–441.

Massey, E.W., & Bullock, R. (1979, January). Peroneal palsy in depression. *Psychiatry Digest, 41*.

McAllister, T.W., & Price, R.P. (1982). Severe depressive pseudodementia with and without dementia. *American Journal of Psychiatry, 139*, 626–629.

McCrae, R.R., Bartone, P.T., & Costa, P.T. (1976). Age, anxiety and self-reported health. *International Journal of Aging and Human Development, 7*, 49–58.

McGarvey, B., Gallagher, D., Thompson, L.W., & Zelinski, E. (1982). Reliability and factor structure of the Zung Self-Rating Depression Scale in three age groups. *Essence, 5*, 141–153.

McNair, D.M. (1979). Self-rating scales for assessing psychopathology in the elderly. In A. Raskin & L.S. Jarvik (Eds.), *Psychiatric symptoms and cognitive loss in the elderly* (pp. 157–168). Washington: Hemisphere.

Montgomery, S.A., & Asberg, M. (1979). A new depressive scale designed to be sensitive to change. *British Journal of Psychiatry, 134*, 382–389.

Nies, A., Robinson, D.S., & Friedman, M.J. (1977). Relationship between age and tricyclic antidepressant plasma levels. *American Journal of Psychiatry, 134*, 790–793.

Okimoto, J.T., Barnes, R.F., Vieth, R.C., Raskind, M.A., Inui, T.S., & Carter, W.B. (1982). Screening for depression in geriatric medical patients. *American Journal of Psychiatry, 139*, 799–802.

Payne, E.C. (1975). Depression and suicide. In J.G. Howells (Ed.), *Modern perspectives in the psychiatry of old age* (pp. 290–312). New York: Brunner/Mazel.

Pearse, J. (1974). Mental change in Parkinsonism. *British Medical Journal, ii*, 445.

Perris, C. (1966). A study of bipolar (manic-depressive) and unipolar recurrent depressive psychoses. *Acta Psychiatrica Scandinavica, 194*, 1–89.

Pfeiffer, E. (1977). Psychopathology and social pathology. In J.E. Birren & K.W. Schaie (Eds.), *Handbook of psychology and aging* (pp. 650–671). New York: Van Nostrand Reinhold Co.

Pfeiffer, E. (1980). The psychosocial evaluation of the elderly patient. In E.W. Busse & D.G. Blazer (Eds.), *Handbook of geriatric psychiatry* (pp. 275–284). New York: Van Nostrand Reinhold Co.

Pfeiffer, E., & Busse, E.W. (1973). Mental disorders in later life—affective disorders: Paranoid, neurotic and situational reactions. In E.W. Busse & E. Pfeiffer (Eds.), *Mental illness in later life* (pp. 199–232). Washington: American Psychiatric Association.

Plutchik, R. (1979). Conceptual and practical issues in the assessment of the elderly. In A. Raskin & L.F. Jarvik (Eds.), *Psychiatric symptoms and cognitive loss in the elderly: Evaluation and assessment techniques* (pp. 19–38). New York: Hemisphere.

Post, F. (1962). *The significance of affective symptoms in old age*. Maudsley Monograph 10. London: Oxford University Press.

Post, F. (1965). *The clinical psychiatry of late life*. Oxford: Pergamon.

Post, F. (1975). Dementia, depression, and pseudodementia. In D.F. Benson & D. Blumer (Eds.), *Psychiatric aspects of neurological disease* (pp. 99–120). New York: Grune & Stratton.

Raskin, A. (1979). Signs and symptoms of psychopathology in the elderly. In A. Raskin & L.F. Jarvik (Eds.), *Psychiatric symptoms and cognitive loss in the elderly: Evaluation and assessment techniques* (pp. 3–18). New York: Hemisphere.

Raskin, A., & Sathananthan, G. (1979). Depression in the elderly. *Psychopharmacology Bulletin, 15*(2), 14–16.

Rehm, L.P. (1980). Assessment of depression. In M. Hersen & A.S. Bellack (Eds.), *Behavioral assessment* (pp. 246–295). New York: Pergamon.

Rossman, P.L. (1969). Organic diseases resembling functional disorders. *Hospital Medicine, 5*, 72–76.

Roth, M. (1955). The natural history of mental disorders in old age. *Journal of Mental Science, 101*, 281–301.

Sakalis, G., Gershon, S., & Shopsin, B. (1974). A trial of Gerovital-H3 in depression during senility. *Current Therapeutic Research, 16*, 59–63.

Salzman, C., & Shader, R.I. (1979). Clinical evaluation of depression in the elderly. In A. Raskin & L.F. Jarvik (Eds.), *Psychiatric symptoms and cognitive loss in the elderly* (pp. 39–72). Washington: Hemisphere.

Schwab, J.J. (1966). A study of the somatic symptomatology of depression in medical inpatients. *Psychosomatics, 6*, 273.

Schwab, J.J. (1976). Depression among the aged. *Southern Medical Journal, 69*, 1039–1041.

Schwab, J.J., Holzer, C.E., & Warheit, G.J. (1973). Depressive symptomatology and age. *Psychosomatics, 14*, 135–141.

Seligman, M.E.P. (1975). *Helplessness: On depression, development and death.* San Francisco: W.H. Freeman.

Shinfuku, N. (1981). Depression in old age. In T.A. Ban, R. Gonzalez, A.S. Jablensky, N.A. Sartorius, & F.E. Vartanian (Eds.), *Prevention and treatment of depression* (pp. 63–68). Baltimore: University Park Press.

Sloane, R.B. (1980). Organic brain syndrome. In J.E. Birren & R.B. Sloane (Eds.), *Handbook of mental health and aging* (pp. 554–590). Englewood Cliffs, NJ: Prentice-Hall, Inc.

Smith, W.J. (1978). The etiology of depression in a sample of elderly widows: A research report. *Journal of Geriatric Psychiatry, 11*, 81–83.

Snaith, R.P. (1981). Rating scales. *British Journal of Psychiatry, 138*, 512–514.

Soldo, B.J. (1980). America's elderly in the 1980s. *Population Bulletin* (Vol. 35, No. 4). Washington: Population Reference Bureau, Inc.

Spitzer, R.L., Endicott, J., & Robins, E. (1978). Research diagnostic criteria: Rationale and reliability. *Archives of General Psychiatry, 35*, 773–782.

Stenback, A. (1980). Depression and suicidal behavior in old age. In J.E. Birren & R.B. Sloane (Eds.), *Handbook of mental health and aging* (pp. 616–652). Englewood Cliffs, NJ: Prentice-Hall, Inc.

Steuer, J. (1980). Depression, physical health, and somatic complaints in the elderly: A study of the Zung Self-Rating Depression Scale. *Journal of Gerontology, 35*, 683–698.

Strassman, G. (1957). Unrecognized intracranial lesions in mentally sick patients over the age of 60. *Geriatrics, 12*, 350–354.

Taylor, J.B., Carithers, M., & Coyne, L. (1976). MMPI performance, response set, and the "Self-Concept Hypothesia." *Journal of Consulting and Clinical Psychology, 44*, 351–362.

Todhunter, E.N. (1976). Lifestyle and nutrient intake in the elderly. In M. Winick (Ed.), *Nutrition and aging* (pp. 119–127). New York: John Wiley & Sons.

Verwoerdt, A. (1973). Emotional responses to physical illness. In C. Eisdorfer & W.E. Fann (Eds.), *Psychopharmacology and aging* (pp. 169–181). New York: Plenum Press.

Verwoerdt, A. (1976). *Clinical geropsychiatry.* Baltimore: Williams & Wilkins.

Verwoerdt, A. (1980). Anxiety, dissociative and personality disorders in the elderly. In E.W. Busse & D.G. Blazer (Eds.), *Handbook of geriatric psychiatry* (pp. 368–380). New York: Van Nostrand Reinhold Co.

Verwoerdt, A. (1981). *Clinical geropsychiatry* (2nd ed.). Baltimore: Williams & Wilkins.

Waskow, I.E. (1981, June). *The psychotherapy of depression collaborative research program: The first year experience.* Symposium presented at the meeting of the Society for Psychotherapy Research, Aspen.

Weinberg, J. (1975). Geriatric psychiatry. In A.M. Freedman, H.I. Kaplan, & B.J. Sadock (Eds.), *Comprehensive textbook of psychiatry/II* (Vol. 2, pp. 2405–2420). Baltimore: Williams & Wilkins.

Whanger, A.D., & Wang, H.S. (1974). Vitamin B_{12} deficiency in normal aged and elderly psychiatric patients. In E. Palmore (Ed.), *Normal aging* (Vol. 2, pp. 63–73). Durham, NC: Duke University Press.

White, P.D. (1971). Cardiovascular disorders. In E.V. Cowdry & F.U. Steinberg (Eds.), *The care of the geriatric patient* (pp. 51–58). St. Louis: C.V. Mosby Co.

Wigdon, B.T., & Morris, G. (1977). A comparison of 20 year histories of individuals with depressive and paranoid states. *Journal of Gerontology, 32*, 160–163.

Wiggins, J.S. (1966). Substantive dimensions of self-report in the MMPI item pool. *Psychological Monographs, 80* (22, No. 630).

Willmuth, L.R. (1979). Medical views of depression in the elderly: Historical notes. *Journal of the American Geriatrics Society, 27*, 495–498.

Wilson, S.A.K., & Bruce, A.N. (1955). *Neurology* (2nd ed.). Baltimore: Williams & Wilkins.

Winegardner, J. (1981). *A comparison of cognitive, affective, and life experience correlates of depression in young adults and the aged*. Unpublished doctoral dissertation, University of Montana, 1981.

Winokur, G. (1973). The types of affective disorders. *Journal of Nervous and Mental Disease, 156*, 82–90.

Winokur, G., Morrison, J., Clancy, J., & Crowe, R. (1973). The Iowa 500: Familial and clinical families favour two kinds of depressive illness. *Comprehensive Psychiatry, 14*, 99–107.

Woodruff, R.W., Murphy, C.E., & Herjanic, M. (1967). The natural history of affective disorders I. Symptoms of 72 patients at the time of index hospital admission. *Journal of Psychiatric Research, 5*, 255–263.

Yesavage, J.A., Brink, T.L., Rose, T.L., Lum, O., Huang, V., Adey, M., & Leirer, V.O. (1983). Development and validation of a geriatric depression scale: A preliminary report. *Journal of Psychiatric Research, 17*, 37–49.

Zarit, S.H. (1980). *Aging and mental disorders: Psychological approaches to assessment and treatment*. New York: Free Press.

Zemore, R., & Eames, N. (1979). Psychic and somatic symptoms of depression among young adults, institutionalized aged and noninstitutionalized aged. *Journal of Gerontology, 34*, 716–722.

Zung, W.W.K. (1965). A self-rating depression scale. *Archives of General Psychiatry, 12*, 63–70.

Zung, W.W.K. (1967). Depression in the normal aged. *Psychosomatics, 8*, 287–292.

Zung, W.W.K. (1970). Mood disturbances in the elderly. *Gerontologist, 10*, 2–4.

Zung, W.W.K. (1972). The depression status inventory: An adjunct to the self-rating depression scale. *Journal of Clinical Psychology, 28*, 539–543.

Zung, W.W.K. (1980). Affective disorders. In E.W. Busse, & D.G. Blazer (Eds.), *Handbook of geriatric psychiatry* (pp. 338–367). New York: Van Nostrand Reinhold Co.

Zung, W.W.K., Gianturco, D., Pfeiffer, E., Wang, H.S., Whanger, A., Bridge, T.P., & Potkin, S.G. (1974). Pharmacology of depression in the aged: Evaluation of Gerovital-H3 as an antidepressant drug. *Psychosomatics, 15*, 127–131.

Zung, W.W.K., & Green, R.L. (1973). Detection of affective disorders in the aged. In C. Eisdorfer & W.E. Fann (Eds.), *Psychopharmacology and aging* (pp. 213–224). New York: Plenum Press.

Chapter 4

Cognitive Impairment and Cognitive Disorders in the Aged: Assessment and Management

Burgeoning interest in the elderly's cognitive functioning disorders since the 1950s reflects growing recognition of the fact that such problems pose the most formidable challenge presented by the elderly population around the world. As more of the elderly survive into their eighth and ninth decades, a growing number of those with cerebral degenerative disease inevitably experience cognitive functioning disorders. Dementia and delirium, the main cognitive disorders, are most common among the elderly. Medical editorials (e.g., *British Medical Journal*, 1978; Jolley, 1981) speak of dementia as a "quiet epidemic," one posing the greatest problem to modern society in terms of transient and progressive cognitive disorders.

Disorders of cognitive functioning is a collective term that refers to a variety of conditions causing cognitive impairment. Since the 1950s there has been a sufficient research impetus to isolate some of the problematic issues in the differential diagnosis of disorders such as senile dementia, organic brain syndrome, reversible dementias, senile psychosis, and pseudodementia. In view of the clinical and medical usefulness of distinguishing cognitive disorders from cognitive changes of normal aging, geriatric research is beginning to study progressive impairment of the intellect (i.e., attention, learning, and memory) separately from subgroups of impairments of cognitive abilities that are transient and selective rather than global and progressive.

As research is beginning to generate a better understanding of the causes of severe cognitive loss in the elderly, there has been more impetus to making differential diagnosis between the relatively mild and benign changes, especially minor decrements of memory and intellect, from the more severe and pathological disruptions of function. Another recent shift has been toward diagnosing reversible and irreversible causes of cognitive loss and impairment. For clinical utility the reversible conditions are categorized as those associated with acute brain syndromes, delirium, depression, stress, and cognitive disturbance frequently caused by chronic alcoholism, or drugs and toxicity. The nonreversible conditions by contrast are those generally originating from multi-infarct dementia, which affects the central nervous system, and Alzheimer's disease, which causes primary neuronal degeneration. Despite their clinically observed heterogeneity the most characteristic feature of irreversible disorders is progressive impairment of cognition, that is, attention, learning, and memory. Additional frequent symptoms include hallucinations, delusions, aphasias, difficulty in abstraction, emotional lability, and depression (Eisdorfer & Cohen, 1978).

The prevalence of cognitive disorders in the elderly is reported to vary from 1 percent to 7 percent for severe dementias (Kay, 1977) and from 2.6 percent to 15 percent for mild dementia. Overall, 10 percent to 18 percent of the older population is estimated to suffer moderate cognitive losses. The cumulative lifetime risk to each individual today of becoming severely demented may be as high as 20 percent. This figure must be interpreted with the knowledge that persons with severe dementia require almost total care. A serious disruption of memory and intellect is extremely disabling not only for the afflicted individuals; it can cause a severe disruption in the daily lives of relatives and families caring for the demented older person. Cognitive loss may be one of the major factors leading to nursing home placements. The National Nursing Home Survey (1977) estimated that 50 percent of nursing home patients had significant cognitive impairments, especially decrement of memory and intellect. This does not include persons who are in more formal institutions or those with dementing illnesses who continue to live at home. The latter group may, in fact, comprise the majority of persons with mild dementia syndromes (Kay, 1977). Overall the risk for cognitive impairment arising from cognitive diseases shows a sharp increase with advancing age.

In some instances, however, this has led most clinicians to assume the presence of dementia without sufficient supporting evidence. Lezak (1976), for example, notes that signs of memory defects, disorientation, or psychomotor slowness were all too frequently diagnosed as cerebral degenerative manifestations of dementia when in fact some of these impairments were a reflection of early-life depression (of a primary depressive nature) and manifested themselves in a reduction of intellectual functioning over a long time.

Irreversible cognitive impairments resulting from dementia are one of the most common expectations of practitioners about aging. Once the diagnosis of cognitive impairment has been made, it is typically assumed that the condition will deteriorate with ever-increasing levels of impairment. Because of this stereotypic expectancy it is not surprising that in the United States psychiatrists and clinicians diagnose brain syndromes far more frequently than they do depression, alcoholism, or alterations in metabolism. Of equally great concern is the fact that there is little attempt to identify potentially treatable aspects of the cognitive disorder.

One of the first major tasks for clinicians working with the elderly is to distinguish between cognitive impairment and dysfunction as a consequence of normal aging as opposed to pathological cognitive deterioration that accelerates the process of aging. A second major task of the clinician is to differentiate between the reversible and irreversible variants of the cognitive impairment and to examine the treatable and untreatable aspects. A number of issues concerning the distinction between the irreversible and reversible variants of cognitive impairment, discussed by Eisdorfer and Cohen (1978), deserve specific mention. First, some variants that are viewed to be nonprogressive, the so-called acute brain syndromes, may be of acute onset at first, but if not treated adequately, such disorders may lead to more permanent structural damage in the brain. Second, treatability is distinguished from reversibility in all of the disorders causing cognitive impairment. Eisdorfer and Cohen (1978) note that in the case of nonreversible disorders the presence of coexisting problems may exacerbate the cognitive disorder. Thus the additional coexisting problem, such as a chronic infection, may constitute a component of the disorder that is reversible and can be treated. Third, there may be a wide variability in apparent functional capacity seen in the presence of an identifiable loss of brain substance.

It is hoped, therefore, that with accurate differential diagnosis, appropriate strategies can be developed for working with the cognitively impaired elderly and their families. Diagnostic entities in organic impairment and cognitive disorders resulting from these are not very satisfactory, but a broad classification is necessary to assessment and evaluation. Organic brain disorders are presumed to be closely linked to emotional reactions of depression, anxiety, and confusional states that may contribute to several forms of cognitive impairment. Extension of knowledge regarding the underlying causes, nature, and course of cognitive impairment in the elderly, development of new forms of treatment for the reversible conditions, and management strategies for the irreversible conditions may offer a great deal of hope for those afflicted with mental impairment.

This chapter, therefore, discusses the current conceptual understanding of cognitive disorders and their causes. It focuses primarily on organic brain syndrome, focal brain damage, depression, and delirium as causative factors in cognitive impairment. In addition, relevant psychodiagnostic measures for the assessment of the afflicted client's mental status, neuropsychological status, and level of intellectual functioning are discussed. Relevant clinical, behavioral, and psychological information on etiology and the course of cognitive disease is presented to assist the practitioner. The chapter describes the step-by-step procedures necessary to the assessment of the senile dementias and other reversible dementias. Specific aspects of functional assessment procedures as they pertain to cognitively impaired elderly are also briefly reviewed. Finally there is a brief discussion of the management procedures that may be useful in caring for the cognitively impaired elderly and in improving some treatable areas of the afflicted individual's cognitive dysfunctioning.

MAJOR FACTORS UNDERLYING COGNITIVE IMPAIRMENT IN LATE LIFE

Senile Dementia

The most difficult task in the differential diagnosis of cognitive impairment is the distinction between dementia and the effects of normal aging (Reifler, Larson, & Hanley, 1982). There has been considerable dispute about whether the senile dementia condition exists as a disease. This and other etiological considerations have been exhaustively discussed by Levy and Post (1982). They isolated the problematic issues of dementia: the distinction from depression, the distinction from normal aging, and the attempt to attribute the senile dementia condition to extracerebral causes.

Symptomatic Manifestations

Mortimer, Schuman, and French (1981) use the term *dementia* to refer to a clinical disorder of significantly deteriorated mental functioning resulting from organic brain disease. They recognize that other features such as chronicity, irreversibility, persistent disorientation as to time and place, and diffuse cerebral lesions are often, although not always, seen in senile dementia. Particularly in the early stages of dementia when severe changes in memory, intellectual functioning, orientation, judgment, or effect are not present, recognition of dementia may be difficult, and errors in classification often result (Wells, 1979).

In a relatively broad definition *dementia* refers to an unusual loss of intellectual function as evidenced by a noticeable decline in specific cognitive abilities (Post, 1975). According to Post the basic clinical features may include depression and failing memory. As the disease progresses, these lapses in memory increase in frequency and begin to affect all other affective, biological, and behavioral capacities. Senile dementia has a slow and gradual onset and may be difficult to recognize at an early age (Levy & Post, 1982, p. 166). Disorientation is usually the first defect and this is often noted in unfamiliar circumstances. Social judgment and bodily care may begin to deteriorate. However, patients initially seem unaware of the extent and severity of their cognitive functioning and they frequently employ a variety of stratagems to conceal their disabilities from other persons (Wells, 1979). In time, more extensive impairments develop, and the afflicted person may not be able to perform even the most basic tasks, for example, eating or dressing. The salient point about dementia is that it refers to a global deterioration in all aspects of mental functioning, including memory, general intellect, emotional attributes, and distinctive features of personality (Roth, 1976, 1980).

The global nature of dementia makes it a constellation of clinical features in which memory for both recent and past events may become void and restricted to a few jumbled recollections. In intellectual functions abstract thinking is particularly vulnerable even in those elderly who were alert and intellectually competent earlier. Most patients are unable to discern common themes or essential differences (Roth, 1971). They cannot apply experience to new situations or separate the significant from the trivia. According to Roth (1980) the inability to grasp what is happening to them leads to false ideas. These are technically delusions, but evidence of their falsehood is not rejected as in schizophrenia and senile psychosis but merely is not understood. The personality is grossly affected, acquiring undesirable traits such as meanness, tactlessness, and impulsiveness. Deviant conduct formerly held in check may be released because of an inability to inhibit or control.

Once the dementia sets in, the loss of intellectual function may be rapid. This sets this syndrome apart from memory loss in normal aging, when the memory fails gradually. There may be an insidious, sudden, and indeterminate onset observed with conditions such as cerebrovascular insufficiencies (Joynt & Shoulson, 1979). The best assurance of clinical diagnostic accuracy is close attention to the insidious onset of the disease, gradual progression of symptoms, lack of focal neurologic signs in the early stages, and characteristic mental symptoms of the Alzheimer's disease patient (Hutton, 1981). When dubious cases are encountered, it is probably prudent not to include them in the irreversible dementia.

The prevalence figures for dementia in old age vary from 3 percent to 14 percent overall but jump to 20 percent among those in the eighth or ninth decade of life, when many elderly are in hospitals and have other chronic illnesses that unfortunately confound the diagnosis of dementia. Community surveys, however, have found the overall prevalence of senile dementia to be relatively low (Gurland, 1980) with approximately 4 percent of people over the age of 65 showing distinct symptoms of dementia (Mortimer, Schuman, & French, 1981). More women than men have dementia (Gurland, Dean, Cross, & Golden, 1980) although this difference is probably related to women's greater longevity into the eighth and ninth decade rather than to a higher susceptibility to the disease.

Characteristic Contrasts of Multi-Infarct Dementia and Alzheimer's Disease

With regard to classification and the clinical diagnosis of dementia, Roth (1971, 1976) has demonstrated characteristic contrasts in the natural course of senile dementia and other forms of brain disease. The most common type of dementia has been termed *senile dementia of the Alzheimer's type* (SDAT) and is characterized behaviorally by loss of memory and orientation and cortical atrophy, neuronal loss, neurofibrillary tangles, and plaques. This type of dementia was originally described as *presenile dementia* as the age of onset was estimated before 65 years. Recent investigations (Roth & Myers, 1976), however, suggest that pathological changes characteristic of Alzheimer's disease occur after 65 years of age.

Although careful clinical and pathological analysis has not distinguished any differences in the abnormal structures in the brain peculiar to Alzheimer's disease and other forms of senile dementia, there are some marked contrasts noted in the causes and course of Alzheimer's disease and another major type of dementia labeled *multi-infarct dementia*. In the latter type of dementia the person suffers a series of small strokes, presumed to be caused by pieces of plaque on artery walls breaking off and traveling to the brain (Hachinski, Lassen, & Marshall, 1974).

Emotional changes such as depression are variable, indeed markedly so in the case of multi-infarct dementia. Special attention is merited by features reflecting fallout such as loss of the finer aspects of social tact, judgment, and sensibility. Also in this category are the fading of concern for others, narrowing of interest, and increasing preoccupation with self (Roth, 1980). The same negative features of intellectual and emotional functioning are also seen in diffuse cerebral degenerative disease. As no valid or useful measures are available to identify their exact origins, the detection of symptoms of Alzheimer's disease as distinguished from multi-infarct dementia entails subjective judgments. This does not make them any less important.

For many years cerebrovascular problems were regarded as the primary cause of brain syndromes in the elderly. The cognitive problems of aging were blamed on hardening of the arteries (Roth, 1955). Current neuropathologic data (Terry & Wisniewski, 1973, 1977), indicate, however, that only 15 percent to 25 percent of irreversible dementias are clearly due to cerebrovascular compromise, and greater than 50 percent of the irreversible dementias are the result of primary neuronal alterations. The rest are of mixed type with both multi-infarct and Alzheimer's characteristics or are caused by other rare diseases. The differential diagnosis of dementia from other psychiatric and physical illness becomes increasingly complex since dementia can be a major clinical finding in a variety of conditions (Haase, 1977), which may include diffuse degenerative diseases of the brain such as Parkinson's disease and Huntington's chorea, metabolic and vascular disorders, toxins, and nutritional deficiency diseases (Hutton, 1981). Accurate diagnosis is of great importance since a number of these conditions may respond to specific treatments. Furthermore, accurate identification of Alzheimer's disease and dementia, although they are not likely to respond to therapeutic measures, still permits appropriate counseling of those caregivers of institutions providing supportive therapies.

In tracing the natural course of the types of irreversible brain syndromes, it has been noted that senile dementia is characterized by a stepwise course while Alzheimer's shows gradual deterioration and markedly shortened life expectancy. The diagnosis of primary neuronal degeneration (of the Alzheimer's variant) can be made when there is evidence of progressive mental deterioration, characterized initially by attentional problems and memory loss and eventually in more or less total loss of orientation as to time, place, and person (Eisdorfer & Cohen, 1978).

In the early stages of Alzheimer's disease, accurate medical diagnosis may be difficult since no tests provide a definitive diagnosis (Libow, 1977; National Institute of Aging Task Force, 1980). There is the difficulty in the differential diagnosis of the manifestations of primary depression and dementia (Nott & Fleminger, 1975). The prevalence of depression is so high that even a small proportion of erroneous judgments substantially expands the assumed prevalence of dementia (Roth, 1980). Careful history taking protects against this hazard because the majority of progressive cerebral degenerative disorders commence insidiously with a history extending for years, whereas depressive illnesses are usually of no more than weeks' or months' duration. Any physical illness factors or depressive disorder factors should therefore be eliminated before establishing a clear clinical diagnosis of dementia.

In both Alzheimer's disease and multi-infarct dementia the treatment may produce little alteration in the progressive nature of the disorder although life expectancy may be slightly increased by intensive care (Gruenberg, 1977). Thus the major value of differential diagnosis is to indicate something about the natural course of the disorder and the clear origin, if any, of the disease so that the progressive disability associated with the disorder can be pinpointed and improved care provided to the afflicted elderly patient.

There are various theories about the etiologies of these diseases. Aluminum metabolism and zinc poisoning have been the subject of speculation as possible causes (Crapper, Krishnan, & Dalton, 1973). Latent viruses have been implicated as the cause of brain changes in Alzheimer's dementia (Gajdusek, 1977; Traub, Gajdusek, & Gibbs, 1977); immune and autoimmune processes have been studied by Nandy (1977) and Perry, Perry, Blessed, and Tomlinson (1977) to explain deficits observed in the cholinergic system in the brain of Alzheimer's patients.

Genetic theories have been spurred by findings of Mortimer, Schuman, and French (1981). Larsson's data support the hypothesis that senile dementias are inherited by an autosomal dominant mode of inheritance with a 40 percent penetrance by age 90. These investigators reported a relative risk of 4.3 for the development of senile dementia among first-degree relatives of persons (i.e., children and siblings) with this disease compared to the general population. Larsson, Sjogren, and Jacobson (1963) have implicated a major dominant gene in the transmission of senile dementia and a polygenic inheritance for Alzheimer's disease. Roth's (1980) data note a relationship between multi-infarct dementia and the incidence of stroke and heart disease, although no explanation is known on why these risk factors lead to dementia in some persons and not in others.

The evidence reviewed thus far suggests that an accurate medical diagnosis of Alzheimer's disease is difficult and can be established only after morphological findings at postmortem. Since it does not have a pure diagnostic entity separate from other dementias, it is subject to frequent diagnostic classification and treatment errors and may be representative of many behavioral disorders and depressive symptoms.

From a neuropathological standpoint there is little to distinguish Alzheimer's disease and dementia. The same neurochemical abnormalities are observed in both. Incapacitating and irreversible cognitive impairment, emotional lability, and functional incapacity occur in both. Behavioral and cognitive manifestations of both Alzheimer's disease and multi-infarct dementia are reliably related to brain pathology and can be used to determine the presence of disease. Blessed, Tomlinson, and Roth (1968) have shown that beyond a certain minimum the density of plaque formation is positively correlated with the extent of cognitive loss. In the later stages patients with Alzheimer's disease can show marked restlessness and aphasia, affective lability, and eventually a total lack of knowledge of self and surroundings. The electroencephalogram (EEG) may show generalized slowing of the alpha rhythm and slow wave activities. The computerized axial tomography (CAT) scan may show general cortical atrophy in both the multi-infarct and Alzheimer's type dementias (Eisdorfer & Cohen, 1978). Fortunately for diagnostic utility, patients with cognitive impairment and disorientation due to other psychiatric or medical factors (such as depression or viral and bacterial infections) do not show the same widespread buildup of senile plaques as witnessed in the brain of dementia patients. According to Levy and Post (1982) for purposes of clinical utility Alzheimer's disease and senile dementia are one and the same thing.

Reversible Dementias

Pseudodementia: Diagnostic Considerations

A serious problem of the clinician is the differential diagnosis of dementia and pseudo-dementia. The latter has less clearly defined features and is attributed to divergent etiologies. The syndrome of pseudodementia is the subject of increasing attention and interest due in part to the diagnostic challenge it presents to clinicians working with the elderly. According to McAllister (1983) the syndrome is particularly common in the elderly and often presents the greatest therapeutic dilemma. Goldstein and McHugh (1978) focus on the problem of pseudodementia in which the manifest cognitive manifestations resemble those of the senile dementias but in which the causes of these impairments are viewed to be stemming from treatable conditions. *Pseudodementia* is a syndrome in which dementia is mimicked or caricatured by functional psychiatric illness, most often depression (Wells, 1979). A critical distinction lies in the presumption that pseudodementia is without associated or coexisting cerebral dysfunction.

Post (1975), on the basis of his clinical experience with psychogeriatric patients and depressed elderly, wrote that even experienced clinicians could not always discern whether they were dealing with an emotional disorder or cerebral dysfunction when the onset was acute. However, he emphasized the diagnostic importance of symptoms in order to establish whether pseudodementia exists alone or coexists with other cerebral dysfunctions. Therefore pseudodementia symptoms of depression in elderly patients need careful diagnostic attention. Pseudodementia symptoms not only confound the issues of depression and the aging processes of brain functioning but also oversimplify the division between affective and cognitive illness (Shraberg, 1978). Generally speaking, however, the reversible dementia label to pseudodementia implies that the clinical presentation is nonprogressive and that depression, not so much brain syndrome, is the primary factor in the cognitive impairment (Caine, 1981, p. 1359).

Wells (1979) has provided the most thorough examination of the problem of pseudodementia as differentiated from true dementia and also depression in the aged. Wells notes that the patient with pseudodementia reports (1) a more recent onset of symptoms that can be dated, (2) rapid progression of symptoms after onset, (3) recognition of and emphasis on the disability, (4) more pervasive affective change, and (5) more frequent don't know answers to mental status questions. Wells notes that the pseudodementia elderly patients in particular provide more frequent documentation of a previous depressive or affective disorder that is typically congruent with more current affective changes such as irritability, insomnia, severe dysphoria, withdrawal, and lassitude. Compared with the performance of the true dementia patient, the psychological performance of the pseudodementia elderly on the Wechsler Adult Intellectual Scale (WAIS) is variable. One of the important distinguishing features of the pseudodementia elderly patient is the relatively well-preserved attention span and concentration skills. Also of great interest to the differential diagnosis of reversible and nonreversible dementias is the study of pseudodementia in relation to other psychiatric and cerebral dysfunctions.

Wang (1980) regards the pseudodementia label to be most unsatisfactory since in diagnosis it may obscure the existence of some underlying physiological and metabolic changes that could help to understand those whose dementia is reversed and those who become progressively more demented. Furthermore, the cognitive impairment and metabolic disturbances in pseudodementia are often indistinguishable from those in degenerative central nervous system diseases and organic brain diseases most often seen in late-life dementias (McAllister & Price, 1982, p. 628).

McAllister (1983) has reviewed a number of smaller series and case reports that collectively delineate the variety of associated illnesses seen along with pseudodementia. He groups these clinical presentations into two categories, those that report on pseudodementia alone and those that coexist with cerebral dysfunction from other causes.

With respect to the first category pseudodementia has been diagnosed as existing without associated cerebral dysfunction. In these circumstances the pattern of intellectual impairment is a subcortical one, sparing higher cortical functions (Caine, 1981). Retarded depression and hysterical conversion reaction may present a pseudodementia (Friedman & Lipowski, 1981), and the abnormal dexamethasone suppression test (DST) may be useful in establishing the presence of pseudodementia.

With respect to the second category of pseudodementia, that is, coexisting with cerebral dysfunction, the weight of the evidence from small series reports suggests that marked diffused cognitive impairment in persons with a history of primary degenerative dementia may sometimes be judged secondary to a superimposed depressive illness. McAllister and Price (1982) found that patients having marked diffused cognitive impairment without underlying organic brain disease responded to ECT treatment.

In McAllister's (1983) view these reports highlight the often atypical nature of depressive illness or subacute deterioration in patients with coexisting neurological disorders or chronic cerebral dysfunction. The weight of the evidence suggests that depressive illness is frequently associated with cognitive deficits. When these two coexist, the chances are that by excluding depression as a treatable cause of the subacute deterioration, the cognitive deficits can also be reversed.

This leads to the question of whether pseudodementia is in fact distinguishable on clinical grounds from dementia. One of the reasons for this confusion is that pseudodementia does not represent a single, homogeneous syndrome and often coexists with other primary psychiatric illnesses (McAllister, 1983). Since there are no clearly accepted diagnostic criteria for diagnosing pseudodementia and for distinguishing it from dementia, it is to be expected that at times the clinical picture presented by a patient may best fit a depressive dementia; at times there may be features suggestive of a delirium. Therefore, at this point it is difficult to conclude anything definite about depressive pseudodementia. History taking of the patient is most important to accurate diagnosis of pseudodementia, and Well's (1979) differential diagnostic criteria may be of significance.

The prognosis for patients with a pseudodementia (tentatively defined as a depression-induced organic mental disorder) appears to be good. Once it is established that the cognitive impairment or deficits are depression-induced, the cognitive deficits resolve completely with appropriate treatment of the psychopathology and are not predictive of a more severe illness, high relapse rate, or unmasking of a dementing illness (McAllister, 1983). In patients having coexisting organic or functional illness, the degree of cognitive clearing depends on the extent of deficit caused by the organic or psychiatric illness.

Other Unidentified Variants of Brain Syndrome

Cognitive impairments that arise from a variety of unidentified dementing or disease processes are sometimes referred to as *organic brain syndrome* associated with impairment in the function of brain tissue. Some elderly may show cognitive impairment in conjunction with a number of risk factors such as focal neurologic signs, signs and symptoms of retinal or brachial arteriosclerosis, and a history of hypertension and diabetes. These patients have an identified history of blackouts or strokes. According to Rivera and Meyer (1975) these small strokes and cerebrovascular insufficiencies may give rise to brain syndrome. Careful diagnosis may show profound softening in several areas of the brain. A number of clinicians (e.g., Tomlinson, Blessed, & Roth, 1970) have suggested a variable course in the development of the brain syndrome. Patients may show temporary partial remissions and long lucid intervals followed by exacerbations that keep families of the afflicted in a state of keen uncertainty as to the prognosis. Weinberg (1975) refers to these brain syndromes as occurring in three forms:

1. Focal brain damage. *Focal brain damage* is a less common source of cognitive impairment. As in some of the other unidentified variants of cognitive impairments, focal brain damage is attributed to head trauma, strokes, and tumors of the brain. Unlike the course of dementias, the onset of the symptoms is usually abrupt, but the impairment of cognitive abilities is selective rather than global and is not necessarily progressive. Unless there is a clear evidence of tumor or strokes, it is difficult to diagnose focal brain damage with any degree of certainty. However, the distinction between focal damage and dementia is significant. With early diagnosis and treatment, medical interventions can prevent further brain damage.

2. Acute brain syndromes. Sometimes when the onset of cognitive dysfunction is rapid and without signs of overwhelming anxiety, florid delusions, or hallucinations, it is important to probe for a physical cause underlying the acute behavioral change (i.e., acute brain syndrome). Acute brain syndromes may be exacerbated by a variety of factors. Principal among these are structural causes (e.g., normal pressure hydrocephalus, a syndrome that can be corrected by relieving the increased cerebral spinal fluid) or drugs and the use of various antipsychotic, antidepressant, and anti-Parkinsonian agents (Weinberg, 1975).

   Hypoglycemia, congestive heart failure, infections, and other metabolic factors may frequently be causes of acute brain syndrome. In the aged it may reveal a reversible disorder precipitated by nutritional deficiencies or anemias and may manifest itself in symptoms of restlessness or active delirium. Correction of these metabolic and medical causes may often eliminate confused and disoriented behavior of many elderly whose previous caloric intake, thyroid insufficiency, and general neglected state may have been significantly serious so as to produce apathy, confusion, depression, etc. There are not consistent or characteristic neuropathological findings in acute brain syndrome. In all cases the presence of acute brain syndrome may be taken as evidence of the simultaneous presence of developing chronic brain syndrome if prompt treatment is not undertaken.

   The majority of those who develop the acute syndrome have a good chance of recovery in cognitive functioning. Social and behavioral functioning may improve dramatically when the physical cause underlying the acute brain syndrome (e.g., an infection, toxicity from drugs) is identified and corrected.

3. Chronic brain syndrome. This brain syndrome suggests that some diffuse brain damage has taken place before the emergence of chronic brain syndrome. Often senile brain changes are presumed to be causative factors in the production of the syndrome even though the patient may not show any neurological impairment signs and no

history of a stroke. Senile plaques in the cortical layers of the brain are present in most cases, and there is marked atrophy or cellular changes in the central nervous system, suggesting a substantial measure of irreversibility in the brain syndrome (Blazer, 1982). The symptoms commonly appear in the elderly after the age of 70 and are similar to those of senile dementia. The elderly person may pass slowly from normal old age to senile psychosis with no abrupt change (Weinberg, 1975). According to Weinberg early features of the chronic brain syndrome are errors in judgment, decline in personal care, an impairment in capacity for abstract thought, a lack of interest, and apathy. Emotional reactions commonly include depression and irritability, and as deterioration progresses, medical symptoms and organic dysfunction signs and paranoid tendencies also become exacerbated.

Delirium

The term *delirium* is less clearly defined than acute brain syndrome and has a heterogeneous and multifactorial etiology that makes it difficult to distinguish delirium from acute confusional states, clouded states, acute brain failure, or pseudosenility. To clear up this semantic muddle, Lipowski (1983) proposes that the label *delirium* be used exclusively for those transient global cognitive disorders that may occur at any age and that are judged to be of organic etiology. *Delirium* is therefore defined as an organic brain syndrome characterized by global cognitive impairment of abrupt onset and relatively brief duration (usually less than one month).

Symptomatic Manifestations and Causative Underlying Factors. Delirium, as differentiated from dementia, is by definition transient and is treatable and reversible. This should not obscure the fact that in the elderly it is often the most common herald of the onset of physical illness or a prelude to death or probably less often to dementia (Lipowski, 1983, p. 1427). It is reported that 33 percent of 4,000 patients exhibiting delirium died within a month. Bedford (1959) and Millar (1981) reported that 10 percent to 15 percent of elderly surgical patients became delirious after surgery and died. Etiology of delirium in elderly persons is typically multifactorial. The most common physical illnesses associated with delirium include congestive heart failure, pneumonia, infections, dehydration, sodium depletion, and cerebrovascular accidents (see Hodkinson, 1973; Seymour, Henschke, & Cape, 1980). Aging processes and impairment of vision and hearing predispose the elderly to delirium. Lipowski (1980a, 1980b) has observed that brain damage and disease, especially vascular and degenerative, increase predisposition to delirium.

The aging brain is highly vulnerable to hypoxia of any origin. The central cholinergic system is affected by aging with resulting reduction in acetylcholine synthesis (Gibson, Peterson, & Jenden, 1981). Since adequate functioning of this system is needed for normal memory, learning, attention, etc., its deficiency is likely to predispose to delirium (see Table 4–1, adapted from Lipowski, 1983, describing common organic causes of delirium).

These changes related to aging and cerebral disease are compounded by additional factors such as decreased capacity for homeostatic regulation and reduced resistance to stress. Sleep loss and fatigue may play a contributing role in delirium with increased general susceptibility to disease. With the ingestion of high-powered medication and drugs during illness, delirium is especially likely to be induced when several anticholinergic drugs are administered simultaneously. Disease impaired mechanisms of drug metabolism render the elderly highly susceptible to drug-induced delirium (Lipowski, 1980a, 1980b). Initially several causative organic factors are implicated in delirium, but their deliriogenic effect is

Table 4–1 Common Organic Causes of Delirium

Cause	Type
Drugs	Diuretics, sedative-hypnotics, analgesics, antihistaminics, antiparkinsonian agents, antidepressants, neuroleptics, cimetidine, digitalis glycosides
Alcohol intoxication or withdrawal	
Cardiovascular disorders	Congestive heart failure, myocardial infarction, cardiac arrhythmias, aortic stenosis, hypertensive encephalopathy, orthostatic hypotension, subacute bacterial endocarditis
Infections	Pneumonia, urinary tract infection, bacteremia, septicemia, cholecystitis, meningitis
Metabolic encephalopathies	Electrolyte and fluid imbalance; hepatic, renal, and pulmonary failure; diabetes and other endocrine diseases; nutritional deficiency (especially of vitamin B complex); hypothermia and heat stroke
Cerebrovascular disorders	Transient ischemic attacks, stroke, chronic subdural hematoma, vasculitis
Cerebral or extra-cranial neoplasm	
Trauma	Head injury, surgery, burns, hip fracture

Source: From "Transient Cognitive Disorders in the Elderly" by Z.J. Lipowski, 1983, *American Journal of Psychiatry, 140,* p. 1431. Copyright 1983 by American Psychiatric Association. Adapted by permission.

---

frequently precipitated in the elderly by such psychological stresses as bereavement, relocation, and dislocation or by a deficit in auditory and visual inputs (Lipowski, 1980a).

Not only does the delirium syndrome pose surgical and medical threats and diagnostic challenges to the physicians and surgeons, it also gives rise to global disturbance of cognition, which baffles the minds of clinicians. In elderly persons especially, delirium must be regarded as a grave prognostic sign of cognitive disorganization in response to physical illness and trauma or in response to psychological stresses. Etiologic organic factors could be identified in 80 percent to 95 percent of reported cases of clinically diagnosed delirium in the elderly (Purdie, Honigman, & Rosen, 1981). Despite the heterogeneity of organic disorders observed, there were core features of cognitive disorders in perception, thinking, and memory. Lipowski (1983) notes that perception in delirium is frequently marked by reduced ability to discriminate and integrate precepts or to distinguish them from imagery, dreams, and hallucinations. The patient may perceive objects to be too big (macropsia), too small (micropsia), and misshapen. About half of the patients experience both auditory and visual hallucinations at night. Stationary objects may be perceived as moving or flowing together and objects appear to be far away.

Thinking is also disorganized and fragmented in terms of ability to reason, use abstract concepts, judge, problem solve, and plan action. The elderly delirious person is likely to have impoverished and incoherent thought processes and may on occasion appear to have all of the core features of senile dementia.

Memory is impaired in all aspects of registration, retention, and retrieval. Although both immediate and long-term recall are impaired, memory for recent events is more impaired than is remote memory. Unless delirium coexists with dementia, the person is likely to have relatively intact remote memory for both personal and public events.

Delirium, short-lived though it may be, has a characteristically fluctuating effect on attention, which becomes disordered in all of its main aspects: alertness, responsiveness to stimuli, selectiveness, and directiveness (Lipowski, 1983). The victim of delirium has difficulty in shifting attention at will or in directing mental processes. Abnormalities of attention and disordered wakefulness are often directly responsible for the cognitive disorganization of the patient. Sleep disorders and attentional disorders exacerbate disruption in cognitive processes, obstruct communication, and may contribute to temporary disorders of the patient's psychomotor behaviors.

Diagnosis of Delirium: Assessment Considerations

Diagnosis of delirium involves two essential steps. The first step involves a recognition of the syndrome in terms of course and outcome. Delirium comes on acutely over a few hours or days, often first appearing at night. It usually clears up completely in one to four weeks. Lipowski (1983) notes that it tends to last longer in the elderly than in younger patients.

A delirium patient can be recognized by the predominant tendency to be hyperactive during the night and then switching quickly to hypoactivity. Both speech and nonverbal behavior are disordered and may range from catatonia to lethargy to incessant aimless activity and vocalization. Speech may be slurred; tremors, such as asterixis, may be observed especially in drug withdrawal delirium. Autonomic reactions, especially sympathetic nervous system hyperarousal, dilated pupils, tachycardia, and sweating may occur in conjunction with fear and hyperactivity (Lipowski, 1980a). Disordered wakefulness, fragmented sleep with dreaming, and hallucinations disturbing the sleep are one of the most characteristic distinguishing features (Lipowski, 1980b).

The second step in diagnosis involves a recognition of the syndrome in terms of its causes. This involves an assessment of the clinical features. The patient's cognitive functions of memory, learning, and attention need to be evaluated through direct observations or cognitive testing. Causative factors such as medical drugs the patient has ingested and evidence of physical illness, either acute or chronic, with acute exacerbation need to be scrutinized for their deliriogenic potential or effects.

The choice of assessment tools must depend on the clinician's judgment but must include a psychological, physical, and medical assessment to scrutinize cognitive functions and mental status, blood chemistry, toxic drug screen, and urinalysis. The EEG is often a sensitive and reliable indicator of cerebral metabolism generally and of its derangement in delirium in particular (Engel & Romano, 1959). However, Lipowski (1983) notes that in the elderly the diagnostic value of the EEG may be limited by the fact that generalized slowing is seen not only in delirium but also in primary degenerative dementia.

Differential Diagnosis of Delirium versus Dementia and Organic Brain Syndromes

Such differential diagnosis may at times be difficult, limited by the fact that in the elderly, delirium is often superimposed on dementia so that we have the manifestations of an organic brain syndrome that also features global cognitive impairment. Table 4–2 adapted from Lipowski (1983) may assist the reader in the differential diagnostic process.

As Lipowski (1983) notes, the symptoms of dementia and delirium are sometimes indistinguishable since it is frequently found that dementia and delirium coexist in a significant number of hospitalized demented patients (*Journal of Royal College of Physicians,* 1981). The two syndromes overlap with respect to deficits in memory, thinking ability, complex hallucinations, confabulations, etc. (Table 4–2).

As a general rule, information about the mode of the onset of the disorder (whether abrupt or insidious) and about the nature and duration of symptoms (Tables 4–1 and 4–2) is crucial

Table 4–2 Differential Diagnosis of Delirium and Dementia

Feature	Delirium	Dementia
Onset	Rapid, often at night	Usually insidious
Duration	Hours to weeks	Months to years
Course	Fluctuates over 24 hours; worse at night; lucid intervals	Relatively stable
Awareness	Always impaired	Usually normal
Alertness	Reduced or increased; tends to fluctuate	Usually normal
Orientation	Always impaired, at least for time; tendency to mistake unfamiliar for familiar place or person	May be intact; little tendency to confabulate
Memory	Recent and immediate impaired; fund of knowledge intact if dementia is absent	Recent and remote impaired; some loss of common knowledge
Thinking	Slow or accelerated; may be dreamlike	Poor in abstraction, impoverished
Perception	Often misperceptions, especially visual	Misperceptions often absent
Sleep-wake cycle	Always disrupted; often drowsiness during the day, insomnia at night	Fragmented sleep
Physical illness or drug toxicity	Usually present	Often absent, especially in primary degenerative dementia

Source: From "Transient Cognitive Disorders in the Elderly" by Z.J. Lipowski, 1983, *American Journal of Psychiatry, 140*, p. 1432. Copyright 1983 by American Psychiatric Association. Adapted by permission.

---

for clinical diagnosis of delirium. A patient who by all accounts has functioned well intellectually, then suddenly develops a cognitive-attentional disorder that fluctuates in severity over a short period and becomes worse at night, is suffering from delirium unless proven otherwise by other laboratory and psychological tests.

Acute and fluctuating worsening of cognitive functioning in a patient known to be suffering from a gradual progression of cognitive impairment (dementia) should suggest the onset of delirium superimposed on dementia. The delirium aspect then constitutes a component of the dementia that is definitely treatable. As a general rule this should lead to medical management in which there should be a further scrutiny of infection, drug toxicity, etc., which may have contributed to a worsening of the disorientation, bewilderment, and incoherence of the dementia patient.

When psychotic symptoms may be part of the dementia, more frequently the accompanying hallucinations and delusions are manifestations of delirium (Kapnick, 1978). Delirium and dementia may be superimposed on the elderly patient's history of longstanding psychosis. Whatever the cause of the hallucinations and delusions, the delirium symptoms constitute a reversible component of the chronic mental disorder or the dementia of the elderly patient and should be treated as such. As is clear from the foregoing discussion, differential diagnosis of delirium and dementia is often complicated by the concurrence of other cognitive disorders stemming from depression, stress-induced acute cerebral function, and psychosis.

In clinical practice the often difficult task of differentiating cognitive disorganization occurring in delirium from depression-induced incoherence and from dementia-related cognitive impairment will be experienced by clinicians with growing frequency, as the number of very old persons will predictably increase. This will lead to a greater prevalence of dementia, delirium, and depression in those elderly who survive into their eighth and ninth decade of life. Furthermore, there is likely to be a greater incidence of the coexistence of dementia, delirium, depression, and cerebral insufficiency as a function of age (Waxman, Carner, Dubin, & Klein, 1982).

Depression: Differential Diagnosis of Depression versus Dementia

Depression as a major contributing factor to cognitive impairment can be particularly difficult to distinguish on clinical grounds from dementia and other organic brain syndromes. In the elderly all these states can present a picture of neglect, lack of verbal communication, apparent low effect and loss of memory, psychomotor retardation, and withdrawal from activities and can create the impression of dementia. Kenny (1979) recommends the formulation of some psychodynamic notions as to why certain depressive behaviors are going on and to decide on the basis of both the psychodynamic and clinical-medical picture as to whether the primary contributing factor in the cognitive impairment is depression or whether depression symptoms are a concomitant of dementia. Clinical depression may exist in such instances and should be considered a causative factor in cognitive disorganization if depressive symptoms last more than six weeks, if weight loss is significant, and if sleep is disrupted. If worthlessness and guilt are expressed, the symptoms of cognitive confusion may be more reflective of clinical depression than dementia.

There is no clear-cut and objective way to assess the degree to which neglect by others, rejection of the caregivers, poor motivation of the patient, or emotional needs contribute to a given level of observed cognitive impairment in relation to observed depression. Practitioners and clinicians should consider the possibility that both diagnoses coexist, that both dementia and depression are dynamic and fluctuating processes, and that the severity of one or both may affect the functioning of the patient. Depression may often worsen the true dementia and therefore while treatment of depression may not correct the cognitive impairment, it may possibly lead to symptomatic improvement in the patient. Notwithstanding the clinical utility of this hypothesis, clinical assessment of depression, when coexisting with cognitive impairment, is difficult. The clinician may proceed to treat the elderly patient on the basis of a clinical hypothesis of cognitive impairment, but the hypothesis to some extent can be tested only by the patient's response to treatment.

As noted by Gurland (1980), sometimes far-reaching actions are taken as a result of a report that an old person has exposed self and others to danger, for example, by virtue of leaving a gas stove lit and unattended. It is sometimes concluded that this behavior is a token of progressive dementing process resulting in memory loss and cognitive disorders. A full cognitive functioning assessment, however, may often reveal that such behaviors are due to a reversible condition such as depression. While such lapses of attention when associated with depression do not necessarily cause concern in younger adults, they must be taken more seriously in older persons. Systematic assessment must determine whether such attentional lapses are indeed normal accidents or whether they might indicate depressive withdrawal or progressive cognitive impairment (Gurland, 1980).

Perhaps one of the greatest difficulties in the diagnosis of depression in the elderly is presented by institutionalized patients who show both severe depression symptoms and cognitive impairment. Many patients with dementias caused by neuropathological factors show depressive symptoms in the early stages and serious cognitive impairment at a later stage. Moreover, many depressed elderly complain of memory loss, which is mistakenly viewed to be a symptom of approaching dementia in elderly patients. Some studies (e.g., Kahn, Zarit, Hilbert, & Niederehe, 1975) have found that complaints about poor memory do not reflect the severe type of memory impairment characteristic of the dementia patients but are more likely to reflect the depressed person's overreportings of complaints and self-criticisms. Miller and Lewis (1977) have developed a spatial memory recognition task in which older persons with depression did not show an impairment in memory processing in contrast to those with brain syndrome. The extent of memory complaints in dementia patients, however, is inversely related to severity of symptoms. In the later stages of the dementia, memory loss is so severe that the afflicted person may have no awareness of the memory loss and hence there are no complaints (Kahn et al., 1975). However, in those cases where depression responds to antidepressant treatment, the cognitive symptoms may diminish. It has been observed that when dementia is not present, cognitive symptoms due to depression will lessen as mood improves (Kiloh, 1961).

Unfortunately the pervasiveness of depression observed in a variety of circumstances, in diverse forms, and across a range of severity of cognitive impairment makes it difficult to distinguish clinical depression and dementia. Raskind (1976) has reported that at least 9 percent of those referred to the Older Adults Outreach Program with a cognitive disorder presumed to be associated with senile dementia were in fact manifesting a clinical depression. While a depression may be difficult to detect immediately, persistent and careful interviewing will clarify its presence. Since depression is so intricately linked with dementia in the early stages, it has been suggested that depression and dementia are not actually exclusive conditions (Post, 1975; Epstein, 1976). Only history taking of the client can indicate whether there has been a gradual and progressive cognitive impairment with accompanying depression or whether the depression has existed without a progressive cognitive impairment. Information regarding work accomplishments and educational achievements are useful to assess premorbid functioning and difficulties in activities of daily living. A careful history obtained from a relative is important to the evaluation of a genetic component in the cognitive disorder.

ASSESSMENT PROCEDURES IN COGNITIVE DISORDERS

The complex task of differential diagnosis presupposes the clinician's knowledge of the distinguishing features of the various syndromes (i.e., dementias, reversible and irreversible, delirium, depression) of cognitive disorders and cognitive impairment. It highlights the need for prompt and accurate assessment steps and procedures. Although geropsychologists and mental health practitioners for the elderly may not be able to assist with laboratory tests, they can play a key role in preliminary but salient assessment procedures outlined by Zarit and Zarit (1983) in Table 4–3.

It is recommended that with the first suspicion of dementia the practitioner conduct a psychosocial and mental status evaluation of the patient by means of an individual structured interview with the patient in surroundings where the patient cannot fall back on the assistance of the spouse or other family member in providing specific information (Zarit & Zarit, 1983; Lipowski, 1975). In cases of mild to moderate severity of dementia the clinician must attempt to assess the patient's level of motivation, intellectual deficits, affective states, and accessibility to environmental supports. Such criteria are relevant initially to diagnosis and classification and later to intervention and management (Lipowski, 1975). In the case of severely impaired elderly, similar assessment will not be possible and information about the client must be obtained from the referring family.

Table 4–3 A Summary of Assessment Procedures

	Dementia	Delirium	Reversible Dementia	Focal Brain Damage	Depression	Normal Aging
1. Current Symptoms						
a. Complaints of memory problems	Reported by others; patient often unaware	Patient often denies problems	Reported by others; patient often unaware	Patient may complain of memory loss	Patient usually complains of memory problems	Patient may complain of memory loss
b. Types of memory problems reported	Major—interfere with activities of daily living	May be selective and variable; major activities disrupted	Major—interfere with activities of daily living	Specific functions more affected (e.g., spatial but not verbal abilities or vice versa)	Mild, mostly due to inattention	Mild increase in normal forgetting (e.g., names)
c. Hallucinations and delusions	Paranoid accusations sometimes present with mild memory loss; illusions in severe cases	Sometimes vivid hallucinations and well-developed delusions are present	Not described well in the literature	Absent	Absent, except in extremely severe cases	Absent
2. History						
a. Onset	SDAT: insidious multi-infarct: sometimes sudden	Usually sudden	Not described well in the literature	Sudden; associated with brain trauma	Coincides with life changes; onset often abrupt	Reactions to normal life changes; no specific aging pattern
b. Duration	Months or years	A few days or weeks	Not described well in the literature	Dates from incident	At least 2 weeks; can be several months or years	

c. Progression	SDAT: gradual multi-infarct; stepwise	Prodromal symptoms become severe in a few days	Not described well in the literature	Not progressive	Not progressive	Minimal change over long periods of time
d. Fluctuations	SDAT: little multi-infarct; some daily fluctuation, usually worse in evening	Can be extreme, even from hour to hour	Not described well in the literature	Little	Typically worse in the morning	Mild situational fluctuations
3. Tests						
a. Mental Status Questionnaire (MSQ)	2 or more errors	Connotative errors may be present	2 or more errors	Usually 0 or 1 error, unless damage is severe	Usually 0 or 1 error	Usually 0 or 1 error
b. Face-hand	Errors after 4th trial	May make errors after 4th trial	Errors after 4th trial	No, or unilateral, errors	No errors after 4th trial	No errors after 4th trial
c. Neuropsychological	Severe global deficit	Selective impairment, especially attention	Not described well in the literature	Only certain abilities affected, depending on site of damage	Normal aging pattern; speeded tests may be lower	Normal aging pattern
d. Memory and behavior problems checklist	Mild to extensive impairment	Mild to extensive impairment	Not described well in the literature	Usually only a few problems present	No, or a few, problems	No, or a few, problems
e. Caregiver's burden	Mild to severe	Not determined	Mild to severe	Absent or mild	Mild to severe	If present, related to longstanding relationship problems or physical disability

Source: From *Clinical Geropsychology: New Directions in Assessment and Treatment* (pp. 40–47) by P.M. Lewinsohn and L. Teri (Eds.), 1983, Elmsford, NY: Pergamon Press, Inc. Copyright 1983 by Pergamon Press, Inc. Reprinted by permission.

- Step 1 in the assessment (Table 4–3) recommended by Zarit and Zarit (1983) is an examination of the current symptoms of memory problems, disorientation, and the presence of hallucinations and delusions.

- Step 2 is taking a history of the nature and course of the syndromes in terms of onset, duration, progression, and fluctuation of the cognitive disorders.

- Step 3 is instituting a mental status and neuropsychological status examination to determine the extent and severity of the cognitive impairment that occurred as a function of the organic brain disease. Because no single medical or psychological test unequivocally proves the presence of dementia, evidence from various sources must be evaluated. It is best to begin with evaluating cognitive impairment by seeking information and feedback from the target client and the family members or friends. After appropriate history taking through interviewing procedures, the presence of dementia-related cognitive impairment can be confirmed or disconfirmed through cognitive testing including mental status examination and neuropsychological testing (Table 4–3).

When the concurrent presence of cognitive impairment and acute or chronic physical illness presumed to be related with the cognitive impairment is seen or suspected, the search for causative factors must start at once. A number of potential errors can be avoided, principally the following.

It must never be assumed a priori that a patient's cognitive impairment is due to a reported physical illness or life change or psychosocial stress. Thus, it should not be assumed that the cognitive disorder is transient and will subside. For many elderly patients, cognitive disorders become more serious unless forestalled by early detection and effective treatment of the syndrome. Conversely it is a grave error to treat the cognitive impairment as an integral part of the dementia in elderly patients just as it would be a serious error to attach the label of *senile dementia* to a patient suffering only from delirium.

It is also a grave error to ignore the superimposed symptoms of delirium on a demented patient since the delirium is a treatable component in a patient with an irreversible dementia. By alleviating delirium symptoms through appropriate treatment of the causative factors (Table 4–1), it is possible to improve the behavioral functioning of the demented patient. Such misdiagnoses are not uncommon and may cause disastrous consequences for the elderly patients and their families (Libow, 1973; Glassman, 1980).

As suggested by a number of clinicians (Zarit & Zarit, 1983; Lipowski, 1982; Liston, 1982), it is important to consider the evolution of the patient's cognitive disorder symptoms over time as well as behaviors and cognitive performance at the time of the examination. This procedure (Table 4–3) is critical to making a differential diagnosis and assessment of the various organic brain syndromes. The different syndromes carry different prognostic and diagnostic implications. In the elderly especially, efforts to treat promptly the reversible components of the dementias, acute brain syndromes, focal brain damage, and delirium can avoid the risk of chronic brain syndromes. The elderly patient would also be spared the risk of being branded as demented if, for example, a prompt diagnosis of acute brain syndrome or delirium is established. Efforts to isolate the deliriogenic effects of medication and psychotropic drugs so frequently consumed by the elderly can also assist in the differential diagnosis of dementia and delirium.

With respect to a differential diagnosis of the reversible and irreversible dementias, the psychological cost associated with diagnostic errors are indeed crucial. Failure to diagnose accurately means that in many elderly patients the treatable components are untreated. The potential error of incorrectly labeling an older person as *demented* is called a Type II error, which can have serious negative consequences for the individual (Kahn & Miller, 1978).

- Step 4 in the assessment is a comprehensive medical test. Appropriate medical evaluation should always be recommended whenever even minimal evidence suggests that cognitive impairment may be due to a reversible condition. If a medical assessment fails to establish a reversible condition, then no real damage is done (see Type I error in Kahn and Miller, 1978). It is not uncommon for mildly impaired elderly to go without a medical test for many years. When symptoms of cognitive impairment suggest the presence of delirium, a preexisting dementia, or acute brain damage, the person should be promptly referred for a medical evaluation by a physician who is knowledgeable about the medical aspects of dementia and other related brain syndromes. The types of common organic causes producing reversible impairments are listed in Table 4–1. Determination of the effects of drugs, cardiovascular disorders, infection, metabolic encephalopathies, and brain damage by means of medical assessment should be done because timely arrest of these problems may improve the cognitive impairment. The presence of substantial cognitive impairment does not hold any specific implications for somatic treatment approaches. The main concern prognostically is in making the medical diagnosis.

McAllister (1983, p. 532) suggests guidelines that may direct assessment of the dementias contributing to cognitive impairment. These guidelines overlap considerably with assessment procedures listed in Table 4–3. However, for the sake of completeness, they are enumerated here again.

1. Results of bedside mental status examination should be reported and specified in detail with attention to cognitive tests such as orientation, recall, calculations, naming, and simple spatial-temporal relationships.
2. Wherever possible, a neuropsychological test battery such as the Halstead-Reitan should be administered.
3. DSM-III criteria for dementia and delirium should be applied to each patient, and mention should be made of the extent of clouding of consciousness and confusional states.
4. Ancillary diagnostic tests such as CAT scan should be instituted as part of the medical diagnostic workup for dementia. Cortical atrophy and correspondingly enlargement of the ventricles and sulci (as assessment through the computerized axial tomography scans) have been found to correlate with measures of impairment in dementia patients (Caird, 1977; Fox, Topel, & Huckman, 1975). The CAT scan does not conclusively tell us about the significance of the degree of atrophy since some degree of cortical atrophy is normal in late life (Caird, 1977). An important diagnostic use of the CAT scan is to rule out a tumor as a factor contributing to cognitive impairment. Other ancillary aids such as EEG, dexamethasone suppression test (DST), and CSF examinations have sometimes proved promising tools in diagnosis.

Signs of physical illness such as fever or asterixis should suggest delirium. The patient's level of awareness tends to fluctuate irregularly. If doubts persist about whether delirium or pseudodementia is present, the amobarbital interview may be advised. Severely disordered cognitive performance tends to normalize under amobarbital unless dementia is also present, and DST results are likely to be abnormal if a major depressive disorder underlies the transient cognitive disorder in the absence of advanced primary dementia or inanition (McAllister, Ferrell, Price, & Neville, 1982).

Once a body of data that incorporates this assessment information has been accumulated and integrated, it should be possible to confirm more reliably the presence of dementia as contributing to the cognitive impairment. If it is confirmed on the basis of compelling evidence from cognitive testing, neuropsychological assessment, and medical assessment that the person has dementia, only then must this diagnosis be discussed with the elderly person's family or caregiver.

5. When the dementia is confirmed, the assessment should provide the patient's family accurate information about the difficulties that the cognitive impairment is likely to cause in the person's daily functioning. It would be ethically desirable to inform the family that there are no effective medical treatments for dementia. However, the usefulness of planning psychosocial interventions for the dementia patient should be positively stressed so that neither patient nor the family is left with a sense of therapeutic nihilism.

6. Once it is determined that a patient has dementia, a functional assessment of the patient's current capacities and deficits is important to the planning of effective intervention. The diagnosis of dementia and the results of the cognitive tests are not a sufficient basis for planning intervention for the individual client. There are wide variations in the functional capacities that individual patients are able to retain. Some may experience a rapid decline in self-care tasks and be totally disoriented, agitated, and incontinent while others may maintain some social skills and self-care habits. Families of the afflicted patient may also vary in terms of their problems and personal and financial resources for helping to care for the dementia patients. All these factors should be evaluated in a functional assessment and will guide the therapist in designing interventions for dementia patients and their families.

COGNITIVE TESTING

Cognitive testing has played an important role in psychiatric evaluation for a number of years. Since it is designed to provide a relatively rapid description of a patient's mental capacity, such testing is essential for confirming or disconfirming the presence of deficits typical of dementia (i.e., deficits in orientation, memory, and judgment). Cognitive functions of orientation, memory, and judgment are specially vulnerable to impairment with chronic brain syndromes. Thus these examinations have been viewed as critical (in combination with other diagnostic medical procedures) to evaluation and assessment of organic brain syndromes. There are two traditions in the literature on assessment of dementia. The first is conducting a mental status examination based on observations of the clinical practitioner, and the other is using test batteries to assess the neuropsychological status of the patient. Each of these approaches has its own strengths and limitations. The two approaches can be applied in conjunction in order to improve the overall reliability of assessment.

Mental Status Tests

As noted by Salzman, Kochansky, and Shader (1972), mental status examinations involve systems of categories that structure the reporting of clinical categories frequently witnessed in brain syndrome clients: appearance and behavior, speech, thought content, mood, orientation, insight, and judgment. However, in clinical settings there is some variability in the categories included and in the specific questions posed by the examiner to assess the functioning relevant to each category (Kochansky, 1979).

Although there is no consensus as to the contents of mental status examinations, Kahn, Goldfarb, Pollack, and Peck (1960) note that from the vantage point of the geriatric client there is a distinct advantage in tapping relatively overlearned and straightforward information so that two or more errors can conclusively indicate significant cognitive impairment (Zarit, Miller, & Kahn, 1978). Several standardized mental status examinations have been developed, and although there is considerable overlap with respect to psychological functions included and the method (i.e., tasks and items) of assessment, virtually all mental status examinations (Pfeiffer, 1975; Kahn et al., 1960; Plutchik, Conte, & Lieberman, 1971) assess the patient's orientation in the three spheres by asking direct questions about time, place, and person (Where are you? What is today's date? How old are you? What is the name of the president of the country?). All assess psychomotor functioning with a writing task, drawing task, etc., and some tests include calculations, naming objects, spelling backward, and recall tests. Other clinicians (e.g., Kahn and associates) supplement their mental status questions with a test of perception of double, simultaneous stimulation, the face-hand test developed by Fink, Green, and Bender (1952). The essential objective always is to confirm or disconfirm the presence of dementia.

Several problems arise when the clinician uses mental status examinations to help make subtle distinctions of organic disease and functional and affective disorders in the aged patients. Although depression, delirium, and dementia responses to the mental status examination are difficult to distinguish, Kahn and Miller (1978) suggest a few clinical differences that may be observed and may assist in differential diagnosis.

First, depressed older persons rarely make errors on mental status examinations despite frequent complaints about memory loss. If elderly clients with severe depressive symptoms are found to score in the impaired range on mental status examination, this should be viewed as an indication that the person has a dementia in addition to depression. Reifler, Larson, and Hanley (1982) have reported on the coexistence of dementia-related cognitive impairment and depression in geriatric outpatients. Another alternative interpretation is that the individual is not concentrating or attending to the questions because of altered mood. Folstein, Folstein, and McHugh (1975) observed that it is not unusual for depressive, disordered patients (because of altered mood) to make the same kinds of errors in their mini mental state examination as are usually seen in dementia patients. They also demonstrated in these patients the return of the mini mental state examination toward normal following effective treatment of depression. Thus history and previous course of treatment for affective disorders and moods will clarify the role of depression in these cases.

Second, on the mental status examination the delirium patient may make specific errors that distinguish this type of patient from the dementia patient. According to Lipowski (1983) the delirium patient is always mildly disoriented in time and, in more severe delirium, disoriented also for place and person. One essential difference should be noted: most dementia patients will try to answer mental status questions but will get them wrong. Delirium-disoriented patients by contrast tend to misidentify unfamiliar places and persons as familiar ones (Levin, 1945). Delirium patients practically never lose the sense of personal identity and may therefore be able to answer questions such as "What is your name?" and "How old are you?" Delirium patients sometimes respond to connotative aspects of questions (Kahn & Miller, 1978). For example, when asked, "Where are you?" a delirium-disoriented person may say "in a hotel" but give the hotel the name of a hospital. Some patients may say they are in a hospital with the same name, located in a different part of the town, or they may say they were in a different part of the town the night before. These responses reflect a tendency of the delirium-disoriented patient to minimize illness and stimuli associated with it (Weinstein & Kahn, 1955).

Further, a significant body of literature suggests that the brain-injured person with a focal brain injury will not generally make errors on a mental status examination. The weight of the evidence suggests that while brain injury and brain damage are frequently associated with cognitive disorientation, this disorientation is not of a diffuse global nature. Thus, whenever someone with a history of trauma is seen to score in the cognitively impaired range, two possibilities should be considered. One is that the person has brain injury coexisting with cerebral dysfunction. Another consideration is that although the person showed little or no progression of symptoms immediately following the injury, the worsening of the symptoms at a later stage indicates that there may be some other secondary problem (in addition to the original brain injury), which could be contributing to the individual's overreporting of cognitive impairment. Whenever there is the coexistence of brain injury and depression, the patient may overreport episodes of memory loss, even though the actual functioning has not changed. Thus evaluating the course of symptoms, both clinically and medically, can help to identify the treatable aspects of the cognitive impairment.

The issue of differential diagnosis, based on mental status tests, is usually treated as an either-or issue. Rarely is there a follow-up assessment to determine whether there is any change in the lucid periods. Without making a periodic assessment, most mental status problems of the elderly (i.e., forgetfulness, amnesia, and confusion) are conveniently attributed to senile deterioration.

Neuropsychological Status

The Wechsler Adult Intelligence Scale (WAIS) and Halstead-Reitan battery have been extensively used with the elderly to assess impairment in verbal-performance cognitive functioning. The WAIS and Halstead-Reitan battery represent broad-band approaches to neuropsychological assessment which use complex tasks relying on the elderly's ability to integrate different types of cognitive functionings (Boll, 1981). Albert (1981) recommends that narrow-band tests focusing on discrete and simpler constructs such as attention, memory, and preservation should be used with cognitively impaired elderly since these independent cognitive functions are the ones most affected in dementia patients. Furthermore, the narrow-band tests would be less likely to cause overload on the resources of the elderly person.

The neuropsychological approach has more potential for identifying early cases of dementia. However, a number of clinical cautions with regard to the use of cognitive tests with older patients are essential.

In summary, our present tools fall short of evaluating the cognitive processes affected in senile dementia. Results of studies using clinical neuropsychological tests suggest that such evaluation does not reveal much about the extent of the deficits, the availability of alternate capacities, and the elderly individual's ability to control environmental demands. A neuropsychological evaluation of the cognitively impaired elderly may be useful in developing rehabilitation programs for the elderly person's specific cognitive deficits and changes in behavior. The end result may be a program of retraining tailored to the individual to mobilize available skills, assets, and resources.

MANAGEMENT OF THE SENILE DEMENTIA ELDERLY AND PSYCHOSOCIAL APPROACHES TO THE CARE OF CLIENTS

At the outset it is necessary to mention that treatment possibilities for senile dementia patients are limited, and care for the basic illness is unknown. Figure 4–1 illustrates the process of intervention that is generally recommended for senile dementia patients.

Lindsley (1966), who contrasts therapy with prosthetics, contends that prosthesis assumes the unchangeable quality of the basic condition of illness and seeks a measure whose permanent application will counteract the disability associated with the condition. This concept of prosthesis has significant application to the care of senile dementia patients who are sufficiently impaired that they will rely permanently on others for supervision and assistance with daily tasks. In discussing management and psychosocial and environmental intervention for dementia patients therefore, we shall generally be speaking of prosthetic care in which there is the search for effective means of counteracting the functional disabilities of the brain syndrome clients.

The prevailing approach to the treatment of patients with dementia is strictly custodial, and families are often advised by professionals to place the dementia patients in a nursing home for the aged. But nursing homes for the aged are often a poor alternative and, being overcrowded and understaffed, are ultimately not able to offer adequate psychosocial care to the elderly individual. Dementia-afflicted elderly relocated in nursing homes and institutions are frequently unable to adjust to new environments. They are frequently tranquilized to alleviate behavioral problems, and neither prosthetic nor therapeutic approach to care is practiced.

Furthermore, Brody (1978) has reviewed evidence suggesting that there are concentrations of demented elderly in a poorly regulated genre of residences, boardinghouses, and foster homes. Unknown numbers undoubtedly live alone in scattered residences with no one to care for their daily needs. These data show clearly the considerable need for effective management of these demented elderly and intervention programs for their care and support.

Clinical observations have suggested four factors that may be important in determining reasonable bases for interventive efforts. First, it is a reasonable assumption that there is no medical treatment for senile dementia. However, Kahn (1975) provides compelling evidence for the notion that while the biological aspects of dementia may not be modifiable, some of the psychological and social problems may be alleviated with intervention.

Second, it would not be reasonable to expect that interventive efforts will benefit the patient to the extent of restoring cognitive functioning or reversing the organic brain damage. Third, growth of any kind is more likely if the environment of the senile dementia patient is so structured that the external demand on the individual is metered so as to be only incrementally greater than the level of demand to which the individual has contemporaneously adapted (Lawton & Nahemow, 1973).

Alternatives to institutionalization must be sought so that more structured training can be given in noncustodial settings to caregivers to help them provide prosthetic (as opposed to

Figure 4–1 Process of Intervention for Senile Dementia Elderly

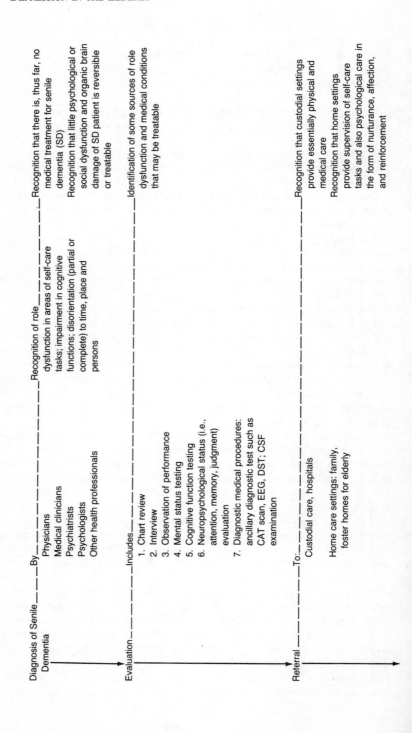

Diagnosis of Senile Dementia —— By ——
Physicians
Medical clinicians
Psychiatrists
Psychologists
Other health professionals

—— Recognition of role dysfunction in areas of self-care tasks; impairment in cognitive functions; disorientation (partial or complete) to time, place and persons

—— Recognition that there is, thus far, no medical treatment for senile dementia (SD)
Recognition that little psychological or social dysfunction and organic brain damage of SD patient is reversible or treatable

Evaluation —— Includes ——
1. Chart review
2. Interview
3. Observation of performance
4. Mental status testing
5. Cognitive function testing
6. Neuropsychological status (i.e., attention, memory, judgment) evaluation
7. Diagnostic medical procedures: ancillary diagnostic test such as CAT scan, EEG, DST; CSF examination

—— Identification of some sources of role dysfunction and medical conditions that may be treatable

Referral —— To: ——
Custodial care, hospitals

Home care settings: family, foster homes for elderly

—— Recognition that custodial settings provide essentially physical and medical care
Recognition that home settings provide supervision of self-care tasks and also psychological care in the form of nurturance, affection, and reinforcement

Treatment by
Caregivers —————— Provide training to caregivers in use of
medication (pharmacologic aids,
vitamin regimens), use of physical
prosthetic aids; use of step-by-step
instructional programs, mnemonic
devices, and memory recognition
tasks that caregivers can use with
impaired elderly members

Activities —————— Goal of maintaining function in areas
of self-care (bathing, dressing,
eating) and maintaining interest in
the surroundings

Goal —————— Recognition that the goal of treatment
is not to improve or cure but to
arrest further psychomotor decline,
avoid excessive disability, and, if
possible, to delay institutionalization
of SD patient

Recognition that caregivers
themselves will need continuing
counseling, training, and social and
emotional support in order to care
for the SD patient

Termination —————— When patient is no longer capable of
any functioning or self-care

Referral of SD patient to hospital or
other custodial services

custodial) care for the elderly dementia patients. The focus of these prosthetic programs would be primarily on the caregivers and to a lesser extent on the dementia patient. Some patients who are not severely impaired may on occasion benefit from brief counseling sessions, but too much focus on trying to teach or change the patient may tend to exceed the incremental goals that the dementia patient can reasonably be expected to achieve. The more productive approach would be to help caregivers identify realistic and practical changes for the cognitively impaired elderly that will lower the burden on the family caregiver.

By caring for the dementia patients in settings such as the home, it may be possible for the caregiver to supervise the care in such a way that the elderly patient does not become more disabled. Kahn (1975) addresses this issue of excess disability. If care is provided by the family in the home, a considerable number of elderly may be helped to retain some measure of self-care functions or social skills. Not all dementia patients are so cognitively impaired that they cannot maintain, for a while at least, some useful self-care habits of dressing, grooming, or eating. A program of intervention can help to reduce the burden on the primary caregiver and thereby delay or prevent institutionalization of the dementia patient.

Fourth, intervention programs must include a number of supports for the caregiver. Because of the continuing dependence of the dementia patient on others for supervision with daily tasks, caregiving places enormous physical, emotional, and financial demands on family members (Adams, Caston, & Danis, 1979). Therefore, supports for caregivers may be solicited either from paid sources such as social agencies or from other professional sources that may contribute to the nursing, nutritional, pharmacologic, and psychological aspects of intervention. As noted by Lawton (1980), when we are talking about individuals with human needs (and in the case of dementia-afflicted individuals, the burdened family members who function as primary caregivers), the total armamentarium of help resources must be mobilized. All financial, psychosocial, and environmental support must be considered as useful components of the biopsychosocial phenomenon of caring for the demented elderly person.

Clinical observations suggest that the ability of the caregivers to accept help from outside sources, including the judicious use of medication, pharmacologic aid, and physical prosthesis, varies with the caregiver's stability and personal-emotional endurance, the amount of knowledge and information about the nature and course of the senile dementia disease, and the degree of interest and involvement of the professionals in the burden of caring for the dementia patient (Zarit, Gatz, & Zarit, 1981; Zarit, Reever, & Bach-Peterson, 1981).

Alternatives to Custodial Care

As research is generating better understanding of the grave limitations and negative consequences of a custodial care system for demented elderly, there has been more impetus in considering alternatives to nursing home and institutional custodial care for the elderly. Zarit and associates (Zarit, Gatz, & Zarit, 1981; Zarit, Reever, & Bach-Peterson, 1981; Zarit, 1982) are staunch advocates of home care and pioneers in the study of home care for the elderly dementia patients. Their clinical work has focused on finding ways of lowering the strain and relieving some of the burden on family caregivers in such situations. Some of their preliminary findings suggest that elderly patients receive better care at home. Usually a particular family member functions as the primary caregiver for a community-residing patient. Typically this person is the spouse or daughter and occasionally other relatives of the afflicted elderly such as siblings or friends.

Some families, through counseling and the assistance of agencies, can be helped to bear the burden of a demented relative and to work creatively to keep that relative outside an institution. For others the burden on the family for dealing with dementia is far greater than the burden of dealing with a physical illness (Lawton, 1980, p. 279).

Zarit and his colleagues have stressed that we must take the needs of the family into account too, no matter how much we may favor the use of noninstitutional treatment resources. They have designed a research instrument—a burden interview—to assess the strain from the burden of caregiving (Zarit, Reever, & Bach-Peterson, 1981). This instrument assesses the extent to which caregivers perceive caregiving activities to have affected their health, emotional adjustment, social life, and financial status. A similarly designed measure has been initiated by Lawton (1971), which assesses intact ability of the patient in instrumental daily activities and personal abilities to prepare food, manage medication, and remain in the community without excessive assistance from others. Through the caregiver's reactions to a behavioral checklist it is possible to identify current areas of caregiving that are most problematic to caregivers and can be the focus in intervention and management of the dementia patient.

Intervention procedures focus on treatment programs and techniques for providing information about dementia, creative problem-solving for problems or troubles of the client, and support to the primary caregivers of the dementia patient. Caregivers' questions about the nature, causes, and course of the dementia illness can be handled by providing them with literature available from the local Alzheimer's foundations or from the National Institute of Aging information office and other information about the advisability of drug and vitamin regimens for the patient. Caregivers need to be informed about techniques for dealing with repetitive questions and common complaints of the patient. Caregivers can occasionally devise clever stratagems for stimulating memory by providing useful clues such as mnemonic devices, recognition tasks, and step-by-step methods of instructing the patient in task performance. As much as possible, caregivers should try to build solutions to the patient's problems on the basis of the patient's habits, personality, needs, etc. It is important that a caregiver be able to combat the problem of social isolation and lack of stimulation for the patient. If possible, some participation in pleasant activity, some social interaction with others, however marginal, should be encouraged.

Effective management of the demented patient will often impose a sufficient strain on caregivers that they will need one-to-one counseling for their own mental health needs and support for working through their own feelings of conflict, guilt, and blame vis-á-vis the elderly relative. Some cities have local support groups for families of patients with Alzheimer's disease.

Eventually caregivers may decide that they can no longer care for the patient at home. Once the decision to institutionalize the patient is made, the caregiver may need professional help in selecting an appropriate institution or nursing home for the elderly person. Caregivers must not be allowed to become guilty about institutionalizing their elderly, although the goal of intervention is to prevent institutionalization as long as possible.

Controlled evaluations of these programs for caregivers have not been done. These intervention programs are predicated on the assumption the treatment does not alter the course of the dementing illness, but better home care can occasionally improve the life expectancy of the patient. There is evidence that it can improve the quality of life for the patient who can continue to live in the familiar and empathic environment of the home.

PSYCHODIAGNOSTIC TESTS OF COGNITIVE IMPAIRMENT AND COGNITIVE FUNCTIONING

While detailed neuropsychological assessment need not be done in every case, such assessment may be critical when there is a question as to differentiation between depression, organic brain disease, cognitive impairment reflective of depression and anxiety, or cognitive impairment resulting from brain damage. However, in many instances elderly clients will not warrant the time expended in administering tedious batteries of mental status examination or cognitive impairment.

Memory and information tests are particularly useful, and performance on these tests often relates to pathological changes (Blessed et al., 1968) to measures of atrophy (Jacoby & Levy, 1980) and to outcome (Whitehead, 1976). More detailed cognitive assessment would be appropriate to explore more complex issues when these are clinically relevant and when misdiagnosis of dementia is a real possibility (Bergmann, Kay, & Foster, 1971). Woods (1982, p. 90) suggests that a detailed cognitive assessment may be warranted when a patient has apparently recovered from a confusional state and when it may be necessary to assess the degree of residual impairment. Before a detailed cognitive assessment is carried out, it is useful to consider what the results will contribute to the management of the case (Whitehead, 1976). Many tests have been reviewed by Kramer and Jarvik (1979). Some of the more common tests for examining the elderly person's pattern of abilities are critiqued here.

Tests of Cognitive Functioning

Such tests may be useful to the clinician for administration to elderly patients who present a problem of differential diagnosis between dementia, temporary depression, and functional disorders.

Wechsler Adult Intelligence Scale (WAIS)

The WAIS (Wechsler, 1955) is the intelligence test most widely used. Savage, Britton, Bolton, and Hall (1973) have shown that its standardization holds up well on elderly people in the United Kingdom. With regard to intellectual performance as measured by the WAIS, Raven's Progressive Matrices, and other tests of intellectual performance, cross-sectional data have long suggested a decline with age (Doppelt & Wallace, 1955) irrespective of intelligence level and without reference to SES status or residential situations.

Siegler (1980) describes in some detail the structure of the WAIS. This test is organized into two major components, verbal and performance intelligence, with several subtests, six verbal and five nonverbal. Siegler (1980, p. 181) concludes that verbal intelligence tends to increase until the sixties and then falls off gradually, but there is a sharp decline in performance intelligence after the forties. Verbal abilities are maintained considerably longer by the elderly than nonverbal abilities, an almost two decades' difference. In contrast the abilities that require speed for optimal performance are related to aging processes manifest much earlier in life (i.e., declines are seen between the ages of 30 and 50 years). The administration of the WAIS alone has not been helpful to clinicians in making differential diagnosis of depression and functional disorders or depression and dementia (Miller, 1980). Probably the most useful result of administering a highly reliable test of general intelligence like the WAIS is that it gives a good basis for the measurement of any decline should diagnosis remain in doubt (Miller, 1980). Britton and Savage (1966) have developed and standardized a useful short form of the test: Raven's Colored Progressive Matrices and Vocabulary Scales can be used to measure performance and verbal intellectual levels respectively; however, they lack the variety of task performances demanded by the full WAIS. In their favor they are relatively simple and quick to administer.

A number of indexes of cognitive impairment have been suggested, based on the well-documented differential effect of age on WAIS subtest scores. Most of these involve some variation on Wechsler's (1938) Deterioration Quotient (DQ). The DQ is calculated by summing the age-corrected scaled scores for the WAIS verbal and performance subtests that hold with age (i.e., vocabulary, information, object assembly, picture completion) and those that don't hold with age (i.e., digit span, similarities, digit symbol, block design). The DQ is of help to the clinician in that it expresses the amount of deterioration in excess of that expected in the normal aging process (Crook, 1979). Unfortunately Botwinick and Birren (1951) and other investigators have found that the DQ is an inadequate index of cognitive decline.

Tests of Verbal Ability

Wang (1980) suggests a number of verbal ability tests that are less time-consuming than the verbal subtests in the WAIS and are designed to be a more effective substitute:

1. The Quick Test. This test developed by Ammons and Ammons (1962) is a test of verbal ability, chiefly vocabulary. Wang (1980) suggests caution in using the Quick Test since it emphasizes recognition vocabulary that may decline more slowly than active vocabulary items included in the WAIS. However, it is a quick procedure for screening out dementia patients.
2. The Shipley Institute of Living Scale (Shipley, 1940, 1946). This test can be easily administered to the elderly and has the advantage of being brief and not imposing too much stress on elderly clients, who tend to approach traditionally designed problem-solving measures of intelligence with less confidence and more apprehension. However, Wang (1980) believes that this test, when used alone, is open for serious questions as it has not been standardized on a broad spectrum of elderly subjects with diverse socioeconomic status, education, or geographical position.
3. Mill Hill Vocabulary Scale. This (Raven, 1943) is a brief index of the best verbal intellectual level attained and can be used to measure verbal intellectual levels. This multiple-choice, 80-word, long-term recall test has been found sensitive to dominant hemisphere damage (Lansdell, 1968). There is considerable debate regarding the suitability of this test to assess brain damage in the elderly. As a gross measure of cognitive impairment in verbal recall, the test has been reported to be quite effective.

Tests of Verbal Learning Tasks

These tests are perhaps the most satisfactory for separating organic and depressive-dysfunctional states. Miller (1980) recommends a few tests of vocabulary learning and memory that reflect more sophisticated developments specifically designed for use with geriatric populations. A common principle in learning tests has been to take a set of words that the subject is unable to define and to teach their meanings by a set procedure. The test paper is based on the first 10 consecutively failed words from the vocabulary test of the WAIS (Walton & Black, 1957) and the subject is taught the meanings of these words by a set procedure. Cross-validation studies have substantially confirmed that such tests of learning are independent of the subject's prior knowledge, socioeconomic status, or performance ability. Description of the three tests suggested in this section are essentially adapted from Miller's (1980) recommended considerations for the cognitive assessment of the older adult:

1. Inglis Paired Associate Learning Test. This (Inglis, 1959) is one of the earliest learning and memory tests devised specifically for use with the elderly. This has two parallel forms and requires the subject to learn three pairs of otherwise unrelated words. Inglis (1970) regards this test as well-established in the geriatric field, and successful results in differentiating organics, functionals, and normals have been reported with the paired associate learning test (Caird, Sanderson, & Inglis, 1962; Parsons, 1965). Motivation may lead to improved scores, but it is not always clear whether the change reflects heightened capacity or an increase in rate of production. Leech and Witte (1971) were able to change the elderly's learning response to a paired associate task by offering cash rewards. Botwinick (1973) suggested that older people may be at least as motivated and involved in a learning test as younger people but may focus on inappropriate aspects of a test. The implication is that it may not be as critical to vary the amount of motivation for older persons as it is to help in the productive challenging of it. Poor performance in the Inglis paired associates task has identified organic problems in studies comparing older functionally and organically impaired individuals (Caird, Sanderson, & Inglis, 1962).

2. The Modified Word Learning Test (MWLT). MWLT (Bolton, Savage, & Roth, 1967) has been shown to separate organics and other patients with little overlap (Walton & Black, 1957; Walton, White, Black, & Young, 1959) and to correlate with objective signs of brain damage (Walton & Black, 1957). According to Miller (1980) it correctly discriminates a high proportion of those elderly with functional disorders, although it does less well in classifying those with brain disease. Also as noted by Miller (1980), a limitation of this test, which it shares with other tests of similar learning, is that it starts to misclassify the nonorganic subjects when used with patients whose basic intelligence level is associated with mental retardation.

3. The Synonym Learning Test (SLT). This (Kendrick, Parboosingh, & Post, 1965) is designed for use with a geriatric population and has potentials for showing differential declines with age but more importantly differential sensitivity to brain damage. The SLT is based on the Mill Hill Vocabulary Test (Raven, 1943), which Davies (1968) concluded is an index of the best intellectual level attained since age does not lower it but brain damage does. Orme (1957) also found that the SLT (based on the Mill Hill test) was able to discriminate organic from elderly normals and elderly depressives and has an advantage over the Mill Hill test in that procedures used for teaching words unknown to the client are quite unambiguously defined.

As noted by Miller (1980) the SLT does not stand on its own merits but should be used in conjunction with the Digit Copying Test (DCT) (Clement, 1963), Digit Code Test (Clement, 1963), and Progressive Matrices (Raven, 1938), which are also useful measures of psychomotor speed on simple tasks. Kendrick (1967) has demonstrated that an extremely high level of diagnostic efficiency (90 percent) can be obtained in distinguishing organic and depressive disorders when the SLT and DCT are administered on two occasions six weeks apart.

One of the major limitations noted by Kendrick (1967) in administering the SLT is that elderly subjects find it stressful to continue and will refuse to continue until the learning criterion has been reached. In order to combat this difficulty, Gibson and Kendrick (1976) have devised the Object Learning Test (OLT), in which subjects can rely on remembering pictures of common words. This preliminary version of the learning test is quicker to administer, is more readily accepted by the elderly, and to date indicates a 90 percent diagnostic discrimination accuracy in geriatric patients (Kendrick, Gibson, & Moyes, 1978, 1979).

Conclusions

The tests described so far are only a few which, as clinical measures of verbal learning and memory, have been minimally successful in differentiating between dementia-related cognitive impairment and functional disorders in the older patients. Erickson and Scott (1977) recommend further exploration with the use of many similar tests for differential diagnosis between depressive disorders and organic disorders including dementia. The techniques available for the elderly are open to criticism. They are often too difficult, and too stressful, often exposing the elderly subjects to too many failures. They emphasize deficits rather than abilities, often contain materials irrelevant to the elderly's stage of life, and are not sufficiently sensitive to change (Woods, 1982, p. 93) or treatment effects. Other difficulties in cognitive testing arise from easy fatigability, sensory impairments, and withdrawal of elderly patients, which have an impact on the memory and performance.

Despite the difficulties, Roth and Kay (1962) recognized that psychological tests are valuable for weighing diagnostic decisions and for alerting the clinician to the frequent possibility of a misdiagnosis of cognitive impairment in the elderly. Increasing efforts are being made to develop measures of cognitive function that are technically more adequate and more appropriate for impaired aged individuals (e.g., Dana, White, & Merlis, 1970).

Tests for Organicity

Psychologists have attempted to develop standardized procedures to assess specific organic impairment. Many of these procedures are particularly applicable to geriatric patients. While the Wechsler Intelligence Test is frequently utilized as a measure of organic impairment, its one major limitation is that the estimate of organic impairment is based on a discrepancy between the verbal and performance scores. A lower performance than verbal IQ, and higher scores on the vocabulary and picture completion tests have been alleged to be more typical of dementia, but these features can also be found to be in a substantial proportion of cases with functional disorders (McFie, 1975; Miller, 1977a, 1977b). In fact, Whitehead (1973a) was unable to discriminate between elderly depressives and dements on the basis of the pattern of WAIS subtests scores. Wang (1980, p. 27) notes that although many elderly show differences between verbal and performance scores, it is quite possible that these differences can to a large measure be accounted for by current occupation and other social and economic responsibilities.

Thus it is important to consider other tests that, though measures of cognitive impairment, show a better potential for assessing specific organic impairment. Some tests that may be useful in monitoring change in selected elderly subjects are critiqued here:

Benton's Revised Visual Retention Test

This test involves both visual and graphic reproduction requiring subjects to draw figures from memory after 10- and 5-second exposures, to copy the figures as accurately as they can, and to draw them after a 10-second exposure followed by a 15-second delay. The various design-copying tests, for example, the Visual Motor Gestalt Test (Bender, 1946) and Graham and Kendall's (1960) Memory for Designs Test, are aimed at detecting organic brain damage and focus on visual perception, visual memory, and visuoconstructive skills. These tests do not place the same stress on the subject as the verbal learning tests and, used along with other tests of cognitive impairment, have potential value for discriminating between organic and nonorganic cognitive disorders in the elderly. The Benton's Revised Visual Retention Test shows a progression until middle life, when it has plateaued, and subsequently it is followed by a decline in efficiency of performance in the more advanced years. Although the authors acknowledge the usual age sensitivity of the test with lower age ranges, they suggest that other external attentional factors may overshadow the influence of age beyond the age of 75.

Wechsler Memory Scale

The *Wechsler Memory Scale* (Wechsler, 1945) primarily taps memory functions, both recent and remote, but does not assess other areas of cognitive performance such as attention and concentration. The Wechsler Memory Scale has been much criticized, and certainly its use to provide a single memory quotient cannot be recommended (Woods, 1982). Several clinicians and researchers (e.g., Whitehead, 1973b; Russell, 1975) have adapted the test so that there is a measure of delayed recall. Using geriatric samples, Skilbeck and Woods (1980) identified three factors that denote memory changes in the elderly: (1) verbal learning and current orientation factor, (2) concentration factor, and (3) visual recall factor. Some normative memory data on elderly subjects are available (e.g., Hulicka, 1966; Klonoff & Kennedy, 1966; Cauthen, 1977). All of these tests suffer from the fact that they do not take into consideration the individual occupational status and educational attainments, which materially affect the elderly person's test performance.

Bender Visual Motor Gestalt Test

The *Bender Visual Motor Gestalt Test* (BIP) (Bender, 1946) is the most commonly used perceptual motor test for assessing organic function. It consists of nine designs presented singly to the subject, who is allowed unlimited time (within reason) to complete the test, which usually involves 5 to 10 minutes of testing time.

The test has demonstrated effectiveness in distinguishing organic impairment from psychiatric disturbance. When dementia is secondary to a widespread process such as Alzheimer's disease or cerebrovascular disease, drawings of the elderly patients appear abnormal, over- or undersized, displaced upward, with many corrections, and with simple broken lines (Kramer & Jarvik, 1979).

This procedure according to Wang (1980) has been augmented by the Background Interference Procedure (BIP) (Canter & Straumanis, 1968), which seems to increase the sensitivity of the Bender Gestalt in discriminating organic brain damage from functional problems. The BIP is also believed to be less influenced by such factors as intelligence, affective status, and age. Several observers suggest that when a single test must be used, the Bender Gestalt is most appropriate since it has developed a fairly reliable scoring method for identifying brain damage.

Halstead-Reitan Tests

Halstead-Reitan Tests (Halstead, 1947; Reitan & Davison, 1974) are a battery of several tests including the Halstead Neuropsychological Battery and the Reitan's Trailmaking Test (TMT). A Halstead Impairment Index can be derived from a score based on 10 discriminating tests in the Halstead battery. Wang (1980) speculates that this impairment index has some limitations, as it has not been clearly standardized on a basis that includes age as a determining factor. Similarly the Trailmaking Test is one of the scales included in the Halstead Impairment Index, but it has also been used alone as an index of brain damage in the young adult. A severe limitation concerning its use with the elderly is the demanding length of administration. Both the Bender Gestalt and the WAIS have been reported to show better discriminatory power than the Halstead-Reitan for comparing persons with brain damage and those with psychiatric diagnoses.

As with other measures of psychoneurologic impairment, Wang notes that better validation data obtained from elderly subjects are necessary to gaining a full understanding of their usefulness. In general only simple neuropsychological tests can be used, and the results of these must be interpreted with clinical judgment with regard to the overall pattern of abilities of the elderly person.

Bender's Face-Hand Test

Bender's Face-Hand Test (FHT) (Bender, Fink, & Green, 1951) is a neurological test of particular value in the diagnosis of organic disorders. It is a test of double simultaneous tactile stimulation. The subject is touched simultaneously on one hand and one cheek and has to report where touched. The test is done initially with the patient's eyes closed and later, if necessary, with the eyes open. The examiner touches the patient simultaneously on the cheek and the dorsum of the hand, contralaterally and ipsilaterally, in a specific order so as to include at least 10 trials. Errors made by the patient after the four initial demonstration trials are considered presumptive evidence of brain damage. Responses that are considered errors include not reporting the touch to the hand and localizing the hand touch to the cheek or to the knee. The indications are that the scores obtained on the Bender Face-Hand Test give worthwhile levels of discrimination between organic and functional disorders. One of the advantages of the FHT is its insensitivity to education or intelligence. Also, normally dull persons or anxious adults are allowed an opportunity to get accustomed to the format of the test and their expected role in it, without a scoring penalty. Once oriented, most people, regardless of anxiety states, perform normally. The test is widely used as a gross measure of organic impairment. While it may miss mild brain damage, it is not likely to yield false positives (Kramer & Jarvik, 1979). However, like many neuropsychological tests, the Face-Hand Test could benefit from better standardization on geriatric patients. Kramer and Jarvik recommend its use only in conjunction with or as an adjunct to other tests of organic impairment or mental status examination scales.

Mental Status Examinations in Geriatric Assessment

Mental status examination has traditionally been a procedure designed to provide a relatively rapid description and diagnosis of a person's mental functioning and capabilities and emotional state with respect to agitation, confusion, disorientation, and anxiety. However, descriptions of psychological functions included under mental status examination and the method (i.e., tasks and items) of assessment need to be expanded and updated in view of the increasingly important role that mental status examination is playing in the clinical assessment of psychogeriatric clients. Some of the more well-known, reliable, and valid mental status examinations are critiqued and evaluated here in terms of their previous success with geriatric samples:

Short Portable Mental Status Questionnaire

Short Portable Mental Status Questionnaire (SPMSQ): This 10-item, mental status questionnaire (Pfeiffer, 1975) has been validated on 997 elderly persons residing in the community and on smaller samples of referred and institutionalized inpatients. Since clients in the advanced age group (65 and older) are at a high risk for cognitive impairment in terms of orientation in place, space, and time, an inability to give satisfactory answers to straightforward questions relating to day and date or place (e.g., date, month, and year; subject's age; name of the city in which subject resides; mother's maiden name) must immediately raise suspicions of an organic disorder of some kind (Williams, 1970). For this reason the presence and degree of cognitive deficit in regard to orientation, long- and short-term memory, and information necessary for activities of daily living must be ascertained.

On the basis of test administration to a large community population of elders, standards of performance have been established for intact mental functions, mild organic impairment, moderate and severe organic impairment (see Pfeiffer, 1975). These levels of intellectual functioning are intended to aid in concrete clinical decision making regarding capacity for self-care. Thus it is assumed that persons scoring in the intact range (0–2 scores) are from an intellectual-cognitive point of view entirely capable of self-care. Three or more errors on this scale are indicative of some degree of organic impairment. The implication is that those persons scoring in the severely impaired range (7 to 10 errors) may indicate organic syndrome and in all probability require continuous supervision of their activities. Such an instrument would aid in quickly arriving at a psychiatric diagnosis when organic brain syndrome is the patient's primary problem or when the patient's basic medical or psychiatric condition is compounded by the coexistence of organic impairment. Thus it provides the clinician with a gross measure of overall mental status as opposed to localized organic malfunctioning.

According to Pfeiffer (1980) the test is sensitive to educational attainment, which materially affects test performance. Unlike the Kahn-Goldfarb Mental Status Questionnaire (Kahn et al., 1960), which was standardized on institutional populations of the elderly, the present test of mental status has been standardized on community samples. Hence it is more suited to office and outpatient clinic assessments. The test is not capable of distinguishing between reversible organic brain deficit (delirium) and irreversible organic brain deficit (dementia). However, as suggested by Pfeiffer, it can be used repeatedly, over days, weeks, and months, to follow quantitatively the course of drug-induced delirium or of senile dementia.

Clifton Assessment Schedule

The *Clifton Assessment Schedule* (CAS): This scale (Pattie & Gilleard, 1979) has been devised to assess psychogeriatric subjects in a brief, reliable procedure. It assesses information and orientation, mental ability and psychomotor functioning with a writing task. Its items dealing with orientation of time and place are virtually identical to those used in other mental status examination scales such as the Mental Status Questionnaire (MSQ) (Kahn et al., 1960). However, the CAS has the advantage of brevity and has been used with elderly chronic patients both by clinicians and psychiatric nurses. It measures various aspects of cognitive functioning and is specifically sensitive to very impaired patients, who must be guarded against premature discharge from hospital, or those who might need continuous care and supervision (Pattie & Gilleard, 1975).

Geriatric Interpersonal Evaluation Scale

Geriatric Interpersonal Evaluation Scale (GIES): This (Plutchik et al., 1971) is a more recently developed test designed to assess the degree of cognitive functioning of highly regressed patients through the use of a semistructured interview, which focuses on the patients' ability to relate to the environment and the interviewer. It also measures the elderly clients' perceptual-motor ability and, like the CAS, assesses orientation (in this particular instance through a drawing task, i.e., figure reproduction), immediate and remote memory, and verbal and quantitative cognitive functions. Its major advantage is that it has also been used in studies of geriatric psychopharmacology and is a useful index of change due to pharmacology treatment. The presence of a clinician in the semistructured interview is useful to accurate diagnostic testing. The use of this scale is recommended for highly regressed inpatients (Kochansky, 1979).

Other widely used tests of mental status that essentially assess orientation and examine various aspects of elderly clients' behavior such as appearance, effect and thought processes include the Quantified Mental Status Scale (Rockland & Pollin, 1965), Mental Status Examination Record (Spitzer & Endicott, 1971), and Mental Status Checklist (Lifshitz, 1960). All these scales have the advantage of brevity. However, like many mental status tests, these scales could benefit from better standardization on geriatric patients. No single scale of mental status examination is deemed sufficient for diagnostic purposes. Their use is recommended only in conjunction with or as an adjunct to other batteries of cognitive assessment or neuropsychological tests. Clinical considerations in the use of mental status examinations were discussed in Chapter 2.

Conclusions

Although a few adequately reliable and valid mental status examination scales specifically developed for aged population scales have been available to geriatric clinicians and psychiatric nurses, their sensitivity to the effects of social isolation, emotional withdrawal, and severe grief reactions has been limited. Many problems involved in the psychological evaluation of elderly patients with cognitive or organic impairment still require resolution.

SUMMARY

This chapter has discussed problems related to differential diagnosis of a number of brain disorders that lead to cognitive impairment in varying degrees. The assessment of these brain disorders, some with irreversible effects on cognitive functioning, is probably the most difficult and challenging task facing the practitioner. Accurate evaluations are rather difficult, and the potentials for misdiagnosis are considerable. Thus careful identification and assessment of the reversible and irreversible invariants of dementia, and an accurate medical assessment of the treatable and untreatable components of senile dementia, acute brain syndrome, and delirium, are crucial to treatment of the factors that have led to the cognitive disorders.

Assessment procedures that enhance the possibilities for a better identification of divergent types and causes of brain disorders have been outlined. In senile dementia no medical approaches have been found that can effectively halt the progressive deterioration in cognitive functioning. Prosthetic interventions for care of the demented elderly have been discussed. Treatment of elderly with dementia can be successful if it is focused on appropriately managing the behavioral disturbances and cognitive dysfunctioning associated with the brain syndrome. Programs of home care for demented elderly can be of considerable help in delaying institutionalization and in allowing the impaired elderly to continue living in the familiar and empathic environment of the home. This is possible by providing support to family caregivers and in giving them information, education, and counseling for dealing with the practical problems of caring for demented elderly persons.

REFERENCES

Adams, M., Caston, M.A., & Danis, B.C. (1979). *A neglected dimension in home care of elderly disabled persons: Effects on responsible family members.* Paper presented at the meetings of the Gerontological Society, Washington, DC.

Albert, M.S. (1981). Geriatric neuropsychology. *Journal of Consulting and Clinical Psychology, 49*, 835–850.

Ammons, R.B., & Ammons, C.H. (1962). The quick test: Provisional manual. *Psychological Reports, 11*, 11–161.

Bedford, P.D. (1959). General medical aspects of confusional states in elderly people. *British Medical Journal, 2*, 185–188.

Bender, L. (1946). *Instructions for the use of the Visual Motor Gestalt Test.* New York: American Orthopsychiatric Association.

Bender, M.B., Fink, M., & Green, M.A. (1951). Patterns in perception on simultaneous tests of face and hand. *Archives of Neurology and Psychiatry, 56*, 355–375.

Bergmann, K., Kay, D.W.K., & Foster, E. (1971). A follow-up study of randomly selected community residents to assess the effects of chronic brain syndrome and cerebrovascular disease. *Proceedings of the 5th World Congress of Psychiatry*, Mexico. Amsterdam: Excerpta Medica.

Blazer, D.G. (1982). *Depression in late life.* St. Louis: C.V. Mosby Co.

Blessed, G., Tomlinson, B.E., & Roth, M. (1968). The association between quantitative measures of dementia and of senile change in the cerebral gray matter of elderly subjects. *British Journal of Psychiatry, 114*, 797–811.

Boll, T.J. (1981). Assessment of neuropsychological disorders. In D.H. Barlow (Ed.), *Behavioral assessment of adult disorders* (pp. 45–86). New York: Guilford.

Bolton, N., Savage, R.D., & Roth, M. (1967). The Modified Word Learning Test and the aged psychiatric patient. *British Journal of Psychiatry, 113*, 1139–1140.

Botwinick, J. (1973). *Aging and behavior.* New York: Springer.

Botwinick, J., & Birren, J.E. (1951). The measurement of intellectual decline in the senile psychoses. *Journal of Consulting Psychology, 15*, 145–150.

British Medical Journal. (1978). Dementia: The quiet epidemic (editorial). *British Medical Journal, 2*, 1374–1375.

Britton, P.G., & Savage, R.D. (1966). A short form of WAIS for use with the aged. *British Journal of Psychiatry, 112*, 417–418.

Brody, E.M. (1978). *The formal support network: Congregate treatment setting for residents with senescent brain function.* Presented at the Conference on the Clinical Aspects of Alzheimer's Disease and Senile Dementia, National Institute of Mental Health, Bethesda, MD, December.

Caine, E.D. (1981). Pseudodementia: Current concepts and future directions. *Archives of General Psychiatry, 38,* 1359–1364.

Caird, F.I. (1977). Computerized tomography (Emiscan) in brain failure in old age. *Age and Aging, 6*(suppl.), 50–51.

Caird, W.K., Sanderson, R.E., & Inglis, J. (1962). Cross-validation of a learning test for use with elderly psychiatric patients. *Journal of Mental Science, 108,* 368–370.

Canter, A., & Straumanis, J.J. (1969). Performance of senile and healthy older persons on the BIP Bender test. *Perceptual Motor Skills, 28,* 695–698.

Cauthen, N.R. (1977). Extension of the Wechsler Memory scale norms to older age groups. *Journal of Clinical Psychology, 33,* 208–211.

Clement, F. (1963). Une epreuve rapide de mesure de l'efficience intellectuelle. *Revue de Psychologie appliquee, 13,* 1215.

Crapper, D.R., Krishnan, S.S., & Dalton, A.J. (1973). Brain aluminum distribution in Alzheimer's disease and experimental neurofibrillary degeneration. *Science, 180,* 511–513.

Crook, T.H. (1979). Psychometric assessment in the elderly. In A. Raskin & L.F. Jarvik (Eds.), *Psychiatric symptoms and cognitive loss in the elderly* (pp. 207–220). Washington: Hemisphere.

Dana, L.A., White, L., & Merlis, S. (1970). A new approach to measuring short-term memory in geriatric subjects: A pilot study. *Psychological Reports, 27,* 8–10.

Davies, A.D.M. (1968). Measures of mental deterioration in aging and brain damage. In S.S. Chown & K.F. Riegel (Eds.), *Interdisciplinary topics in gerontology. Vol. 1. Psychological functioning in the normal aging and senile aged* (pp. 78–90). New York: Karger.

Doppelt, J.E., & Wallace, W.L. (1955). Standardization of the Wechsler Adult Intelligence Scale for older persons. *Journal of Abnormal & Social Psychology, 51,* 312–330.

Eisdorfer, C., & Cohen, D. (1978). The cognitively impaired elderly: Differential diagnosis. In M. Storandt, I.C. Siegler, & M.F. Elias (Eds.), *The clinical psychology of aging* (pp. 7–42). New York: Plenum Press.

Engel, G.L., & Romano, J. (1959). Delirium, a syndrome of cerebral insufficiency. *Journal of Chronic Disorders, 9,* 260–277.

Epstein, L.J. (1976). Depression in the elderly. *Journal of Gerontology, 31,* 278–282.

Erikson, R.C., & Scott, M.L. (1977). Clinical memory tests: A review. *Psychological Bulletin, 84,* 1130–1149.

Fink, M., Green, M.A., & Bender, M.B. (1952). The face-hand test as a diagnostic sign of organic mental syndrome. *Neurology, 2,* 48–56.

Folstein, M.F., Folstein, S.E., & McHugh, P.R. (1975). "Minimental state": A practical method for grading the cognitive state of patients for the clinician. *Journal of Psychiatric Research, 12,* 189–198.

Fox, H.H., Topel, J.L., & Huckman, M.S. (1975). Use of computerized tomography in senile dementia. *Journal of Neurology, Neurosurgery and Psychiatry, 382,* 948–953.

Friedman, M.J., & Lipowski, Z.J. (1981). Pseudodementia in a young Ph.D. *American Journal of Psychiatry, 138,* 381–382.

Gajdusek, D.C. (1977). Unconventional viruses and the origin and disappearance of Kuru. *Science, 197,* 943–960.

Gibson, A.J., & Kendrick, D.C. (1976). The development of a visual learning test to replace the SLT in the Kendrick Battery. *Bulletin of the British Psychological Society, 29,* 200–201.

Gibson, G.E., Peterson, C., & Jenden, D.J. (1981). Brain acetylcholine synthesis declines with senescence. *Science, 213,* 674–676.

Glassman, M. (1980). Misdiagnosis of senile dementia: Denial of care to the elderly. *Social Work, 25,* 288–292.

Goldstein, M.F., & McHugh, P.R. (1978). Dementia syndrome of depression. In R. Katzman, R.D. Terry, & K.L. Bick (Eds.), *Alzheimer's disease, senile dementia and related disorders* (pp. 87–93). New York: Raven Press.

Graham, F.K., & Kendall, B.S. (1960). Memory for Designs Test: Revised General Manual. *Perceptual and Motor Skills, 11,* 147–188. Monograph Supplement 2-VII.

Gruenberg, E. (1977). The failures of success. *Milbank Memorial Fund Quarterly, 55*(1), 3–24.

Gurland, B.J. (1980). The assessment of the mental health status of older adults. In J.E. Birren & R.B. Sloane (Eds.), *Handbook of mental health and aging* (pp. 671–700). Englewood Cliffs, NJ: Prentice-Hall, Inc.

Gurland, B.J., Dean, L., Cross, P., & Golden, R. (1980). The epidemiology of depression and delirium in the elderly: The use of multiple indicators of these conditions. In J.O. Cole & J.E. Barrett (Eds.), *Psychopathology in the aged* (pp. 37–62). New York: Raven Press.

Haase, G.R. (1977). Diseases presenting as dementia. In C.E. Wells (Ed.), *Dementia* (pp. 27–67). Philadelphia: Davis Co.

Hachinski, V., Lassen, N., & Marshall, J. (1974). Multi-infarct dementia: A cause of mental deterioration in the elderly. *Lancet, 2*, 207–210.

Halstead, W.C. (1947). *Brain and intelligence*. Chicago: University of Chicago Press.

Hodkinson, H.M. (1973). Mental impairment in the elderly. *Journal of the Royal College of Physicians, 7*, 305–317.

Hulicka, I.M. (1966). Age differences in Wechsler Memory Scale scores. *Journal of Genetic Psychology, 109*, 135–145.

Hutton, J.T. (1981). Results of clinical assessment for the dementia syndrome: Implications for epidemiologic studies. In J.A. Mortimer & L.M. Schuman (Eds.), *The epidemiology of dementia* (pp. 62–69). New York: Oxford University Press.

Inglis, J. (1959). A paired associate learning test for use with elderly psychiatric patients. *Journal of Mental Science, 105*, 440–448.

Inglis, J. (1970). Memory disorder. In C.G. Costello (Ed.), *Symptoms of psychopathology* (pp. 95–133). New York: John Wiley & Sons.

Jacoby, R.J., & Levy, R. (1980). Computed tomography in the elderly 2. Senile dementia: diagnosis and functional impairment. *British Journal of Psychiatry, 136*, 256–259.

Jolley, D. (1981). Acute confusional states in the elderly. In D. Coakley (Ed.), *Acute geriatric medicine* (pp. 175–189). London: Croom Helm.

Journal of Royal College of Physicians. (1981). Organic mental impairment in the elderly, *15*, 141–167.

Joynt, R.J., & Shoulson, I. (1979). Dementia. In K.M. Heilman & E. Valenstein (Eds.), *Clinical neuropsychology* (pp. 475–502). New York: Oxford University Press.

Kahn, R.L. (1975). The mental health system and the future aged. *Gerontologist, 15*(1, pt. 2), 24–31.

Kahn, R.L., Goldfarb, A.I., Pollack, M., & Peck, A. (1960). Brief objective measures for the determination of mental status in the aged. *American Journal of Psychiatry, 117*, 326–328.

Kahn, R.L., & Miller, N.E. (1978). Assessment of altered brain function in the aged. In M. Storandt, I.C. Siegler, & M. Elias (Eds.), *The clinical psychology of aging* (pp. 43–69). New York: Plenum Press.

Kahn, R.L., Zarit, S.H., Hilbert, N.M., & Niederehe, G. (1975). Memory complaint and impairment in the aged. *Archives of General Psychiatry, 32*, 1569–1573.

Kapnick, P.L. (1978). Organic treatment of the elderly. In M. Storandt, I.C. Siegler, & M.F. Elias (Eds.), *The clinical psychology of aging* (pp. 225–251). New York: Plenum Press.

Kay, D.W.K. (1977). The epidemiology and identification of brain deficit in the elderly. In C. Eisdorfer & R.O. Friedel (Eds.), *Cognitive and emotional disturbance in the elderly* (pp. 11–26). Chicago: Year Book Medical Publishers.

Kendrick, D.C. (1967). A cross-validation study of the use of the SLT and DCT in screening for diffuse brain pathology in elderly subjects. *British Journal of Medical Psychology, 40*, 173–178.

Kendrick, D.C., Gibson, A.J., & Moyes, I.C.A. (1978). The Kendrick battery: Mark II. *Bulletin of the British Psychological Society, 31*, 177–178.

Kendrick, D.C., Gibson, A.J., & Moyes, I.C.A. (1979). The revised Kendrick battery: Clinical studies. *British Journal of Social and Clinical Psychology, 18*, 329–340.

Kendrick, D.C., Parboosingh, R.C., & Post, F. (1965). A synonym learning test for use with elderly psychiatric subjects: A validation study. *British Journal of Social Clinical Psychology, 4*, 63–71.

Kenny, A.D. (1979). Designing therapy for the elderly. *Drug Therapy, 9*, 49–64.

Kiloh, L.G. (1961). Pseudo-dementia. *Acta Psychiatrica Scandinavica, 37*, 336–351.

Klonoff, H., & Kennedy, M. (1966). A comparative study of cognitive functioning in old age. *Journal of Gerontology, 21*, 239–243.

Kochansky, G.F. (1979). Psychiatric rating scales. In A. Raskin & L.F. Jarvik (Eds.), *Psychiatric symptoms and cognitive loss in the elderly* (pp. 125–156). Washington: Hemisphere.

Kramer, N.A., & Jarvik, L.F. (1979). Intellectual changes in the elderly. In A. Raskin & L.F. Jarvik (Eds.), *Psychiatric symptoms and cognitive loss in the elderly* (pp. 221–271). Washington: Hemisphere.

Lansdell, A.C. (1968). Effects of temporal lobe ablations on two lateralized deficits. *Physiology and Behavior, 3*, 271–273.

Larsson, T., Sjogren, T., & Jacobson, G. (1963). Senile dementia: A clinical, socio-medical and genetic study. *Acta Psychiatrica Scandinavica* (supple.), *167*, 1–259.

Lawton, M.P. (1971). The functional assessment of elderly people. *Journal of the American Geriatrics Society, 19*, 465–481.

Lawton, M.P. (1980). Psychosocial and environmental approaches to the care of senile dementia patients. In J.O. Cole & J.E. Barrett (Eds.), *Psychopathology in the aged* (pp. 265–278). New York: Raven Press.

Lawton, M.P., & Nahemow, L. (1973). Ecology and the aging process. In C. Eisdorfer & M.P. Lawton (Eds.), *Psychology of adult development and aging* (pp. 619–674). Washington: American Psychological Association.

Leech, S., & Witte, K.L. (1971). Paired-associate learning in elderly adults as related to pacing and incentive conditions. *Developmental Psychology, 5*, 180.

Levin, M. (1945). Delirious disorientation: The law of the unfamiliar mistaken for the familiar. *Journal of Mental Science, 91*, 447–450.

Levy, R., & Post, F. (1982). The dementias of old age. In R. Levy & F. Post (Eds.), *The psychiatry of late life* (pp. 163–175). Oxford: Blackwell Scientific Publications.

Lezak, M.D. (1976). *Neuropsychological assessment*. New York: Oxford University Press.

Libow, L.S. (1973). Pseudosenility: Acute and reversible organic brain syndrome. *Journal of the American Geriatrics Society, 21*, 112–120.

Libow, L.S. (1977). Senile dementia and "pseudosenility": Clinical diagnosis. In C. Eisdorfer & R.O. Friedel (Eds.), *Cognitive and emotional disturbances in the elderly* (pp. 75–88). Chicago: Year Book Medical Publishers.

Lifshitz, K. (1960). Problems in the quantitative evaluation of patients with psychoses of the senium. *Journal of Psychology, 49*, 295–303.

Lindsley, O.R. (1966). Geriatric behavioral prosthetics. In R. Kastenbaum (Ed.), *New thoughts on old age* (pp. 41–60). New York: Springer.

Lipowski, Z.J. (1975). Organic brain syndromes: Overview and classification. In D. Benson & D. Blumer (Eds.), *Psychiatric aspects of neurologic disease* (pp. 11–35). New York: Grune & Stratton.

Lipowski, Z.J. (1980a). *Delirium: Acute brain failure in man*. Springfield, IL: Charles C Thomas.

Lipowski, Z.J. (1980b). Delirium updated. *Comprehensive Psychiatry, 21*, 190–196.

Lipowski, Z.J. (1982). Differentiating delirium from dementia in the elderly. *Clinical Gerontologist, 1*, 3–10.

Lipowski, Z.J. (1983). Transient cognitive disorders (delirium, acute confusional states) in the elderly. *American Journal of Psychiatry, 140*, 1426–1436.

Liston, E.H. (1982). Delirium in the aged. *Psychiatric Clinic of North America, 5*, 49–66.

McAllister, T.W. (1983). Overview: Pseudodementia. *American Journal of Psychiatry, 140*, 528–533.

McAllister, T.W., Ferrell, R.B., Price, T.R.P., & Neville, M.B. (1982). The dexamethasone suppression test in two patients with severe depressive pseudodementia. *American Journal of Psychiatry, 139*, 479–481.

McAllister, T.W., & Price, T.R.P. (1982). Severe depressive pseudodementia with and without dementia. *American Journal of Psychiatry, 139*, 626–629.

McFie, J. (1975). *Assessment of organic intellectual impairment*. London: Academic Press.

Millar, H.R. (1981). Psychiatric morbidity in elderly surgical patients. *British Journal of Psychiatry, 138*, 17–20.

Miller, E. (1977a). The management of dementia: A review of some possibilities. *British Journal of Social and Clinical Psychology, 16*, 77–83.

Miller, E. (1977b). *Abnormal ageing*. Chichester: John Wiley & Sons.

Miller, E. (1980). Cognitive assessment of the older adult. In J.E. Birren & R.B. Sloane (Eds.), *Handbook of mental health and aging* (pp. 520–536). Englewood Cliffs, NJ: Prentice-Hall, Inc.

Miller, E., & Lewis, P. (1977). Recognition memory in elderly patients with depression and dementia: A signal detection analysis. *Journal of Abnormal Psychology, 86*, 84–86.

Mortimer, J.A., Schuman, L.M., & French, L.R. (1981). Epidemiology of dementing illness. In J.A. Mortimer & L.M. Schuman (Eds.), *The epidemiology of dementia* (pp. 3–23). New York: Oxford University Press.

Nandy, K. (1977). Immune reactions in aging brain and senile dementia. In K. Nandy & I. Sherwin (Eds.), *The aging brain and senile dementia* (pp. 181–196). New York: Plenum Press.

National Institute of Aging Task Force (1980). Senility reconsidered. *Journal of the American Medical Association, 244*(3), 259–263.

National Nursing Home Survey (1977). *National Nursing Home Survey: United States (1973–1974).* Washington: Government Printing Office.

Nott, R.N., & Fleminger, J.J. (1975). Presenile dementia: The difficulties of early diagnosis. *Acta Psychiatrica Scandinavica, 51*, 210–217.

Orme, J.E. (1957). Non-verbal and verbal performance in normal old age, senile dementia and elderly depression. *Journal of Gerontology, 12*, 408–413.

Parsons, P.L. (1965). The mental health of Swansea's old folk. *British Journal of Preventative Social Medicine, 19*, 43–58.

Pattie, A.H., & Gilleard, C.J. (1975). A brief psychogeriatric assessment schedule: Validation against psychiatric diagnosis and discharge from hospital. *British Journal of Psychiatry, 127*, 489–493.

Pattie, A.H., & Gilleard, C.J. (1979). *Manual of the Clifton Assessment Procedures for the Elderly (CAPE).* Sevenoaks, Kent, England: Hodder & Stoughton Educational.

Perry, E.K., Perry, R.H., Blessed, G., & Tomlinson, B.E. (1977). Necropsy evidence of central cholinergic deficits in senile dementia. *Lancet, 1*, 189.

Pfeiffer, E. (1975). A short mental status questionnaire for the assessment of organic brain deficit in elderly patients. *Journal of American Geriatrics Society, 23*, 433–441.

Pfeiffer, E. (1980). The psychosocial evaluation in aging. In E.W. Busse & D.G. Blazer (Eds.), *Handbook of geriatric psychiatry* (pp. 275–284). New York: Van Nostrand Reinhold Co.

Plutchik, R., Conte, H., & Lieberman, M. (1971). Development of a scale (GIES) for assessment of cognitive and perceptual functioning in geriatric patients. *Journal of the American Geriatrics Society, 19*, 614–623.

Post, F. (1975). Dementia, depression, and pseudodementia. In D.F. Benson & D. Blumer (Eds.), *Psychiatric aspects of neurological disease* (pp. 99–120). New York: Grune & Stratton.

Purdie, F.R., Honigman, T.B., & Rosen, P. (1981). Acute organic brain syndrome: A review of 100 cases. *Annals of Emergency Medicine, 10*, 455–461.

Raskind, M. (1976). *Community-based evaluation and crisis intervention.* A paper presented at the Workshop on Aging, New York, October.

Raven, J.C. (1943). *The Mill Hill Vocabulary Scale.* London: Lewis.

Raven, J.C. (1938). *Progressive matrices.* London: Lewis.

Reifler, B.U., Larson, E., & Hanley, R. (1982). Coexistence of cognitive impairment and depression in geriatric out-patients. *American Journal of Psychiatry, 139*, 623–626.

Reitan, R.M., & Davison, L.A. (1974). *Clinical neuropsychology: Current status and applications.* Washington: Winston.

Rivera, V.M., & Meyer, J.S. (1975). Dementia and cerebrovascular disease. In J.S. Meyer (Ed.), *Modern concepts of cerebrovascular disease* (pp. 135–158). New York: Spectrum.

Rockland, L.H., & Pollin, W. (1965). Quantification of psychiatric mental status: For use with psychotic patients. *Archives of General Psychiatry, 12*, 23–28.

Roth, M. (1955). The natural history of mental disorders in old age. *Journal of Mental Science, 101*, 281–301.

Roth, M. (1971). Classification and aetiology in mental disorders of old age: Some recent developments. In D.W.K. Kay & A. Walk (Eds.), *Recent developments in psychogeriatrics: A symposium, British Journal Psychiatry Special Pub. no. 6* (pp. 1–18). Ashford, England: Headley Brothers.

Roth, M. (1976). The psychiatric disorders of later life. *Psychiatric Annals, 6*, 417–444.

Roth, M. (1980). Senile dementia and its borderlands. In J.O. Cole & J.E. Barrett (Eds.), *Psychopathology in the aged* (pp. 205–232). New York: Raven Press.

Roth, M., & Kay, D.W.K. (1962). Psychoses among the aged. In H. Blumenthal (Ed.), *Aging around the world: Medical and clinical aspects of aging* (pp. 74–96). New York: Columbia University Press.

Roth, M., & Myers, D.H. (1976). The diagnosis of dementia. In T. Silverstone & B. Barraclough (Eds.), *Contemporary psychiatry* (pp. 87–99). Ashford, England: Headley Brothers.

Russell, E.W. (1975). A multiple scoring method for the assessment of complex memory functions. *Journal of Consulting and Clinical Psychology, 43*, 800–809.

Salzman, C., Kochansky, G.E., & Shader, R.I. (1972). Rating scales for geriatric psychopharmacology—A review. *Psychopharmacology Bulletin, 8*, 3–50.

Savage, R.D., Britton, P.G., Bolton, N., & Hall, E.H. (1973). *Intellectual functioning in the aged*. London: Methuen.

Seymour, D.G., Henschke, P.J., & Cape, R.D.T. (1980). Acute confusional states and dementia in the elderly: The role of dehydration/volume depletion, physical illness and age. *Age Ageing, 9*, 137–146.

Shipley, W.C. (1940). A self-administering scale for measuring intellectual impairment and deterioration. *Journal of Psychology, 9*, 371–377.

Shipley, W.C. (1946). *Institute of Living Scale*. Los Angeles: Western Psychology Services.

Shraberg, D. (1978). The myth of pseudodementia: Depression and the aging brain. *American Journal of Psychiatry, 135*, 601–603.

Siegler, I.C. (1980). The psychology of adult development and aging. In E.W. Busse & D.G. Blazer (Eds.), *Handbook of geriatric psychiatry* (pp. 169–221). New York: Van Nostrand Reinhold Co.

Skilbeck, C.W., & Woods, R.T. (1980). The factorial structure of the Wechsler Memory Scale in samples of neurological and psychogeriatric patients. *Journal of Clinical Neuropsychology, 2*, 293–300.

Spitzer, R.L., & Endicott, J. (1971). An integrated group of forms for automated psychiatric case records. *Archives of General Psychiatry, 24*, 540–547.

Terry, R.D., & Wisniewski, H. (1973). Ultrastructure of senile dementia and of experimental analogs. In C. Gaitz (Ed.), *Aging and the brain* (pp. 89–116). New York: Plenum Press.

Terry, R.D., & Wisniewski, H.M. (1977). Structural aspects of aging of the brain. In C. Eisdorfer & R.O. Friedel (Eds.), *Cognitive and emotional disturbance in the elderly* (pp. 3–9). Chicago: Year Book Medical Publishers.

Tomlinson, B.E., Blessed, G., & Roth, M. (1970). Observations on the brains of demented old people. *Journal of the Neurological Sciences, 11*, 205–242.

Traub, R., Gajdusek, D.C., & Gibbs, C.J. (1977). Transmissible virus dementia: The relation of transmissible encephalopathy to Creutzfeldt-Jakob disease. In W.L. Smith & M. Kinsbourne (Eds.), *Aging and dementia* (pp. 91–146). New York: Spectrum.

Walton, D., & Black, D.A. (1957). The validity of psychological test of brain damage. *British Journal of Medical Psychology, 20*, 270–279.

Walton, D., White, J.G., Black, D.A., & Young, A.J. (1959). The modified word learning test—a cross validation study. *British Journal of Medical Psychology, 22*, 213–220.

Wang, H.S. (1980). Diagnostic procedures. In E.W. Busse & D.G. Blazer (Eds.), *Handbook of geriatric psychiatry* (pp. 285–304). New York: Van Nostrand Reinhold Co.

Waxman, H.M., Carner, E.A., Dubin, W., Klein, M. (1982). Geriatric psychiatry in the emergency department: Characteristics of geriatric and non-geriatric admissions. *Journal of the American Geriatrics Society, 30*, 427–432.

Wechsler, D. (1938). Mental deterioration: Its measurement and significance. *Journal of Nervous and Mental Disease, 87*, 89–97.

Wechsler, D. (1945). A standardized memory scale for clinical use. *Journal of Psychology, 19*, 87–95.

Wechsler, D. (1955). *Manual for the Wechsler Adult Intelligence Scale*. New York: Psychological Corp.

Weinberg, J. (1975). Geriatric psychiatry. In A.M. Freedman, H.I. Kaplan, & B.J. Sadock (Eds.), *Comprehensive textbook of psychiatry* (Vol. 2, pp. 2405–2420). Baltimore: Williams & Wilkins.

Weinstein, E.A., & Kahn, R.L. (1955). *Denial of illness*. Springfield, IL: Charles C Thomas.

Wells, C.E. (1979). Pseudodementia. *American Journal of Psychiatry, 136*, 895–900.

Whitehead, A. (1973a). The pattern of WAIS performance in elderly psychiatric patients. *British Journal of Social & Clinical Psychology, 12*, 435–436.

Whitehead, A. (1973b). Verbal learning and memory in elderly depressives. *British Journal of Psychiatry, 123*, 203–208.

Whitehead, A. (1976). The prediction of outcome in elderly psychiatric patients. *Psychological Medicine, 6*, 469–479.

Williams, M. (1970). Geriatric patients. In P.J. Mittler (Ed.), *The psychological assessment of mental and physical handicaps* (pp. 319–339). London: Methuen.

Woods, R. (1982). The psychology of ageing: Assessment of defects and their management. In R. Levy & F. Post (Eds.), *The psychiatry of late life* (pp. 68–113). Oxford: Blackwell Scientific Publications.

Zarit, J. (1982). *Predictors of burden and distress for caregivers of senile dementia patients.* Unpublished doctoral dissertation, University of Southern California, Los Angeles.

Zarit, J., Gatz, M., & Zarit, S.H. (1981). *Family relationships and burden in long-term care.* Paper presented at the meetings of the Gerontological Society, Toronto, Ontario.

Zarit, S.H., Miller, N.E., & Kahn, R.L. (1978). Brain function, intellectual impairment and education in the aged. *Journal of the American Geriatrics Society, 26,* 58–67.

Zarit, S.H., Reever, K.E., & Bach-Peterson, J. (1981). Relatives of the impaired elderly: Correlates of feelings of burden. *Gerontologist, 21,* 158–164.

Zarit, S.H., & Zarit, J. (1983). Cognitive impairment. In P.M. Lewinsohn & L. Teri (Eds.), *Clinical geropsychology: New directions in assessment and treatment* (pp. 38–80). New York: Pergamon.

Chapter 5

Assessment of Stress Reactions and Coping Behavior in Old Age

Since the 1950s the subjective psychological reactions to stress among the elderly have emerged as the central concern of gerontology reflected both in the empirical research and major thesis of the determinants of stress and in chronic stress as a determinant of behavior. The study of stress assumes special significance for older adults because of the frequency and intensity of stressful life events that they may experience during a life stage when their economic, physical, social, and psychological resources are limited (Rosow, 1967). Recent studies in gerontology have therefore moved from descriptions of the disabilities of older adults to analyses of the stress mechanisms that underlie these changes. Cellular theories of aging and genetic theories propose that chemical changes, accumulation of waste materials, and cumulative effects of trauma and stress to the body cause disease and injury to the organism.

Stress may accelerate the aging process over a given time, and it is generally accepted that aging postmaturity is associated with a gradual decline in many psychological functions (Botwinick, 1973). Stress may impair the reserve capacity of the organism and compromise ability to respond. Especially in the elderly such decline may form the bases of several losses, cognitive and intellectual, not entirely understood so far.

In accord with this interest much effort has been expended on developing various psychological perspectives for studying the effects of stress on the elderly and toward examining distinct dimensions that are determinants of stress disorders. Efforts are also being made, from a therapeutic point of view, to study stress in the elderly from a variety of psychological perspectives.

Therefore it is the aim of this chapter to develop comprehensive conceptual and theoretical frameworks for understanding the impact of stress on the elderly, to discuss definitional issues of stress and explore the psychological and physiological mechanisms that mediate the negative impact of life stress on the elderly, to examine various perspectives and strategies of coping adopted by the elderly to achieve the person-environment fit, and finally to discuss tools and clinical procedures for assessing stressful life events and the availability of social support networks.

IMPACT OF STRESS ON THE ELDERLY

A summary of the effects and consequences of stress in the elderly is presented in Exhibit 5–1. The impact of stress can be understood from a number of perspectives. These

Exhibit 5–1 Effects and Impact of Stress on the Aged

1. *Subjective (Affective) Effects*

   Anxiety; agitated depression; loss of motivation; anhedonia or loss of interest; frustration and irritability; guilt and shame; nervousness; loneliness and feelings of self-pity; low self-worth; somatic concerns; extreme worries about the future in regard to health, finances, and social resources; feelings of mistrust and paranoia

2. *Cognitive Effects*

   Delusions of thought disorders without noticeable loss of memory or consciousness; disorientation and frequent forgetfulness; increase in mental blocks; loss of integration in thinking with lowered comprehension and clarity of expression; relative loss of vocabulary; easy distractibility; inability to make decisions; incapacity for persistent concentration or problem solving; hypersensitivity to criticism

3. *Health Effects*

   Cardiovascular disorders; circulatory insufficiency; myocardial infarction; diabetes mellitus; increased susceptibility to pulmonary and renal failure and to dizziness, faintness, and delirium. Chest and back pains; gastric motility, dyspepsia, diarrhea; insomnia and disturbed sleeping involving nightmares; frequent urination especially at night

4. *Physiological Effects*

   Gastric hyperfunction; hyperglycemia or elevated blood sugar levels; hypertension resulting in increased heart rate and blood pressure; hot spells; dryness of mouth; loss of energy; chronic fatigue; difficulty in breathing; prolonged loss of sensation in limbs; sudden loss of visual or auditory acuity

5. *Behavioral Effects*

   Increasing degree of psychomotor retardation or impaired motor function; increasing subordination, dependency, and withdrawal; reduction in acting out behaviors; diminishing aggression; functional deficiencies in communication including impaired speech; loss of appetite; increased use of alcohol or tranquilizers; restlessness, agitated random pacing; repetitive activity and repetitive dialogue; incapacity for routine tasks such as dressing, cooking, or minor chores; accident proneness (falling, slipping, spilling); increase in attention-seeking behaviors such as crying, sobbing, trembling; hypochrondriacal symptoms

Note: A complex interaction of subjective, cognitive, health, and physiological effects in terms of frequency, duration, and accumulation is assumed to precipitate the severe forms of behavioral effects.

perspectives are useful not merely in examining the immediate impact of stressful events but also in helping to explain the disorientation, disorganization, or the kind of pathogenesis immediately following a period of stress, and the psychic regression that follows as a long-term response to the stress. Titchener and Ross (1974) have identified the following psychological perspectives for understanding the impact of stress:

- A psychodynamic perspective attempts to understand the meaning of the stressful experiences for the individual person at both the conscious and unconscious level.

- An adaptive perspective is concerned with the nature of the relationship of the stressed individual with the environment, including the human and nonhuman aspects of the environment. Adaptations required of older persons may range from a new life style posed by retirement to learning to cope with the death of a loved one, to changes in daily living created by change in financial conditions, physical disability, and loss of social status.

- A psychogenetic perspective is concerned with examining the effects of experience on the response to impact and the process of reconstitution. (For further details on these threefold approaches, see Titchener & Ross, 1974.)

The value of these three approaches to the understanding of general psychological functioning in the elderly is significant mostly for purposes of reconstitution and treatment of the stressed elderly. Conceptions and descriptions of stress in the elderly as seen from these perspectives are based on clinical experience with the elderly and from the reports of experience of clinicians who have done psychotherapy with those stressed elderly with whom they were familiar in the prestress situation.

Psychodynamic Aspect

This aspect is concerned with the immediate impact of stress. The primary problem with regard to the reactions of many elderly to stress is the lack of meaning when it happens. Many elderly women, although prepared for widowhood, went through a period of anticipatory grief, yet still felt an absence of meaning regarding the bereavement (see Ujhely, 1963; Clayton, 1973). This external meaninglessness is the special challenge to coping with the stress. The external meaninglessness of the loss may contribute to the feelings of helplessness but must be assimilated and worked through before reintegration can begin.

As with all age groups but especially with the elderly, the situation of helplessness (as an aftermath of stress and bereavement) may have special implications and impact because of the diminution of physical strength and self-control in the aged. Such concerns about personal helplessness may dovetail with other serious concerns about deterioration of social and family roles (Rosow, 1974). Whereas a physically healthy and relatively active adult may understand the feelings of helplessness as temporary and simply get help where and whenever necessary, many physically ill elderly and those with rapidly depleting mental and physical energies may interpret the sense of helplessness following trauma as a permanent failure and become increasingly depressed and anxious.

Many elderly who are basically trusting, those who are flexibly confident of their interactions with friends and family members, or others who are cognizant of the strength of their role within the family may be accepting of their emotional dependency or even physical injury following a stressful accident. Other elderly, with a high sense of invulnerability or with conflicts over basic trust in friends and family, may interpret the stressful event as a deprivation beyond endurance and may become depressed and angry. Many elderly widowers have been observed to interpret the death of the spouse as a deprivation beyond toleration. Lacking confidence in their own capacities to continue without the role of husband, provider, and protector, many elderly men may become increasingly depressed and anxious. These elderly widowers with fundamental concerns about self-image may interpret the stress of the spouse's death as a personal failure. Thus the significance of the stress may be formed from unconscious needs and thoughts. These assigned meanings, arising from the depths of personality, may interact with prestress fears and anxieties about personal identity and strongly influence the poststress processes of reconstitution in the elderly widower.

The external meaninglessness of the spouse's death may cause many elderly who face this stress to create their own meaning for what has happened, often without regard to external reality. The survival guilt may make many elderly widows or widowers prone to angry self-condemnation, aggression, or agitation as a reflection of a powerful need to assign conscious meaning to stressful events and often to restore the loss by psychological means.

Adaptive Aspect

The understanding of the adaptive aspect of stress reactions is important with respect to the stages of reorganization, reintegration, and reconstitution. As noted by Titchener and Ross (1974, p. 47), the nature of the relationship of the individual to environment and other persons may be most central to the individual's adaptive reactions to the stress. The individual's sense of environment and patterns of human relations are the resources for responding to stress and for recovering from the impact of acute trauma.

Especially for the elderly individuals who have encountered trauma or stress, resuming meaningful relations during or after stress is a powerful resource for reorganization. For many elderly who have encountered stresses such as serious illness, bereavement, or separation from friends and family, meaningful communication with other humans restores structure and redefines the self. In the poststress period, relationship to reality is effectively restored through these connections with others.

Stress is an isolating experience for individuals at all ages, but it is a particularly solitary experience in old age. Following stress, the elderly are prone to sensing their environment in two extreme ways: hostile and friendly. This interpretation of friendly or hostile environment derives in large part from the past expressions, actions, and interactions of those who are in a relationship of trust with the elderly. The elderly's functions of adaptations may be revitalized by the warmth, assurance, and integrating power of personal interchange, or conversely, the potential connections among the fragmented parts of the self may be irreversibly shattered in a hostile environment. The responding capacity of the stressed individual is more likely to be eroded by isolation, loneliness, neglect, apathy, and stimulus deprivation in the formal structure. From this point of view any state of rejection following the stress or traumatic situation may permanently damage the elderly individual's capacity to accept the stress or loss or may damage the motivation to be restored physically or psychologically to a condition of recovery after the impact phase of a traumatic situation.

Psychogenetic Aspect

Titchener and Ross (1974) theorize that the psychogenetic perspective of stress contributes to a psychodynamic, developmental understanding of major aspects of the personality. First to be considered is the ego-functioning of the prestress and premorbid personality. Such an assessment would allow an estimate of the strength and weaknesses that the ego of the individual has to meet the stress. Second to be considered are the individual's particular emotional sensitivities and fragilities dating back to childhood and infancy (see Exhibit 5–2).

Such an assessment would uncover emotional and material deprivations and losses experienced in earlier life. The assumption is that recollections of helplessness conditions occasioned by stress in adulthood can be an extremely important factor in the elderly individual's capacity to accept physical and emotional losses and trauma in later life. Titchener and Ross (1974) speculate that the nature of the stimulus barrier, its resilience, and points of weakness are derived from early family experiences and from the protection that the family could afford the distressed individuals as they developed their own stimulus barrier (p. 48).

This twofold conceptualization of the psychogenetic determinants of stress reactions has special implications for the elderly. First, it signifies that the elderly's capacity to have a basic trust (in their family members, social support members, and medical and mental health practitioners) may provide strength for relieving the helplessness during and after the

---

Exhibit 5–2 Assessing Precursors and Precipitators of Stress Reactions
in the Aged

1. *Health Factors*
   Multiple health problems; chronic conditions such as coronary heart condition, high blood pressure, pernicious anemia, kidney failure; painful conditions such as arthritis, chest and back pain, asthma; threatened body-integrity resulting from surgery, accidents and loss of bowel control; genetic factors causing inability to control autonomic arousal; focal brain damage and diseases such as Cushing's disease, Parkinson's disease, Alzheimer's disease

2. *Personal-Social Factors*
   Gradually depleting financial resources; sudden loss of psychological role through adverse change, retirement, or disability; multiple social, economic, or personal losses; loss of spouse; loss of loved ones; family breakup; family relationships lacking in warmth and nurturance; forced disengagement as a result of external influences; loneliness and depression; predisposition to self-injurious behaviors

3. *Developmental and Early-Life Factors*
   Early childhood deprivations and losses such as loss of parents; divorce, separation, and family breakup in the early growing years; physical and psychological abuse in the early growing years; history of childhood illness and ill health; overprotective family environment; conflict-ridden family environment; history of depression, neurotic anxieties, and paranoid tendencies; dependent life style, anxiety traits, and emotional sensitivities

4. *Environmental and Ecological Factors*
   Environmental rejection combined with a concomitant decline in physical and financial resources; decline in social support and nurturant relationships; reduced social interaction; marked social isolation and sensory deprivation especially in the case of elderly who have held active and stimulating leadership positions; remoteness from health and medical facilities; and lack of proper health and medical care in previous instances of illness and disease

Note: A complex interaction of health, personal-social, developmental, and environmental factors in terms of their frequency, duration, and accumulation is assumed to precipitate the severe forms of stress.

impact phase of a traumatic situation (Erikson, 1959). Second, it suggests that an important first step in reconstitution of the elderly (after the immediate impact phase of stress situations) is the bringing together of the past sensitivities, the developmental cognitive factors, and the current internal resources.

Sometimes the trauma becomes a screen on which the patient projects all previous problems (Glover, 1929). We usually see in elderly clients whose histories include evidence of such significant emotional breakdowns before the traumatic event that a physical illness in old age becomes a screen on which the person projects family problems, problems of self-doubt, and problems of social rejection. This concept of the traumatic event as a screen for past problems explains why old age often becomes a stage of life in which physical illness, in addition to presenting medical problems, becomes a common psychic stress, especially in many dependent-type elderly, leading to a much enhanced and regressive investment in the self.

The death of a spouse is also a particularly potent stress agent even in those elderly who may have anticipated the death of the spouse for many years. Nevertheless, the knowledge and recognition that the loss of the spouse implies that the elderly survivor has to face a drastically altered environment may be a particularly strong precursor of stress and a potent stress agent (see Exhibit 5–2). The elderly individual may unconsciously lapse into a state of narcissistic regression, and various depressive, psychosomatic, and hypochondriacal symptoms may follow these stresses (Epstein, 1976).

Titchener and Ross (1974) note that suicidal intent leading to trauma or chronic stress does not lessen the psychological effects of impact, even though the individual intended to do harm. This observation may have special implications for suicidal elderly who experience great stress following an incomplete suicidal act and who may often revert to a narcissistic withdrawal state following the trauma. Suicidal acts, however, do not lessen problems of recovery. It may appear temporarily as if the suicidal elderly has reached a resolution to the problem, but in a majority of cases it has been shown that elderly with suicidal intent may use one recent stressful or aversive event on which to project a number of other depressive-emotional conflicts or problems of adjusting with family. Some suicidal reactions to stress are not episodic or repetitive but may develop from situations of intense personal conflict with a family member. They may also develop from losses, changes in relationship during old age, and religiosity resulting in much depression, hopelessness, and anomie for the elderly individuals (Fry, 1984).

PHYSIOLOGICAL ASPECTS OF STRESS

Numerous studies have found a significant relationship between the elevation of life stresses and a wide range of physiological responses mediated through a large number of biological mechanisms. Renner and Birren (1980) note that when an individual is confronted with stressors that present a threat, cause frustration, or demand dealing with crises or emergency, certain physiological and psychological reaction patterns are set up to allow the individual to adapt and protect the self. Wolff (1950, p. 1064) postulated that individuals involved in continual feelings of stress, emotional deprivation, and lack of support may experience considerable gastric hyperfunction in the stomach. A variety of gastrointestinal disorders may result due to the prolonged adaptive use of the gastrointestinal tract to cope with provoking or threatening situations. In old age in particular, other bodily adaptive patterns may result in cardiovascular disease, circulatory insufficiency, hypertension, and a variety of metabolic diseases (see Exhibit 5–1).

As noted by Renner and Birren (1980), past and current stressful life experiences may act as catalysts to alter a person's susceptibility to stress-related diseases, and this susceptibility presumably increases with aging. Gellhorn and Kiely (1973) and Kiely (1976) have drawn attention to a number of psychosomatic disorders that may appear in old age as a direct effect of stresses. It is suggested (Kiely, 1976) that of the two neurobiological systems, the trophotropic system and the ergotropic system, it is difficult to determine which may become more dominant in creating stress-related psychiatric disorders in the elderly.

Mediated by changes in the reticular formation, hypothalamus, the limbic system, and the higher cortical regions, the ergotropic system "is characterized by alerting, arousal, excitement, increased muscle tone, and sympathetic nervous activity, and the release of catabolic hormonal products" (Kiely, 1974, p. 518). In contrast the trophotropic system, in order to conserve energy and permit withdrawal, raises its perceptual stimulus threshold and is thus characterized by decreased skeletal muscle tone, increased parasympathetic nervous function, and the circulation of anabolic hormones" (Kiely, 1974, p. 518).

In old age the stress-related psychiatric symptoms could result from either system acting independently or simultaneously and be manifest in symptoms of anxiety, agitated depression, and delusions of thought disorders without loss of memory or consciousness (Kiely, 1976, p. 2759). Kiely (1976) has argued that the elderly are more prone to delirium symptoms and agitated depression because of their increased susceptibility to cardiac, pulmonary, or renal failure, which may lead to cerebral inefficiency. The following stress-related reactions are frequently noted in the elderly. (See Exhibit 5–1 for summary of effects of stress on the aged.)

Stress Reactions and Reduction in Aggression

In examining the elderly's physiological responses to stress, a number of authors (e.g., Henry, 1976; Henry & Ely, 1976; Henry & Stephens, 1977) postulate that when the organism perceives the stressor or threat to involve defeat, failure, loss of status, inability to fulfill expectations, or loss of control, the predominating physiological response does not involve the sympathetic adrenal medullary chain but rather the pituitary adrenal cortical system. Henry (1976, p. 67) claims that with increasing age there is a shift in the type of response evoked under circumstances of stress, challenges, or threats imposed on the elderly persons. As the person ages, the stress response may shift from a preponderance of the active, acting-out, sympathetic adrenal medullary mode toward a greater participation of the adrenal cortical mode. "This shift would be reflected in the elderly's decreasing sense of control, of subordination with diminishing aggressiveness, and of an increased bottling up of emotions as aging progresses" (p. 67).

The reduction of aggressive behavior in old age may often mistakenly be viewed as adaptation and adjustment to aversive stimuli in the environment. Reis, Ross, Brodsky, Specht, and Joh (1976) and Henry (1976) emphasize the need for stress research and for practitioners working with elderly clients, to take into account the factor of age when outward symptoms of withdrawal, subordination, and diminished affective responses are seen in elderly clients under circumstances of supposedly high stress, anxiety, and threat.

Evidence (Everitt & Burgess, 1976) suggests that a substantial part of the regulation of the aging process may be centered in the hypothalamus and the related pituitary-endocrine axis. The declining ability of the organism to undergo regenerative processes in the brain is related to declining regulatory processes in the central nervous system and hormonal systems. Renner and Birren (1980) postulate that such breakdown phenomena are concomitant with aging and are accelerated under chronic or persistent stress.

Stress Reactions and Endocrine Changes

Ordy and Kaack (1976, p. 290) have emphasized the need to take into account the endocrine disorders that tend to increase with age and stress. These researchers note that endocrine changes involving the hormone insulin may result in diabetes mellitus, which increases in incidence with age. Other endocrine disorders that may also result from functional disregulation of the hypothalamus and of hypothalamic misinformation of the organism (Frolkis, 1976, p. 630) involve vascular and metabolic complications that may be due to changes in the thyroid hormones. All such endocrine disorders have a good prognosis if detected in time but if neglected over prolonged periods of stress, may permanently reduce the adaptive abilities of the elderly individual and lead to age-related pathological disorders such as hypertension, myocardial infarction, atherosclerosis, and diabetes mellitus—abnormalities related to such disorders as Cushing's syndrome (see Exhibit 5–1).

Blood pressure increases with age and may result in hypertension with subsequent coronary arterial disease or cerebral vascular disease. Although a variety of factors may be involved in the endocrine disorders in old age, Renner and Birren (1980) caution that they are not merely age-related disorders. In their experience these disorders are also stress-related diseases that tend to have a greater incidence among older persons. These authors maintain that the hormones involved (e.g., renin, angiotensin, and aldosterone) are the hormones of stress, and therefore the illnesses of old age are not just the expression of peripheral constitutional effects but heavily involve the endocrine and neuroendocrine systems. It is suggested that stressful events and the mismanagement of external stressful events may contribute sufficiently to internal stressful consequences so as to exacerbate disease symptoms in the elderly.

Stress Reactions and Adaptation Energy

Selye has been a primary force in propounding the discovery of a triphasic general adaptation syndrome (alarm reaction, stage of resistance in which there is an increased capacity for the organism to respond, and exhaustion stage), which also implies a severe decline in the organism's adaptation energy. In the final stage, that is, the exhaustion stage, the ability of the organism to adapt to the stressors is weakened considerably as a function of the pituitary adrenal cortical responses to stress. The release of such diverse hormones as adrenocorticotropic hormone (ACTH) is normally regulated by the central nervous system (CNS), which in turn is regulated by the hypothalamus. It is suggested that such conditions as chronic and persistent stress impose continual wear and tear on the organism's physiological responses. If there is a decreased regulatory effectiveness in the CNS and ANS, common in old age, the elderly person's continued subjection to stressful psychosocial stimuli will impose wear-and-tear effects on the physiological structures. Thus continued exposure to stressful stimuli in old age combined with general aging factors may account for greater disease symptoms as well as decremental performance patterns such as slower reaction times and decline in learning and cognitive abilities.

Although the stress response is specific for each individual depending on genetic endowment and past experiences of the individual, the reactions of stress are powerful enough in old age so as to utilize great amounts of adaptation energy and result in diseases primarily from pituitary hormone imbalances. Furthermore, as Renner and Birren (1980) note, not only may the individual's emotional or mental health state affect the onset of these diseases, but the existence of such disease states as hypertension commonly associated with very high tension, agitation, and anxiety levels may in turn affect the mental states of the people concerned (Exhibit 5–1).

One of the important implications of this notion of stress induction is that the process of aging will be accelerated with continued exposure to stressful stimuli. Since exacerbation of disease states may be modulated by stressful events, it follows that every encounter with such a stressful event may use up considerable ratios of the adaptation energy, of which there is only a fixed amount (Selye & Tuchweber, 1976, 1978). Renner and Birren's (1980, p. 321) analysis of senescent decline in capacity to respond implies that an older person may show greater stress-related disease in a period in which the number of stressful events themselves may decline but consume considerable amounts of adaptation energy to adapt to even little stresses.

Life Stress and Disease

Investigation has been directed at the toll of diverse life stresses in the origin and course of physical or mental illness. With advancing age, there is apparent increase in the relative incidence of deaths due to diseases suspected of being related to stress (e.g., diseases of the heart, cancer, and cerebrovascular diseases, mainly strokes). Studies in psychosomatic medicine also show that social-psychological stress has been implicated in a wide variety of old age diseases (Moos, 1977; Selye, 1976; Hurst, Jenkins, & Rose, 1979).

The results of numerous studies (e.g., Holmes & Rahe, 1967; Rahe, Biersner, Ryman, & Arthur, 1972) indicate that clusters of life events and transitions precede the onset of illness and that with increasing age there is presumed loss of physiologic adaptability to cope with the stressful life events. A number of other studies (e.g., Henry & Ely, 1976; Henry & Stephens, 1977; Schally, Kastin, & Arimura, 1977) have also supported the claim that disease may develop or be exacerbated by the continual exposure to stress that would increase the output of stress hormone. Bessman (1976) refers to the specific and nonspecific physiological and biochemical reactions that occur to some degree in all humans under various conditions of stress. According to his biphasic approach the pathological consequences of stress in the first phase include hyperglycemia, ketonemia, and eventually diabetic ketoacidosis. Consequences of the second phase of stress additionally involve breakdown of protein and liberation of amino acids, causing elevated blood sugar levels. Eventually, as Bessman (1976) notes, the uncontrolled mechanisms of the biphasic processes of stress simulate the conditions of diabetes.

A number of other studies (e.g., Andres & Tobin, 1977; Burgess, 1976) note that with increasing age the body's metabolic preparation to meet the threat or stress becomes increasingly ineffective and the machinery becomes less and less adaptive and efficient. Thus Bessman's biphasic theory has special applicability to old age. It implies that elderly persons who are under stressful situations are particularly vulnerable to a diabetic condition, the onset of which is considered to be related to stressful conditions. With regard to the physiological mechanisms that mediate stress reactions, many issues of physiological responses to stress and many issues of pharmacology effects on physiological stress are hitherto quite unclear and will need considerable research.

PSYCHOLOGICAL DISORGANIZATION AND REGRESSION AS AN ADAPTIVE RESPONSE TO STRESS

In many elderly the disorientation and changes in perception that follow stress may not be as self-limiting as they might be at younger ages. Often there is a loss of integration of thinking and fragmentation, which lowers comprehension and clarity of expression of thoughts. The disorganization may take the form of distortions in thinking, memory disturbance, and incapacity to understand a situation and to perceive clearly what is happening. Some of these symptoms may closely resemble the disorganization reflected in brain damage or brain impairment cases in which there are similar symptoms of blunting of awareness, disturbance in perception, and defects of judgment. The potentials for misdiagnosis may have serious implications. While some degree of disorganization is expected in all elderly experiencing a traumatic event, the greater concern of the clinician and the family members is with the degree of cognitive and perceptual impairment in some elderly and the duration of such disorders. Unfortunately, whether resulting from misdiagnosis or neglect, the longer-term disorganization effect sensitizes the individual to all other types of adverse happenings in the environment. Over the long term the reconstitution of the elderly client is considerably hampered, and the number of traumatic events with which the elderly must learn to adjust increase in significant proportions (Amster & Krauss, 1974).

While psychic regression in behavior, feeling, and mental function is often the most adaptive reaction of the elderly individuals faced with traumatic loss, illness, or other severe trauma, it is still the intrapsychic process least understood by family and friends of the elderly, who are likely to become upset by the elderly individual's regressive behaviors. Many elderly, as a part of this psychic regression (which is often narcissistic in nature), may resort to either dependent or aggressive ways of relating, adjusting, communicating, problem solving, and behaving. As noted by several observers of the psychic regression following trauma, regression is at first a means of resilience that helps the afflicted individual to resist the overwhelming stimuli accompanying the trauma. Later it may become a fixed pattern that may prevent a resumption of the more mature responses (Grinker & Spiegel, 1945; Titchener, 1970; Ross, 1966). While this regressive tendency may have less of an effect on the already diminishing ego functions of the afflicted elderly, all efforts must be made to work toward the reversibility of the regressive process.

ASSESSMENT OF POSTSTRESS ADAPTATION

Assessment of Psychosocial and Cognitive Factors

Reconstitution and poststress adaptation of the elderly client will involve a step-by-step assessment of many psychosocial aspects of adaptation such as the following.

Assessing Life Stress as Related to Depression

A number of authors (e.g., Miller, Ingham, & Davidson, 1976; Plutchik, Hyman, Conte, & Karasu, 1977; Rahe & Arthur, 1978; Blazer, 1980) have drawn attention to the relationship between stressful life events, psychological depression, and medical illness. Also, it has been widely assumed that individuals differ in their vulnerability to stress, and thus the relationship between life stress and affective disorders is higher for some subsets of individuals than others (Meehl, 1962; Rosenthal, 1970; Zubin & Spring, 1977).

Goodstein (1981) notes that by the nature of sheer longevity the elderly face multiple stresses acting in tandem across social, psychologic, and biologic parameters. Therefore, in any systematic approach to assessment, Goodstein advocates a study of the elderly individual's stresses in the social sphere, personal-emotional stresses, and increased susceptibility to stress due to altered physiologic function and metabolic aging. In addition to the overlap of stresses in various life spheres, a number of authors assume that the individual's responses to these stresses depends on other factors of psychosocial functioning such as previous ego-strength and coping styles, present support systems, and type of previous health care provided (Busse, 1971; Pfeiffer, 1971; Eisdorfer, 1977), which will influence the elderly individual's future adaptation (Exhibit 5–2).

Therefore a study of stress factors and the social support systems available to the elderly is always of clinical interest to social gerontologists. The assumption is made that stress contributes to depression and depressive disorders by depleting the reserve capacity of all organisms. (See Osgood's 1985 model of stress, depression, and suicide.) Verwoerdt (1981) proposes that psychological decompensation may occur as a result of accumulated and cumulative stress states, hastening in the elderly individuals a process of withdrawal, depressive regression, and reduced perception of the pain of organismic stress.

Meier-Ruge (1975) notes that with advancing years and advancing stress adaptation the protein synthesis balance of the aging brain is affected, resulting in some degree of change in metabolic activity. Gradually, repeated and persistent stress may result in irreversible cognitive, physical, and affective impairment symptoms. Gaitz and Varner (1980, p. 384) propose that metabolic disturbance may explain at least partially the development of pseudodementia, a condition associated with advancing years. It may be that psychological and social stress factors are first implicated in anxiety states of the elderly and subsequently implicated in some forms of pseudodementia in the elderly.

The assessment of stress factors, both predisposing and precipitating (Exhibit 5–2 and Table 5–1), should take into account the reduced adaptive capacity of the elderly individual. How much lessened adaptivity there may be depends on the number of stresses occurring for the individual and the stress adaptiveness of the individual in terms of personality and life style. Conceivably, then, extremes of isolation and withdrawal during stress may be effective adaptive strategies in late life. During stress many elderly may even manifest apparent cognitive impairment often related to the emotional state but may retain few or none of these signs of withdrawal when the stress fades or is reduced.

Assessing Personality and Life-Style Correlates

A number of authors (e.g., Chiriboga & Cutler, 1980; Bergmann, 1972; Siegel, Johnson, & Sarason, 1979) have examined the relationship between stress adaptiveness and personality types, emotional states and life styles of the elderly. A general conclusion emerging from the literature is that certain personality types with certain characteristics show a greater degree of tension, exertion, and unadaptive responses to stress events. It is therefore suggested that the elderly individual's lifelong personality traits represent a set of constants that will determine the individual's affective states following exposure to stressful events.

Rosen (1961) in examining life style refers to the sum total of drive and ego. He defines *life style* as a "progressing synthesis of form and content in an individually typical manner and according to the individual's sense of appropriateness" (p. 447). Thus according to Rosen style is one of the most constant aspects of expressive activity in the individual. Berezin (1972b, p. 486) observes that a commitment to a way of life linked to the

Table 5–1 Assessment of Coping Styles and Coping Resources

Assessing Coping Styles		Assessing Coping Resources
Adaptive	*Unadaptive*	

(Characterized by flexibility, purposiveness, and organization)	(Characterized by rigidity, constraint, and excessiveness)	1. *Health Factors:*
		  a. Positive factors include high-level energy, stamina, determination, and sound cognitive and sensory functioning.
		  b. Adverse factors include physical illness, low stamina, fatigue, low resistance, organic problems, physical handicaps, cognitive impairment, respiratory problems, gastric motility, and partial or total loss of visual and auditory acuity.

1. Individuals' use of instrumental strategies whereby they take action; initiate change; control and manipulate the stressful environment; adopt an information-seeking, direct action, and problem-solving orientation.	4. Individuals' use of escapist resolution of problem strategies whereby they refuse to talk about the problem and deny that they are stressed.	

2. Individuals' use of intrapsychic strategies whereby they seek psychological solutions to problems of stress in their environment (cognitive reappraisals of stressful events; acceptance of their limitations).	5. Individuals' use of resigned helplessness strategies: taking on the sick role or being helpless and letting others handle the stressful event.	2. *Psychological Factors*
		  a. Positive factors include high self-esteem and traits of assertiveness and aggressiveness, ability to introspect, high levels of hope and motivation to deal with common stresses of old age: role loss, family conflict, grief and bereavement, and economic loss.
		  b. Adverse factors include traits of dependency, passivity, anomie, low self-esteem, and pessimism.

3. Individuals' use of affective strategies aimed at reducing emotional distress through crying or appealing to others for help in stressful circumstances. Individuals admit that such strategies may be effective in releasing tension and reducing stress.		3. *Social Factors*
		  a. Positive factors include high levels of income, education, and density of active and reactive social network and effective interpersonal skills, enabling the person to relate to influential others, seek information, and take direct action.
		  b. Adverse factors include poverty, illiteracy, and lack of human relatedness.

Note: A complex interaction of unadaptive coping styles and deficits in health, psychological and social resources is assumed to precipitate severe forms of stress.

personality style becomes stabilized and is usually unaltered by circumstances of daily routine. However, if unusual life events (e.g., a major loss) deprive an elderly individual of the opportunity to continue with a style of life, the aged individual will respond with severe stress and distress, often leading to depression and dysphoria (Bergmann, 1972).

Personality characteristics acquired earlier in life functioning may predispose certain older individuals to resort to certain life-style functionings that may serve as effective adaptive strategies in later life. Gaitz and Varner (1980) speculate, for example, that older persons who were labeled *paranoid, hostile,* or *aggressive* in their earlier years may often have learned to do without social activity and intimate relationships. Therefore such individuals in old age may continue in a self-contained and self-sufficient modal style.

The theory of disengagement advanced by Cumming and Henry (1961) is a similar concept that views the aging individuals as withdrawing from intense or stressful involvement or engagement in their social world while at the same time permitting society to disengage them from intense transactions. By contrast proponents of activity theory (see Maddox, Busse, Siegler, Nowlin, Palmore, & Cleveland, 1977; Neugarten, 1964) have argued that good adaptation in later life is more often a function of a high level of activity. More recent research review has found a positive association of activity and well-being. Butler (1975) notes, however, that each elderly person must individually determine what has been attained in a lifetime of learning and adapting; the elderly must conserve strength and resources wherever and however necessary and adjust creatively to stresses and losses of the aging experience.

Thus, from the perspective of the mental health practitioner, disengagement is neither to be encouraged nor discouraged. Because of the wide range of physical abilities, past experiences with life stresses, and past successes or failures in adapting to losses, the path toward disengagement or continuing involvement will vary from one individual to another.

Chiriboga and Cutler (1980) suggest that the practitioner's assessment of the elderly individual's life-style patterns before the encounter with life stressors would facilitate the prediction of how the individual would manage stress. For example, some people might have been stress avoiders in their earlier years, whereas others may have enjoyed the stimulation and exhilaration of braving new experiences. In assessing the individual's depression and affective functioning in the context of late-life stresses, the practitioner may find it especially significant to examine long-term patterns of individuals' responses to stressful circumstances within a continuity framework (Fiske, 1980; Renner & Birren, 1980).

In regard to adaptation to late-life stresses, Blazer (1982, p. 94) notes that although older people appear to experience fewer stressful events, the question has not been addressed as to whether this particular cohort of older adults may have had a longstanding life style of stress avoidance or whether the apparent decrease in exposure to life events is a function of the environmental management of stresses organized and provided by the social support network (Nuckolls, Cassel, & Kaplan, 1972). Hence, Blazer (1982) suggests that a detailed assessment of the social support networks is important to understanding the stress preoccupations reported by the elderly.

The age transition studies of Fiske (1980) and Renner and Birren (1980) have particular relevance to stress and aging. According to Fiske (1980, p. 354) the timing of stressful events and circumstances accounts for variations in the way the elderly respond to stress. Important dimensions include stresses of early life, slowly accumulating stress, a steady stream of new and concurrent pressures occurring at the same time, sudden or precipitating stress, and finally the anticipation of stresses to be encountered in the future.

Fiske (1980) contends that many elderly who underwent a barrage of problems and events in several spheres of their lives are thought to be the least susceptible to precipitating stress that triggers mental disturbance, depression, and physical illness. Unlike people who have had a great many stressful experiences in their early or middle years, it is conceivable that these elderly individuals adopted life styles that protected them from stress. Thus the relation of the individual to stresses in the environment is at the crux of understanding the behavior of the elderly and at the crux of identifying some of the personal or environmental variables that make for successful aging or coping in old age.

Renner and Birren (1980) suggest four categories of personality coping styles that play a significant role in determining how one deals with stressful circumstances and the degree of emotion or psychological significance one associates with particular events:

1. The environmental stress amplifiers, the personalities that on being exposed to a stressful stimulus, however trivial, amplify the distressful situation and magnify the stressful implications surrounding routine circumstances.
2. The environmental stress dampeners or insulators, the personalities that avoid events that may be stressful. Such individuals minimize the significance of any stressful events both in terms of behavioral reactions and verbal responses. Categories 1 and 2 may apply to the elderly individuals' behavioral tendencies and provide some measure of the emotional, symbolic, or psychological significance that they may associate with particular events.
3. The internal stress amplifiers, those individuals whose coping styles lead to heightened emotional arousal, which can be of long duration, even in response to apparently minor crises.
4. The internal stress dampeners or insulators, whose coping style allows them to reduce the intensity and duration of physiological arousal in response to stress. These personalities on being exposed to stressful stimuli, however severe, tend to dampen or reduce their significance.

The last two categories, which relate to the individuals' internal or physiological responses, reflect the intensity, frequency, and duration of emotional arousal in response to stressful events. One of the important implications of this notion of stress for the elderly is that the process of aging will be accelerated with continual emotional arousal responses to stressful stimuli.

Recent studies have investigated actual coping strategies that middle-aged and older adults have used or could use in specific stressful situations (see Birren, 1969). Lazarus (1975a, 1975b) and Stenback (1975) have emphasized the importance of cognitive restructuring, which can be used by individuals when confronted with a stressful situation. Birren (1969) and Birren and Renner (1980) refer to psychological defenses such as relaxation therapy and assertive training, which can be used to regulate the amount of autonomic nervous system (ANS) arousal. Knowledge of such management procedures could enable internal stress dampening styles of coping to generate less arousal than those who internally amplify stressful stimuli.

Assessing Genetic and Constitutional Factors as Related to Late-Life Stress

In examining the parameters of late-life stress, Bergmann (1972) noted that constitutional and genetic factors influence the quality and quantity of the individual's autonomic arousal in the presence of stress stimuli. The suggestion is that some individuals may be genetically predisposed to anxiety state or depressive affective states. Similarly it has been suggested that individuals who experienced physical illness in early life and became fatigue-prone might resort to a longstanding dependent life style (Exhibit 5–2). Such individuals are more likely to avoid social stressors and accept or actively seek protection and nurturance from the social network during stressful periods in their advanced years.

Bergmann (1972) concludes that genetic factors and early environmental experience may to a very large measure determine the motivations and ability of elderly persons to succumb to or withstand the stresses of old age (Exhibit 5–2). It is suggested by a number of authors (e.g., Bergmann, 1972; Gaitz & Varner, 1980; Siegel, Johnson, & Sarason, 1979) that the influence of psychosocial factors as stressors may be somewhat overemphasized and overrated. When the effects of psychosocial stressors are examined in the elderly, the strain, tension, and duress usually attributed to social stressors may be in many cases the byproducts of genetic and physical disorders in early life that continued into later years and seriously affected the elderly individuals' stress reactions.

Assessing Psychic Precursors of Late-Life Stress

While it is expected and accepted that emotional pressures are part of everyone's daily experience, Dowd and Brooks (1978) suggest that the elderly experience a deep anomie that is often accompanied by a conscious estrangement from their social institutions and their environment and this anomie is both actual stress and stressful. Thus, according to Seeman (1976) more consideration should be given to abstract concepts such as alienation and anomie that the elderly experience. Seeman found six parameters of alienation that were assumed to be stressful to the elderly in particular: these are feelings of powerlessness, meaninglessness, normlessness, cultural estrangement, social isolation, and self-estrangement. Using these parameters, Martin, Bengtson, and Acock (1974) found that these stressors were higher in old age than during middle age. These authors postulated that the feelings of alienation combined with a concomitant decline in physical and psychological resources are a more erosive loss of support in old age. The interaction of these parameters may therefore be particularly stressful in later years of life. Given what may be the narrower limits of the adaptive capacity in old age, even a small amount of psychic stress may have a stronger and more protracted impact on the older person (Renner & Birren, 1980, p. 330). Thus one of the important implications of studying the psychic components of stress in the elderly is the matter of sensitizing professionals to the potential outcomes of anomie and loss of meaning for life.

Distinguishing Results of Stress from Precipitators of Stress

Gaitz and Varner (1980, p. 382) draw the clinician and practitioner's attention to the significance of distinguishing between the stressor (that which induces the stressful state) and the result of stress. Thus with respect to the elderly, depression and the related concomitants such as anxiety, grief, and somatic concerns all may represent results of stress, while inevitable life events in the later years such as retirement, reduced income, family breakup, reduced social interaction, and sensory deprivation are more appropriately the stressors (Exhibit 5–2). As noted by a number of authors (e.g., Eisdorfer, 1977; Gaitz & Varner, 1980; Verwoerdt, 1976), the manifestations of both depression and stress as seen in the elderly are varied and cover a range of emotional, physical, and behavioral symptoms.

However, results of stress may also become stressors in themselves if they are not altered or mitigated in some way (Gaitz & Varner, 1980).

Concerning depression and stress in the elderly, the picture is rather complex in that both the precursors (Exhibit 5–2) and consequences of stress (Exhibit 5–1) manifest themselves in depressive symptoms. Although it may be assumed that depression will subside when the environmental stressors cease or are eliminated, remission in depression in the elderly may be very slow or depression may become chronic if the stressors have been allowed to persist. Lloyd's (1980a, 1980b) review of the literature on stressful life events and their relationship with depression shows that the dimensions of loss and separation, loss of activity, and insufficiency of pleasant life events are both the predisposing and precipitating life events that contribute to stress and depression (Grauer, 1977).

Assessing Cognitive and Perceptual Functioning in Poststress

There is an interaction between stress factors and cognitive deterioration of the elderly necessitating a systematic assessment of cognitive functioning in the etiological picture of stress (Savage, 1975). Wechsler (1958) was concerned with deterioration in the intellectual capacities of the aged and found that some subtests (e.g., comprehension, object assembly, and vocabulary) of the adult intelligence scale (WAIS) hold up with age while others (e.g., speeded tasks, arithmetic, and abstract reasoning tasks such as block design and similarities) decline with stress. Cath (1976) and Jarvik and Blum (1971) present a more balanced view of the issues involved in the cognitive decline and regressive phenomena in the stressed elderly. They support the idea that elderly subjects tend to be uneven in their functioning with some abilities showing signs of deterioration and decline during stress and distress and other abilities staying stable.

However, in any psychosocial evaluation of the elderly's functioning following crises or stress events, the measured extent of deficit or lack of deficit may be a function of the specific ability assessed. Other authors (e.g., Savage, 1975) who emphasize the malfunctional aspects in poststress functioning focus more on the regressed thought and behavior that is evident in the elderly and may be a definite indicator of stress, not to be confused with organic impairment of the brain.

Horowitz (1980) notes that under stress the prototypical anxious person might likely become considerably impaired in motor, perceptual, and interpretive functions. Shapiro (1965) notes a lack of sharp focus of attention and a corresponding lack of factual detail plus distractibility and incapacity for persistent or intense concentration. Shapiro regards these patterns as relatively fixed, perhaps the result of constitutional predisposition and earlier life experiences. Other analysts regard them more likely during stress. With respect to the elderly, either position is acceptable since both allow us to assume a fixed baseline of cognitive-perceptual style and an intensification of such patterns during stress. It is not uncommon for a general defective style of representation of perception, thought, and emotion to emerge in many elderly in the poststress period. This may lead to observable disorders in interpersonal relations, traits, and communication styles, not to be confused with organic brain syndrome or irreversible regressive behaviors. According to Horowitz (1980, p. 376) short-order patterns of information-processing style may be adversely affected. The clinician's observations of the elderly's flow of thoughts and communication may reveal global disruption of attention, unclear or incomplete representations of ideas and feelings, possibly with lack of details.

In terms of traits the clinician's observations in interviews with the distressed elderly client may reveal many attention-seeking behaviors, including childlike demands or aggressive demands for attention. There may be many inconsistencies in apparent attitudes and fluid changes in mood and emotion. Horowitz (1980) notes that as with all age groups, observation of elderly clients under stress shows that they often regress to victim-aggressor or child-parent repetitive interpersonal relationships. Similarly a number of other authors (e.g., Sobel, 1980; Fenichel, 1945; Camaron, 1967) note that losses of various kinds— death of a loved one, ill health, threatened body integrity, reduced cerebral and physiological reserve, and environmental deprivation (which constitute the powerful enemies)—may distort perceptions of reality and precipitate regression in the cognitive, perceptual functioning. Horowitz (1980) cautions practitioners that these are typically hysterical responses to stress and should be treated as such. However, as certain gerontologists (e.g., Palmore, 1980; Pfeiffer, 1980) note, prolonged periods of stress may contribute to more observable loss of cognitive dysfunctioning and may permanently affect the interpersonal relations of the elderly. Even after the stresses have been eliminated, many functional deficits in communication, attention-seeking behaviors, and cognitive dysfunctioning may persist awhile or even indefinitely.

Other mediating factors that influence the relationship between stress and depressive disorders may be the aging brain, genetic factors, concomitant disease states, depleting social and financial resources, and psychological traits and defenses (Gaitz & Varner, 1980) and ageism. Hence, practitioners working with elderly clients need to be more cognizant of stressful life events, as mediating precipitating or causative factors in depression in the elderly.

Practitioners should consider also the role of cultural differences in the elderly's responses to life stresses and strains. Because of the cultural awkwardness and uneasiness in knowing how to comfort grieving elderly people, or how to seek comfort, the elderly are often forced to fall on their own resources in times of life stress. For all these reasons the elderly are at greater risk for being victims of ageism-related stressful events (Butler, 1975; Perlin & Butler, 1963). In this connection there is the need for assessing individual life stressors as opposed to universal general stressors, which may have little relevance to the individual life style and psychosocial assets or deficits of the elderly client.

Assessment of precipitating stressful events can uncover information that is often critical for the treatment of depression. As Gaitz and Varner (1980, p. 388) note, "early recognition and intervention to neutralize or at least minimize the effects of stressors carries with it the promise of avoiding later stressful impairment or dysfunctioning."

COPING IN OLD AGE

Verwoerdt (1981, p. 369) defines *coping* as that state between the organism and the environment that allows the organism to conform to the reality of the external world while at the same time allowing activity directed toward change. Similarly Lazarus and Launier (1978, p. 311) define *coping* as "efforts, both action oriented and intrapsychic, to manage (that is, to master, tolerate, reduce, minimize) environmental and internal demands and conflicts among them which tax or exceed a person's resources." Among the important features of such a definition is that reference to taxing demands limits the concept of coping to stressful transactions rather than to adaptations in general. Second, the definition is process oriented, as opposed to more structural definitions that are keyed to generalized dispositions or styles or to hierarchies of coping and defensive mechanisms. Third, it is broader than many traditional delineations of the function of coping in that it admits to an action or problem-solving function as well as that of regulating the emotional response (Coyne & Lazarus, 1980).

In considering these conceptualizations of coping they allow for two main functions: the alteration of the ongoing person-environment relationship (instrumental or problem-oriented) and the control of stressful emotions (emotional regulation). They also allow for two main approaches: adaptive and unadaptive. Verwoerdt (1976) stresses the notion that whether coping is adaptive or maladaptive depends on the type and intensity of the defenses that the individual brings into the later years as well as on their appropriateness to the situation.

Verwoerdt (1981, p. 34) suggests that adaptive coping techniques imply a reestablishment of an equilibrium in the environment that was disturbed due to a stressful event such as a loss or physical illness frequently encountered in old age. The adaptive coping presupposes that the individual is cognitively aware of the stressful loss or illness and will take reasonable action or initiative in seeking assistance, support, or medical intervention. Conversely the maladaptive coping behavior implies that the individual prolongs or aggravates the problem or stressful situation by not dealing with it but rather avoiding it, denying the presence of a problem or a stressful situation or expressing bodily overconcern about it.

Implicit in Verwoerdt's (1981) discussion of coping behavior and strategies is the notion that coping strategies learned earlier may not be appropriate in the poststress environment. The capacity for coping with stress is a function of the ego and the elderly individual's degree of success in coping will depend very much on the postadaptational assets and liabilities that the individual brings to the late-life functioning (Table 5–1).

The aged person who has to cope with a multitude of losses in the face of declining physical and mental energies often has to adapt to new ways of coping (Zetzel, 1966). First, the usual ways of coping, especially the high-energy defenses, may have to be replaced. The active mastery approach, for example, may have to be replaced by acceptance and the capacity to resign oneself to the realities of the environment so as to avoid prolonged agitation, frustration, and bitterness (Zetzel, 1966).

High-energy individuals who have been accustomed to dealing with crises through active and aggressive mastery strategies may feel especially vulnerable in old age, when certain considerations of energy conservation require the individual to let go and to give in. Such high-energy individuals may find it hard to give up the fight and may cling to an independence and an aggressive coping that may have been appropriate in the past but has lost its usefulness. Such personalities perhaps were action-prone or tended to act out. Old-age decline in energies may interfere with their habitual activities, and the adequacy of their impulse controls may correspondingly deteriorate with old age. Such elderly may respond to stress and crises by becoming angry and frustrated and may need to learn new techniques of low-energy coping patterns.

By contrast low-energy individuals who in their previous functioning relied largely on coping patterns requiring little energy, may feel quite comfortable with the regressive modes of adaptation frequently required or encountered in old age (Verwoerdt, 1981). Such individuals may revert to dependent, submissive, and disengaged modes of adaptation, frequently reinforced in old age. On the other hand, if such elderly are faced with the challenge or stress of moving to a new environment, they may find their low-energy coping styles inadequate for meeting the demands of the new situation. When such an adjustment is unavoidable, the individual must function in a dissonant milieu. Stress and discomfort are assumed to follow (Stern, 1970). The elderly individual may feel especially vulnerable to environmental incongruence and may find it especially problematic to be placed in an environment where a high-energy, active mastery approach is expected.

The practitioner or clinician can assess the elderly individual's capacity for coping by exploring the individual's manner of coping with stress in the past, the objective signs of achievement in the past, and the subjective sense of satisfaction with identified life phases (e.g., occupational career, parenthood, widowhood).

THE PERSON-ENVIRONMENT CONGRUENCE MODEL

Also significant in the various definitions of coping and coping approaches is the essential position of French, Rodgers, and Cobb (1974), who define *coping* as the individual's effort to create congruence between self and the environment. The congruence model of person-environment interaction has its historical antecedents in Lewin's (1951) notion that behavior is a function of the relationship between the person and environment. Murray (1938) has postulated that many times this congruent relationship may be interrupted by catastrophic and stressful life events such as losses, illness, segregation, and discomfort. Depression and agitation are assumed to follow. However, all these authors underscore the notion that whenever there is a lack of congruence or discontinuity between the individual's needs and life situations, either due to a reduction in the coping capabilities or coping resources (e.g., when there is an illness or loss of social support) or due to a change in the environment (e.g., in a move to a big city or to an institution), then various adaptive strategies are evoked to increase the degree of fit between the person and the environment (Kahana & Kahana, 1982).

A conceptualization of congruence that has special significance for elderly persons was developed by Kahana (1975) and tested by Kahana and associates (Kahana, Liang, & Felton, 1980) to study the effects of seven environmental dimensions—segregation, congregation, institutional control, structure, stimulation, effect, and impulse control—on the morale of the institutionalized individuals. The results of this study suggest that the proposed congruence model is a valid one and that individuals are most likely to seek out aspects of the environment that reduce their stresses and anxieties or in turn facilitate their coping with the demands, constraints, and excesses of the environment. Moos (1974) has emphasized how many individuals in their later years may acquire personal strivings toward environmental mastery and competence while other individuals who had isolated themselves from social interactions may seek active support from the social-support system to assist them in their coping (Hogue, 1976).

Psychologists studying coping have focused on adaptive and unadaptive (or defensive) strategies and processes used for handling everyday life stresses as well as major life crises and transition (Alker, 1968). Haan (1963) describes adaptive strategies as characterized by a flexibility in orientation and a quality of purposive and positive problem-solving. Adaptive behavior according to Haan (1969) is an approach to life marked by fluid responsiveness to external and internal states. People noted for their coping abilities and adaptiveness are in touch with what is coming as well as what is past and can act in self-directed ways because they have a firm grasp of reality. In studying the etiology of mental illness in later life, Haan observes a distinction between adaptive behavior on the one hand and defensive and disorganized behavior on the other hand. It is suggested that defensive behavior is not grounded in reality and is often unrelated to a public sense of what is happening. The individual engages in somewhat compelled and rigid behavior—behavior that is somewhat pushed from the past—and in this respect is characterized by disorganization and the use of unadaptive strategies that rely heavily on avoidance, escape, and denial.

Both kinds of coping strategies—adaptive and unadaptive—(Table 5–1) are assumed to be prompted by conflicts and stress experienced by the elderly persons. In the one case, however, there is the suggestion that the elderly individual will use an instrumental approach to modify the situation if possible. In the case of the unadaptive approach, however, there is the suggestion that the elderly person will resort to defensive or avoidance behaviors because of the limited personal and environmental options open in old age. This concept of adaptability rests on positive perceptions of health and self-efficacy as rooted in aspects of intellectual and physical capacities and environmental limitations or assets (Kuypers, 1980).

In defining *adjustment* and *coping* in the elderly, Savage (1975) notes that there are many difficulties in pinpointing the key ingredients. They are undoubtedly multidimensional concepts both in terms of definition and etiology. The concept of *adjustment* is related to equilibrium described as the balance in the person's interaction with the external environment or a balance within the person's own internal system (Linn, 1979). Equilibrium in the elderly, therefore, denotes the idea of satisfaction, enhancement, and growth. It suggests that coping, not unlike adjustment, is a process rather than a state. In adjustment the emphasis is more on the idea of satisfaction of personal and social needs within and beyond the immediate environment. Coping by contrast implies the idea of tension reduction in the person-environment interaction.

Whether coping is adaptive and instrumental or unadaptive and defensive will depend on the adaptational patterns and coping strategies that were used by the elderly persons in their earlier years (Exhibit 5–2). Some studies (e.g., Neugarten, 1964; Reichard, Livson, & Peterson, 1962) have suggested that information about the personality types provides a better prediction of how these individuals will cope with stress, anxiety, or changes in their later years.

Others have argued the aged person's external support networks are influential factors in predicting the coping capacity of the elderly individual (Table 5–1). The elderly individual who has greatly diminished capacities for adjusting to changes (e.g., moving to a new residence, institutional placement) may be able to adapt gradually and remain in a familiar environment only if family members or friends move in supportively when greater physical dependence is unavoidable for an elderly member.

Kahana and Kahana's (1982) longitudinal study identified five basic coping styles that were used by institutionalized elderly to deal with problematic situations (see the summary description of coping styles in Table 5–1). These coping styles ranged from very helpless styles with reported inability to cope with their life situations to creative problem-solving coping styles characterized by flexibility, purposiveness, and organization. Each style has a characteristic approach strategy:

1. Instrumental strategies. According to Kahana and Kahana (1982) persons adopting this style of coping seek to modify their situation in order to make it more congruent with their needs. They might use sufficient energy to identify and define the problematic situation and engage in specific behaviors to deal with the problem. These are elderly individuals who may actively try to change their environment by themselves by being assertive and demanding or they may seek assistance from friends and

families in order to accomplish the necessary change. In both cases the coping strategies are adaptive, and the objective is the reestablishment of an equilibrium between themselves and the environment.

2. Intrapsychic strategies. According to Kahana and Kahana (1982) intrapsychic strategies are used by individuals who are low-energy individuals not sufficiently motivated to change the environment. Such individuals may recognize that they have a problem or that a conflict exists between themselves and others in the environment. However, rather than actively trying to change the environment or assertively seeking assistance in doing so, some individuals will seek a psychological solution to the problem. These individuals will reduce the cognitive dissonance elicited by the situation by making cognitive accommodations within themselves. They will resort to defensive reappraisals representing cognitive maneuvering to reduce distress rather than to assess accurately the troubled person-environment relationship with a view to changing it. They may focus on other aspects of the environment in order to forget the conflicting aspects or might actually change their needs and preferences to fit in with the new environment. Thus, eventually these individuals may succeed in repressing the existence of a conflict so that it is no longer outwardly observable.

3. Affective strategies. In this coping approach, efforts to master, tolerate, or minimize the incongruence are not action-oriented or intrapsychic. Rather, coping efforts are aimed at reducing emotional distress and maintaining a satisfactory affective expression of their concern, stress, or anxiety. However, the affective expression or display of emotions is not used as part of an instrumental or psychological solution but becomes an end in itself. In the acute phases of stress and anxiety the affective expression in the form of crying may be effective in releasing tension or in recognizing the reality of a harm, loss, or threat that cannot be easily modified.

4. Escapist resolution of the problem. Coping with extreme stress often involves an acute phase in which efforts are unadaptively directed toward getting involved in other irrelevant activities, avoiding the problem, or denying it. According to Kahana and Kahana (1982) elderly individuals may resort to escape strategies such as excessive sleeping, excessive eating, or excessive consumption of alcohol. Such activities may be of assistance in reducing emotional distress and temporarily distorting the impact of the stressful event. However, as with individuals using affective strategies, individuals using escapism resolution seldom reach the reorganization phase in which the harm, loss, or threat is recognized and coping efforts are focused on altering the troubled person-environment relationship. Thus incongruence becomes a permanent feature of the person-environment interaction.

5. Resigned helplessness. Some individuals, whether submissive, dependent, or emotionally distant in their previous functioning, may take on the sick role and may use the illness defense to cope with stressful events over which they feel they have no control.

Time perspective alterations may be an influential factor in determining the elderly individual's adaptive and coping capacities. A number of authors (e.g., Blazer, 1982; Verwoerdt, 1981; Zarit, 1980) observe that there are specific alterations in the time perspective with advancing age. Some individuals may get desperate about time running out, may suddenly become action prone, and may tend to act out in the presence of any so-called obstacles or hindrances in the way of their habitual activity. However, they may not have sufficient energy to maintain the independent facade too long. Others whose habitual life style was one of submissiveness, dependence, and courteousness may resent being on good behavior in their later years and may act sometimes with physical aggression in the presence of any stressors. Conflicts may develop because the aggressiveness or independence is not genuine and therefore difficult to maintain. Thus late-life coping patterns may bring into sharper profile patterns of adaptational assets and liabilities that had existed throughout life.

ASSESSMENT OF COPING RESOURCES IN LATE LIFE

A model of coping is suggested in which three groups of resources may be considered in predicting the extent of the person-environment congruence that will be achieved. These are summarized in Table 5–1. The first group of resources is concerned with health as measured by the level of physical functioning and cognitive functioning. According to Lieberman and associates (i.e., Lieberman, 1965; Lieberman & Coplan, 1970; Lieberman, 1975; Tobin & Lieberman, 1976) the cognitive and physical resources act as a threshold, with those with poor resources being unable to adapt. Successful coping is negatively influenced by health factors such as organic problems, mental retardation, physical handicaps, and the degree of cognitive impairment and organic brain syndrome. Verwoerdt (1981) notes that individuals who cannot comprehend a problem that needs resolution or who lack the physical capacity to respond efficiently will clearly be limited in their attempts at coping and will need to rely heavily on social support and direct assistance. Thus, the most common index of unadaptive coping in this group of resources is physical illness.

The second group of resources is concerned with psychological strengths, which are a combination of personal coping strategies, personality style, and psychic ego-strengths. Coping, in this context, is indexed by measures of self-esteem, activity, and life satisfaction. Adaptation and coping in crises involve traits of being assertive and aggressive. In addition to having an aggressive personality constellation, what may be particularly useful in old-age coping is the ability to maintain the self-system and levels of hope and ability to introspect. These are important parameters of coping that will often help many physically feeble elderly to withstand a major medical crisis or a major social-emotional loss (Lieberman, 1975). Siegler (1980, p. 206) notes that an important dimension of coping in old age is the motivation of the individual to deal with the types of problems commonly seen in later life (role loss, family conflicts, decline in social support, death and bereavement, and somatic concerns).

Thus the most common index of poor coping in late life is lack of self-esteem, hope, and motivation to persevere. Elderly persons with low psychological resources are more likely to experience stress events and more likely to respond unadaptively.

The third group of resources is that of social resources measured as a combination of income, education, and density of social networks. Social networks and social supports are seen as critical to coping and adaptation in late life. A perusal of the literature points to the immense value of social support systems and networks in ameliorating the negative outcomes of stressful life situations and in promoting stress-adaptational outcomes.

Cath (1976) notes that social networks are a product of the elderly person's own efforts at object and person relationships. With advancing age, however, the human relatedness of earlier years may become increasingly difficult. Individuals in late life may lose contact with social networks developed in their earlier years. Conversely the individuals who had limited social interactions in their earlier years, who isolated themselves, or who had seldom provided help to others are unlikely to have access to social-support networks that are at the root of much of our health and sanity in later years.

Berghorn and Shafer (1979) found that in frail elderly, with poor physical health and low psychological resources, the social support and environmental resources mitigated against the effects of personal impairments on their coping in later life. Caplan (1974) and Cath (1976) found that the assistance of the formal social provider services and the informal assistance of families and friends greatly assisted in attenuating the harmful effects of daily stress and crisis situations. Thus in assessing the social support resources of the elderly in stressful times, it is important to take count of both the formal and informal networks and systems and to provide awareness of accessibility to services and supports not previously tapped at times of crisis.

Other specific parameters that need to be assessed are the elderly individual's own cognitive and psychological resources for conducting an information search on the services available, taking direct action necessary to changing a stressful environment (e.g., unpleasant home surroundings, restrictive institutional setting, isolated dwelling place), and assessing options for self-control, instrumental actions, and expressive activity. Many elderly individuals may experience increasing inability to effect control over their emotions and their instrumental behaviors and may thus convince themselves that they have reduced options or alternatives for instrumental activity.

Verwoerdt (1981) observes that the high-energy defensive patterns the individuals were able to use to deal with primary anxiety of the earlier years may decline in energy production. The elderly individual may need the help of the social support resources to conserve energy and to master and control other useful individuals in the environment in order to bring about instrumental change in the environment. Thus the person-environment fit may have to be achieved more by modifying the environment through adaptive use of the energies in the environment rather than energies in the self.

CLINICAL ASSESSMENT OF STRESS AND COPING

The use of life-event inventories for the assessment of stress has been hitherto confined to research and research-related outcomes of stress. Nevertheless, as Kahana, Fairchild, and Kahana (1982) have noted, life-event inventories may provide useful adjunct information for the clients interviewed in the clinical settings (see Kahana, Fairchild, & Kahana, 1982, for a detailed review of the life-event measures).

Consideration of information about recent life events, environmental stresses, and life-crises events provides important background for clinicians in establishing a diagnosis of stress reactions. From a cost-effectiveness position the use of life-event measures is therefore strongly advocated. These measures will easily provide to the clinician or therapist information about certain stressful events such as widowhood, retirement, major losses, and relocation and the individual's perceptions of the good, bad, or neutral nature of the environmental changes experienced.

Basic information about individuals' perceptions and experiences of crises obtained through life-event inventories must, however, be evaluated more comprehensively and intensively in the clinical interview. As Kahana and Kahana (1983) note, the comprehensive evaluation must include information about early trauma, cumulative and repeated life crises, as well as comprehensive data about recent life events.

All of the data about the stressed individual obtained from the life-event measures must subsequently be evaluated in terms of the needs, preferences, and options of the individual who has experienced crisis events. In addition, information about the individual client's personal modes of coping with stress should be obtained.

Analyzing multiple interviews obtained over several months, Golden (1982) distinguished three modes or styles of coping—confrontation, denial, and avoidance—that suggested important implications for the elderly's adaptation to stress. The confrontational style, according to Golden, involved the investment of major effort to cope with the expression of resentment, guilt, and sadness; turning to intimate confidants; and the use of strategies that magnified or extended the experience of valued emotions and helped to bring stressful episodes to closure. Denial involved basic suppression of emotion initially, and eventual repression of negative emotions. In the denial approach there was an investment of major effort in "undoing," "making amends," and the persistent seeking of the experience of elation, perhaps as a buffer to distress. The avoidant style involved consistent suppression of negative emotion reflected in psychosomatic symptoms such as headaches and indigestion. There was an investment of major effort to cope with feelings of blame and the infrequent achievement of psychological closure in stressful episodes.

In clinical assessment of stress, Golden suggests that attention be directed not merely to major sources of stress but also to the stressed individual's coping style, and which forms of anticipatory coping—confrontational, denial, or avoidance—are used to deal with stressful environmental conditions.

In determining the degree of change that the elderly individual may be required to make in the poststress stage (e.g., moving to an institutional setting, relocating with the adult children), information about the individual's anxieties and fears and hopes and expectations will also be necessary. Coping and adjustment in late life must be assessed in terms of the effects of change and loss on the person-environment fit. Pearlin (1980) has suggested that age or change alone does not influence emotional well-being, even when change is brought about voluntarily. The extent of actual deterioration of life circumstances and the degree of hardship in key conditions of living are the major factors in the variation of the person-environment fit. Therefore, environmental and situational changes presumed to increase fit and thereby reduce stress must be considered. Second, whatever happens is given meaning and personal significance by the patterns of commitment and beliefs about the self and world. Lazarus and DeLongis (1983) therefore stress the significance of considering the elderly individual's valued ideals and goals, and the choices or sacrifices they are prepared to make in their long-standing commitments. Encounters that threaten important commitments are most likely to lead to appraisals of greater threat and stress and to increase the elderly individual's overall vulnerability to stress. In order to ensure that the person-environment fit is a sound one, baselines of commitments, obligations, sense of meaningfulness, and failure of ambitions and dreams must be considered. Excessive reordering of priorities and expectations in old age are most likely to lead to appraisals of fear and stress. Some elderly individuals may continue to struggle with change for a while, but most will soon experience a decline in morale and endangered health produced by the rearguard action against change (Lazarus & DeLongis, 1983).

In order to ensure that the person-environment fit is a sound one, all aspects of the environmental demands, constraints, and limitations must be explained to the elderly client. The individual's perceptions of the environmental demands must also be considered. Studies (e.g., Kahana, Liang, & Felton, 1980) have suggested that even impaired elderly are able to articulate their needs, preferences, and perceptions concerning the salient aspects of their living environment. An attempt must be made to explain to the client the potential benefits of the environmental intervention or change necessitated by the crisis event. Thus the final person-environment fit must be based on information about the verbalized needs of the client and the test data obtained from all professionals and semiprofessionals involved, family members, and other informants.

RECONSTITUTIONAL MEASURES FOR AMELIORATING STRESS

The model of stress as viewed in this section is appropriately broadened to encompass all tensional states resulting from stress situations or events. These concomitant states involve complex patterns of responses characterized by subjective feelings of depression, apprehension, or tension, accompanied by or associated with physical activation or arousal (Spielberger, 1972).

Symptoms of stress are often indistinguishable from symptoms of illness or organic disorders. However, most of the stress-related problems or disorders are more amenable to counseling, therapy, or treatment than are affective disorders or brain syndromes. It must be assumed, therefore, that most stress-induced discomforts, pains, or physiological symptoms are treatable and reversible. Thus, it is all the more important that the counselor, therapist, or caregiver be able to identify the psychodynamics of the stress reactions and to recognize these as the concomitants of stress rather than physical illness or medical problems.

It must be recognized also that stress may be experienced by the elderly person in all or one of various domains of the environment:

- interpersonal environment: friends, family, cultural tradition that surround or affect the elderly individual
- physical environment: living quarters, climate, or weather conditions (heating, cooling, etc.) that surround or affect the individual
- mental environment: the individual's negative or positive thoughts, feelings, and cognitions
- physiological environment: bodily phenomena such as nervous system, gastrointestinal system, glands, or sensory organs

Disorders in any of these domains may produce a generalized psychological and physiological experience of severe anxiety, discomfort, or pain resulting from a high stress level.

In the elderly the arousal response patterns may lead to elevation in blood pressure, respiration problems, or gastric motility and somatic behavioral responses such as tremors, speech disruption, motor inhibition, or disruption of performance. The caregiver or therapist needs to be aware that many stressed elderly may have little awareness of the hyperaroused states of their physiology. A most significant factor in the elderly is that a stressed person may experience too little sensation (numbness) or too much sensation (extreme agitation) and at the same time may not experience certain discomforts, such as chest pain, that may be potentially dangerous.

Other psychodynamics require the caregiver's or counselor's immediate attention. Many elderly may become extremely withdrawn after a stressful event. For example, an elderly woman may shift into a regression in which she is like a child, dependent on her husband or adult children for every basic need or function. Alcohol addiction may sometimes reach a peak after a stressful event, especially if the elderly client had become used to consuming alcohol as an attempt at self-treatment of stress and anxiety.

If stresses become severe enough, many elderly exhibit psychomotor retardation symptoms and overt slowing in response speed, memory, and integrative functions. Stress reactions may take the form of functional disorders, but if the onset of these symptoms follows a stressful event, these disorders should be distinguishable from others resulting from physical illness or organic brain syndrome.

Britton (1967) urges clinicians to remember that mild functional disorders in the elderly following stress episodes may be precursors of regression in performance. However, he advises that such regression in performance on intellectual tasks or physical tasks does not necessarily imply competence deficit or that decline in functioning is irreversible. Functional confusion in the elderly may diminish if steps are taken to counter the stress and depression (Levin, 1964) and strengthen the social support network.

Wedin (1977) speculates that initially the more simplistic and primitive cognitive responses of withdrawal and isolation may reflect the elderly person's adaptive effort to simplify the environment and render it less threatening. Silk (1971) supports this view and postulates that decline in the functional capacities of the elderly, including decline in cognitive functioning, occurs in the service of the individual's attempt to adapt to the internal and external changes that the person may be undergoing. Elderly adults may revert to less-advanced reasoning as an habitual response to stress and as an easier way of thinking under pressure of threat and anxiety (Denney & Wright, 1976). Wedin (1977) acknowledges that the primitive cognitive responses may have superior anxiety-reducing responses. Hence allowing the elderly to withdraw temporarily may serve a therapeutic purpose.

This interpretation has useful implications for the practitioners working with geriatric clients. Sobel (1980) advocates that the therapist working with the regressed later-life client can prevent further cognitive deterioration by not interfering with the elderly's egocentric modes of adaptation or avoidance style of coping.

In the attempt to determine whether the regressive reactions are reversible, the therapeutic counter must focus on asking for details, encouraging the elderly to talk and to provide verbal labels for the feelings of stress and anxiety. Additionally the therapeutic counteractants to stress in the elderly must encourage production, repetition, and clarification of fears for the present and future.

Therapeutic Efforts Aimed at Improving Coping

Reactions to stress are widely recognized as one of the most frequent reasons for emotional disturbances that have an onset late in life (Butler & Lewis, 1977). Timely recognition and management of stress reactions and appropriate intervention can be of great assistance in helping the elderly to make successful adjustment in the later years.

Rosow (1967, 1974) has argued that adaptive capacities of older persons are considerably diminished partly as a function of age but primarily as a function of frequent and major readaptations stemming from age-related factors such as retirement, bereavement, illness, and decline in social and economic status. Rosow (1963, 1967, 1974) observes that in coping with actual or threatened role and status losses, older people find alternatives to previous patterns of social participation, seek new associations, prevent or overcome excessive restrictions on their needs, and look upon their condition with some degree of philosophical detachment in order to continue to regard themselves with dignity. Rosow (1963) writes that the negative impact of retirement, widowhood, declining health and income, and loss of fulfilling roles must be "further qualified by the subjective meaning or impact of the change or lack of change observed" (p. 217). Thus, as Lazarus and DeLongis (1983) observe, it is not merely the objective change associated with age, but its subjective significance and meaning that affect adaptation, especially in the later years.

A number of therapeutic modalities are suggested for helping older persons who are stressed, unable to cope, and show symptoms of succumbing to stresses.

One-to-One Counseling

There are many good reasons for providing one-to-one counseling for the stressed individual. Many elderly are unable to recognize signs and symptoms of stress and stress-related disorders and without one-to-one counseling may blindly accept these symptoms as a confirmation of age-related physical and cognitive deterioration. Many elderly after bereavement and stressful losses may experience a regression in performance and an intrapsychic pain that can be treated only through one-to-one counseling. Kelly, Snowden, and Munoz (1977) see the increase in social support in face-to-face counseling as a key ingredient in intervention for stress. Furthermore, one-to-one counseling and therapeutic strategy may profitably include explicit attempts aimed at helping the older person utilize alternative coping strategies. Although systematic guidelines concerning therapy for stress reactions among the elderly are largely absent, Butler and Lewis (1977) recommend the potential usefulness of short-term insight-oriented therapy consisting of a series of 15-minute sessions to resolve stress and grief reactions. Sifeos (1982) has provided some evidence that psychoanalytically oriented one-to-one counseling holds promise for elderly with intrapsychic concerns.

Support Networks

The firm but supportive reactions of the individuals in the environment of the elderly to the relative helplessness of the elderly subjects will greatly determine the degree of psychological healing and of adaptation in recovery from stress. Through the warmth and support of the family and in the psychological milieu of the family, physician, clergyman, or mental health practitioner, the afflicted elderly can be helped to restore feelings of confidence and trust in self and others. The restoration of both kinds of confidence seems linked with recovery from stress. As noted by Titchener and Ross (1974), when the members of the treatment team are sensitive to these aspects of healing and when family members are trained to intervene with caution, it is possible to restore the elderly individuals' effectiveness of communication and the modes of emotional expression and self-regulation.

In many elderly, depression may arise from a sense of actual or perceived loss after stress and trauma. It may also arise from the feelings of powerlessness, disappointment, and personal weakness, which many elderly experience in conjunction with declining physical and mental energies. Such feelings of powerlessness are especially enhanced during stress. Many elderly fear that following major crises or trauma they will be completely useless to others, a complete burden and strain on their families, and totally incompetent and ineffective in managing their affairs. The impact of the stress or trauma appears to elicit these doubts most intensely. Reassurance, encouragement, and social support are known to be linked with recovery from stress. The elderly need to be assured that a decrease in the sense of personal control at a time of stress does not necessarily reflect a decrease in personal well-being and that reliance on others during a period of stress is more strongly associated with adjustment. Coping is influenced by whether the elderly person is able to accept these beliefs and respond favorably to the help and support of others. What is being suggested here is consistent with a cognitive approach to coping with stress, specifically, that many of the age-related changes in stress result, in part, from a shift in how events are appraised by an elderly person rather than solely from changing circumstances (Lazarus & DeLongis, 1983).

An alternative conceptualization of stress that needs to be emphasized with the elderly is the one that focuses on daily hassles as distinguished from dramatic, change-centered life events. In old age the frequency of hassles such as misplacing or losing things, not having enough time with the family, filling out forms, and concern about physical energy are transient but vital concerns. Unfortunately, these daily hassles are irritating, frustrating, and distressing enough that many elderly cannot distinguish them from the stress of change-centered life events such as bereavement, loss, and grief. If the elderly are not helped to separate the daily hassles and to evaluate them more lightly and less dramatically, the daily hassles may establish as strong a relationship to health outcomes and morale as do major life events.

One-to-one counseling and the assurance of emotional support can give most elderly the self-confidence they need to cope successfully with the daily hassles.

Problem-Solving Training

The counselor's assistance in behavioral analysis and record keeping often helps the stressed client to identify antecedents and consequences of problems, which in turn suggest possible interventions. A common problem with stressed clients is sleeplessness at night and fatigue and confusion at other times. Many elderly suffering from stress and trauma may become agitated and confused and ill prepared to focus on problem-solving activities or strategies that signal concentration and attention. However, a key ingredient in intervention for stress reactions in the elderly is giving them a problem-solving orientation (Haley, 1976). The most frequently used techniques are

- behavioral analysis of the problem,
- mobilization of the human resources and environmental supports, and
- information seeking and taking direct action.

Because solutions to problems of stress are unique, the counselor should be concerned with helping elderly individuals understand the problem-solving process and not with reaching a particular solution. The process may involve assisting the emotionally upset and stressed elderly client to evaluate the following aspects of the stress-related situation:

- What information does the person already have?
- What course of action has been tried?
- What aspects of action did not work?
- What is the person willing to try because it might work?
- How much support and assistance would the person like to receive from others?
- What kind of solution to the problem is the person seeking?
- What aspects of the self or the environment need to be changed in order to manage the stressful transaction?

An important aspect of problem solving is the recognition that there is no right solution for problems causing stress and that strategies for dealing with stress responses will vary from situation to situation and also from person to person, depending on previously learned ways of coping. A cognitive problem-solving approach that helps clients to identify and examine their thoughts is often useful (Beck, Rush, Shaw, & Emery, 1979). Elderly persons become upset over small problems that are readily seen as having no important consequences. Because of a certain rigidity in thinking, many elderly may have difficulty in distinguishing important and relevant from unimportant and irrelevant outcomes. A detailed breakdown of outcomes and consequences and an examination of the essential from the insignificant consequences would be helpful to the emotionally upset client in evaluating the changes that need to be made and in concentrating on problem-solving activities.

Alternate Modes of Coping

A key ingredient in intervention for stress reactions in the elderly is teaching them alternate modes of coping. Lazarus and Launier (1978) have identified four coping modes, each of which has specific implications and applications when working with an elderly clientele. According to Lazarus and Launier modes of coping (information seeking, direct action, inhibition of action, and intrapsychic modes) are included within two main functions—the instrumental and the emotional-regulatory—and all four can deal with the self and the environment (Table 5–2).

Information Seeking. Information seeking and information giving have the obvious instrumental function of providing the elderly client a basis for action to change a stressful transaction. Seligman (1975) has argued that older persons experience intense feelings of lessened competence and increased helplessness following stressful episodes. The latter feelings have been attributed to the elderly experiencing uncontrollable situations, that is, those stressful events in which outcomes are independent of a person's behavior. Therefore, Kiyak (1978) has argued that one way to help the elderly diminish symptoms of stress and anxiety is to teach them effective coping skills that can lead to an enhanced sense of environmental control and mastery over the environment. Therapeutic effort with such individuals may involve the use of such strategies as information seeking, which has the effect of making a person feel better by making the stress event seem more under control (Janis, 1968). In stressful situations most elderly may bolster a difficult decision and feel better about it by seeking more information from various sources on how to deal with the stressful event. The following cases illustrate this point.

Client 1. Mrs. M.'s 50-year-old widowed son died, leaving two young motherless children. Mrs. M. was most distressed and felt completely unable to care for the grandchildren. She became quite ill and showed symptoms of dizziness, mental confusion, and loss of physical balance. In one-to-one counseling, Mrs. M. was encouraged to seek more information from child welfare services, from her son's legal advisor about the family's financial assets, and from the insurance company about insurance benefits and coverages. All this information seeking helped Mrs. M. to feel more in control. Within a short period her physical energy was restored and she was more cognitively alert.

Client 2. Mrs. W. had serious chest pains following her husband's death but was most reluctant to see a doctor because she wanted to avoid a diagnosis. She became agitated and nervous, lost appetite, and within a few days became quite run down. With the support of friends and confidants Mrs. W. was persuaded to make an appointment with a specialist and

Table 5–2 Coping Classification Scheme

Instrumental Focus	Temporal Orientation			
	Past-present		Future	
	Functions			
Self	1. *Altering the troubled transaction (instrumental)*	2. *Regulating the emotion (palliation)*	1. *Altering the troubled transaction (instrumental)*	2. *Regulating the emotion (palliation)*
	Coping modes			
	a. Information seeking	a. Information seeking	a. Information seeking	a. Information seeking
	b. Direct action	b. Direct action	b. Direct action	b. Direct action
	c. Inhibition of action	c. Inhibition of action	c. Inhibition of action	c. Inhibition of action
	d. Intrapsychic	d. Intrapsychic	d. Intrapsychic	d. Intrapsychic
	Functions			
Environment	1. *Altering the troubled transaction (instrumental)*	2. *Regulating the emotion (palliation)*	1. *Altering the troubled transaction (instrumental)*	2. *Regulating the emotion (palliation)*
	Coping modes			
	a. Information seeking	a. Information seeking	a. Information seeking	a. Information seeking
	b. Direct action	b. Direct action	b. Direct action	b. Direct action
	c. Inhibition of action	c. Inhibition of action	c. Inhibition of action	c. Inhibition of action
	d. Intrapsychic	d. Intrapsychic	d. Intrapsychic	d. Intrapsychic
	Appraisals			
	Harm		Threat or challenge; maintenance	
	Thematic character			
	Overcoming, tolerating, making restitution, reinterpreting past in present		Preventive or growth-oriented processes	

Source: From *Perspectives in Interactional Psychology* (p. 312) by L.A. Pervin and M. Lewis (Eds.), 1978, New York: Plenum Publishing Corporation. Copyright 1978 by Plenum Publishing Corporation. Reprinted by permission.

to seek accurate information about her condition and possible courses of action to take. Her condition was serious, requiring bypass surgery. However, seeking accurate information about postsurgery outcomes and consequences was useful. The necessary social support and accurate information gave Mrs. W. the mental control and self-confidence she needed for undergoing surgery.

Direct Action. Various forms of direct action are also located within various coping factors. Such action can be instrumental, as in phoning a friend for advice and seeing a lawyer for legal and financial concerns, or designed to regulate an emotion, as in taking a prescribed tranquilizer or engaging in muscle relaxation. Direct action can also be employed to alter oneself (e.g., exercising self-control in diet, stopping smoking) or to change the environment (e.g., seeking action against the residence manager, complaining to the food services about unnutritional food).

Thus, taking direct action helps clients to cope better by mobilizing resources and by feeling more in control of environmental factors that affect their lives. Gal and Lazarus (1975) stress the importance of the availability and utilization of active behaviors in coping. They suggest that active coping results in more desirable psychological and social outcomes that help to negate previous learned helplessness responses. This positive role of activity is especially salient in those circumstances when the active behavior undertaken is functionally related to the stress situation. The following case illustrates this point.

Client 3. Mr. L. at age 72 suffered a serious financial loss. His accountant, who was also a long-time friend and confidant, misappropriated his funds. Mr. L. was shattered by the loss. He became withdrawn and uncommunicative. He refused to eat, could not sleep, and had severe tremors in his hands. In a one-to-one counseling interaction Mr. L.'s counselor advised that he should take a specific course of action. After consulting with a lawyer and financial specialist, Mr. L. outlined a specific course of action for himself, which involved his examining the records, going over the receipts and payments, reading materials, seeking more information from the accountant. Within a few weeks Mr. L.'s self-confidence was restored. He felt he had a much better understanding of how the losses occurred and how he could come to grips with the problem. The therapeutic strategies of taking direct action and seeking information made him feel stronger and in control of the stressful outcomes.

Inhibition of Action. Therapeutic efforts with stressed clients often involve the use of such strategies as inhibition of action. Since every direct action carries reality or moral constraints and danger, inhibition of action performs the instrumental function of regulating emotion and exercising restraint. The following case illustrates this point.

Client 4. Mr. P. came for counseling. He seemed very agitated and said he had been having anxiety attacks. He said that he had worked for 40 years in a high-pressure executive position and never had time for his family. He complained that he had to be constantly on the move or be active and doing something because he had anxiety attacks whenever he was not active. As a result he felt that he could not allow himself a moment to sit still and think. A few days before his seeking counseling his wife threatened to leave him. Mr. P. immediately felt he ought to take a series of actions to stop this. Therapeutic efforts with Mr. P. involved urging him to lower his stimulation level by inhibition of action. Through insight therapy Mr. P. was led to recognize that he was too highly stimulated at all times, that he used up too much energy in aimless stimulation and consequently had little energy to devote to interpersonal interactions, intimate relationships, etc. Mr. P. came to realize that he must gradually disengage from overactivity.

Intrapsychic Coping Modes. These modes of coping fall within the other previous modes of information seeking, direct action, and inhibition of action. Included are all cognitive processes designed to regulate the emotions by making the person feel better (Lazarus & Cohen, 1978; Lazarus & Launier, 1978). In short the person says to oneself statements that make the person feel better. Such intrapsychic processes can have an instrumental value when an elderly client tries self-encouragement, self-reinforcement, and self-assurance or seeks assurance from others. The following case illustrates the point.

Client 5. Mr. O. at age 78 was a leader in the community and engaged in many community service programs. He had been frequently called on to make speeches and deliver addresses. In the last two or three years he had not been presenting himself very well and was becoming more and more distraught. He could not sleep at night, he was losing weight, and his speech was becoming confused. He was afraid that his whole world was collapsing. He sought counseling for his loss of self-confidence, nervousness, and keen anxiety. Mr. O. was taught strategies such as relaxation and desensitization. In cognitive restructuring he reinforced himself as follows: I am not helpless; I have done a lot for this community. There is no danger to my family; I do not have any brain disorder or mental confusion. The people in the community care for me greatly.

As much as possible, any therapeutic efforts with the stressed elderly person should build on the person's habits and cognitive style, rather than learning new skills, for example, assertiveness, reeducation, or retraining. The key to all situations is to get the client willing to try relaxation therapy, to try to communicate with support groups, and to try problem-solving therapy with the help of supportive individuals and in sheltered environments. A number of other innovative therapeutic approaches appear to hold promise for helping elderly clients with their stress reactions. Most of these programs (e.g., Beck, 1982; Langer & Rodin, 1976) have predicated their therapeutic concepts on the assumption that a majority of the elderly persons are both motivated and capable of coping with the stressful aspects of their lives by enhancing control, exercising more options for control and responsibility, and acquiring more environmental mastery over stressful events and life situations.

More elderly cohorts are taking initiative in coping with negative situations that they encounter in community settings or institutional living. Furthermore, encouragement to elderly persons to engage in direct action and information seeking has the effect of

- Reducing the high degree of uncertainty or ambiguity that typically characterizes the institutional environments of the elderly. (A possible reason is that when other persons control the environment, the elderly become victims of uncertainty about what will happen, when it will happen, and what the outcome will be.)
- Reducing the degree of appraised threats from people and objects in the environment.
- Reducing conflict between the information seeker and other persons in the environment. (The concept of conflict is central to psychological stress but direct action and information seeking reduces the conflict.)
- Reducing the degree of helplessness that the elderly person typically feels in stressful conditions. (The concept of helplessness is central to the traditional clinical emphasis on the elderly client's mode of coping through dependency.)

Through psychotherapeutic intervention, Selye (1980) and Sobel (1980) also emphasize the significance of augmenting the individual's inner resources and remobilizing the cognitive energies through techniques of relaxation therapy, cognitive restructuring, and stress management.

In brief, stress management training involves teaching the elderly client how to avoid unnecessary stressors such as family conflicts, not allow neutral events to become stressors, develop a proficiency (e.g., relaxation skills) in dealing with conditions that are unavoidable, and seek relaxation or diversion from the demand of stressful events (Selye, 1980, p. 141). In addition, stress management requires elderly individuals to learn how to recognize overstress—when they have exceeded the limits of their adaptability—and also to determine when the environment is boring, deprived, and socially constricted. The ultimate goal is to strike a balance between the person's needs and preferences on the one hand and the demands and stresses of the environment on the other hand.

ASSESSMENT OF LIFE EVENTS

Some of the more frequently used scales are discussed here.

Social Readjustment Scale

Verwoerdt (1976) has used the Holmes and Rahe's Social Readjustment Scale (SRE) (Holmes & Rahe, 1967) approach to measuring life events. Because of its easy administration and understandability this scale has been extensively used to quantify some of the stressor events inherent in psychosociobiological loss. The Holmes and Rahe scale studies the relative impact of 43 life events in an attempt to quantify the importance of life changes. In clinical practice it is regarded a convenient measure of the cumulative effects of life changes. Subjects are asked to indicate whether they experienced a given event during the recent past and if so, to specify the number of times. Thus subjects are required to rate each event in terms of the degree of social readjustment each event would require. A total life-stress score for the SRE is obtained by determining the events (e.g., death of a spouse, losing a job) experienced by the subject and summing the life changes associated with these events. As Gaitz and Varner (1980) observe, many of these events in the SRE are more likely to occur late in life and there is also a greater likelihood of more psychosocial losses accumulating as one grows older. The SRE, similar to the Zung Self-rating Depression Scale, is used as a screening instrument to study social stress, mental illness, and stress responses of subjects (Holmes & Masuda, 1974).

Geriatric Scale of Recent Life Events

Other unique stressful losses often encountered by the elderly include a shortened time-perspective, decline in health, victimization, and crime. These items are included in the Geriatric Scale of Recent Life Events (GSRLE), which focuses on events more common in later life (Kiyak, Liang, & Kahana, 1976). The GSRLE is predicated on the notion of cumulative stress effects in aging and the notion that stressful life events contribute to the aging process. This scale requires respondents to indicate a percentage of change a given event would produce in an individual's usual way of life.

Life Experiences Survey

Using the Holmes and Rahe approach to measuring life events, Sarason, Johnson, and Siegel (1978) developed the Life Experiences Survey (LES), which also attempts to assess the individual's perceptions of life stresses experienced in the recent past. This 47-item self-report measure, when compared to the GSRLE and to the SRE, has the advantage of providing change scores for both positive and negative life events. Scores on the LES are relatively unaffected by the subject's current mood states. Life events on the LES can also be rated as good, bad, or neutral. Subjects can also be required to state the degree to which the life event affected their functioning, the extent to which they expected the event to happen, and the degree of control the respondent had over the events.

Cautions in Using Psychometric Measures of Stress Factors

Unfortunately the use of the preceding scales is fraught with methodologic problems, and the use of life events as a measure of stress in the elderly poses additional difficulties. As Jenkins, Hurst, and Rose (1979) have noted, all of the life event measures of stress use a retrospective method. Poor memory for life events is often a major concern with elderly persons who may be at particular risk for forgetting and covering up for poor memory. Therefore, when the life-events approach is used with the elderly, it should be confined to recalling relatively recent events. In addition, older persons may put more distance between themselves and events that are potentially invasive and may have difficulty in rating the degree of change readjustment or strain resulting from the various life events.

In using a life-events approach with depressed individuals, care should be taken to differentiate events that are a consequence of a disorder or disruption as opposed to being a potential cause. If one assumes that clustering of events is important, then Monroe (1982) reminds us of the significance of causal sequencing. This notion implies that certain events may trigger off other events. For example, chronic physical illness in an elder may lead to loss of employment, which may in turn lead to reduced contact with others and reduced activity.

As noted by Monroe (1982), the order in which events occur may determine the severity of the personal distress. Under normal circumstances the event of retirement for an elderly person is assumed to subsume other events such as lowered income, loss of role, and decreased social contact. However, if loss of role is caused by psychosocial factors other than retirement (e.g., disability or illness) and eventually is followed by retirement, the significant life event that is a stressor is not retirement but the event that caused the loss of role. Given such wide considerations in assessment practices, the use of life events as a measure of stress in the elderly should be used with caution.

Despite the serious shortcomings inherent in the study of life-events approach, Yamamoto and Kinney (1976) recommend the scales for purposes of a preliminary screening and assessment of life-event stressors. These authors found the life-stress scores to be better predictors of stressful effects than scores derived from other self-reporting measures generally used in interview procedures. However, these authors underscore the importance of using only those contents that have particular relevance for specific age groups and ensuring that events can be seen by the respondent as being, as far as possible, independent events. Such events should be considered only in terms of their relationship with event accumulation and disorders.

Particularly promising for future clinical use are the Holmes and Rahe Social Readjustment Scale and the Life Experiences Survey, which include subjective evaluations of the perceived stressfulness of specific life events as rated by older persons. Also recommended is the Geriatric Scale of Recent Life Events, which can be useful to the clinician in assessing the total number of stressful events commonly experienced in late life.

According to Lazarus and DeLongis (1983), an alternative approach to conceptualizing and measuring stress, one that supplements the life events strategy, focuses on daily hassles. DeLongis, Coyne, Dakof, Folkman, and Lazarus (1982) argue that daily hassles often have a stronger relationship to health outcomes than do major life events because daily hassles are *proximal* measures of stress whereas life events are *distal* measures. Hassles, therefore, make a distinct contribution to adaptational consequences such as health and morale status. The two approaches serve supplementary roles in the measurement of stress in the elderly (DeLongis et al., 1982).

Lazarus and associates (Lazarus & DeLongis, 1983; DeLongis et al., 1982) designed a hassles scale to assess the frequency and severity of daily hassles as contributors to stress. They found this strategy of measuring stress to be more useful than that of life events in predicting adaptational outcomes such as morale, psychological symptoms, and somatic illness (DeLongis et al., 1982).

The measurement of coping is one of the weak links in efforts to study coping in late life. Hitherto, evaluative measures of stress have attempted to assess coping as a trait or style, but such one-shot measures have been inadequate in assessing adaptation, or in predicting how well the elderly will react across a variety of stressful transactions. Limitations in the measurement of stress and coping represent one obstacle to understanding. The current emphasis on major life events as the sole measure of stress, and the treatment of coping as a static trait reflects the grave inadequacy in the assessment of stress (Lazarus & DeLongis, 1983). Lazarus and DeLongis (1983), therefore, emphasize the significance of observing coping in diverse contexts. They recommend using life-event stress inventories in conjunction with the Hassles Scale (DeLongis et al., 1982) and Ways of Coping Checklist (Folkman & Lazarus, 1980) that inquires about what an individual thought, felt, and did in several stressful encounters. This approach to stress measurement is a major advance in that it attempts to examine how elderly people, appraising a misfit, use different types of coping processes depending on the type of stressful encounter—for example, work-related, health-related, or loss- and grief-related. The importance of a process perspective to assessment of stress may be even greater in the study of the aged because of the continual presence of stressful events and widespread losses of roles and relationships (Lazarus & DeLongis, 1983; Lazarus, Averill, & Opton, 1974).

SUMMARY

This chapter has reviewed major theoretical perspectives (e.g., psychodynamic, psychogenetic, and physiological) of stress reactions in the elderly and has examined the physical, psychological, and cognitive functioning correlates of stress reactions. Although age is generally assumed to play an important role in determining how a person reacts to stress, the extent to which age-related physiological changes may affect the elderly person's reaction to stress is not clear.

In examining the relationship of stress and aging, it has been observed that with age the metabolic machinery becomes less adaptive and efficient, and therefore internal stress amplifier personalities may exacerbate their own disease conditions such as diabetic ketoacidosis. It is as if a perception and appraisal of a threat lead to a metabolic and emotional arousal preparation to meet the threat. It has been suggested that hypertension, which increases with age, in turn increases the incidence of cardiovascular diseases in old age. Renner and Birren (1980) note that prolonged autonomic arousal will have greater harmful effects among older persons who after stressful experiences take longer to return to basal homeostatic levels.

Much data support the hypothesis that patterns of behavior including performance in areas of intellectual and cognitive functioning are linked to ongoing stress and disease states in the elderly. Conversely there is evidence to support the notion that many disease and predisease states related to stress are seen independent of aging. The relationship between stress and old age and stress as a basis for accelerating aging is also a reasonable hypothesis but one that is unproven and needs more empirical study.

One of the problems adding to the complexity of assessing stress in the elderly is that many of the process variables customarily included in stress research—such as impaired behavioral performance and cognitive distortions and emotional problems—frequently occur with increasing age independent of an apparent stress situation (Eisdorfer & Wilkie, 1977). As a consequence, it is often difficult to determine whether aging per se or stress is the causative factor in the disorders and cognitive, physical and emotional reactions of many elderly.

In assessing stress reactions of the elderly and in observing the consequences of stress on the psychological and physical health of the elderly, we must carefully examine not only the major life events and crises but also the degree of person-environment fit. This conceptualization of the person-environment fit clearly includes stressors that affect the elderly on an ongoing basis as well as major or sudden events. As a consequence it is often difficult to determine whether a specific event caused the stress or whether the overall intensity of the person-environment misfit or incongruence in an elderly person may be seen as a source of continual stress. This has been one of the major methodological problems in assessing stress in many elderly who may be continually in a state of transition from one stressful event to another—from retirement to social relocation, loss of status, loss of social support, and finally impending death.

We must carefully examine temporal aspects of the stresses as well as qualitative aspects of the type of stresses faced by older clients in order to make the best uses of the available resources for the problems of the aged. The implications of a relationship between stress and aging and between stress, disease, and cognitive disorganization in the aged go well beyond theoretical interest. An understanding of the potential causes and consequences of mediating stresses on the behavior of the elderly carries with it the potential for effective stress management and intervention at both the prestress and poststress stages, not only at the behavioral but also at the physical-somatic level. The chapter has also briefly discussed clinical methods of evaluating stress and coping. It has critiqued a few life-event measures and inventories for assessing stress. Various reconstitutional measures for ameliorating the impact of stress on the elderly have been described and discussed with illustrative case histories.

REFERENCES

Alker, H.A. (1968). Coping, defense and socially desirable responses. *Psychological Reports, 22,* 958–988.

Amster, L.E., & Krauss, H.H. (1974). The relationship between life crises and mental deterioration in old age. *International Journal of Aging and Human Development, 5,* 51.

Andres, R., & Tobin, J.R. (1977). Endocrine systems. In C.E. Finch & L. Hayflick (Eds.), *Handbook of the biology of aging* (pp. 357–378). New York: Van Nostrand Reinhold Co.

Beck, A., Rush, D., Shaw, B.F., & Emery, G. (1979). *Cognitive therapy of depression: A treament manual.* New York: Guildford.

Beck, P. (1982). Two successful interventions in nursing homes. *Gerontologist, 22,* 378–383.

Berezin, M.A. (1972). Psychodynamic considerations of aging and the aged: An overview. *American Journal of Psychiatry, 128,* 1483–1491.

Berghorn, F.J., & Shafer, D.E. (1979). *Support networks and the frail elderly.* Paper presented at the 32nd Annual Meeting of the Gerontological Society, Washington, DC.

Bergmann, K. (1972). Personality traits and reactions to the stresses of ageing. In H.M. Van Praag & A.F. Kalverboer (Eds.), *Ageing of the central nervous system: Biological and psychological aspects* (pp. 162–182). Haarlem, Netherlands: DeErven F. Bohn N.V.

Bessman, S.P. (1976). The philosophic basis for the artificial pancreas. Excerpta Medica International Congress Series no. 403 Endocrinology. Proceedings of the 5th International Congress of Endocrinology. *Exerpta Medica, 2,* 576–577.

Birren, J.E. (1969). Age and decision strategies. In A.T. Welford & J.E. Birren (Eds.), *Decision making and age* (pp. 23–36). New York: S. Karger.

Blazer, D.G. (1980). The epidemiology of mental illness in late life. In E.W. Busse & D.G. Blazer (Eds.), *Handbook of geriatric psychiatry* (pp. 249–271). New York: Van Nostrand Reinhold Co.

Blazer, D.G. (1982). *Depression in late life.* St. Louis: C.V. Mosby Co.

Botwinick, J. (1973). *Aging and behavior.* New York: Springer.

Britton, D. (1967). Mental state, cognitive functioning, physical health, and social class in the community aged. *Journal of Gerontology, 22,* 517–520.

Burgess, J.A. (1976). Diabetes mellitus and aging. In A.V. Everitt & J.A. Burgess (Eds.), *Hypothalamus, pituitary, and aging* (pp. 497–510). Springfield, IL: Charles C Thomas.

Busse, E.W. (1971). Biologic and sociologic changes affecting adaptation in mid and late life. *Annals of Internal Medicine, 75,* 115–120.

Butler, R.N. (1975). Psychotherapy in old age. In S. Arieti (Ed.), *American handbook of psychiatry* (Vol. 5, 2nd ed., pp. 807–828). New York: Basic Books.

Butler, R.N. & Lewis, M.I. (1977). *Aging and mental health: Positive psychosocial approaches* (2nd ed.). St. Louis: C.V. Mosby Co.

Camaron, P. (1967). Ego strength and happiness in the aged. *Journal of Gerontology, 22,* 199–202.

Caplan, G. (1974). *Support systems and community mental health.* New York: Behavioral Publications.

Cath, S. (1976). Functional disorders. In L. Bellak & T.B. Karasu (Eds.), *Geriatric psychiatry* (pp. 141–172). New York: Grune & Stratton.

Chiriboga, D.A., & Cutler, L. (1980). Stress and adaptation: Life span perspectives. In L.W. Poon (Ed.), *Aging in the 1980s: Psychological issues* (pp. 347–362). Washington: American Psychological Association.

Clayton, P. (1973). Anticipatory grief and widowhood. *British Journal of Psychiatry, 122,* 47–51.

Comfort, A. (1956). *The biology of senescence.* New York: Holt, Rinehart & Winston.

Coyne, J.C., & Lazarus, R.S. (1980). Cognitive style, stress perception, and coping. In I.L. Kutash & L.B. Schlesinger and Associates (Eds.), *Handbook on stress and anxiety* (pp. 144–158). San Francisco: Jossey-Bass.

Cumming, E., & Henry, W.E. (1961). *Growing old: The process of disengagement.* New York: Basic Books.

DeLongis, A., Coyne, J.C., Dakof, G., Folkman, S., & Lazarus, R.S. (1982). Relationship of daily hassles, uplifts, and major life events to health status. *Health Psychology, 1,* 119–136.

Denney, N.W., & Wright, J.C. (1976). Cognitive changes during the adult years: Implications for development and research. In H. Reese (Ed.), *Advances in child development and behavior* (Vol. 11, pp. 213–224). New York: Academic Press.

Diagnostic and Statistical Manual of Mental Disorders (DSM-III) (1980). Washington: American Psychiatric Association.

Dowd, J.J., & Brooks, F.P. (1978). *Anomie and aging: Normlessness of class consciousness.* Paper presented at the 31st Annual Scientific Meeting of the Gerontological Society, Dallas, November.

Eisdorfer, C. (1977). Stress, disease, and cognitive change in the aged. In C. Eisdorfer & R.O. Friedel (Eds.), *Cognitive and emotional disturbance in the elderly* (pp. 27–44). Chicago: Year Book Medical Publishers.

Eisdorfer, C., & Wilkie, F. (1977). Stress, disease, aging and behavior. In J.E. Birren & K.W. Schaie (Eds.), *Handbook of the psychology of aging* (pp. 251–275). New York: Van Nostrand Reinhold Co.

Epstein, L.J. (1976). Depression in the elderly. *Journal of Gerontology, 31,* 278–282.

Erikson, E. (1959). *Identity and the life cycle. Psychological issues* (Vol. 1, no. 1). New York: International Universities Press.

Everitt, A.V., & Burgess, J.A. (Eds.). (1976). *Hypothalamus, pituitary and aging.* Springfield, IL: Charles C Thomas.

Fenichel, O. (1945). *The psychoanalytic theory of neurosis.* New York: Norton.

Fiske, M. (1980). Tasks and crises of the second half of life: The interrelationship of commitment, coping, and adaptation. In J.E. Birren & R.B. Sloane (Eds.), *The handbook of aging and mental health* (pp. 337–373). Englewood Cliffs, NJ: Prentice-Hall, Inc.

Folkman, S., & Lazarus, R.S. (1980). An analysis of coping in the middle-aged community sample. *Journal of Health and Social Behavior, 22,* 219–239.

French, J., Rodgers, W., & Cobb, S. (1974). Adjustment as person-environment fit. In G.V. Coelho, D.A. Hamburg, & J.E. Adams (Eds.), *Coping and adaptation* (pp. 316–333). New York: Basic Books.

Frolkis, V.V. (1976). The hypothalamic mechanisms of aging. In A.V. Everitt & J.A. Burgess (Eds.), *Hypothalamus, pituitary and aging* (pp. 614–633). Springfield, IL: Charles C Thomas.

Fry, P.S. (1984). Development of a geriatric scale of hopelessness: Implications for counseling and intervention with the depressed elderly. *Journal of Counseling Psychology, 31,* 322–331.

Gaitz, C.M., & Varner, R.V. (1980). Adjustment disorders of late life: Stress disorders. In E.W. Busse & D.G. Blazer (Eds.), *Handbook of geriatric psychiatry* (pp. 381–389). New York: Van Nostrand Reinhold Co.

Gal, R., & Lazarus, R.S. (1975). The role of activity in anticipating and confronting stressful situations. *Journal of Human Stress, 12,* 4–20.

Gellhorn, E., & Kiely, W.F. (1973). Autonomic nervous system in psychiatric disorder. In J. Mendels (Ed.), *Biological psychiatry* (pp. 235–261). New York: John Wiley & Co.

Glover, E. (1929). The screening function of traumatic memories. *International Journal of Psychoanalysis, 10,* 90–93.

Golden, G. (1982). *Coping with aging: Denial and avoidance in middle-aged care-givers.* Unpublished doctoral dissertation, University of California, Berkeley, CA.

Goodstein, R.K. (1981). Inextricable interaction: Social, psychologic and biologic stresses facing the elderly. *American Journal of Orthopsychiatry, 51,* 219–229.

Grauer, H. (1977). Depression in the aged: Theoretical concepts. *Journal of the American Geriatrics Society, 25,* 447–449.

Grinker, R.R., & Spiegel, J.P. (1945). *Men under stress.* New York: Blakiston (McGraw-Hill).

Haan, N. (1963). Proposed model of ego functioning: Coping and defense mechanisms in relationship to IQ change. *Psychological Monographs, 77*(8), 1–23.

Haan, N. (1969). A tripartite model of ego functioning values and clinical research applications. *Journal of Nervous and Mental Disease, 148,* 14–30.

Haley, J. (1976). *Problem-solving therapy.* San Francisco: Jossey-Bass.

Henry, J.P. (1976). Understanding the early pathophysiology of essential hypertension. *Geriatrics, 31,* 59–72.

Henry, J.P., & Ely, D.L. (1976). Biologic correlates of psychosomatic illness. In R.G. Grennel & S. Galay (Eds.), *Biological foundations of psychiatry* (pp. 945–985). New York: Raven Press.

Henry, J.P., & Stephens, P.M. (1977). *Stress, health and the social environment. A sociobiologic approach to medicine.* New York: Springer-Verlag.

Hogue, C.C. (1976). *Support systems: A model for research and services to older Americans.* Unpublished paper presented at the National Gerontological Society Meeting, New York, October 15.

Holmes, T.H., & Masuda, M. (1974). Life change and illness susceptibility. In B.S. Dohrenwend & B.P. Dohrenwend (Eds.), *Stressful life events: Their nature and effects* (pp. 45–72). New York: John Wiley & Sons.

Holmes, T.H., & Rahe, R.H. (1967). The social readjustment rating scale. *Journal of Psychosomatic Research, 11,* 213–218.

Horowitz, M.J. (1980). Psychoanalytic therapy. In I.L. Kutash & L.B. Schlesinger and Associates (Eds.), *Handbook of stress and anxiety* (pp. 364–391). San Francisco: Jossey-Bass.

Hurst, M.W., Jenkins, C.D., & Rose, R.M. (1979). The relation of psychological stress to onset of medical illness. In C.A. Garfield (Ed.), *Stress and survival: The emotional realities of life-threatening illness.* St. Louis: C.V. Mosby Co.

Janis, I.L. (1968). Stages in the decision making process. In R. Abelson & E. Aronson (Eds.), *Theories of cognitive consistency: A source book* (pp. 577–588). Chicago: Rand McNally.

Janis, I.L. (1974). Vigilance and decision making in personal crises. In G.V. Coelho, D.A. Hamburg, & J.E. Adams (Eds.), *Coping and adaptation* (pp. 139–175). New York: Basic Books.

Jarvik, L.F., & Blum, J. (1971). Cognitive declines as predictors of mortality in twin pairs: A 20-year longitudinal study of aging. In E. Palmore & J.C. Jeffers (Eds.), *Prediction of life span* (pp. 199–211). Lexington, MA: D.C. Heath.

Jenkins, C.D., Hurst, M.W., & Rose, R.M. (1979). Life changes: Do people really remember? *Archives of General Psychiatry, 36,* 379.

Kahana, B., & Kahana, E. (1983). Stress reactions. In P.M. Lewinsohn & L. Teri (Eds.), *Clinical geropsychology: New directions in assessment and treatment* (pp. 139–169). New York: Pergamon.

Kahana, E. (1975). A congruence model of person-environment interaction. In P.G. Windley & G. Ernst (Eds.), *Theory development in environment and aging* (pp. 181–214). Washington: Gerontological Society.

Kahana, E., & Kahana, B. (1982). Environmental continuity, discontinuity, futurity and adaptation of the aged. In G. Rowles & R. Ohta (Eds.), *Aging and milieu: Environmental perspectives on growing old* (pp. 205–228). New York: Academic Press.

Kahana, E., Fairchild, T., & Kahana, B. (1982). Measurement of adaptation to changes in health and environmental changes among the aged. In R. Mangen & W. Peterson (Eds.), *Research instruments in social geronotology: Clinical and social psychology* (Vol. 1, pp. 145–159). Minneapolis: University of Minnesota Press.

Kahana, E., Liang, J., & Felton, B. (1980). Alternative models of person-environment fit: Prediction of morale in three homes for the aged. *Journal of Gerontology, 35,* 584–595.

Kelly, J.G., Snowden, L.R., & Munoz, R.F. (1977). Social and community interventions. *Annual Review of Psychology, 28,* 323–361.

Kiely, W.F. (1974). From the symbolic stimulus to the pathophysiological response: Neurophysiological mechanisms. *International Journal of Psychiatry in Medicine, 5,* 517–529.

Kiely, W.F. (1976). Psychiatric syndromes in critically ill patients. *Journal of the American Medical Association, 235,* 2759–2761.

Kiyak, H.A. (1978). Person-environment congruence models as determinants of environmental satisfaction and well-being in institutions for the elderly. Doctoral dissertations Detroit, Wayne State University.

Kiyak, A., Liang, J., & Kahana, E. (1976). *A methodological inquiry into the schedule of recent life events.* Paper presented at Symposium on Life Events, American Psychological Association, New York.

Kuypers, J.A. (1980). Ego functioning in old age: Early adult life antecedents. In J. Hendricks (Ed.), *Being and becoming old* (pp. 111–132). Farmingdale, NY: Baywood Publishing.

Langer, E., & Rodin, J. (1976). The effects of choice and enhanced personal responsibility: A field experiment in an institutional setting. *Journal of Personality and Social Psychology, 34,* 191–198.

Lazarus, R.S. (1975a). The self-regulation of emotions. In L. Levi (Ed.), *Emotions—Their parameters and measurement* (pp. 47–67). New York: Raven Press.

Lazarus, R.S. (1975b). Psychological stress and coping in adaptation and illness. In S.M. Weiss (Ed.), *Proceedings of the National Heart and Lung Institute Working Conference on Health Behavior* (Basye, May 12–15, 1975, pp. 199–214, DHEW Publication no. NIH 76–868). Washington: Government Printing Office.

Lazarus, R.S., Averill, J., & Opton, E. (1974). The psychology of coping: Issues of research and assessment. In G.V. Coelho, D.A. Hamburg, & J.E. Adams (Eds.), *Coping and adaptation* (pp. 249–315). New York: Basic Books.

Lazarus, R.S., & Cohen, J.B. (1978). *Theory and method in the study of stress and coping in aging individuals.* Paper presented at Symposium 5, Society, Stress and Disease, Stockholm, June 1976.

Lazarus, R.S., & DeLongis, A. (1983). Psychological stress and coping in aging. *American Psychologist, 38,* 245–253.

Lazarus, R.S., & Launier, R. (1978). Stress-related transactions between person and environment. In L.A. Pervin & M. Lewis (Eds.), *Perspectives in interactional psychology* (pp. 287–327). New York: Plenum Press.

Levin, S. (1964). Depression in the aged. The importance of external factors. In R. Kastenbaum (Ed.), *New thoughts on old age* (pp. 179–185). New York: Springer.

Lewin, K. (1951). *Field theory in social science.* New York: Harper.

Lieberman, M.A. (1965). Psychological correlates of impending death: Some preliminary observations. *Journal of Gerontology, 20,* 181–190.

Lieberman, M.A. (1975). Adaptive processes in late life. In N. Datan & L. Ginsberg (Eds.), *Lifespan developmental psychology: Normative life crisis* (pp. 135–139). New York: Academic.

Lieberman, M.A., & Coplan, A.S. (1970). Distance from death as a variable in the study of aging. *Developmental Psychology, 2,* 71–84.

Linn, M.W. (1979). Assessing community adjustment in the elderly. In A. Raskin & L.F. Jarvik (Eds.), *Psychiatric symptoms and cognitive loss in the elderly* (pp. 187–206). New York: Hemisphere.

Lloyd, C. (1980a). Life events and depressive disorder reviewed. I. Events as predisposing factors. *Archives of General Psychiatry, 37,* 529.

Lloyd, C. (1980b). Life events and depressive disorder reviewed. II. Events as precipitating factors. *Archives of General Psychiatry, 37,* 541.

Maddox, G.L., Busse, E.W., Siegler, I.C., Nowlin, J.B., Palmore, E., & Cleveland, W.P. (1977). Stress and adaptation in later life: Symposium presented at Gerontological Society, San Francisco. Abstracted in *Gerontologist, 17,* 5 (pt. 2), 139.

Martin, W.C., Bengtson, V.L., & Acock, A.C. (1974). Alienation and age: A context-specific approach. *Social Forces, 53,* 266–274.

Meehl, P.E. (1962). Schizotaxia, schizotypy, schizophrenia. *American Psychologist, 17,* 827–838.

Meier-Ruge, W. (1975). From our laboratories. *Triangle, 14,* 71–72.

Miller, P.M., Ingham, J.G., & Davidson, S. (1976). Life events, symptoms and social support. *Journal of Psychosomatic Research, 20,* 515–522.

Monroe, S.M. (1982). Life events assessment: Current practices, emerging trends. *Clinical Psychology Review, 2,* 435–453.

Moos, R. (1974). Psychological techniques in the assessment of adaptive behavior. In G.V. Coelho, D.A. Hamburg, & J.E. Adams (Eds.), *Coping and adaptation* (pp. 334–399). New York: Basic Books.

Moos, R. (1977). *Coping with physical illness.* New York: Plenum Press.

Murray, H.A. (1938). *Exploration in personality.* New York: Oxford University Press.

Neugarten, B.L. (1964). Personality change over the adult years. In J.E. Birren (Ed.), *Relations of development and aging* (pp. 176–208). Springfield, IL: Charles C Thomas.

Nuckolls, K.B., Cassel, J., & Kaplan, B.H. (1972). Psychosocial assets, life events and psychiatric symptomatology: Change as undesirable. *Journal of Health & Social Behavior, 95,* 431–441.

Ordy, J.M., & Kaack, B. (1976). Psychoneuroendocrinology and aging in man. In M.K. Elias, B.E. Eleftheriou, & P.K. Elias (Eds.), *Special review of experimental aging research: Progress in biology* (pp. 255–299). Ellsworth, ME: Ellsworth American.

Osgood, N.J. (1985). *Suicide in the elderly: A practitioner's guide to diagnosis and intervention.* Rockville, MD: Aspen Systems Corp.

Palmore, E. (1980). The social factors in aging. In E.W. Busse & D.G. Blazer (Eds.), *Handbook of geriatric psychiatry* (pp. 222–248). New York: Van Nostrand Reinhold Co.

Paykel, E.S. (1974). Life stress and psychiatric disorder: Applications of the clinical approach. In B.S. Dohrenwend & B.P. Dohrenwend (Eds.), *Stressful life events: Their nature and effects* (pp. 135–149). New York: John Wiley & Sons.

Pearlin, L.I. (1980). The life cycle and life strains. In H.M. Blalock (Ed.), *Sociological theory and research: A critical approach* (pp. 349–360). New York: Free Press.

Perlin, S., & Butler, R.N. (1963). Psychiatric aspects of adaptation to the aging experience. In J.E. Birren, R.N. Butler, S.W. Greenhouse, L. Sikoloff, & M.R. Yarrow (Eds.), *Human aging: A biological and behavioral study* (pp. 159–191). (USPHS Publ. no. 986). Washington: Department of Health, Education, & Welfare.

Pfeiffer, E. (1971). Psychotherapy with elderly patients. *Postgraduate Medicine, 50,* 254–258.

Pfeiffer, E. (1980). The psychosocial evaluation of the elderly patient. In. E.W. Busse & D.G. Blazer (Eds.), *Handbook of geriatric psychiatry* (pp. 275–284). New York: Van Nostrand Reinhold Co.

Plutchik, R., Hyman, I., Conte, H., & Karasu, T.B. (1977). Medical symptoms and life stresses in psychiatric emergency-room patients. *Journal of Abnormal Psychology, 86,* 447–449.

Rahe, R.H., & Arthur, R.J. (1978). Life change and illness studies: Past history and future directions. *Journal of Human Stress, 4,* 3–15.

Rahe, R.H., Biersner, R.J., Ryman, D.H., & Arthur, R.J. (1972). Psychosocial predictors of illness behavior and failure in stressful training. *Journal of Health and Social Behavior, 13,* 393–397.

Reichard, S., Livson, F., & Peterson, P.C. (1962). *Aging and personality: A study of 87 older men*. New York: John Wiley & Sons.

Reis, D.J., Ross, R.A., Brodsky, M., Specht, L., & Joh, T. (1976). Changes in catecholamine synthesizing enzymes in ganglia, adrenal medulla and brain of aged rats. *Federation Proceedings, 35,* 486.

Renner, V.J., & Birren, J.E. (1980). Concepts and issues of mental health and aging. In J.E. Birren & R.B. Sloane (Eds.), *Handbook of mental health and aging* (pp. 3–33). Englewood Cliffs, NJ: Prentice-Hall, Inc.

Rosen, V.H. (1961). The relevance of style. *International Journal of Psychoanalysis, 42,* 447–557.

Rosenthal, D. (1970). *Genetic theory and abnormal behavior*. New York: McGraw-Hill Book Co.

Rosow, I. (1963). Adjustment of the normal aged: Concept and measurement. In R. Williams, C. Tibbits, & W. Donahue (Eds.), *Processes of aging* (Vol. 2, pp. 195–223). Atherton Press.

Rosow, I. (1967). *Social integration of the aged*. New York: Free Press.

Rosow, I. (1974). *Socialization to old age*. Berkeley: University of California Press.

Ross, W.D. (1966). Neuroses following trauma and their relation to compensation. In S. Arieti (Ed.), *American handbook of psychiatry* (Vol. 3, pp. 131–147). New York: Basic Books.

Sarason, I.G., Johnson, J.H., & Siegel, J.M. (1978). Measuring the impact of life changes: Development of the Late Life Experiences Survey. *Journal of Consulting and Clinical Psychology, 46,* 932–946.

Savage, R.D. (1975). Psychometric techniques. In J.G. Howells (Ed.), *Modern perspectives in the psychiatry of old age* (pp. 397–420). New York: Brunner/Mazel.

Schally, A.V., Kastin, A.J., & Arimura, A. (1977). Hypothalamic hormones: The link between brain and body. *American Scientist, 65,* 712–719.

Seeman, M. (1976). Empirical alienation studies: An overview. In R.F. Geyer & D.R. Schweitzer (Eds.), *Theories of alienation* (pp. 265–305). Leiden, Germany: Martinus Nijhoff Social Sciences Division.

Seligman, M.E.P. (1975). *Helplessness: On depression, development and death*. San Francisco: W.H. Freeman.

Selye, H. (1976). *The stress of life* (2nd ed.). New York: McGraw-Hill Book Co.

Selye, H. (1980). The stress concept today. In I.L. Kutash, L.B. Schlesinger & associates (Eds.), *Handbook on stress and anxiety* (pp. 127–143). San Francisco: Jossey-Bass.

Selye, H., & Tuchweber, B. (1976). Stress in relation to aging and disease. In A.V. Everitt & J.A. Burgess (Eds.), *Hypothalamus, pituitary and aging* (pp. 553–569). Springfield, IL: Charles C Thomas.

Selye, H., & Tuchweber, B. (1978). *Stress and aging*. Paper presented at Symposium 5, Society, Stress and Disease, Stockholm, June 1976.

Shapiro, D. (1965). *Neurotic styles*. New York: Basic Books.

Siegel, J.M., Johnson, J.H., & Sarason, I.G. (1979). Mood states and the reporting of life changes. *Journal of Psychosomatic Research, 23,* 103.

Siegler, I.C. (1980). The psychology of adult development and aging. In E.W. Busse & D.G. Blazer (Eds.), *Handbook of geriatric psychiatry* (pp. 169–221). New York: Van Nostrand Reinhold Co.

Sifeos, P. (1982). Psychoanalytic therapy with the aged. Paper presented at National Institute of Mental Health Conference on Psychodynamic Research Perspectives on Development, Psychotherapy and Treatment in Late Life, Baltimore, November 5–8.

Silk, S. (1971). *The breakdown of cognitive functions in senile dementia*. Unpublished doctoral dissertation, Yeshiva University, NY.

Sobel, E.F. (1980). Anxiety and stress in later life. In I.L. Kutash, L.B. Schlesinger & associates (Eds.), *Handbook of stress and anxiety* (pp. 317–328). San Francisco: Jossey-Bass.

Spielberger, C.D. (1972). Anxiety as an emotional state. In C.D. Spielberger (Ed.), *Anxiety: Current trends in theory and research* (Vol. 1, pp. 23–49). New York: Academic Press.

Stenback, A. (1975). Psychosomatic states. In J.G. Howells (Ed.), *Modern perspectives in the psychiatry of old age* (pp. 269–289). New York: Brunner/Mazel.

Stern, G. (1970). *People in context*. New York: John Wiley & Sons.

Titchener, J.L. (1970). Management and study of psychological response to trauma. *Journal of Trauma, 10,* 974–980.

Titchener, J.L., & Ross, W.D. (1974). Acute or chronic stress as determinants of behavior, character, and neurosis. In S. Arieti & E.B. Brody (Eds.), *American handbook of psychiatry. Vol. 3, Adult clinical psychiatry* (2nd ed., pp. 39–60). New York: Basic Books.

Tobin, S., & Lieberman, M.A. (1976). *Last home for the aged*. San Francisco: Jossey-Bass.

Ujhely, G.B. (1963). Grief and depression: Implications for preventive and therapeutic nursing care. *Nursing Forum, 5*, 23–35.

Verwoerdt, A. (1976). *Clinical geropsychiatry*. Baltimore, MD: Williams & Wilkins.

Verwoerdt, A. (1981). *Clinical geropsychiatry* (2nd ed.). Baltimore: Williams & Wilkins.

Wechsler, D. (1958). *The measurement and appraisal of adult intelligence*. Baltimore: Williams & Wilkins.

Wedin, R.W. (1977). *The effects of experimental stress on measures of Piagetian intelligence in concrete operational children*. Unpublished doctoral dissertation, Long Island University, Long Island, NY.

Wolff, H.G. (1950). *Life stress and bodily disease—A formulation*. In H.G. Wolff, S.G. Wolf, & C.C. Hare (Eds.), Life stress and bodily disease. *Proceedings of the Association for Research in Nervous and Mental Diseases* (pp. 1069–1094). Baltimore: Williams & Wilkins.

Yamamoto, K.J., & Kinney, O.K. (1976). Pregnant women's ratings of different factors influencing psychological stress during pregnancy. *Psychological Reports, 39*, 203–214.

Zarit, S.H. (1980). *Aging and mental disorders: Psychological approaches to assessment and treatment*. New York: Free Press.

Zetzel, E.R. (1966). Metapsychology of aging. In M.A. Berezin & S. Cath (Eds.), *Geriatric psychiatry: Grief, loss, and emotional disorders in the aging process*. New York: International Universities Press.

Zubin, J., & Spring, B. (1977). Vulnerability—A new view of schizophrenia. *Journal of Abnormal Psychology, 86*, 103–126.

Chapter 6

Functional Disorders in the Elderly: Description, Assessment, and Management Considerations

Functional disorders of late life can be most appropriately viewed as a continuum of overlapping clusters. According to Post (1982) these functional disorders do not exist as separate entities, each with their own distinct and separate etiology. The disorders overlap just as the syndromes do. For practical reasons, however, it is still fitting to set functional disorders apart from disorders or conditions related to the deterioration or disease of the brain. This section reviews the etiology of several disorders that have a high prevalence in old age and present a complex symptomatology because of several conditions being coexistent.

Busse and Blazer (1980) attempt to distinguish functional disorders related to biological functioning from other functional disorders related to intrapsychic and psychosocial functioning. They agree, however, that determining the relative contribution of intrapsychic factors, psychosocial factors, psychosomatic factors, somatopsychic factors, and physical factors to the development of physical symptomatology or psychological malfunctioning is a difficult task for the clinician working with older adults. This lack of sharp lines of demarcation is reflected in discussing the functional disorders of late life as a series of conditions representing serious disruptions in the psychic adjustment and physical symptomatology of late life. For a clearer understanding, especially of functional conditions that are a potent factor in psychological malfunctioning and breakdown, this section looks at various late-life disorders, including late-life anxieties, paranoid states, hypochondriasis, alcoholism, and suicidal tendencies. In reviewing these disorders, attention is given to the specific relationship to old age and the context of aging. The problems to be discussed are considered functional, that is, having no identified organic basis (Post, 1982; Zarit, 1980). The syndromes cannot be viewed as separate illnesses or as necessarily having one underlying etiology. Immediate distinction among the disorders is not possible or sought.

In assessing symptoms such as pain, somatic complaints, sleep disorders, and psychosexual disorders (disorders in sexual functioning when psychological factors are of major etiologic significance), a tentative distinction is made between these symptoms and disorders of psychosocial adjustment. However, many disorders of psychological adjustment may arise secondary to physical disorders, for example, affective disorders that are often precipitated by various types of physical illness.

Psychosocial factors frequently play an etiologic role in the development of many physical conditions of the elderly. Hypertension is the most important of these conditions in the elderly, and hypochondriasis is the presentation of physical symptoms or complaints not explainable on the basis of demonstrable organic findings.

A summary of the major categories of functional disorders and their leading symptoms is presented in Table 6–1. In order to make appropriate suggestions for the management of various functional disorders, the major psychosocial factors that are assumed to be contributing to the initiation, exacerbation and perpetuation of these conditions are reviewed in Table 6–1. For example, in the management of alcoholism in the elderly, the psychosocial stresses contributing to the development of this condition may play an important etiologic role that should be understood by the clinician. Treatment might in fact be radically different for two persons with problems of alcohol abuse. Clinically, in the vast majority of functional disorders a few diagnostic differences between types of disorders may be easily observed. Where the immediate distinction is not possible, this is often due to two or more functional disorders being coexistent.

For convenience, only those functional disorders more commonly prevalent among the elderly than at other stages of the life cycle are discussed here. Significant steps and measures necessary to the assessment and management are also described separately in detail for each of the disorders.

AFFECTIVE DISORDERS

It is generally accepted that affective disorders are a serious problem in the elderly. Affective illnesses as a rule have a sudden onset and are precipitated by various types of loss or physical illness. Few causative relations exist between affective illnesses and chronic brain syndrome, and as noted by Weinberg (1975), affective symptoms are rarely prodromal features of the dementias of old age and rarely linked causatively with other functional disorders. The highest first incidence of affective disorders occurs between the ages of 55 and 65 years and regardless of the neurotic or psychotic symptoms of the affective disorders, the onset follows closely traumatic events such as various kinds of loss—loss of status, loss of family member through death, loss of job, and threatened loss of limbs or organs through illness or surgery (see Table 6–1). Such precipitants occur more frequently in later-life and in late-onset depression. Clinical practitioners in geriatrics have reported that, as is true of depression, affective disorders in the elderly generally do not take the same form that they do in younger persons.

Zung and Green (1973), for example, presented data from Zung's Self-Rating Anxiety Scale (Zung, 1971), that show the normal elderly population has higher baseline values for symptoms of anxiety and anxiety-related affective disorder symptoms than do normal young adults. In addition Gershon (1973), who discussed antianxiety agents for the elderly, observed a number of differences in the anxiety symptomatology of the elderly subjects compared to the younger age group. Gershon concluded that the aged have different host qualities for psychiatric disorders, and the symptomatology seen in them "may not fit automatically within the established systems of classification developed for a younger age group" (p. 184).

There may be genetic explanations for such late-onset depressive reactions. Affective disorders do respond favorably to electroconvulsive therapy and in the recent past antidepressant drugs, especially the tricyclics, have been fairly effective in the treatment of depressive reactions (Table 6–1). The following subtypes need some attention because of their common occurrence in late life.

Table 6–1 Major Categories of Functional Disorders in the Aged in Which Psychosocial Factors Play an Etiologic Role

Major Categories of Functional Disorders	Psychosocial Precipitators and Precursors	Therapeutic Considerations and Management of Disorders
1. *Affective Disorders* -Anxiety states showing acute anxiety accompanied by symptoms of guilt, agitation, hostility, threat, and sleep disturbance. -Depletion anxiety; restless stress, irritability, loss of appetite, dependency and depression, weight loss. -Helpless anxiety with loss of control. -Chronic anxiety.	-Psychosocial losses such as loss of status, loss of loved ones, organ loss. -Series of traumatic and precipitant events including illness, surgery, and major transitions. -History of neurotic symptoms.	-Affective disorders may respond favorably to electroconvulsive therapy, antidepressant therapy, antianxiety medication. -Supportive psychotherapy is always recommended as an adjunct to antidepressant therapy and should be aimed at helping client to resolve feelings of rejection, guilt, trauma, and depression.
2. *Chronic Fatigue States* -Lack of energy. -Lack of motivation and interest. -Hypersomnia.	-Emotional frustration. -Lack of gratification and satisfaction. -Depression resulting from retardation in metabolic activity.	-Rule out the possibility of physical illness or medical causes. -Recommend balanced diet of rest, recreation, and interesting activity allowing for elderly clients having reduced vigor, reduced agility, and reduced motivation for learning of new skills. -Open up opportunities for satisfying accomplishments and prospects for social gratifications and interpersonal interactions.
3. *Hypochondriasis* -Inordinate preoccupation with bodily functions and concern about the presence of disease. For example, the person has serious concerns about organs of ingestion and digestion, perceives self to be ill when there are no indicators of organic problems or physical ailment. -Apprehensions about terminal diseases such as cancer, cardiac arrest, and obstructive pulmonary disease.	-Depression, interpersonal conflict, and unhappiness. -Lack of social support, positive appreciation, and encouragement in the social environment. -Grief and bereavement. -Dependent personality traits and anxiety patterns accompanied by guilt and conflict.	-Rule out possibility of medical disorders and physical illness. -Mild medications such as mild antidepressants or tranquilizers. -Focus on health-related activities such as physiotherapy, biofeedback, mild exercises, short visits to the physician or medical clinician. -Encourage group therapy to help client deal with issues of unresolved guilt and subconscious need for acceptance, comfort, and support. -Encourage socially oriented group activities to help shape the client's social skills, to enlarge sources of social reinforcement, and to enhance self-concept.

Table 6–1 continued

Major Categories of Functional Disorders	Psychosocial Precipitators and Precursors	Therapeutic Considerations and Management of Disorders
4. Sleep Disorders -*Insomnia:* Insufficient sleep accompanied by mild disorientation as to time place and persons; poor and disordered sleep patterns sometimes accompanied by nightmares and hallucinations. -*Hypersomnia:* Excessive sleeping.	-Adjustment to new environment, new relationships and changes in physiological and metabolic body functioning. -Arthritic pain may cause sleep disturbances. -Loneliness, grief, depression and general decline in morale; low degree of contact with relatives and friends. -Physical disorders such as congestive heart, obstructive pulmonary disease, and shortness of breath.	-Rule out sleep disorders caused by organic syndromes and physical disorders such as congestive heart, obstructive pulmonary disease, hyper- or hypothyroidism, alcohol and drug dependencies. -Judicious use of mild tranquilizers to induce sleep in conjunction with a psychological regimen of guided program of sleep hygiene, pleasant activities, exercise, and relaxation therapy. -Judicious use of stimulants for hypersomnia including a psychological regimen of guided program for increasing the client's level of activity and degree of social interactions with family and friends.
5. Alcohol Abuse a. *Behavioral effects:* Inability to conduct routine tasks; behavioral manifestations of anger, hostility, aggression; trembling and "shakes." b. *Psychological effects:* Impairment in intellectual functioning and cognitive judgments; debilitating hangovers, blackouts, massive loss of recent memory, and perceptual impairment. c. *Physical effects:* Impairment in functioning of lungs, heart, liver, and kidney; severe nutritional deficiencies, anemia, weight loss, abdominal pain, and diabetes; chronic alcoholism leading to brain damage. d. *Interpersonal effects:* Problems and conflicts with family, friends, and neighbors; belligerence associated with drinking; problems with the police.	*Reactive factors:* -Depression resulting from bereavement, divorce, loss of spouse, loss of occupational role, lowering of social status leading to loss of power and control. -Physical illness and associated disabilities and physical handicaps. -Social deprivation resulting from social isolation, boredom, loneliness, and alienation from friends. -Bodily pain and discomfort. -Previous history of drinking as a means of coping with environmental stresses.	-Assess whether excessive drinking has situational determinants (for example, recent stressful events, recent stressful adjustment, or illness) or whether excessive ingestion is chronic, habitual, and addictive. -Assess client's sources of stress (both internal and external), anxiety, guilt, and rejection. -Assess client's existing coping behaviors and threshold of stress. -Intervention, based on individual assessment of client may take the following forms: a. Antidepressant therapy for situational depression, anxiety, and stress. b. Hospitalization, treatment of alcohol withdrawal and long-term addiction treatment for chronic alcoholism. c. Psychotherapy or one-to-one counseling (as an important adjunct to a

Table 6–1 continued

Major Categories of Functional Disorders	Psychosocial Precipitators and Precursors	Therapeutic Considerations and Management of Disorders
		pharmacologic regimen) should be aimed at helping the elderly client deal with problems of guilt, loneliness, depression, and incapacity for social relatedness.
		d. Group therapy and family therapy (as an important adjunct to individual therapy) should be aimed at providing the client moral support and ego-strength and at enhancing the social network system.
		-Participation in alcohol anonymous groups and other self-help groups should be encouraged.
		-Behavior therapy, along aversion therapy lines, may be necessary in extreme cases.
6. *Paranoid States*		
-Suspiciousness, lack of trust behaviors, accusations, and exaggerated perceptions of persecution and wrongdoing by friends and family.	-Sensory losses such as deficits in hearing and visual acuity; deficits in memory and cerebral functioning.	-Rule out possibilities of medical disorders, organic brain damage, or psychoses contributing to paranoia.
-Delusions and hallucinations of bodily harm, theft, and persecution usually without thought disorders or cognitive impairment.	-Stress arising from major adjustments or extreme losses.	-Assess hearing impairment and loss of visual acuity.
-Hypochondriacal symptoms.	-Aloneness and isolation against a background of self-centeredness, self-involvement, and long hospitalization.	-Assess mental status of client.
	-History of economic insecurity.	-If paranoid states are present in the absence of organic brain damage and psychoses the following interventions are suggested:
	-Long-term self-perceptions of inadequacy, inferiority, and low self-esteem.	a. Individual psychotherapy aimed at providing moral support and social reinforcement and providing an atmosphere for gaining client's trust.
	-Stressful experience of physical abuse, burglary, housebreaking, or robbery.	b. Judicious use of medication (e.g., phenothiazines).
	-Organic brain damage or previous psychotic conditions.	
7. *Psychosexual Disorders*		
-Expressions of fear over failing sexual capability with aging.	-High incidence of depression; anxiety states.	-Education of the elderly in healthy sex life and biological changes occurring with aging.
-Expressions of guilt over a desire for active sexual life in old age.	-Chronic fatigue state.	-Natural estrogen sulfate replacement therapy for women with dyspareunia symptoms.
-Tension and depression.	-Marginal physical health and disease states such as diabetes, obesity, injury to spinal discord may lead to secondary impotence.	-A physical health regimen of balanced diet and exercise.
-Painful sexual intercourse or dyspareunia in females.	-Self-medications such as	

Table 6–1 continued

Major Categories of Functional Disorders	Psychosocial Precipitators and Precursors	Therapeutic Considerations and Management of Disorders
-Abrupt decline of interest in sexual activity. -Difficulty in ejaculation. -Secondary impotence.	sedatives, sleep medication, and phenobarbital ingredients can induce sexual dysfunction or secondary impotence.	-A psychological health regimen of pleasant activity, recreation, and relaxation. -Practitioner's willingness to explore and discuss elderly clients' problems, concerns, and fears regarding sexual dysfunction with aging. -Psychological intervention for amelioration of guilt, anxiety, and fears associated with sexual activity in old age.

Anxiety States

An anxiety neurosis is characterized by increased muscular tension, sleep disturbance, restlessness, headaches, and a vague sense of impending disaster. Such anxiety neuroses are quite common in later years. At times, acute anxiety may emerge in the elderly persons because of guilt feelings resulting from hostility toward friends or family when they fail to meet their needs. Anxiety in the elderly is frequently associated with the possibility of emotional deprivation or a threat to security. McCrae, Bartone, and Costa (1976) report that anxiety in the elderly has been found to be associated with a denial of one's physical problems. Since physical illness and realistic anxiety producing situations are more common in later life, Verwoerdt (1980) emphasizes that various subtypes of anxiety states such as acute traumatic anxiety, chronic neurotic anxiety, helplessness anxiety, and anxiety depression manifest themselves in the elderly and need to be diagnosed more specifically. In terms of phenomenology Verwoerdt (1976, pp. 152–158) notes that the elderly are most susceptible to the following major groupings of anxiety:

- Depletion anxiety or insecurity about loss of external supplies and possible isolation and loneliness. Such anxiety is an integral part of late-life depressions. Verwoerdt (1976, 1980; 1981) postulates that these reactions develop in response to the elderly's diminishing ability to screen and ward off unwanted stimuli through earlier mechanisms of selective inattention and other forms of diversion. This type of anxiety accompanies depression when the psyche is overwhelmed by an influx of external and internal stimuli too great to be mastered, as in catastrophic reactions of brain damaged patients or informational overload. Clinically it represents an adjustment mechanism at a time in later life when the ego is relatively weak and unable to deny feelings of dependency and depression. Milder cases show symptoms of restlessness and irritability, but the severe cases show depressive reactions such as withdrawal, loss of appetite, distortion, and misinterpretations.
- Helplessness anxiety in the elderly is generated by a potential or actual loss of control or mastery. As noted by Verwoerdt (1976), the elderly's anxiety may be based on the apprehensions that others will not be available when they need help from them. Helplessness anxiety is felt as loss of self-confidence and shame and may thus be

experienced as a concomitant of depression. Most clinicians would agree, however, with Zung and Green (1973) in describing helplessness anxiety as general feelings of apprehension and uncertainty that are not attached to any specific or real external danger.

- Anxiety depression is often difficult to distinguish from a depressive disorder in that acute anxiety and depression are inextricably mixed in the experiences of the elderly. Gershon (1973) and others have described typical burdens (e.g., physical impairments, ability, and capacity losses) that are frequent precursors first of depression and later of depressive anxiety in the elderly. He also hypothesized that depressive features frequently accompany anxiety states in the elderly and that anxiety in the aged may often take the form of "rather primitive body focused type" (Gershon, 1973, p. 184) associated with somatic symptoms that are often indicative of masked depression (e.g., pain, failing bodily functions). Anxiety depression implies that the elderly person has experienced a series of traumatic and precipitant events that may cause the person to reach a breaking point and to despair and be extremely fearful in the anticipation of additional misfortunes.

- Chronic neurotic anxiety in the elderly is generally a carryover from earlier days and may not be associated with any specific precipitant factors or events. Varying degrees of depression are usually present with the anxiety, and the accompanying agitation due to chronic anxiety may be difficult to differentiate from agitated depression, which is closely related to specific precipitants of depression. Such chronic anxiety mixed with depressive symptomatology is often seen in elderly clients and may be hard to distinguish from acathisia (Verwoerdt, 1976).

Some of the best-known scales commonly used to assess anxiety symptoms in the elderly are critiqued and evaluated here in terms of their utility in geriatric anxiety and psychopharmacology.

Anxiety Assessment Scales

Hamilton Anxiety Scale (HAMA)

This (Hamilton, 1959) is a 14-item scale intended for use with patients already diagnosed as suffering from neurotic anxiety states—not for assessing anxiety in patients suffering from other functional or organic disorders (Guy, 1976, p. 195). The scale has items that assess affective, cognitive, and behavioral (i.e., interview behavior) dimensions. The 14 items cluster into general anxiety, somatic anxiety, and psychic anxiety factors (Hamilton, 1959). Although the validity and reliability of the HAMA have not been extensively explored for the elderly samples, Covington (1975) and Kirven and Montero (1973) noted that the scale was sensitive to geriatric psychopharmacology treatment effects.

Zung Anxiety Status Inventory (Zung ASI) and the Zung Self-Rating Anxiety Scale (Zung SAS)

According to Zung (1971) both the ASI and SAS were designed specifically for the assessment of anxiety as a disorder rather than as a trait or feeling state. Like the HAMA, the Zung ASI is intended for adults with a diagnosis of anxiety neurosis. Like the HAMA, it has items that assess somatic anxiety symptoms and affective dimensions. Although data concerning validity and reliability of the Zung ASI and SAS are limited, Zung has offered data (Zung et al., 1974) that suggest the scale may have adequate validity and reliability for purposes of assessing geriatric psychopharmcological (i.e., Gerovital H3) effects of anxiety.

Profile of Mood State (POMS)

This (McNair, Lorr, & Droppleman, 1971) is a brief inventory of mood states that provides mood distress scores on six mood factors such as confusion-bewilderment, tension-anxiety, and fatigue-energy. While reliability and validity data are limited and the scale items have not been standardized on populations of the elderly, LaForet, Sidd, and Waterman (1974) found a considerable degree of success in applying the scale to elderly presurgery patients ages 60 to 85 who showed significant decrease postsurgery on some of the six mood factors of the POMS. Similarly Salzman and Shader (1972) showed that the POMS was sensitive to psychopharmacological treatment effects on the elderly patients' fatigue factor of the POMS. These results suggest that further work using the POMS could be of considerable use in the assessment of anxiety among geriatric subjects.

The use of anxiety scales in geriatric psychopharmacology studies have also indicated that anxiety symptoms are decreased by the use of some antianxiety drugs. Antianxiety agents including benzodiazepines, barbiturates, alcohol, and diphenylmethanes, if effective, will decrease both psychological anxiety and muscle tension but do not alter psychotic symptomatology (Gershon, 1973; Piland, 1979). However, Kapnick (1978) suggests that the use of these drugs should be greatly discouraged in the elderly because of the ease of overuse and the potential of somewhat serious withdrawal problems.

Conclusions and Management Considerations

None of the observer rating scales or self-report scales in use with the elderly have in fact been standardized on the elderly, and therefore they do not focus exclusively on symptoms of anxiety most frequently experienced by the aged. The critical question of whether the face of anxiety in the elderly differs significantly from that in other age groups cannot be assessed by means of the existing anxiety scales. Some observer rating scales used on elderly samples for specific studies have drawn attention to some of the implicit differences in anxiety measurements for the elderly and younger samples. Zung and Green (1973), for example, presented data from Zung's Self-Rating Anxiety Scale (ZSAS) that indicate that the normal elderly population has higher baseline values for symptoms of anxiety than do normal younger populations. Lehmann and Ban (1969) indicated that intrapsychic conflicts are rarely central to the anxiety seen in the elderly. By contrast, anxiety, agitation, and restless tension in the elderly are said to be most often associated with some physical disorder and to take the forms of sleeplessness, hypochondriacal fears concerning body organs, anorexia, etc. Finally, the tendency noted for normal elderly subjects to deny feelings of depression, as compared to younger adults, is also apparent for feelings of anxiety and tension. In a specific study using the Taylor Manifest Anxiety Scale (Taylor, 1955) and the Tension Factor of the Profile of Mood States (McNair, Lorr, & Droppleman, 1971), Salzman and Shader (1972) observed that normal elderly subjects, 60 years and older, scored significantly lower on anxiety and tension factors than normal volunteers 21 to 35 years of age.

While Verwoerdt (1976, 1981) has provided a thoughtful classification of anxiety in the elderly, geriatric researchers have been unable to meet the methodological challenge of developing a single all-purpose scale that systematically operationalizes the various dimensions of anxiety implicit in Verwoerdt's classification or in Salzman and Shader's construct of anxiety. Such an age-specific all-purpose scale would be of immense value for assessing anxiety in the elderly.

There is little evidence of how anxiety responses change over time. There is some question in particular about whether anxiety-related disorders are exacerbated with aging. While some authors consider anxiety a problem of old age, others do not distinguish between old-age anxiety and depression in their conceptualization of the assessment procedures or their management. Based on clinical impressions it is hard to distinguish anxiety states from depressive states. In part, this lack of information reflects the imprecision in the current diagnostic categories and systems. The practitioner should be aware that those elderly persons whose anxiety disorders begin in old age have a significantly increased prevalence of physical ill-health and disability.

It has been suggested that the autonomic overactivity caused by anxiety may have a deleterious effect on the long-term prognosis of cerebrovascular and ischemic heart disease, making control of anxiety reactions extremely important. There is also some evidence that regardless of diagnostic category, acutely ill elderly persons with anxiety disorders require longer to recover from physical health problems than do other patients not showing anxiety reactions (Bergmann & Eastham, 1974). Prompt psychotropic or psychological treatment of anxiety speeds recovery and reduces mortality in elderly persons who are otherwise not victims of dementia.

Weinberg (1975) observes that chronic neurotic anxiety potentials are ever present in the lives of the elderly who have few environmental supports. Weinberg stresses that anxiety neurosis reactions in the elderly should be recognized as a danger signal for something more serious that may supervene. The elderly person chooses not to withdraw from any experiencing of feelings and through the expression of an acute anxiety state may draw attention to personal needs for security and assistance. In many cases effective avoidance of stressful situations and instruction in coping skills may be the solution to effective control of anxiety.

CHRONIC FATIGUE STATES

Because of the prevalence of many physically debilitating illnesses in old age, it is difficult to separate the origins of psychological and physical chronic fatigue states in the elderly. Indeed it is normal for elderly persons to tire quite easily and to recover more slowly than younger persons. However, it is important to assess whether fatigue states are associated with known physical illness. If they are not, chronic fatigue states in the elderly may be a result of emotional frustration, lack of gratification, and depression resulting from retardation in metabolic activity. While easy fatigability is common in the elderly, the clinician should be able to assess, with the help of the elderly person's family, whether fatigability varies with the prospect of gratification and the potential for satisfying accomplishments. Although the direct effect of fatigue states on the physical well-being of the elderly is not well understood, it would be a mistake to meet these fatigue states (unless they are related to known physical causes) in older people with advice for rest cures or prolonged vacations. Weinberg (1975) suggests a balanced diet of rest, recreation, and interesting occupation, making allowance for the reduced vigor, agility, and learning capacity of the elderly patient (Table 6–1).

HYPOCHONDRIASIS

Hypochondriasis is the inordinate preoccupation with one's own bodily functions or the concern that one or another specific disease is present. It is an especially common disorder in the aged, and the symptoms are directed mostly to the organs of ingestion and digestion. Symptoms of the gastrointestinal tract, heart, and circulatory system interfere with all other activities, including interpersonal relationships. Verwoerdt (1976) suggests that the older the person grows, the more experience the person has had with physical illness, surgery, and accidents, which then become the focus of attention. Blazer (1982) proposes that social isolation, to which the elderly are prone, may increase a tendency toward hypochondriasis.

According to Goldstein and Birnbom (1976) hypochondriacal behavior can be considered to have two features. First, the person perceives oneself to be ill when there is no objective indication of an organic problem or physical ailment. Second, reassurance and information about the person's health status are ineffective in reducing these concerns. In fact the hypochondriacal patient resolutely resists any suggestion that the illness complaints have a psychological origin and are not related to health problems.

Goldstein and Birnbom (1976) together with Pilowsky (1970) have divided hypochondriasis into primary and secondary syndromes, both of which are a notable problem among the elderly. According to these authors primary hypochondriasis is the situation in which principal symptoms involve somatic complaints without any other accompanying psychiatric diagnosis. By contrast secondary hypochondriasis diagnosis applies to those patients who manifest significant degrees of depression (DeAlarcon, 1964) or anxiety in addition to their health concerns. Pilowsky reports that those hypochondriasis patients classified as secondary appear to have had more severe anxious patterns of behavior and had made a suicide attempt.

Psychologically it is believed that this concern is tied in with an unconscious expression of the person's dependency needs. The concern is an expression of the desire to be taken care of. By the unconscious use of physical symptoms tied in with anxiety, conflict, apprehension, and unhappiness, the older person often attempts to regain attention, affection, and sometimes domination. Mechanic (1972) proposes that many elderly consider somatic complaints more desirable to report than emotional distress. In the elderly especially, bodily concerns help to save face when one is beset by failures, uncontrollable situations, and inability to achieve success (Busse, 1976), and flight into a sick role can be an excuse for not coping with problems or stresses (Blazer, 1982, p. 207). Clinical experience indicates that the condition is more frequent among older women (Busse, Barnes, & Dovenmuehle, 1956) and is characterized by fears and worries about the body, which are grossly exaggerated (Strain & Grossman, 1975) (Table 6–1).

Attempts to determine the etiology of hypochondriacal symptoms and to understand the self-absorption of the hypochondriacal patients have not been fruitful. Because of the prevalence of chronic health problems in old age, many complaints about aches and pains and discomfort may in fact have an organic basis. Whether the elderly have an excessive preoccupation about potential cancer, cardiac problems, digestive problems, and the like cannot be accurately determined. Hypochondriacal symptoms are frequently accompanied by overt symptoms of anxiety or depression. Twenty-four percent of those individuals with hypochondriacal symptoms attempted suicide while among those free of symptoms only 7.3 percent attempted suicide. Even though it is likely that hypochondriasis in the elderly is shaped and rewarded through attention, the complaints of hypochondriacal patients should not be dismissed lightly.

Given the high prevalence of physical symptoms in the hypochondriacal patient, Mechanic (1972) proposes that the occurrence of both actual or exaggerated complaints may be difficult to separate in patients with chronic ailments. While patients seldom die of excessive preoccupation with bodily functions, hypochondriacal patients often have depressive disorders, are high suicide risks (DeAlarcon, 1964; Litman & Wold, 1974), and may present many potentially critical situations to the clinician. Thus, elderly patients' health complaints must be investigated seriously. Only after treatable medical disorders have been ruled out should the elderly be confronted with the problem of hypochondriacal concerns.

The elderly person's high bodily involvement is more likely to result from a withdrawal of interests in others and displacement of anxiety. Some form of group therapy with elderly individuals who suffer from chronic symptoms and complaints may be quite valuable with such individuals, if placed in the proper context. Group psychotherapy may be structured to deal with issues of unresolved guilt and to help the bereaved elderly to communicate grief in more nonsomatic ways by providing an atmosphere of comfort, warmth, and support. This approach to the management of hypochondriasis is based on the notion that many elderly have had rather restricted opportunities to learn verbal means of expressing and dealing with grief and distress. Pilowsky (1970) notes that hypochondriacal symptoms are more commonly noted in persons who are less socially educated. Similarly Maddox (1964) found that such persons report receiving little positive appreciation and encouragement. Hence the goal of group therapy with elderly hypochondriacal persons is to help them to focus on alternate ways of expressing the need for reinforcement. Mechanic (1972) suggests similar techniques for providing relief of tension via group work. Regardless of the etiology of their symptoms, these individuals greatly desire understanding on the part of clinicians, family members, and physicians. The following proposed guidelines could be helpful to family members, clinicians, and physicians in their interaction with these individuals (see Busse & Blazer, 1980, p. 405, for details):

- Never try to explain to the patient that symptoms are not caused by an illness. Most persons resolutely resist any suggestion that they are not ill and may insist on various and extensive physical examinations before they abandon their search for a cure of the physical illness. Even direct angry confrontations do not usually have any impact. It is worth emphasizing that the individual may have a serious condition that needs to be monitored and assessed by the physician but that the condition is not critical. A similar approach can be taken by family members who interact with the elderly.

- In considering the consequences of telling the person that there is no physical illness or that medication is not warranted, Busse and Blazer (1980) suggest the physician not venture a clear diagnosis or prognosis of the condition. There can instead be acceptance of the person's symptoms and a suggestion that long-term prognosis is not possible at this juncture.

- Mild medications to be self-administered may be suggested as an indication that an effort is being made to do something to alleviate the patient's symptoms, but treatment should also focus on alternative health-related activities such as physiotherapy, biofeedback, and home activities such as warm baths or massage. (See Table 6–1 for summary.) There are few reports of treatment outcome. Pilowsky (1970) suggests the use of antidepressants for depression with secondary hypochondriasis and minor tranquilizers for primary hypochondriasis.

- Since hypochondriacal persons are greatly distressed by the suggestion that their complaints may have a psychological origin, it is important that patients be seen periodically in a medical clinic setting as opposed to a psychiatric or mental health setting. Patients can be seen for a series of brief visits, and the patient should not be encouraged to elaborate too much on symptoms of distress or discomfort experienced between visits. If the physician is convinced that the ailments are hypochondriacal, the patient should be encouraged to continue brief visits with the physician. The visits over time may be spaced out and the time spent with the patient may be gradually decreased.

- Over time, when the patient has built trust in the physician, there should be a recommendation for some form of psychotherapy in addition to physician visits.

Assessment of hypochondriacal patients for psychotherapy should include their social skills, other resources, and their degree of satisfaction with the social and emotional support systems available. Some form of group work may be used to shape individuals' social skills, enlarge their sources of social reinforcement, and enhance their self-concept.

It has been shown that the hypochondriacal person is likely to have low morale, to be poorly adjusted to the environment, to report past and current periods of depression, and to express feelings of neglect. The loss of self-esteem may therefore be a major feature explaining the intrapunitive personalities among hypochondriacal and physically ill elderly persons. These patients require psychotherapy to adopt a better idea of themselves and their achievements (Bergmann, 1978). Many elderly persons whose hypochondriasis is linked with anger and resentment toward family members have to be helped to harness these feelings into a productive use of family members' help in order to avoid rejection.

Where family members are reinforcing problem behaviors by being critical or ambivalent toward the hypochondriacal patient, they should be involved in the treatment. Goldstein and Birnbom (1976) suggest that simple home tasks for the family and the elderly hypochondriacal patient can be used to build the elderly person's confidence and self-esteem.

Hypochondriasis in the elderly must always be treated as an important sign of psychic and psychological distress. Lifelong hypochondriacal tendencies combined with affective disorders ought to be treated with even greater care because of the complexities of the critical situations they can present to the clinician and physician. Generally speaking, when hypochondriacal complaints appear to rise in later life, there may be an increased risk of suicide but also of serious and perhaps unrelated underlying physical disease of which the elderly person is not otherwise aware (Bergmann, 1978, p. 52).

INSOMNIA AND OTHER SLEEP DISTURBANCES

Insomnia and other sleep disturbances can be a most serious and regrettable symptom in late life. Many elderly persons complain of a variety of sleep disturbances including difficulty in falling asleep, insufficient total sleep, restless sleep, and early morning awakening. Some of these changes in sleep are a part of the expected normal alterations with aging. However, many older persons and their families are concerned that poor sleep or insufficient sleep will lead to serious illness. In old age it has been estimated that at least 50 percent suffer from insomnia (Feinberg & Carlson, 1968; Kahn & Fisher, 1969; Pfeiffer, 1977). The prevalence of sleeping problems among the elderly is more frequently attributed to stressful events, depression, and other affective disorders that affect sleep.

Pfeiffer (1977) stresses the significance of differentiating between changes in sleep patterns that are concomitant of normal aging and those sleep disturbances that are a manifestation of emotional or psychiatric disturbance. Busse and Blazer (1980) make the distinction between sleep disorders of a nonorganic etiology and others of organic etiology. Several types of sleeping disorders can be present individually or in various combinations.

Normal Sleep Patterns in Old Age

In order to understand sleep disturbances that may be linked to either physical illness or major psychiatric conditions of old age, it is important to know the normal sleeping pattern of aging persons. Just as there are pattern changes over all other age groups, old age has its own unique patterns that must be properly understood so that any changes in the expected patterns are not treated as a disease. On an average the elderly require less sleep than younger individuals and on an average elderly persons have more difficulties in sleeping because of the greater frequency of somatic ailments, anxiety, and stress.

Most clinicians are aware that there are four major stages of sleep ranging from light to deep sleep. At stage 1 REM (rapid eye movement) sleep is a stage in which dreams are most likely. Stage 4 sleep, the deep sleep stage in which there is considerable delta activity, has been reported to decrease with age. In elderly subjects deep sleep virtually disappears, and older persons from the age of 50 until 90 require a longer period to fall asleep and generally do not need more than six to seven hours of sleep per night (Kahn & Fisher, 1969; Kales, Beall, & Berger, 1968). Clinicians should be aware that this changed sleep pattern of less deep sleep and more frequent awakenings is the normal pattern for aging persons. There are two or three awakenings during the night from which the older person can easily go back to sleep. Therefore trying to keep an older person asleep for eight hours at a stretch (through the use of sleep medication) is not consistent with the normal pattern of sleeping in later years.

Sleep Disorders of Nonorganic Etiology

These sleep disorders are often associated with initial difficulty that elderly individuals may experience in adjusting to a new environment or to new relationships. Such anxiety disorders may lead to muscle tension, cardiovascular distress, upset stomach, urinary frequency, and especially insomnia (Busse & Blazer, 1980). In the extreme, sleep deprivation accompanied by these anxiety disorders and interruptions of the REM sleep can produce marked behavioral alterations including hallucinations and mild confusion resulting in lack of orientation to time, place, and person. Although such disorientation is only temporary, the symptoms are rather alarming to many elderly persons and their families and can lead to many everyday complications including the strong demand for tranquilizing or hypnotic drugs to induce longer sleep. Such persons are generally found to catnap during the day and to spend a lot of time at night worrying about themselves and their circumstances. The most important procedure in the management of these sleep disorders is the judicious use of increasing the patient's level of activity and adjusting the person's sleeping hours so that less time is spent fretting about the day's events and the anticipated problems of the next day. Although there are regrettably few systematic investigations of treatment for insomnia in old age, the judicious use of minor tranquilizers shortly before bedtime can be of definite benefit (Table 6–1).

Excessive sleep or hypersomnia is also evident in some elderly and is attributed to loneliness, grief, or general decline in morale. An aging factor indicative of the vicissitudes of life connected with increasing loneliness and low degree of personal or intimate contact with relatives or friends appears to be highly correlated with hypersomnia (Table 6–1). Elderly persons who complain more of hypochondriacal symptoms seldom complain of hypersomnia. Excessive sleep in all situations is more likely to be a complaint of family members or the staff of the institution where the elderly might reside. Busse and Blazer (1980) recommend careful evaluation to rule out the organic basis of hypersomnia. Essentially, well elderly persons without gross physical and psychiatric illness but with the loss of intimate relationships and contacts may show symptoms of hypersomnia. Treatment may revolve around the use of mild stimulants and around increasing the patient's level of activity.

Several psychiatric disturbances, especially agitated reactions and transient situational reactions, are also characterized by pronounced sleep disturbances. Depression has also been noted to affect the sleep patterns of the elderly significantly (Mendels & Hawkins, 1968). Slow wave sleep has been shown to be markedly diminished in the depressed, so that persons who are depressed typically spend less time in stages 3 and 4 and show less delta wave activity (Hawkins & Mendels, 1966; Mendels & Chernik, 1975). Some studies report lowered REM sleep in depressed persons while others noted increased levels of REM sleep, but these differences may be due to the organic or inorganic etiology of the depression. Patients with chronic organic mental disorders such as dementia-related depression show less total sleep time and a marked increase in the time spent awake.

The frequency of symptoms of depression complicated by organic mental disorders may significantly affect the reactions of elderly patients to the drugs. The sleep problems among the organically mentally impaired patients do not improve by clinical intervention, and in many cases the use of drugs is contraindicated. By and large, sleep in the elderly depressed is significantly improved by the use of the more sedating tricyclic antidepressants, which increase slow wave sleep (Mendels & Chernik, 1975). As depressed patients improve, their sleep patterns usually return to normal, although some elderly continue to experience problems similar to those reported as concomitant with aging. Whether sleep patterns found in depression are similar to those reported in normal aging is not exactly clear, but after improvement in depression takes place, persons deprived of REM sleep or stage 4 sleep will subsequently increase the amount of time spent in those phases, as if to make up for lost time (Mendels & Chernik, 1975).

Borkovec (1977) refers to other sleep disorders caused by drug dependence and neurological dysfunctions (e.g., sleep apnea) while several other clinicians have addressed the issue of sleep disorders that are secondary to physical disorders. Physical disorders such as congestive heart failure and chronic obstructive pulmonary disease may cause sleep difficulties secondary to shortness of breath and chronic or acute psychogenic pain disorders (Nowlin, 1965). Some pain syndromes (such as fractures of the hip, arthritic pains, and pains secondary to cancers and gastrointestinal infections) more frequently encountered in old age may produce significant disturbing factors in the sleep of many elderly (Table 6–1). Kales, Heuser, Jacobson, Kales, Hanley, Zweizig, and Paulson (1967) have discussed hypothyroidism as a cause of significant changes in the sleep patterns of the elderly, demonstrating a marked decrease in the percentages of stage 3 and stage 4 sleep. These patterns of sleeping improve with treatment of hypothyroidism.

Management of Sleep Disorders

Although there are few systematic investigations of whether some changes observed in the sleep patterns are due principally to aspects of the aging process or due to chronic physical ailments of many elderly, some tentative suggestions can be made for dealing with some of the sleeping problems of the elderly (Table 6–1). Sleep disorders associated with chronic mental disorders such as dementia do not require clinical intervention, but in all cases of sleep problems of the elderly there should be a thorough assessment to rule out disorders caused by organic syndromes, somatic illness, and alcohol or drug dependencies.

A number of important steps in assessment of sleep disturbances can help the clinician to ascertain whether sleeping medications are going to be more effective than psychogenic treatments. More often than not the complaints of sleep disturbances do not stem exclusively from well-defined medical or psychiatric conditions, and disturbances of nonspecific etiology may require treatment or management involving a combination of pharmacology and psychosocial measures. Busse and Blazer (1980) suggest a program of good sleep hygiene that can be beneficial to a majority of elderly whose sleep disorders stem from nonspecific etiology. They suggest a program similar to one proposed by Harris (1977) that includes a form of mild exercise taken during the day but not before bedtime, because the latter will arouse the individual (Kales & Kales, 1970). Other behavioral steps include a light bedtime snack such as warm milk, which is known to mobilize serotonin, which induces sleep. All stimulants (especially coffee) should be avoided at least three to four hours before bedtime.

Another important overriding consideration is that persons with sleep disorders should be evaluated for depression. When depressed effect is present, treatment and management of the sleep problems should focus on the depressive problem rather than on sleep medication, and the objective should be to provide the elderly more insight into their depression. However, rather than just focusing on the depressive symptoms, many depressed elderly similar to nondepressed elderly may also need help in improving their sleeping and waking habits.

The elderly person, for example, should be encouraged to get out of bed at the same time each morning. This regular arousal time appears to strengthen circadian cycling and therefore leads to regular times of sleep onset (Busse & Blazer, 1980), which may help many stressed elderly who cannot return to normal sleeping patterns even after the stress-evoking situations have been improved. Decreasing the time that many elderly spend in bed has also been known to improve the quality of sleep. This improvement may be due to the fact that on an average elderly persons not engaging in any vigorous work require 6.5 hours of sleep, and longer periods of 9 to 12 hours spent in bed is thought related to fragmented and shallow sleep (Harris, 1977). The bedroom should be used at night only, as far as possible, so as to promote the cognitive association between the bedroom and sleep. Coates and Thoresen (1977) suggest that the person should be discouraged from taking naps and at night should get out of bed and go into another room if experiencing difficulties in falling asleep.

General treatment approaches can include attempts to increase the amount of pleasant activity, learning how to relax and deal with tension-producing events and how to enhance interpersonal relationships that will contribute to rewarding and reinforcing interactions (Coates & Thoresen, 1977). These approaches can help to change cognitions of depression and induce mental relaxation during the day and may provide a better emotional readiness for sweet dreams and relaxed sleep in many elderly who feel considerable anxiety during the day.

The treatment of sleep disorders through sleep medication intervention needs to be well considered and evaluated because of the inherent risks associated with the chronic use of nighttime hypnotics. Their chronic use can have many undesirable effects, including tolerance to the drug and physical dependence and daytime retention of some of the drug. Hypnotic drugs commonly prescribed for insomnia suppress the amount of REM sleep leading to daytime delirium, drowsiness, decrease in mental alertness, and loss of equilibrium. Pfeiffer (1977) notes that the older brain is more easily subject to delirium from sedative and hypnotic drugs, which should therefore be used only on a temporary basis. Most of these agents have been proven ineffective and even antagonistic to sleep after two weeks of continual sleep (Harris, 1977). Hartmann (1977) reports the effectiveness of tryptophan in improving sleep in some patients. Tryptophan is a serotonin precursor helping in the initiation and maintenance of sleep. Although little work has been done on the long-term use of tryptophan with sleep problems of the elderly, some of the clinical observations are that low doses appear to induce sleep without producing distortions of physiologic sleep, and the medication is normally ingested in the diet and rapidly metabolized. However, long-term effects of tryptophan need to be studied more thoroughly before extensive use of this drug can be recommended.

Use of antidepressant tricyclic medications usually results in decreased complaints of insomnia in the depressed elderly by increasing slow-wave sleep and controlling depressive symptoms. Flemenbaum (1976), however, cautions that the daily administration of this medication to the elderly at bedtime may lead to nightmares and confusional states. The use of alcohol as a night sedative may enable the tense and anxious person to fall asleep more quickly, but as Harris (1977) notes, the ensuing sleep of these individuals tends to be more fragmented. Furthermore, there is the risk of increased alcohol dependency leading to more confusional states in the elderly.

The elderly are known to self-medicate themselves for sleep difficulties with over-the-counter preparations frequently containing scopolamine, the extensive use of which leads to confusional episodes and even toxic delirium in the aged. Many of these medications should be discouraged. Doses of aspirin are frequently consumed by many elderly as a relief for pain, but the secondary effect of aspirin may be that it increases the brain serotonin level and this induces sleep. The beneficial or detrimental effects of aspirin are hard to evaluate. Because dependencies are built up by chronic users, persons using hypnotic sedatives should be withdrawn only in a medically guided program (Amin, 1976). When some hypnotic drugs are stopped abruptly, a REM rebound often occurs, causing more sleep disturbances than an elderly person is prepared to tolerate. The deleterious effects of some of the low doses of a sedative hypnotic agent may not seriously outweigh the beneficial effects of these medications for many elderly who have taken these medications for many years. Sudden withdrawal of these hypnotics may not be necessary in the case of these elderly chronic users. Busse and Blazer (1980) advocate the careful use of these medications in conjunction with a psychological regimen of a guided program of sleep hygiene.

ALCOHOL ABUSE AND ANXIETY IN THE ELDERLY: SOME DIAGNOSTIC PROBLEMS AND MANAGEMENT CONSIDERATIONS

The problems associated with the diagnosis and management of alcoholism in the elderly have received little attention both clinically and in regard to its relationship with the multiple stresses, adaptations, and anxieties of the elderly. In addition to its prevalence in the aged, especially after bereavement, alcohol may have more deleterious effects on older persons' physical and cognitive functioning than on the young.

According to Blazer (1982) alcohol continues to be the drug most commonly used by the elderly for its central nervous system effect. Butler and Lewis (1973) describe alcohol as a central nervous system depressant. It is not, as many observers believe, a stimulant except as it inhibits cortical control and thereby releases emotional reactions. Since higher intellectual functions are associated with the cortical control, inhibition and impairment of intellectual functions commonly lead to failure in cognitive judgment. In the case of the elderly such failure in judgment may add to other cognitive impairments that may already exist in the aging brain. Thus alcohol may affect muscular control and bodily equilibrium, which may contribute to physical accidents and other injuries in old age.

It is sometimes believed that alcoholic problems have their widest prevalence in middle age between ages 35 and 50 and that alcohol use decreases at advanced ages, when there is a burnout phenomenon. Several studies (e.g., Schuckit & Pastor, 1979; Schuckit, 1977), however, suggest a high prevalence of alcoholic problems (20 percent) among the community elderly and for outpatient elderly.

An important dimension in the assessment of older alcoholics is whether drinking problems were of recent origin or longstanding. Restricting their sample to those persons who had a first psychiatric admission at age 60, Simon, Epstein, and Reynolds (1968) concluded that older alcoholics usually begin to drink heavily in middle age and have a serious drinking problem in old age. On the whole, however, the prevalence of problem drinking seems to be lower in the elderly than in other age groups; still, significant numbers of elderly experience situational problems and difficulties that may precipitate their excessive difficulties to alcohol consumption. The diagnosis of alcohol-related troubles has generally been made on the basis of outside rather than self-report evaluation.

Carruth (1973) comments that in old age, drinking problems include the same nine constellations of symptoms that Cahalan, Cisin, and Crossley (1969) report for the general population. The symptoms, summarized in Table 6–1, include the following:

- symptoms developed as a result of drinking, such as debilitating hangovers, blackouts, memory loss, and "shakes"
- psychological dependence on alcohol, defined as the inability to conduct normal everyday tasks without drinking or planning one's life around drinking
- health problems related to alcohol use, including accidents resulting from drinking
- financial problems related to alcohol use
- problems with spouse or relatives as a result of alcohol use
- problems with friends or neighbors as a result of alcohol use
- problems of handling any tasks as a result of drinking
- belligerence associated with drinking
- problems with the police or the law as a result of drinking

Although survey findings indicate that the extent of alcohol use and alcohol abuse is less, alcoholism still exists and can pose a serious disruption to the life of the older person and affect a large constellation of medical and social service agencies. In view of the many more health problems that the elderly tend to have, the effect of alcohol tends to exacerbate the other existing difficulties. Hence the mediating role of mental ill-health and physical illness in alcohol-related difficulties in old age leads to the reportings of many dire conditions of elderly alcoholics and their need for help. This poses a special concern to the practitioner who is trying to help an older person with alcohol problems or a hospital director faced with a high proportion of hospital admissions consisting of older persons with alcohol-related complications (Mishara & Kastenbaum, 1980).

Alcohol and Physical Health Effects

In discussing the deleterious effects of alcohol on the psychological, cognitive, and medical health, a number of authors (e.g., Gaitz & Baer, 1971; Rosin & Glatt, 1971; Simon, Epstein, & Reynolds, 1968) note that the ill-health effects are greater in older persons than in the young. Wood's (1978) animal studies indicated that with alcohol ingestion older organisms have greater changes in body chemistry and in behavioral coordination. Since most chronic alcoholics subsist on a diet high in carbohydrates and low in thiamine and other B vitamins, alcohol can cause impairment in those organs that are already most impaired by the effects of aging: the lungs, heart, liver, kidneys, brain, and digestive system.

The vitamin deficiencies common among alcoholics more easily lead the elderly to clinical conditions such as anemia and glossitis. The deficiencies may also play a role in creating or intensifying cardiac dysfunction. As Mishara and Kastenbaum (1980) note, nutritional deficiencies beset many old people even apart from alcohol involvement. Inadequate income, depression, loneliness, and the like (nobody to cook for, nobody to eat with) often result in a diet that is not conducive to health. When excessive drinking becomes associated with poor food intake, then vulnerability to a variety of medical problems increases even further. In addition to acquiring symptoms of abdominal pain, weight loss, and diabetes, many elderly may experience incapacitating atrophy and weakness of muscles, with the lower extremities often affected.

On the positive side it is suggested by some observers (see Mishara & Kastenbaum, 1980; Drew, 1968) that moderate use of alcohol may be more positively associated with favorable health status in old age, either because of direct alcohol effects or because moderate use is part of a more health-conducive life style in general. However, even when chronic alcoholism is present in the elderly, clinicians (Drew, 1968; Mishara & Kastenbaum, 1980) are optimistic that many of the physical health problems described can be alleviated or even reversed with some attempt on the part of the elderly alcoholic to abstain or to reduce consumption.

In other words it would be a mistake to assume that old age somehow forecloses the possibility of substantial health improvement or relinquishing a bad habit (Mishara & Kastenbaum, 1980, p. 110). Nevertheless, there is a consensus on the notion that elderly people are somewhat more likely to have multiple medical problems and to be taking more than one kind of medication. This increases the possibility of a variety of alcohol-drug interactions, which are difficult to identify and difficult to manage and control.

Alcohol and Effects on Cognitive-Behavioral Functioning

In regard to cognitive functioning or cognitive impairment as a result of alcohol abuse, a number of authors (e.g., Gaitz & Baer, 1971) note that the extent of cognitive and personality disturbance is greater when alcoholics also have chronic brain damage.

Williams, Ray, and Overall (1973) conclude that those who chronically abuse alcohol beverages tend to show two distinct patterns of mental deterioration, one of which is consistent with general organic brain syndrome, while the other is more closely associated with aging. The finding that alcoholics tend to show both types of impairment was stronger than the trend toward greater impairment with advancing age. Results of this study suggest that elderly alcoholics may be at greater risk for organic brain syndrome because of chronological age and accelerated aging in the mental sphere brought about by alcoholism. The alcoholic elderly in the Williams et al. (1973) study showed more test-measured signs of mental aging than any other age grouping. Results of this study suggest, however, that the organic brain syndrome versus accelerated aging distinction might be an important one to look for.

In presenting a clinical picture of the older patients with a history of alcoholism and chronic brain disease caused by the alcohol, Rosin and Glatt (1971) and Gaitz and Baer (1971) note severe personality disorders. Verwoerdt (1981) notes that chronic alcoholics, usually males and elderly, may manifest extreme jealousy and there may be a serious risk of violent behaviors or depressive symptoms even to the point of suicide. Schuckit and Pastor (1979) note that symptoms such as auditory hallucinations may appear but will clear up following a period of abstinence. They depicted alcoholics, particularly the elderly, as being in a state of confusion and disorientation. Thus, Mishara and Kastenbaum (1980) emphasize the importance of recognizing that a seemingly senile older person who has alcohol-related problems may be reflecting transitory organic brain syndrome that will disappear once the alcohol difficulties are treated (p. 79).

Korsakoff's psychosis is one of the more disabling conditions associated with excessive drinking in the elderly. The mental changes are conspicuous and include massive loss of recent memory, confabulation, poor insight, and behavioral inertia. Mishara and Kastenbaum (1980), while not necessarily associating such psychosis with the elderly alcoholics in particular, note that all of the symptoms of drowsiness, disorientation, and palsies observed with Korsakoff and Wernicke syndromes become more obvious in elderly alcoholics. The explanation for this is that both the Korsakoff and Wernicke syndromes are also related to thiamine and other vitamin deficiencies, which are more frequent correlates of prolonged drinking in the elderly.

In any evaluation or assessment of the cognitive impairment, severe depressive disorders or psychosis-type personality disorders are usually associated with alcoholics. Rosin and Glatt (1971) caution that much of the same symptomatology may often be found in elderly with no alcohol problems. Thus many symptoms such as malnutrition, depressive or aggressive behaviors, or brain damage, often seen in the elderly, should not necessarily be associated with alcohol problems.

Social Correlates of Alcoholism in Old Age

Butler and Lewis (1973) refer to *acute alcoholism* as a state of acute intoxication with temporary and reversible mental and bodily effects while *chronic alcoholism* is the fact and consequence of excessive ingestion and habitual use. Rosin and Glatt (1971) identified different precipitating factors in alcoholism among the elderly, depending on whether onset was in early, middle, or late adulthood. These authors noted that medical illness and stresses associated with old age were often the key precipitants in alcohol abuse among persons who began to drink heavily in middle years or later. Other situational precipitants such as bereavement, retirement, and Alzheimer's-type dementia are also noted in the development of chronic alcoholism for those persons with late onset who began to drink heavily in middle age or later.

One of the major implications of alcoholism in elderly persons pointed out by Gaitz and Baer (1971) is the great strain on family relationships. This strain and the feelings of rejection that the elderly subsequently experience from the family become an added reason for their maintaining the alcoholism and the behavior disorders.

Schuckit (1977) noted that elderly cardiac alcoholic patients had a more general picture of psychiatric difficulty and social dislocation in the group (i.e., higher divorce rate, greater frequency of living alone in a hotel, history of emotional problems).

Rosin and Glatt (1971) have distinguished between two broad categories of factors (primary and reactive) that are known to operate in the drinking of the elderly. The most common primary factors were habitual, excessive drinking patterns, which they attributed to psychological traits of neuroticism, self-indulgence and self-centeredness, and a reliance on alcohol as a psychological support. Rosin and Glatt noted that these psychological factors were most conspicuous in the group of elderly whose drinking was recently exacerbated by physical, mental, or environmental conditions. For example, in six cases these persons had been abstainers until the onset of dementia, which occurred with advancing age and triggered problem drinking. Among the reactive factors Rosin and Glatt (1971) cited bereavement as the most important life circumstance that precipitated excessive drinking. Other important causes of problem drinking were retirement, loneliness, and depression resulting from bereavement or retirement.

Similar findings of psychosocial factors were reported by Wax (1975), who also stressed the importance of social and environmental variables such as alienation from friends and family and loss of spouse as precipitating and maintaining factors in alcoholism among the aged. These findings received support in Lutterotti's (1967) earlier study, which showed that one of the most important factors in old-age alcoholism is the nature of the family situation. Lutterotti's investigation of Italian families showed that alcoholism in old age was often a result of abandonment by family or problems in family life such as separation, divorce, and loss of spouse. A lowering of social status and a feeling of loss of power and control were also cited by Lutterotti as precipitating factors among elderly workers who became alcoholics.

In the Fry (1983) study the findings indicated that personality trait deficits (such as low self-esteem, perceptions of inferiority and disability, perceptions of poor self-control) were strongly linked with anxiety in those depressed elderly who had alcohol-related problems. However, this is not to imply that environmental factors such as social isolation or low income were not present in these elderly, only that the personality factors were quite prominent.

Perceptions of Social Work and Health Agencies concerning Elderly Alcoholics

In regard to social causes of problem drinking Williams and Mysak's (1973) survey of older problem drinkers implied that 79 percent of the social service agency workers and 72 percent of the health agency workers perceived loneliness, loss of spouse, or loss of other meaningful relationships as the most frequently mentioned cause of elderly problem drinkers. The second most frequently mentioned cause was physical and mental deterioration, which was also reported as a major cause by 65 percent of the personnel from health agencies and 48 percent of the workers from social service agencies. Other responses included depression, a sense of worthlessness and rejection, insecurity and anxiety, financial losses, unemployment, or lack of adjustment to retirement.

Studies of individual agencies and institutions suggest that alcohol problems among the elderly may be more prevalent than indicated in nationwide surveys. It is difficult to draw conclusions from studies conducted in specific locations or specific elderly populations. The studies, however, point to the importance of identifying social indicators of alcohol-related problems emerging in the elderly (see Table 6–1 for a review). Studies have shown that older alcoholics have had a history of lifelong patterns of drinking, but distinctly more elderly develop alcohol problems as a reaction to the specific problems of aging and old age.

In the Fry (1983) study feelings of helplessness were often combined with feelings of purposelessness and hopelessness. Those elderly experiencing both helplessness and purposelessness were particularly prone to excessive drinking. In many cases feelings of hopelessness (Fry, 1984) preceded feelings of helplessness, and in many other cases feelings of purposelessness and hopelessness were closely associated with depression and suicidal ideations.

Reviews of the literature indicate that 7 to 21 percent of alcoholics eventually commit suicide, compared to 1 percent of the general population. As Beck, Weissman, and Kovacs (1976, p. 3) point out, "under the influence of alcohol a typical suicide attempter tends to overcome his inhibitions and is more likely to be impulsive and his actions are likely to be more damaging than they would be if he were sober. Thus, the degree of lethality affects not only his intent but the psychological and physiological effects of intoxication." A number of theorists (e.g., Chordorkoff, 1964; Larson, 1978) have argued that alcoholism is often a form of chronic self-destructive suicidal behavior. Moderately severe memory problems, including disorientation to time and difficulty in abstracting and calculating, may add to the cognitive impairment that may already exist in many elderly as a result of cerebral arteriosclerosis and senile brain disease. The elderly patient's severe depression and expressions of hopelessness may dominate the clinical-psychological picture to an extent that many elderly are scared to leave home and venture out.

Stresses as Causative Factors in Alcohol Abuse

While many professionals are reluctant to diagnose alcohol problems (Zimberg, 1975), there is much evidence that when an alcohol problem is diagnosed, many elderly can be helped concurrently to cope more effectively with the stress factors usually precipitating the alcohol problems. It also raises the issue that late-life drinking problems are reactive to stress problems and may respond well to treatment. As Zarit (1980) observes, greater attention to alcohol problems is warranted both because of the long-term ill-health problems and because the prospects for identifying the stress and anxiety associated with alcohol abuse in the elderly appear more favorable.

Relief from stress is often given as a complex potential motive for the use of alcohol in the elderly. Current stressors of financial difficulty, concerns about getting older, losing physical vitality, and the anticipation of becoming more and more dependent on family members are often preconscious stressors that are frequently influential in alcohol abuse on the part of many elderly. As with any other age group the elderly may drink as a result of the combined effects of stressors. In the Fry (1983) study in which semistructured interviews were conducted with 400 moderately to severely depressed elderly, the subjects indicated that they had many problems on their minds—a general worried feeling—when they drank. The findings suggested that one stressor at a time may have relatively little influence on the incidence of drinking, but a large number of stressors in combination had a major impact on the lives of the depressed elderly who resorted to drinking as a means of seeking relief from stress.

The Fry (1983) research findings showed that the idea of stress relief is often formulated in terms of tension reduction when feelings such as tension, stress, and anxiety go largely undifferentiated in elderly subjects. Fry (1983) found that the degree of drinking or alcohol abuse varies with the stages of stress, which are labeled as demand, threat, and exhaustion (Powers & Kutash, 1980). At each stage it was suggested that habituation and addiction developed as the individual increased amounts or frequency of use of alcohol in efforts to extend temporary effects of the drug.

Characteristics of stages identified in the Fry (1983) study were as follows. In the demand stage of stress, elderly individuals were confronted with the prospects of some environmental change (for example, moving to a less preferred place of residence, approaching retirement, facing a medical test). They reported that they felt unable to cope with the actual change or the anticipation of change. They drank mostly to settle their nerves and to feel less depressed. The use of alcohol at this stage fulfilled two primary purposes: temporary relief of strain and avoidance of strain.

Fry's findings suggest that anxiety may frequently act as a significant signal that the individual is not dealing effectively with the external environment. Thirty-two percent of the subjects reported much anxiety about failure. These were elderly individuals who had been long-term abstainers. They began to resort to alcohol to get relief from anxiety. Such elderly individuals, while reducing anxiety at one level, reported that they still experienced considerable psychological strain.

At the threat stage 22 percent of the subjects reported that they felt overwhelmed by the many changes in their lives. They felt threatened by the possibility of having to acquire new coping behaviors such as the use of prostheses and the expectation that they might not adjust.

Thus, the implication for geriatric mental health work is the need to assess the threatening stressors in the lives of the elderly and to attempt to curtail the number of changes in the environment that may be responsible for the introduction of potential stressors. It is suggested that social support networks may have to be solicited in order to help those elderly individuals who at the threat stage resort to drinking because of their perceived inability to cope with changes.

For many elderly persons a sense of loss of resources for action or protection against the threatened life changes may lead them to drinking. Such elderly individuals may need assistance in preparing for change of role, status, or income. They may need specific and symptomatic treatment of disease or illness and nursing aid or medical assistance in order to deal with surgery, surgical corrections, hearing aids, prostheses, or artificial limbs. (See Table 6–1 for management of alcohol abuse procedures.) Environmental stressors that are causing many elderly to resort to alcohol abuse may thus be eliminated by timely assessment of the stressors or the precipitants.

A third group of elderly (2 percent) at the exhaustion stage of stress reported that they felt emotionally and physically exhausted by the thoughts of the number of things that had gone wrong in the recent few years (Fry, 1983). These were elderly whose old-age history revealed several illnesses, hospitalization, surgery, and crippling diseases.

The implications of the Fry (1983) findings are that mental health practitioners and gerontological clinicians who work with geriatric alcoholics may need to identify the exact nature of the anxiety or psychological stress that is causing some abstainers to resort to drinking. A number of points emerge: First, it is important to make some kind of rough assessment of the elderly individual's stage of alcohol dependency. Such an initial assessment can help the practitioner make better judgments for treatment and outcome.

Second, in the case of many elderly who show signs of anxiety and alcohol abuse, it is essential to distinguish clearly the particular forms of anxiety being evaluated. Any action taken should be restricted to just those anxiety forms being assessed. There are a number of important considerations in assessing the relationship between anxiety and alcohol abuse in the aged. Not only is it important to identify specifically the patterns of anxiety (e.g., fear-shame-guilt; fear-distress-anger; fear-anger-dependency) that the elderly individuals show but also to assess the emergence of new or potential stressors when any social action is taken to eliminate certain existing stressors. Alcohol may relieve one stressor, such as feelings of loneliness and rejection, yet lead to the emergence of new stressors such as relating with new persons.

Third, an elderly individual's personality needs, existing coping behaviors, and perceptions of a changing environment all may play key roles in the changes in anxiety levels. The mental health practitioner may be called on not merely to assess the current social functioning of the elderly individual but also to anticipate and evaluate sources of increased anxiety for the future. The relationship between anxiety and alcohol abuse in the elderly may therefore be highly variable depending on personality factors and environmental factors.

Several implications for prevention become clear. If the external stresses in the lives of many elderly are minimized by social change or intervention, alcohol abuse is likely to be reduced. It is doubtful that medical practitioners, sociologists, or politicians can accomplish the task of minimizing stress for the elderly as a whole. However, using "the degree of external stress as a red flag device" for specific families of the elderly can help to deter alcoholism.

The level of internal stress in the elderly also needs to be assessed by mental health professionals especially when the elderly persons present ideas of rejection, loneliness, guilt, helplessness, hopelessness, and giving up. Many elderly may have had depressive tendencies their entire lives and never acted on them. However, in old age, guilt feelings and hopelessness may lead to an increase in anxiety and in individual expectations that alcohol may reduce tension.

More systematic study of elderly alcoholics is needed to determine the optimal treatment approaches both for acute and chronic alcoholic cases. Greater attention to alcohol problems is warranted because of the serious hazards to physical and intellectual health and functioning. By continued study of both external and internal stresses and their vicissitudes the multidetermined causes of alcohol abuse in the elderly will unfold.

Clinical Diagnosis and Assessment of Chronic Alcoholism

Diagnostically it would seem that the elderly alcoholic can be differentiated on the basis of whether primary or reactive factors precipitated the alcohol abuse. Awareness of this distinction is important in regard to treatment. It is important, for example, to ascertain whether the elderly individual is an essential alcoholic with a deficiency in basic coping skills that are inadequate when confronted with overwhelming stress (Knight, 1937; Pattison, 1974). In practice, however, identifying the elderly problem drinker is not an easy task since it is a matter of recognizing not only the symptoms of the disease but also the application of diagnostic criteria. Part of the ambiguity and confusion in the diagnosis of alcoholism is that there are no clearly defined and objective tests used in determining this condition (Barry, 1974, p. 55), with the result that different observers may label the same person as alcoholic or nonalcoholic at different times, in different settings and varying functions.

A set of diagnostic criteria developed by the National Council on Alcoholism (1972) (see Tables 6–2 and 6–3) are the only ones available to assess, even tentatively and speculatively, problem drinking in the elderly. While the criteria are not without problems, they do represent a set of diverse behavioral, psychological, and attitudinal criteria (as opposed to a single criterion) that are generally more reliable and valid for use with the elderly.

It is generally seen that diagnostic level 2 and 3 criteria occur more frequently in elderly problem drinkers. Timiras (1972) observed, for example, that conditions such as brain damage, gastrointestinal disorders, and cardiovascular disease all show greater frequency and intensity in older persons. Similarly the incidence of many of the depressive or mood-cyclic disorders and changes in employment, financial, and marital status are more significantly associated with the elderly. However, one important consideration in the diagnosis of alcoholism in the elderly using diagnostic levels 2 and 3 is that many of the same behavioral, psychological, and attitudinal factors associated with alcoholism are also associated with aging and the effects of old-age illnesses, independent of alcoholism. Thus there is no sharp objective demarcation between the elderly person who does not abuse alcohol and the elderly problem drinker.

Correct diagnosis of alcoholism in the elderly person is heavily contingent on the caregiver's strong suspicions or reportings of problem drinking and the clinical skills of the physician, psychologist, or social worker to distinguish changes associated with aging from symptoms associated with alcohol abuse (Gordon, Kirchoff, & Philips, 1976). The assumption is that these caregivers will be able to identify those elderly who have had a longstanding history of problems with alcohol as opposed to others who resorted to drinking in response to situational stresses.

Thus knowledge of an individual's type of drinking patterns over the life span might serve as a clue in identifying individuals who do and will respond with excessive drinking to most stressful and sometimes even nonstressful situations in daily functioning. This suggests that the major distinction between the chronic problem drinker and the situational alcoholic is that there is evidence of psychopathological causes for excessive drinking in the former case, and in the latter case there are situational changes in the physical and psychological status of the elderly persons that lead them to excessive drinking (Rosin & Glatt, 1971). In the one case, therefore, the physical consequences of prolonged drinking would have had time to build up considerably, resulting in a greater incidence of organic brain syndrome, pathological changes in the central nervous system, and peripheral nervous and other central neurological diseases (e.g., cerebellar cortical degeneration, myelinolysis, Wernicke-Korsakoff syndrome). These disorders are commonly associated with chronic alcoholism (Dreyfus, 1974). In the case of situational alcoholism, on the other hand, the physical consequences of prolonged drinking may not have developed in these individuals.

Generally speaking, frequency and amount of alcohol consumed are other criteria used for distinguishing the problem drinkers from nonproblem drinkers in the normal population (Tables 6–1 and 6–2). However, in the elderly these criteria are not always valid or reliable in that the elderly show a decreased tolerance to alcohol and it takes considerably less alcohol to produce an effect in an elderly person when compared to a younger adult (Rosin & Glatt, 1971). Hence the amount of alcohol consumed by an elderly person may often be overestimated and misreported because of the higher level of alcohol that is registered in the blood, compared to the blood alcohol level of a younger person consuming the same dose.

Table 6–2 Major Criteria for the Diagnosis of Alcoholism

Criterion	Diagnostic Level	Criterion	Diagnostic Level
TRACK I. PHYSIOLOGICAL AND CLINICAL		Fatty degeneration in absence of other known cause	2
A. Physiological Dependency		Alcoholic hepatitis	1
1. Physiological dependence as manifested by evidence of a *withdrawal syndrome* when the intake of alcohol is interrupted or decreased without substitution of other sedation. It must be remembered that overuse of other sedative drugs can produce a similar withdrawal state, which should be differentiated from withdrawal from alcohol.		Laennec's cirrhosis	2
		Pancreatitis in the absence of cholelithiasis	2
		Chronic gastritis	3
		Hematological disorders:	
		Anemia: hypochromic, normocytic, macrocytic, hemolytic with stomatocytosis, low folic acid	3
		Clotting disorders: prothrombin elevation, thrombocytopenia	3
a) Gross tremor (differentiated from other causes of tremor)	1	Wernicke-Korsakoff syndrome	2
b) Hallucinosis (differentiated from schizophrenic hallucinations or other psychoses)	1	Alcoholic cerebellar degeneration	1
		Cerebral degeneration in absence of Alzheimer's disease or arteriosclerosis	2
c) Withdrawal seizures (differentiated from epilepsy and other seizure disorders)	1	Central pontine myelinolysis ⎫ diagnosis ⎬ only	2
		Marchiafava-Bignami's ⎭ possible disease postmortem	2
d) Delirium tremens. Usually starts between the first and third day after withdrawal and minimally includes tremors, disorientation, and hallucinations.	1	Peripheral neuropathy (see also beriberi)	2
		Toxic amblyopia	3
		Alcohol myopathy	2
		Alcoholic cardiomyopathy	2
2. Evidence of *tolerance* to the effects of alcohol. (There may be a decrease in previously high levels of tolerance late in the course.) Although the degree of tolerance to alcohol in no way matches the degree of tolerance to other drugs, the behavioral effects of a given amount of alcohol vary greatly between alcoholic and nonalcoholic subjects.		Beriberi	3
		Pellagra	3
a) A blood alcohol level of more than 150 mg. without gross evidence of intoxication.	1	TRACK II. BEHAVIORAL, PSYCHOLOGICAL, AND ATTITUDINAL	
b) The consumption of one-fifth of a gallon of whiskey or an equivalent amount of wine or beer daily, for more than one day, by a 180-lb. individual.	1	All chronic conditions of psychological dependence occur in dynamic equilibrium with intrapsychic and interpersonal consequences. In alcoholism, similarly, there are varied effects on character and family. Like other chronic relapsing diseases, alcoholism produces vocational, social, and physical impairments. Therefore, the implications of these disruptions must be evaluated and related to the individual and his pattern of alcoholism. The following behavior patterns show psychological dependence on alcohol in alcoholism:	
3. Alcoholic "blackout" periods. (Differential diagnosis from purely psychological fugue states and psychomotor seizures.)	2	1. Drinking despite strong medical contraindication known to patient	1
B. Clinical: Major Alcohol-Associated illnesses. Alcoholism can be assumed to exist if major alcohol-associated illnesses develop in a person who drinks regularly. In such individuals, evidence of physiological and psychological dependence should be searched for.		2. Drinking despite strong, identified, social contraindication (job loss for intoxication, marriage disruption because of drinking, arrest for intoxication, driving while intoxicated)	1
		3. Patient's subjective complaint of loss of control of alcohol consumption	2

Source: From *American Journal of Psychiatry, 129,* p. 129. Copyright 1972 by American Psychiatric Association. Reprinted by permission.

Table 6–3 Minor Criteria for the Diagnosis of Alcoholism

Criterion	Diagnostic Level	Criterion	Diagnostic Level
TRACK I. PHYSIOLOGICAL AND CLINICAL		Indications of liver abnormality:	
A. Direct Effects (ascertained by examination)		SGPT elevation	2
1. Early:		SGOT elevation	3
Odor of alcohol on breath at time of		BSP elevation	2
medical appointment	2	Bilirubin elevation	2
2. Middle:		Urinary urobilinogen elevation	2
Alcoholic facies	2	Serum A/G ratio reversal	2
Vascular engorgement of face	2	Blood and blood clotting:	
Toxic amblyopia	3	Anemia: hypochromic, normocytic,	
Increased incidence of infections	3	macrocytic, hemolytic with	
Cardiac arrhythmias	3	stomatocytosis, low folic acid	3
Peripheral neuropathy (see also		Clotting disorders: prothrombin	
Major Criteria, Track I, B)	2	elevation, thrombocytopenia	3
3. Late (see Major Criteria, Track I, B)		ECG abnormalities	
B. Indirect Effects		Cardiac arrhythmias; tachycardia;	
1. Early:		T waves dimpled, cloven, or	
Tachycardia	3	spinous; atrial fibrillation;	
Flushed face	3	ventricular premature	
Nocturnal diaphoresis	3	contractions; abnormal P waves	2
2. Middle:		EEG abnormalities	
Ecchymoses on lower extremities,		Decreased or increased REM	
arms, or chest	3	sleep, depending on phase	3
Cigarette or other burns on hands or		Loss of delta sleep	3
chest	3	Other reported findings	3
Hyperreflexia, or if drinking heavily,		Decreased immune response	3
hyporeflexia (permanent		Decreased response to Synacthen	
hyporeflexia may be a residuum of		test	3
alcoholic polyneuritis)	3	Chromosomal damage from	
3. Late:		alcoholism	3
Decreased tolerance	3	TRACK II. BEHAVIORAL,	
C. Laboratory Tests		PSYCHOLOGICAL, AND ATTITUDINAL	
1. Major—Direct		A. Behavioral	
Blood alcohol level at any time of		1. Direct effects	
more than 300 mg./100 ml.	1	Early:	
Level of more than 100 mg./100 ml.		Gulping drinks	3
in routine examination	1	Surreptitious drinking	2
2. Major—Indirect		Morning drinking (assess nature of	
Serum osmolality (reflects blood		peer group behavior)	2
alcohol levels): every 22.4 increase		Middle:	
over 200 mOsm/liter reflects		Repeated conscious attempts at	
50 mg./100 ml. alcohol	2	abstinence	2
3. Minor—Indirect		Late:	
Results of alcohol ingestion:		Blatant indiscriminate use of	
Hypoglycemia	3	alcohol	1
Hypochloremic alkalosis	3	Skid Row or equivalent social level	2
Low magnesium level	2	2. Indirect effects	
Lactic acid elevation	3	Early:	
Transient uric acid elevation	3	Medical excuses from work for	
Potassium depletion	3	variety of reasons	2
		Shifting from one alcoholic	
		beverage to another	2

Table 6–3 continued

Criterion	Diagnostic Level	Criterion	Diagnostic Level
Preference for drinking companions, bars, and taverns	2	Late:	
Loss of interest in activities not directly associated with drinking	2	Psychological symptoms consistent with permanent organic brain syndrome (see also Major Criteria, Track I, B)	2
Late:		2. Indirect effects	
Chooses employment that facilitates drinking	3	Early:	
Frequent automobile accidents	3	Unexplained changes in family, social, and business relationships; complaints about wife, job, and friends	3
History of family members undergoing psychiatric treatment; school and behavioral problems in children	3	Spouse makes complaints about drinking behavior, reported by patient or spouse	2
Frequent change of residence for poorly defined reasons	3	Major family disruptions: separation, divorce, threats of divorce	3
Anxiety-relieving mechanisms, such as telephone calls inappropriate in time, distance, person, or motive (telephonitis)	2	Job loss (due to increasing interpersonal difficulties), frequent job changes, financial difficulties	3
Outbursts of rage and suicidal gestures while drinking	2	Late:	
B. Psychological and Attitudinal		Overt expression of more regressive defense mechanisms: denial, projection, etc.	3
1. Direct effects			
Early:		Resentment, jealousy, paranoid attitudes	3
When talking freely, makes frequent reference to drinking alcohol, people being "bombed," "stoned," etc., or admits drinking more than peer group	2	Symptoms of depression: isolation, crying, suicidal preoccupation	3
Middle:		Feelings that he is "losing his mind"	2
Drinking to relieve anger, insomnia, fatigue, depression, social discomfort	2		

Source: From *American Journal of Psychiatry, 129*, pp. 130–131. Copyright 1972 by American Psychiatric Association. Reprinted by permission.

In the final analysis, diagnosis of problem drinking in the elderly has to be attempted on a case-to-case basis. Since the elderly as a group have more serious health problems, are more accident prone, have greater nutritional deficiencies, and suffer more situational traumas, even nonproblem situational drinking may often mimic all the physical, behavioral, and temporary psychological characteristics of chronic problem drinking in younger adults.

Management of Alcohol-Related Problems

Alcoholism is a serious problem in the elderly population, and in many cases the elderly alcoholics have been considered poor candidates for treatment. Gordon and her associates (1976, p. 39) found that most respondents in their study viewed the elderly alcoholics as a virtually hopeless and incurable group, and consequently not one for which special efforts would be beneficial. On the other hand other clinicians (e.g., Schuckit & Miller, 1976) are more optimistic about good medical centers with a team of physicians, social workers, and occupational/recreational therapists being able to deal quite effectively with the alcohol-related disorders of the elderly.

There is an urgent need to increase the clinician's awareness of the general treatment principles, considerations, and modes for dealing with the elderly alcoholics. The appropriate treatment for the alcohol abusers is not substantially different for older alcoholics than for younger ones (Pfeiffer, 1977). However, if it is determined whether primary or reactive factors have precipitated the alcohol abuse, then the general symptomatology and other characteristics for the two types of problem drinkers should be handled differently (Zimberg, 1975). One of the major differences in the overall general management of the elderly is that many older alcoholics compared to younger adults have a number of coexisting physical disorders such as congestive heart failure, hypertension, emphysema, or other disabling diseases. Pfeiffer (1977), therefore, cautions that alcohol withdrawal symptoms can have more serious life-threatening effects in such elderly. Treatment should be approached much more cautiously and conservatively.

Treatment for the situational alcoholic is directed toward helping the elderly person cope with changes in life style. By contrast the treatment focus for chronic alcoholism involves more conventional treatment including psychotropic drugs, psychotherapy, behavior modification and aversion therapy, and therapeutic intervention with the family.

Blazer (1982) is of the view that the depressive states are more common in the elderly, and also risks associated with alcohol withdrawal syndromes are greater. In most instances, therefore, the elderly patient should be admitted to a hospital for withdrawal from alcohol. Only when family support is reliable and family members are most responsible and diligent, can the institution of the therapeutic regimen be entrusted to the family. In most cases, however, hospitalization cannot be avoided.

Chlordiazepoxide is usually the preferred drug in the treatment of alcohol withdrawal and restoration of fluid and electrolyte balance because of its relatively long half-life and cross-tolerance with alcohol. The attending physician will administer initial doses between 50 and 200 mg every six to eight hours, taking into account the weight, alcohol consumption, and age of the person. Administration of the drug will continue for sedation until the delirium, agitations, and hallucinations have improved. Carefully administered and monitored doses are essential in the elderly who are extremely susceptible to problems of memory, dysarthria, ataxia, and drug intoxication developing in the withdrawal process.

Some of the problems and procedures for restoring fluid and electrolyte balance during treatment should be noted. Dehydration is a severe problem. Also nutritional deficiencies such as parenteral vitamin B and thiamine are also common in elderly alcoholics. Therefore intravenous fluids should be supplemented with magnesium, vitamin B, and thiamine.

Psychotherapy is an important adjunct to the pharmacologic regimen for withdrawal and is extremely important to the long-term stress management and coping abilities of the client. Psychotherapy may be especially indicated if alcoholism is judged to be secondary to a recognized emotional conflict that the elderly person is willing to explore (Busse & Blazer, 1980). Withdrawal therapy must be confined to the hospital setting, and psychotherapy may be continued in an outpatient capacity. The psychotherapist must be both firm and supportive and encourage the client to express feelings and concerns about the present and future. After persons have withdrawn successfully from alcohol, they may view their situation quite differently and be more willing to discuss themes of loneliness, depression, uselessness, and physical pain so frequently underlying the elderly's dependency on alcohol. The therapist's skills in interpersonal relationship, empathy, and acceptance are important, but firmness with the client is vital.

Zimberg (1975) suggests antidepressant therapy is an important adjunct to the development of a supportive, socializing relationship, but it should not be started till the person has withdrawn from alcohol and the affective state of the person has stabilized. This is generally one to two weeks after withdrawal. Antidepressant treatment may usually begin with a tricyclic antidepressant, and the patient must be duly warned of the danger of drug and alcohol interaction. If the patient is able to stay alert during the period of abstinence and recognizes the value of antidepressant medication, the continued use of the latter for a period of six to nine months is perfectly safe and adds an inducement for alcohol abstinence. In Zimberg's (1975) approach to antidepressant treatment, medication with antabuse is contraindicated although other clinicians have found it useful to establish a disulfurim (antabuse) contract with the client and one or other family members. In summary, once the acute physiological effects of alcohol withdrawal have been successfully handled and some measure of affective stability has been achieved in the elderly client, further success in treating alcohol disorder and alleviation of any depressive effects are contingent on the active cooperation of the elderly person and the family members.

Therapeutic intervention with the referring family is extremely important. Family therapy is the intervention of choice when family dynamics appear to play a major role in the development of alcoholism (Berensen, 1976). Therapeutic intervention with the family may also be crucial especially in those families where older patients who have been aggressive and dominant members can often intimidate and physically hurt family members who refer the elderly member for treatment and therapy or establish an alliance with the clinician or therapist. Family members may need help and coaching in avoiding conflicts with the elderly alcoholic and also in being firm but supportive during the period of withdrawal and the subsequent period of abstinence. Like the clinician and the client, family members must be given a clear idea of the seriousness of the condition and the need for long-term treatment and supervision of the patient. Family members must be taught how not to compromise with the elderly person in strong urges for alcohol.

Involvement and participation in alcohol anonymous groups are advocated. Zimberg (1975) found that his elderly subjects did not need involvement in Alcoholics Anonymous and that strong support from the family members was useful in accomplishing the same purpose. However, whenever possible, elderly patients should be encouraged to join Alcoholics Synonymous, which can be especially valuable for depressed and lonely persons. Unfortunately many of the self-help groups in terms of interest and orientation are not centered around the immediate needs of the elderly. Age differences among the members and lack of similarity in value orientations present basic problems to many elderly who at best have difficulty in socializing and adjusting to new situations.

Prospects for the accurate diagnosis and treatment of elderly alcoholics, especially those who began their drinking in old age, appear quite favorable. An important factor to consider from a preventive aspect is that problem drinking in late life may in part be due to increase in stressful events, decrease in energy level, restriction in social activities, or reflection of mental and physical impairment. This points to the need of the family members and health-related professionals to be aware of the potential for drug and alcohol abuse in this population.

Obvious though they may be, several recommendations seem necessary at this time. There is a pressing need to develop methods of identifying and finding old problem drinkers. Programs to consider and respond to the specific social, physical, and economic needs of the elderly client are urgently needed. The individual's life style (including ethnic group roots and current affiliations) must also be considered before coming to a conclusion about alcohol use or abuse. Some elderly may have in fact developed patterns of alcohol use throughout their lives that seem to yield no problems to themselves or others. With such individuals, their general health, including any use of drugs and medications, must be considered before coming to a conclusion about the advisability of drinking in old age.

It is important to recognize the social context or sociophysical setting in which the alcohol is consumed. The psychological problems of the isolated drinker need to be the primary focus of therapy and intervention. It is helpful when we can see beyond the problem drinker as such and discover the anxieties, insecurities, family conflicts, and maladaptive behavioral patterns that have led to the alcoholic condition.

PARANOID STATES IN THE AGED

While few systematic estimates of the actual incidence and prevalence of paranoid states in old age are available, a number of authors (e.g., Roth, 1955; Kay, 1963; Fish, 1960) report that 12 to 16 percent of the elderly from psychiatric hospitals had paranoid symptomatology, the onset of which was observed in individuals over the age of 65 years. Since paranoid persons do not generally present themselves for treatment at hospitals, it is conceivable that the only estimates available are based on the numbers of elderly who were forced to treatment by their families.

Paranoid ideation or behavior, while it occurs less frequently than depression in old age, is a common disorder and often has a significant impact. In old age it is rarely seen in pure culture but is common with depression of any severity, and it may signify the emergence of a schizophrenic disorder previously subclinical in its manifestation.

Even though the symptoms of paranoid states in the aged are highly disturbing to others, Pfeiffer's (1977) observation is that such clients do respond well to treatment, and therefore early diagnosis and assessment of this psychiatric disorder is recommended. There appear to be two possibly distinct etiological factors for paranoid disorders in the later years.

At the most general level, paranoid ideation may represent the continuation of a long-term chronic psychosis that originated in early or middle adulthood, and at the most irreversible level they may accompany either acute brain reactions or senile dementia. Two other major factors in the etiology of late-life paranoid states are linked with a history of social adjustment, which has often been poor.

With respect to the first set of etiological factors, Butler and Lewis (1973, p. 52) note that these states are disorders associated with earlier periods of life, presenting a delusion, visually persecutory or grandiose, as the main abnormality. Persons who were hospitalized for a long time may be more suspicious of treatment, especially when previous hospitalization involved unpleasant experiences. Many of these elderly may manifest feelings of hypersensitivity that morbid forces are thwarting them and attempting to harm them. To some extent there is also a uniqueness to the kinds of paranoid reactions and hallucinations that predominate in the elderly and that are often extensions of the earlier suspicions, anxiety, or persecutions, which were felt but kept under ego control. They may tend to exaggerate and misinterpret the most trivial and inconsequential acts of family members who may have given them much support and care and to become suspicious and critical of the motives of many of their friends and caring associates.

At a second level there is a considerable frequency with which paranoid behavior may accompany senile brain disease or dementia (Pfeiffer & Busse, 1973; Young, 1972).

Following persons over a period, Post (1966) confirmed the presence of an organic disorder in 13 of 61 patients with late-life paranoid states. Similarly he reported that 33 of 93 paranoid patients had suspected or actual organic pathologies. However, Tanna (1974) confirmed there is no evidence that all late-life paranoid states are manifestations of senile brain disease. Nevertheless, paranoid reactions are often misdiagnosed as chronic brain syndromes. Especially in old age, cerebral arteriosclerosis, senile brain disease, and other brain diseases may also present paranoid ideas. In later years paranoid ideas may be engrafted on an organic or somatic illness.

With the current wide use of drugs by many hypersensitive elderly patients, paranoid ideas, not unlike those observed in schizophrenia, are sometimes released. Carbon monoxide poisoning, uremia, and other toxic and organic states may present paranoid delusions as well. Predominant symptoms of paranoid reactions may take on the early symptoms of brain pathology, for example, impairment of memory, hallucinations, delusions, and decreased mental vigor. The misdiagnosis of such cases is too often the result of careless examination and unclear diagnostic criteria. Thus the frequency with which paranoid behaviors accompany altered perceptual, cognitive, and physical health functioning suggests the importance of a multidimensional evaluation of the client's functioning including deficits in behavior, deficits in hearing and visual acuity, and deficits in memory and cerebral functioning in order to identify the organic causes, if any, in paranoid clients (see Table 6–1 for summary review of symptoms).

According to Pfeiffer (1977) when paranoid ideation emerges for the first time in later life, it is usually in more circumscribed form than grandiose form. Despite some personality difficulties and suspiciousness and defensiveness, in paranoid states the elderly's contact with reality may remain quite stable. Intellectual functions may not be impaired, and paranoid states may usually be of short duration. According to Tanna (1974, p. 466) the clinical picture consists of delusions and hallucinations, usually without thought disorders. Thus late-life paranoid states are different from the affective psychoses and schizophrenia in which gross affective, volitional, or psychomotor symptoms are the essential problem. There may be an absence of conspicuous thought disorders or other evidence of emotional deterioration typical in schizophrenia. Although the sensorium is clear, the elderly person may fluctuate between feelings of helplessness, derogatory self-statements, and disappointments in the self to feelings of suspiciousness, aggression, and accusations (Pfeiffer, 1977).

In many elderly these paranoid reactions may be in conjunction with associated feelings of depression or agitation. In the elderly such paranoid states tend to occur under adverse conditions or when major dislocation or relocation takes place and often have an understandable basis. Delusions may follow after hospitalization, major surgery, severe hearing loss, partial blindness, or a move to a new neighborhood. Only rarely do the elderly exhibit actual classic paranoia itself, which is marked by an elaborate, well-organized paranoid system in which the person exhibits bizarre imagery or other persecutory symptoms of being controlled by others or having power over others (Pfeiffer, 1977; Tanna, 1974).

A number of etiological factors (see Table 6–1) associated with the onset of paranoid states at any age, implicate the following precursors in the development of paranoid reactions in late life:

• Social isolation. Aloneness and isolation may be primary factors that serve as precipitants. Elderly individuals with a paranoid state in later years may have a background of self-centeredness and self-involvement. They may often be individuals with long-term self-perceptions of inadequacy, inferiority, and low self-esteem. When late-life social isolation, social losses, and constraints in freedom of activity begin to accumulate, the elderly individual may attempt to overcompensate by accusations suggesting a lack of understanding on the parts of others and persecution by others. They are more likely to be elderly females, living alone, having few close relatives and few social contacts. Kay, Cooper, Garside, & Roth (1976) found that the actual onset of paranoid symptoms often followed a period of social isolation brought about by stressful events such as deaths, physical illness, or family conflicts and disagreements.

• Marginal life-circumstances. Kay et al. (1976) and Post (1966, 1973) concluded that many elderly who showed paranoid symptomatology were persons with a history of poor social adjustment and marginal circumstances. They led fairly isolated lives and had few or no successful intimate relationships. Their adjustment to work and other social demands may have been good, but their histories mainly indicate problems in relationships (Post, 1968). When marginal life circumstances were exacerbated by financial losses and economic insecurity, other factors such as retirement became primary precipitating factors in the paranoid states. Feelings of being unwanted or being subjected to annoyances by authorities, especially employers, may also become more intense in the elderly. Interference with one's property, such as thefts of belongings and money, is also quite common in the aged and may reflect paranoid thinking (Post, 1973).

• Sensory losses. Cooper, Garside, and Kay (1976) and Cooper and Porter (1976) noted that often sensory losses, especially hearing impairment, loss of visual acuity, and deafness were closely associated with the onset of paranoid states in the elderly. Thus isolation from human contact and sensory loss that results in misinterpretation of incoming stimuli are perhaps primary precipitating factors (Butler & Lewis, 1973). For example, patients who believed that talk was being directed at them from next door or from the next floor often had a significant hearing loss (Post, 1973). Post regards this as the most common form of paranoid symptomatology in the elderly. Elderly women are affected more than men, although paranoid states are quite common in the elderly of both sexes.

Allen and Clow (1950) identified four types of paranoid reactions in later life:

1. A type that may be called consistent. According to Allen and Clow it is a consistent representation and reflection of the overreactionary annoyances at real physical and environmental limitations, characteristic to some extent of many elderly over the age of 60. Delusions of intruders, thieves, the government, politicians, etc., are often the annoyances that paranoid elderly bring up.

2. A type characterized by episodic paranoid conditions. Someone with a hearing loss may complain that others are talking about the individual. Delusions are sometimes encapsulated or focused on one particular situation or one particular topic like an imaginary prowler in the middle of the night. According to Allen and Clow the prognosis for this type is favorable after remedial or correctional treatment of the sensory impairment.

3. The paranoid type of involutional psychosis, which may represent the continuation of a long-term psychosis that originated in early or middle adulthood. Often the pre-paranoid personality of these elderly may have been characterized by projective defensive patterns. There may have been tendencies to blame others for failures, to be

critical, and to be generally dissatisfied, secretive, and suspicious. Although for many such elderly the vicissitudes of life were managed up to the involutional period, Polatin (1975) notes that the physiological and psychological pressures of the later years may exert an unusual burden on the precarious personality structure. Even minor stressful situations may be interpreted as intolerable pressures exerting a most profound effect. Unfortunately in some elderly living alone with relatively few social contacts, suicide may result from paranoid states accompanied by depression. Other results may be paranoid symptomatology of severe aggression, delusions, and personality deterioration. Here the prognosis is less favorable than in other types of paranoid reactions. Because of the complications arising from earlier psychiatric treatment and paranoid reactions to earlier physicians or clinicians, the psychotic paranoid conditions generally have a rather more unfavorable prognosis.

4. A type displaying a paranoid trend associated with organic brain disease in which the prognosis precludes complete recovery. According to Pfeiffer and Busse (1973) and several other clinicians (e.g., Goodwin & Bunney, 1973; Mendels, Stern, & Frazer, 1976; Schildkraut, 1965) neurochemical correlates of aging and accumulation of waste brought about by toxic levels of medication (Young, 1972) produce acute brain disorders resulting in paranoid reactions.

With or without the presence of the genetic predisposition to organic brain syndrome, paranoid behavior is common in any temporary or acute brain reaction. With an acute origin, both paranoid symptoms and the underlying causal factor may be reversible. Affective disorder paranoid reactions with organic brain syndrome are usually as responsive to treatment as when there is no organic brain syndrome. Late-life paranoia is not usually associated with serious cognitive impairment (Tanna, 1974). In persons with senile dementia, on the contrary, the initial paranoid symptoms may be most ostensible but gradually decline and fade away.

In summary, it is suggested that late-life paranoid states are usually considered distinct from paranoid schizophrenia (Kay et al., 1976; Tanna, 1974); according to past evidence (see Retterstol, 1968) 81 percent of patients with late onset of symptoms had a favorable outcome. Berger and Zarit (1978) conclude that the best of treatment is likely to bring about some amelioration in symptoms, but complete remission is seldom achieved. Therefore, family members need to be made more aware of the relatively poor prospects of psychotherapy or medical treatment with paranoid-state clients.

Diagnosis, Assessment, and Management of Paranoid Disorders

According to Polatin (1975), at any age the overt, gross, and marked paranoid states are easily discernible and recognized by observing and discussing with the subjects their ideas and feelings. Various diagnostic clues can be obtained from a careful evaluation of the elderly person's tendencies such as seclusiveness and self-sufficiency, the tendency to amplify and elaborate on inconsequential and insignificant details. There is a great leaning toward feeling wronged by friends and family, slighted, and ignored. Expressions of active paranoid delusions may emerge to confirm the diagnosis.

Physical examination may generally reveal no causative factors in relation to paranoid states. Most investigators feel that clinicians working with elders who are suspicious and who have fears that they may be robbed, mugged, or assaulted should examine for sensory losses such as deafness, which appears to be slightly more in evidence in the paranoid elderly than in the general population. Delusions may be usually centered around persecution, bodily harm, and theft. There may be a much greater hypochondriacal element.

In the paranoid states there is a greater than average tendency to withdrawal and isolation, but because of the client's fairly intact personality, memory is intact, and no organic defects are observed. By contrast in the symptomatic forms of paranoid states, as in organic brain disease, there are marked forgetfulness, disorientation, and deficits in judgment and effect. Paranoid reactions are notable at first but fade as the organic brain disease develops.

One additional diagnostic consideration is the relationship of paranoid states with depression in the elderly. When both paranoid ideation and depression are present, depression may be a primary precipitant of paranoid states. In those cases antidepressant medication or other treatment of depression appears effective (Young, 1972) for the amelioration of paranoid symptoms.

Treatment: Drug Therapy and Psychotherapy

There are few systematic studies of treatment of paranoid states in the aged. Three general approaches that have implications for the general mental health of the elderly and their increased personal vulnerabilities follow (see Table 6–1 for summary review).

Psychotherapy Approaches

According to a number of authors (Berger & Zarit, 1978; Pfeiffer & Busse, 1973) paranoid states develop essentially because of the elderly client's need for attention and the need for some social stimulation or internal stimulation in the presence of sensory loss and social isolation. Treatment, therefore, should essentially take the form of supportive therapy and reinforcing relationships to counteract the client's suspiciousness, loneliness, hostility, and other paranoid systems. Such provision of attention, social reinforcement, and support can often be provided by the family members. Care must be taken to ensure that the family members check if the paranoid complaints of the elderly have any basis in reality. There are too many cases of elderly who were cheated by unscrupulous vendors, financial agents, businessmen, and estate managers, etc., for family members and relatives to assume de facto that the elderly person's complaints and suspicions are unfounded or delusional.

Social Reinforcement

Beck (1976) proposes a program of social reinforcement for nonparanoid symptoms. He recommends that the therapist help the client understand the consequences of the paranoid reactions in the social relationships. No direct attack should be made on the delusions or suspicions. The therapist or family members should listen intently without arguing about the delusions, minimizing them, or passing any judgment regarding them. Any attempt to argue with the paranoid patient is likely to have negative effects and may precipitate more suspiciousness and mistrust (Goldfarb, 1974). Family members can also be encouraged to take this reflective approach and not to contest the reality of the elderly relative's perceptions. Group work is seldom effective with paranoid persons, and therapy work must focus on the development of a supportive one-to-one relationship with a few significant others who are prepared to give uncritical acceptance to the person and who may over time assume the role of confidants.

Family members should always be encouraged to stay involved. Institutionalization of the elderly person is likely to increase symptomatology and have more negative effects. Although some studies indicate poor prospects for improvement of paranoid states in later years (Tanna, 1974), most reports are optimistic that a majority of persons respond favorably to a combination of medication, interpersonal therapy, and social support. In the patient who has paranoid symptoms in addition to brain syndrome, cognitive impairment may also improve when the paranoid behavior and attendant anxiety are reduced (Eisdorfer & Cohen, 1978).

Medication

Beneficial effects of some adjunct medication, for example phenothiazines, have been reported by Whitehead (1975), and 43 cases of complete remission were reported by Post (1966). A series of reports from the National Institute of Mental Health has indicated that phenothiazine group of drugs is specifically antischizophrenic and not merely effective against target symptoms. The exact dynamic effect of the tranquilizing drugs in producing clinical improvement is not known (Polatin, 1975). Nevertheless, there may be a benefit to maintain patients who have shown improvement on small doses of the drug in order to sustain improvement (Polatin, 1975, p. 1001). The medication program must be an adjunct to the supportive relationship.

While in theory a combination of psychopharmacological and psychotherapeutic treatments is always advocated (Polatin, 1975), in practice the task of coordinating the two forms of treatment often presents problems when the attending professional is not qualified to handle both treatments. One professional's efforts to refer the client to another professional may engender further suspicion or precipitate feelings of rejection and endanger the tenuous trust established between the worker and the elderly person. Therefore, in situations where medical and nonmedical personnel both must become involved, one must continue to serve as a primary caregiver.

Conclusions

Paranoid states cannot be viewed as illnesses, and there is some debate as to whether they should be regarded as minor maladjustments in the elderly (see Goldfarb, 1974), which should be considered only for their nuisance value, or they should be considered as psychiatric disorders with no identified organicity. Because of the limited research available, there is much confusion. Despite these uncertainties there are some useful guidelines for assessment and treatment of paranoid states in late life. The most critical step is to conduct an individual assessment and to determine from the client's history as to whether there has been a pattern of paranoid symptomatology. An important area of assessment is the extent to which the premorbid history of the client indicates social isolation and loneliness. It is important not to stop a diagnostic workup prematurely. An effective interview may be supportive and informal. If the paranoid individual is allowed to talk without confrontation and criticism, the paranoid process may suddenly emerge and become quite florid within a few minutes (Eisdorfer & Cohen, 1978).

Eisdorfer and Cohen advocate a mental status evaluation and assessment of hearing and memory problems since such loss may present with a paranoidlike symptomatology. Psychobiological assessment of sensory loss alone and effective treatment of it may sometimes return paranoid persons to better levels of functioning (Goldfarb, 1974; Polatin, 1975).

Treatment and disposition strategies should consider how disturbing the problem is to the elderly client and to the surrounding environment, especially the family members. It would be an error to rely too heavily on somatic and chemical treatment since medications often have negative side effects. Where there is clear evidence of cognitive impairment and some schizophreniclike illness, hospitalization and chemical treatment with much reduced doses are indicated in such instances. This is particularly the case when the elderly are alone with nobody to supervise their functioning.

OTHER SPECIAL PSYCHOSOCIAL AND MENTAL HEALTH PROBLEMS

Prolonged Bereavement and Grief

Circumstances that foster considerable dysfunctioning but are not seen as a medical problem are death, grief, and bereavement. These are frequent occurrences in old age, but there is clear evidence that prolonged states of grief and bereavement contribute significantly to psychiatric disorders in old age. Since the effects of bereavement and grief are presumed to be more deleterious on the mental and physical health of more older persons than on the young, a separate chapter (see Chapter 9 on Grief, Bereavement and Dying) has been devoted to a discussion of the psychodynamics, management and treatment considerations.

Psychosexual Problems

Sexual problems are not infrequent among aging persons. These include both marital sexual difficulties and sexual problems encountered by the nonmarried. Research work (e.g., Pfeiffer, Verwoerdt, & Davis, 1972) has established that many aging men and women continue to have an active interest in sex, and that many physically healthy aged persons continue an active sex life even in the eighth and ninth decades of life. From a psychosexual point of view, however, the male over age 50 has to contend with one of the great fallacies of our culture in which every man in this age group is arbitrarily defined as sexually impaired (Masters & Johnson, 1970).

Biologically the older woman experiences little sexual impairment as she ages, and most data show that older men are able to control ejaculatory demand in the 50- to 75-year age group far better than younger adults; women continue sexual activity until late in life (Masters & Johnson, 1970). Even if biological factors (such as endocrine function at menopause and decrease in testosterone levels in the elderly male) affect sexual outcomes, there is certainly no evidence that the gradual changes of aging prohibit pleasure in sexual relationships. However, the stereotypes of the sexless older years still abound and may often lead to a curious mixture of problems and concerns among elderly persons in regard to sexual matters. Pfeiffer (1977) notes that these concerns include fears over failing sexual capability and conversely feelings of guilt on the part of those individuals who still have a desire for an active sexual life. There are social expectations that elderly persons should be proper and act their age. Sexual tension may develop as a part of the special efforts to negate their desires for a meaningful heterosexual intercourse. These problems are of real concern to many aging individuals but because of the unwillingness of health care professionals to discuss and explore these issues, a number of psychosexual dysfunctions may surface among elderly males and females.

Sexual Dysfunctioning in the Aging Female

Masters and Johnson (1966) have described in detail the normal changes in the sexual functioning of the aging female. The menopausal female undergoes a drastic change in endocrine function. However, there is no research evidence that these endocrinal changes necessarily have an adverse effect over her sexual functioning in the postmenopausal period. Among the more noticeable physiological changes in late life is the delayed development of vaginal lubrication in the sexual stimulation act. This change is often due to a decrease in elasticity of the vaginal wall. In some cases this problem may lead to bleeding caused by trauma to the vaginal wall during intercourse. Dyspareunia (pain on coitus) is also most commonly caused by the postmenopausal loss of elasticity in the vaginal wall. The bleeding can be treated locally by the application of estrogen cream. Dyspareunia is a common problem in older women, but since elderly women are often most reluctant to share these concerns with their physicians, it is mostly up to the clinician to make close inquiries about the possibilities of symptoms and to make suggestions about medication for this treatable condition.

Estrogen sulfate replacement therapy has made it possible to prevent many of the normal symptoms of menopause and to allow the postmenopausal woman to continue the pleasure obtained from the vaginal and clitoral stimulation. Compared to the younger women, however, there is a noticeable decrease in the orgasmic phase of the sexual response, especially for those in the sixth or seventh decade of life. There is also the expressed need for a quicker resolution of the sexual response. Masters and Johnson (1966) report that the sexual flush decreases in intensity and extent with increasing age. There are more frequent complaints of abdominal pain in the elderly woman. This pain may be secondary to uterine spasms during orgasm. These spasms are to be expected in the postmenopausal woman (Masters & Johnson, 1966). Some of these complaints and concerns can be remedied through natural estrogen replacement therapy although many physicians are reluctant to prescribe estrogen or medroxyprogesterone because of their potential carcinogenic properties. Overall, modern medicine is making it possible to prevent many of the dramatic and sometimes excessive symptoms of menopause so that a majority of aging women need not experience any significant decline in sexual interest and activity until age 70 or more.

Though most of the studies (e.g., Pfeiffer, Verwoerdt, & Wang, 1968; Verwoerdt, Pfeiffer, & Wang, 1969) reveal that there is a general decline in sexual interest and activity in the later years, they also reveal that much of this decline may be secondary to the unavailability of a sexual partner for many widowed elderly women and secondary also to the prejudices about sexual activity in late life. Elderly women, more so than elderly men, are expected by family members and cohorts to demonstrate a decline in sexual activity with advancing age. Sometimes these secondary factors, rather than any pure physiologic bases, may be a contributing factor to sexual dysfunctioning in the aging female. The woman who is expected to be proper and to act her age may resort to other strategies such as masturbation in order to get relief from sexual tension and to be sexually satisfied. These techniques, however, are most inadequate since the basic psychological need during the later years is more for a meaningful heterosexual relationship rather than the sexual activity per se.

With increasing physical disability during old age, frustration and conflict may often arise between the sexual partners and may lead to guilt about sexual activity in old age. Stereotypes of the sexless older years still abound, often causing embarrassment and even shame in the physically disabled elderly woman. Her elderly sexual partner is also embarrassed about his need for sexual activity, and emotional tensions begin to surround the sexual experience. The clinician's reassurance about the appropriateness of sexual activity in old age and explanation of the range of decline in sexual capability in late life can do much to help many elderly couples maintain a healthy sex life. Whenever estrogen replacement is prescribed as an adjunct, the clinician should monitor the treatment and also be careful that other conditions such as diabetes or carcinomas of the vagina are not the contributing factors in painful intercourse or the lack of spontaneous orgasm in the elderly female.

Sexual Dysfunctions in the Aging Male

Minor changes in the sexual performance of males are frequently perceived to be pathological, and a male is more likely than a female to express concern to the clinician concerning loss of interest in sex or fear of inadequate sexual performance. Erectile impotence becomes increasingly prevalent as the male ages (Kinsey, Pomeroy, & Martin, 1948). But psychological factors, more than physiological factors, are of etiologic significance in these disorders and may lead to a form of adjustment disorder or secondary impotence in the male. Many etiologic factors contribute to secondary or psychologically induced impotence in the aging male, principally inheritance factors that may play a causative role in the failure to ejaculate, which may in turn increase emotional tension and decrease spontaneity. The fear of nonperformance in the male may be further compounded by a subsequent fear that he cannot satisfy the female without achieving ejaculation.

Several physical conditions such as diabetes, obesity, injury to the spinal cord, and a general decline in physical health functioning are often associated with a physiologic change in erectile and ejaculatory capacity and a perceived change in sexual potency. However, although these ill-health conditions may temporarily lead to symptoms of sexual dysfunction, many of these symptoms are potentially reversible once the physical health condition has been restored. Malignancy and urologic surgery may also lead to temporary loss of sexual potency, but impotency is not inevitable in these types of surgical manipulations.

The possible adverse effects of several medications and drugs on sexual performance have not been properly examined. Wood (1975) noted that prescribed medications, including hypertensive agents frequently used by the elderly, may produce dysfunction in erectile potency. Other drugs, especially the phenothiazines and anticholinergic drugs, block the sympathetic and parasympathetic innervation of sex organs. Self-medications such as sedatives and sleep medications containing phenobarbital ingredients may also play an important part in the development of sexual dysfunction in late life (Wood, 1975).

Although small quantities of alcohol may stimulate sexual activity in young adults, with increasing age the use of alcohol may have a particularly deleterious effect on the sexual performance of a male whose physical health is marginal. Typically alcohol is used before the sexual act as an escape and tends to increase rather than decrease the elderly male's fear of poor sexual performance.

Secondary impotence may develop following an acute illness such as myocardial infarction or accident such as injury to the back but is usually reversible if the male does not fall into the trap of believing that the initial nonperformance after injury is progressive or permanent. Psychological or psychosocial disorders of various kinds are also important contributors to sexual dysfunction in late life. Among the psychosocial factors that have etiologic significance in secondary impotence of the elderly males are the high incidence of depression, anxiety states, paranoid states, and hypochondriasis. These psychosocial states and others such as chronic fatigue states and lack of stimulation may also result in secondary impotence.

In most cases of secondary impotence the professional's explanations and reassurance of recovery are important. Willingness to explore and discuss such problems and concerns and efforts to alleviate unfounded fears are a first step toward the resolution of the problem (Table 6–1).

Although the elderly are often perceived to be engaging in inappropriate sexual behavior and are the subjects of suspicion and contempt, in fact they are seldom involved in exhibitionism or other types of socially inappropriate sexual responses (Anderson, 1976). Elderly homosexuals do not present any particular types of problems in old age. Their need for touch and closeness is the same as that of the heterosexual elderly, but homosexual elderly do not have the same kind of social supports and affectional and emotional ties that characterize the life style of the heterosexual elderly. In general, therefore, there is more loneliness, social isolation, and unhappiness among homosexual elderly.

Under the category of sexual problems some mention should also be made of the lack of privacy in old age, which often makes it difficult, if not impossible, for many elderly to maintain even a semblance of sex life. Most of the living arrangements of the elderly are such that the rights to privacy are ignored. The frequency of sexual contacts in the absence of privacy declines dramatically. It may well be that new generations of aging individuals will suffer less from unwarranted restraints on their behavior (Pfeiffer, 1977). More education and more willingness on the part of professionals to discuss the elderly's concerns about failing sexual capability, the causes of pain and distress associated with sexual intercourse, and the potential usefulness of estrogen replacement therapy may help to bridge the gap between the natural desire of the elderly to maintain sexual contacts and the difficulties and problems in doing so.

Although it is difficult to draw any firm conclusions concerning the contribution of psychic and psychological factors to the development of impotence in old age, recent evidence has indicated that emotional factors (including guilt, fear, and shame) are among the most important factors contributing to a decline in sexual activity and sexual interest at all age levels, especially in late life. Thus psychological intervention for amelioration of guilt, anxiety, and fears associated with sex need may be a key factor in the management of sexual dysfunctions frequent in late life.

Suicide

According to Pfeiffer (1977) suicidal ideas often accompany severe depressive intervals. They may take the form of relatively passive wishes for death or they may be the starting point for an active plan to commit suicide. Any indications of suicidal ideation among the elderly must be taken seriously. Every year about 10,000 Americans over 60 years of age kill themselves (Miller, 1979). These figures are consistent with earlier estimations (Grollman, 1971; Resnick & Cantor, 1970) and represent about 25 percent of all suicides. Thus suicide among the elderly has occurred at rates more than triple of those experienced in the general population (U.S. Public Health Service, 1974). Alarming as these statistics are, they probably represent a drastic underreporting. Older persons are more likely to be serious in their suicide attempts and more likely to be successful (Gardner, Bahn, & Mack, 1964). The elderly can easily disguise suicide by taking overdoses of drugs, failing to continue with life-sustaining medications, or starving themselves. If incidence of passive suicide is taken into account, it is not surprising that among the elderly the ratio of attempted to successful suicides is 2 to 1 whereas in the younger persons the ratio is 7 to 1.

Indicators of Suicide Potential

These factors are summarized in Table 6–4. Suicide in the elderly represents a major social problem in that about 30 to 50 percent of the elderly persons attempting suicide were quite depressed before the attempt (Gardner, Bahn, & Mack, 1964; Weiss, 1968). This is not to suggest that all depressed elderly are suicidal but rather that suicidal risk is greater among the elderly because of the accompanying and underlying feelings of hopelessness, loneliness, and social isolation (Beck, Kovacs, & Weissman, 1975), which represent the principal pathology of old age (Pfeiffer, 1975; Shanas, 1969). Loneliness and severe depression often accompany the multiple losses experienced by the elderly. Many experience a deep sense of emptiness and meaninglessness. Miller (1979) has described the reaction to these feelings in what he calls "the line of unbearability." With increasing age the line of unbearability is more easily reached because of the absence of hope. Crises are more easily triggered and have been found to increase the risk of suicide in the elderly (Resnick & Cantor, 1970).

A number of psychiatric symptoms have been found to increase the risk of suicide in late life. Many of these signals are symptoms of depression that leave the elderly particularly

---

Table 6–4 Precursors and Indicators of Suicide Potential in the Aged

Precursors of Suicide	*Warning Signs and Signals of Possible Suicide*
Physical health factors: Serious physical illness, especially diagnosis of cancers, carcinomas, dementia, and progressive cognitive impairment	*Physiological and health signs:* Weight loss, change in eating patterns, especially loss of appetite; extreme fatigue; increased concern with bodily functions; change in sleeping patterns particularly acute insomnia; uncharacteristic increase in alcohol consumption
Affective Disorders: A history of depression, loneliness; and functional and psychiatric disorders, including alcoholism, increasing drug dependency, and chronic insomnia	
Psychosocial factors: Prolonged bereavement and grief; social-emotional losses, especially loss of spouse, loss of occupational role, and loss of psychological role as a function of family breakup or family conflicts	*Affective signs:* Change in moods with a noticeable incline in anger, hostility, or depression; increase in expression of fear, irrational anxiety, and uncharacteristic acting-out behaviors
Environmental factors: Interpersonal deprivation; loss of social support and social networks; loss of social involvement and participation; economic difficulties and downward social mobility interacting with loss of social supports	*Cognitive signs:* Increase in confusion and preoccupation; rapid loss of understanding, judgment, or memory; rapid decline in daily task performance and social functioning
	Special behavioral manifestations: Suspicious behaviors such as going out at odd times of the night; sudden interest in church attendance, religion, and funerals, and visiting the physician; a renewed interest in family reunions and resolving family conflicts

vulnerable to suicide. Other factors that increase vulnerability—many of these concomitants of depression—include increasing helplessness and dependency, loss of social roles, bereavement, diagnosis of terminal illness, a serious family conflict, or a major life move or adjustment (Osgood, 1982, 1985; Pfeiffer, 1977).

The risk of suicide has been found greater in elderly persons who are single, widowed, or divorced or experienced a recent loss. Elderly widowers have the highest rate of suicide. Several explanations have been offered for the increased vulnerability of the elderly widowers; the most feasible one is that elderly widowers suffer doubly because they lose not only their role in the family system but their role in the occupational sphere as well (Berardo, 1970; Osgood, 1982).

Alcoholism and acute or chronic brain dysfunctions, especially when accompanied by depression, are other psychiatric symptoms that have been found to increase the risk of suicide. As commonly accepted, alcohol is a depressant and therefore can increase depressive symptoms to a point of unbearability. The intake of alcohol, furthermore, blunts inhibitions about suicide and may also dull the pain resulting from a suicide attempt. However, alcoholism is only one of a whole constellation of risk factors associated with suicide. Quite frequently alcoholism will interact with other factors such as bereavement and loss of social support and meaningful relations to increase the risk of suicide.

Another important factor that is a principal indicator of suicide is the presence of serious physical illness, especially terminal cancers and carcinomas that do not respond to treatment. According to Sainsbury (1962) serious physical illness preceded 35 percent of suicides among older persons. Terminal illnesses among the aged contribute to the suicide more frequently in the aged from lower socioeconomic levels since there are other risk factors such as economic difficulties and an irregular work history, which may have already lowered the person's social and emotional status (Rosow, 1973). Expanding on Rosow's theoretical work, Miller (1979) has identified three major areas of behavioral deviance that are likely to precipitate in the elderly the risk of suicide: (1) negative self-care, (2) inadequate task behaviors, and (3) difficult and conflictual relationship behaviors.

Several psychosocial dimensions are associated with the increased possibility of suicide in old age (see Table 6–4 for summary). Geriatric acts of social deviance and delinquency such as acting out behaviors, excessive self-neglect, and drinking may also be a clue that there is a weak social support system or that there have been some recent losses in terms of physical disability, financial problem, or social and emotional losses. A combination or interaction of these factors may often result in a drastic change in the social environment of the elderly person and increase the risk of suicide.

In attempting to evaluate the significance of the various factors and dimensions contributing to suicide risk in the elderly, evidence from a number of research studies has been collected to show conclusively that a vast majority of older persons committing suicide were severely depressed (Gardner, Bahn, & Mack, 1964). When depression and organic brain syndrome are seen together in elderly persons, increased confusion may cause the depression to subside awhile. However, with cognitive clearing, depressive symptoms may return temporarily, exacerbate hopelessness and feelings of despair, and precipitate a suicide attempt (Lesse, 1967). Finally, a small but significant number of elderly persons who commit suicide have a diagnosed untreatable illness and feel completely hopeless about recovery.

Therefore, suicide attempters in the elderly should be taken doubly seriously, and their incomplete suicide should by no means be taken to imply that they were not serious in their wish to die or that they will not make similar suicidal attempts in the future. Murphy and

Robins (1968) showed that approximately 33 percent of all successful suicides had made a previous attempt and 60 to 80 percent of those who actually committed suicide did in fact communicate their intent to do so. There is indication that 75 percent of elderly persons who killed themselves saw a physician or clergyman before committing suicide (Grollman, 1971; Litman, Curphey, & Shneidman, 1963). Thus contrary to popular belief that persons who talk about suicide will not follow through, among those who talk about suicide 2 to 10 percent will follow through the act of attempting it (Murphy & Robins, 1968). Had the physicians, ministers, or caregivers been more aware of how these individuals were communicating their intent to commit suicide, perhaps the suicides could have been prevented (Pfeiffer, 1977).

Certainly the risk for suicide is increased if the individual makes a gesture or an attempt of suicide regardless of how the intent is communicated and to whom. Communications about intent to commit suicide are not always verbalized and frequently take the form of attempts to reunite with friends and family and say goodbye, put one's house in order, and make one's wishes known about funeral arrangement. Whether intents are communicated directly and verbally or indirectly and nonverbally, intervention must be prompt. A detailed discussion of the risk of suicide in the elderly is beyond the scope of this chapter. The practitioner is referred to Osgood (1985) for a detailed guide to diagnosis and mental health intervention.

Assessing the potential for suicide in older clients involves several steps, principal among which are a prompt attention to many of the behavioral, cognitive, and affective warning signs and signals of possible suicide in the elderly. They are summarized in Table 6–4.

Management Considerations

Major considerations and precautions in handling potential suicides and attempted cases among the elderly are summarized in Exhibit 6–1. If any of the risk factors (and especially a combination of risk factors) described in Table 6–4 is present, steps should be taken to explore with the elderly client whether the person has been contemplating suicide. As spontaneous revelation of suicidal thoughts is not common, a stepwise probe is the best means of assessing the presence of suicidal ideation. For example, the professional may ask the patient if the person has felt that life is not worth living. If so, the person should be asked directly about thoughts of dying or about ending life. If definite plans are presented, it should be determined whether the means for ending life (e.g,. sleeping pills, drugs, implements, or arms) are available or if the client has made a specific movement toward an attempt and what the details and timing of any future plans are (Shneidman & Faberow, 1968). As discussed by Osgood (1982), clinicians and professionals should be seriously concerned if other vulnerability factors (such as loss of social role, bereavement, widowhood, terminal illness, and previous profile of social adjustment and psychiatric symptoms) coexist with depression.

Assessing the potential for suicide in an older person through interviewing assumes a preestablished trust between client and professional through expressions of sincerity, warmth, and genuine concern (Resnick & Cantor, 1970). If not, the client may resent the questions and may decide to become more withdrawn and uncommunicative. If the client shows many of the risk factors indicated, within the time framework available the professional must attempt to establish quick rapport and take actions to overcome the major problems facing the client. The suicidal client can also be asked for reasons for committing suicide or not, as a way of determining the immediate risk of suicidal action. Contrary to

Exhibit 6–1 Management Considerations and Precautions in Handling Potential
Suicidal Elderly

1. Stepwise probe in the interview may be necessary to assessing the presence of suicide
   ideations, as follows:
   -Patient may be asked directly if contemplating hurting self or ending life.
   -If so, it should be determined what means the client was contemplating using and if these
   means are available or accessible to the client.
   -The client's reasons for self-injury or suicide attempt should be determined.
   -The immediate risk of suicidal action should be determined.
2. Suicidal elderly showing symptoms of severe depression or dementia should be viewed as
   being especially at risk for suicidal action, and should be handled as follows:
   -Prompt hospitalization of severely depressed or demented elderly person who has attempted
   suicide.
   -One-to-one supervision and counseling care of the severely depressed elderly.
   -Firm contract with client's adult family member or caregiver to supervise the suicidal
   elderly on a full-time basis.
3. Psychotherapeutic management of the suicidal elderly should include the following measures:
   -Antidepressant medication for relief of depression and withdrawal symptoms is suggested
   so that client may be able to participate in psychotherapy.
   -Supportive counseling (using active listening, empathy, and positive regard techniques) is
   essential in convincing client of being a valuable person.
   -Life-review therapy technique may be effective in helping suicidal elderly come to terms
   with the pessimism of their past and to start anew with the present.
   -Psychotherapy must also include social intervention measures to improve the client's milieu
   and to alter stressful and depressive environmental conditions.
   -Alternate sources of satisfaction, involvement, and gratification should be arranged for the
   client, including continuing contact and interaction with confidants and supportive cohorts.

popular belief, constructive and sensitive inquiry and discussion about suicide does not
antagonize the client nor does it necessarily implant the idea in someone who has not been
considering it (Pokorny, 1968). Unfortunately, negative responses cannot guarantee that
the patient is not at risk for suicide.

Treatment of the suicidal older person with a combination of depression and dementia
with severe depressive symptoms may often require prompt hospitalization since one-to-
one nursing care and supervision may be necessary to reduce the risk of suicide in a
psychiatrically agitated, depressed, and confused elderly who has made attempts at suicide.
Hospitalization ensures that all dangerous weapons and implements and medications have
been removed. Although the patient may insist on maintaining responsibility for life,
frequent checks by the nursing staff are essential, at least for the first few days, which
normally constitute a crisis period.

After clients get over the crisis period and are prepared to enter into a contract for
controlling suicidal impulses, the stringent restrictions can be lifted. A client who does not
have cognitive impairment may be allowed to return home only if family members are
prepared to assume responsibility for meticulous supervision of the elderly person and for
administering medications. The elderly persons with both depression and dementia are

particularly at risk, and as a part of a routine therapy regimen families should be warned of the potential for suicide, but this warning should not be phrased in sensational terms. If a firm contract cannot be worked out with the family to supervise and watch the suicidal elderly on a full-time basis, the clinician must work out a contract with an identified caregiver or confidant, who may be given instructions about the goals, appropriate responses, and limits of the caregiving role.

In cases of depression this will likely involve psychotherapy in addition to arrangement for antidepressant medication. Initially a major goal of the psychotherapist is to provide a first line of contact for the depressed elderly and the assurance that someone cares. Active listening with empathy and restraint from minimizing or even exaggerating the symptoms is a basic technique that can be used by the counselor in helping the person to deal with the life situations that led to feelings of despair and hopelessness. Sometimes reassurance that an individual's depression is self-limiting and that there will be improvement in effects after a while is also helpful (Mintz, 1968).

Much of psychotherapy with the suicidal elderly is in fact psychotherapy for the alleviation of depressive effects and other concomitants of depression. Psychotherapy is therefore supportive and must focus on the feelings of hopelessness rather than on the details of the deprived environmental conditions or on the details of the suicidal action (Beck, 1976; Beck, Kovacs, & Weissman, 1975). Attempts must be made to suggest alternate ways of looking at and thinking about their current life situations and choices other than suicide. This step is particularly important because the motive for suicide develops essentially from feelings of loneliness and isolation and from interpersonal losses. Group psychotherapy as an adjunct to individual psychotherapy also has a beneficial effect.

Feelings of sheer hopelessness and pessimism about personal worth and prospects for the future are often strong motives for the development of suicidal ideation and intent in many elderly (Butler, 1977; Osgood, 1982) but are not easy to change in the postsuicide situation. It has been suggested that a life review is an effective way for helping the client deal with the pessimism and the concomitant feelings of uselessness and lack of self-worth. It is suggested that others become involved with the client in order to provide the necessary continued support. As a first step, however, it is important that the therapist take major responsibility for the control and care of the treatment process.

Blazer (1982, p. 158) emphasizes the importance of the therapist communicating to the client concern and understanding of how bad the person feels or must have felt in order to attempt suicide. The emphasis is therefore first on empathy (I understand how bad you feel); second on perspective (because you are so sad and physically weak, you probably feel mixed up about how your situation really is); third on control (till you get somewhat physically better and feel better, I must decide what is best for you and give you the appropriate treatment), and fourth on giving the client hope (that the depression will pass and then you will be able to take control of yourself again).

Psychotherapy may be long-term or brief, depending on the severity of the client's depression and the extent of hopelessness and despair. If the life situation of the suicidal elderly is such that there is a basis for reality for the hopelessness (such as poverty, social deprivation, and terminal illness), then psychotherapy must also include social intervention measures to improve the stressful and depressive environmental conditions, which may be a major factor contributing to the client's suicidal attempts.

Psychotherapy with severely depressed clients may have to be supplemented by tricyclic antidepressant therapy, which usually lasts two to three weeks. Vigilance of the client with a history of suicide attempts may be necessary for several months following the crisis period.

Treatment of an older suicidal client should be as active, vigorous, involved, and intense as for a younger person. There are several reasons for this. First, the objective is to dispel the myth in the minds of many elderly that their lives are not valuable and therefore not worth saving. Second, even severe depression is self-limiting, and through intimate contact with the therapist and other supportive cohorts many elderly will be able to regain meaning for life. Through contact with other supportive individuals a despairing elderly person is more likely to find alternative sources of satisfaction. Professionals must be vigorous in their efforts to motivate the elderly clients to live in hope and with dignity. Because of the legal and ethical code governing their professional practice, professionals cannot afford to overlook even passive attempts at suicide.

SUMMARY

This chapter has examined some types of functional problems and disorders presented by the elderly and looked at certain potentials and possibilities for management and treatment of these psychological problems and disorders. It is not clear whether these disorders are related to biological factors and physical diseases or whether they are determined by psychosocial factors and eventually have adverse effects on biological functioning. Certainly in some cases (such as psychosexual disorders, alcohol abuse, sleep disorders) the psychological factors are of major etiologic significance but may lead to adjustment disorders. Some clinicians are pessimistic about improvement in the late-life affective disorders in the elderly, while others suggest that with the help of family members and the social network support there can be considerable success. Paranoid states, for example, according to some authors should be treated only for the nuisance value and not as an illness or disease. Success in treating such disorders has been limited because of our limited knowledge. Treatment approaches to these functional disorders should be conservative but systematic and precise. The use of drugs in treatment should be limited.

Suicide is a common problem in the elderly and its potentials are often linked with depressive symptoms and other concomitants of depression such as social isolation, loneliness, and social and economic losses. Psychotherapy for depression, social intervention, and education in the care and understanding of elderly can greatly improve prevention of suicide in the elderly.

Some functional disorders especially alcohol abuse in the elderly originate from stresses caused by psychosocial changes and external factors and stresses produced in the course of adjusting to old age. Management and treatment of reactive alcohol-related disorders should combine a variety of treatment modalities including psychotropic drugs, psychotherapy, and family intervention.

The focus of this chapter can be best appreciated in the context of the field of gerontology. Functional disorders in the elderly are the focus of a great deal of research and active intervention. There is, however, a basic philosophic problem with this burgeoning interest. It is based on a pathologic model, that is, the basic assumption that the elderly have diseases and that we must attempt to palliate those diseases before functional disorders can be rectified. We need to rethink our concept of functional disorders. In clinical care we need to become aware that the aged are people who happen to be old, and some of them have functional disorders that need to be mediated on either an individual or social-familial level but always within a preventive mental health network.

REFERENCES

Allen, E.G., & Clow, H.E. (1950). Paranoid reactions in the aging. *Geriatrics, 5,* 66–73.

Amin, M.M. (1976). Drug treatment of insomnia in old age. *Psychopharmacology Bulletin, 12,* 52–55.

Anderson, W.F. (1976). *Practical management of the elderly.* London: Blackwell Scientific Publications.

Barry, H. (1974). Psychological factors in alcoholism. In B. Kissin & H. Begleiter (Eds.), *The biology of alcoholism* (Vol. 3, pp. 53–107). New York: Plenum Press.

Beck, A.T. (1976). *Cognitive therapy and the emotional disorders.* New York: International Universities Press.

Beck, A.T., Kovacs, M., & Weissman, A. (1975). Hopelessness and suicidal behavior: An overview. *Journal of the American Medical Association, 234,* 1146–1149.

Beck, A.T., Weissman, A., & Kovacs, M. (1976). Alcoholism, hopelessness, and suicidal behavior. *Journal of Studies on Alcohol, 37,* 66–77.

Berardo, F.M. (1970). Survivorship and social isolation: The case of the aged widower. *Family Coordinator, 19,* 11–25.

Berensen, D. (1976). Alcohol and the family system. In P.J. Guerin (Ed.), *Family therapy* (pp. 284–297). New York: Gardner Press.

Berger, K.S., & Zarit, S.H. (1978). Late life paranoid states: Assessment and treatment. *American Journal of Orthopsychiatry, 48,* 528–537.

Bergmann, K. (1978). Neurosis and personality disorder in old age. In D. Isaacs & F. Post (Eds.), *Studies in geriatric psychiatry* (pp. 42–73). New York: John Wiley & Sons.

Bergmann, K., & Eastham, E.J. (1974). Psychogeriatric ascertainment and assessment for treatment in an acute medical ward setting. *Age and Ageing, 3,* 174–188.

Blazer, D.G. (1982). *Depression in late life.* St. Louis: C.V. Mosby Co.

Borkovec, T.D. (1977). *Relaxation treatment of sleep disorders.* Paper presented at the meetings of the American Psychological Association, San Francisco.

Busse, E.W. (1976). Hypochondriasis in the elderly: A reaction to social stress. *Journal of the American Geriatrics Society, 4,* 145–149.

Busse, E.W., Barnes, R.H., & Dovenmuehle, R. (1956). The incidence and origin of hypochondriacal patterns and psychophysiological reaction in elderly persons. *First Pan American Congress on Gerontology,* Mexico City, September 1956.

Busse, E.W., & Blazer, D.G. (1980). Disorders related to biological functioning. In E.W. Busse & D.G. Blazer (Eds.), *Handbook of geriatric psychiatry* (pp. 390–414). New York: Van Nostrand Reinhold Co.

Butler, R.N. (1977). Toward a psychiatry of the life cycle: Implications of socio-psychologic studies of the aging process for the psychotherapeutic situation. In S.H. Zarit (Ed.), *Readings in aging and death: Contemporary perspectives* (pp. 213–224). New York: Harper & Row.

Butler, R.N., & Lewis, M.I. (1973). *Aging and mental health: Positive psychosocial approaches.* St. Louis: C.V. Mosby Co.

Cahalan, D., Cisin, I.H., & Crossley, H.M. (1969). *American drinking practices: A national study of drinking behavior and attitudes* (Monograph no. 6). New Brunswick, NJ: Rutgers Center of Alcohol Studies.

Carruth, B. (1973). Toward a definition of problem drinking among older persons: Conceptual and methodological considerations. In E.P. Williams (Ed.), *Alcohol and problem drinking among older persons* (pp. 272–293). Springfield, VA: National Technical Information Service.

Chodorkoff, B. (1964). Alcoholism and ego function. *Quarterly Journal of Studies on Alcohol, 25,* 292–299.

Coates, T.J., & Thoresen, C.E. (1977). *How to sleep better: A drug-free program for overcoming insomnia.* Englewood Cliffs, NJ: Prentice-Hall, Inc.

Cooper, A.F., Garside, R.F., & Kay, D.W.K. (1976). A comparison of deaf and non-deaf patients with paranoid and affective psychoses. *British Journal of Psychiatry, 129,* 532–538.

Cooper, A., & Porter, R. (1976). Visual acuity and ocular pathology in paranoid and affective psychoses of later life. *Journal of Psychosomatic Research, 20,* 107–114.

Covington, J.S. (1975). Alleviating agitation, apprehension, and related symptoms in geriatric patients: A double-blind comparison of a phenothiazine and a benzodiazepine. *Southern Medical Journal, 68,* 719–724.

DeAlarcon, R. (1964). Hypochondriasis and depression in the aged. *Gerontologica Clinica, 6*, 266–277.

Drew, L.R.H. (1968). Alcohol as a self-limiting disease. *Quarterly Journal of Studies on Alcoholism, 29*, 956–967.

Dreyfus, P.M. (1974). Diseases of the nervous system in chronic alcoholics. In B. Kissin & M. Begleiter (Eds.), *The biology of alcoholism* (Vol. 3, pp. 186–195). New York: Plenum Press.

Eisdorfer, C., & Cohen, D. (1978). The cognitively impaired elderly: Differential diagnosis. In M. Storandt, I.C. Siegler, & M.F. Elias (Eds.), *The clinical psychology of aging* (pp. 7–42). New York: Plenum Press.

Feinberg, I., & Carlson, V.R. (1968). Sleep variations as a function of age in man. *Archives of General Psychiatry, 18*, 239–250.

Fish, F. (1960). Senile schizophrenia. *Journal of Mental Science, 106*, 938–946.

Flemenbaum, A. (1976). Pavor nocturnus: A complication of single daily tricyclic or neuroleptic dosage. *American Journal of Psychiatry, 133*, 570–572.

Fry, P.S. (1983). Social, affective and cognitive mediators of depression in the elderly. Unpublished research funded by a 1983 grant received from the Social Sciences and Humanities Research Council of Canada, Ottawa, Ontario.

Fry, P.S. (1984). Development of a geriatric scale of hopelessness: Implications for counseling and intervention with the depressed elderly. *Journal of Counseling Psychology, 31*, 322–331.

Gaitz, C.M., & Baer, D.E. (1971). Characteristics of elderly patients with alcoholism. *Archives of General Psychiatry, 24*, 372–378.

Gardner, E., Bahn, A., & Mack, M. (1964). Suicide and psychiatric care in the aging. *Archives of General Psychiatry, 10*, 547–553.

Gershon, S. (1973). Anti-anxiety agents. In C. Eisdorfer & W.E. Fann (Eds.), *Advances in behavioral biology: Psychopharmacology and aging* (Vol. 5, pp. 183–187). New York: Plenum Press.

Goldfarb, A.I. (1974). Minor maladjustments of the aged. In S. Arieti (Ed.), *American handbook of psychiatry* (Vol. 3, pp. 820–860). New York: Basic Books.

Goldstein, S.E., & Birnbom, F. (1976). Hypochondriasis and the elderly. *Journal of the American Geriatrics Society, 24*, 150–154.

Goodwin, F.K., & Bunney, W.E. (1973). A psychobiological approach to affective illness. *Psychiatric Annals, 3*, 19.

Gordon, J.J., Kirchoff, K.L., & Philipps, B.K. (1976). *Alcoholism and the elderly.* Iowa City: Elderly Program Development Center.

Grollman, E.A. (1971). *Suicide: Prevention, intervention, and postvention.* Boston: Beacon Press.

Guy, W. (1976). *ECDEU assessment manual for psychopharmacology* (rev. ed., DHEW Publication no. ADM 76-338). Washington: Department of Health, Education, & Welfare.

Hamilton, M. (1959). The assessment of anxiety states by rating. *British Journal of Medical Psychology, 32*, 50–55.

Harris, P. (1977). *The sleep disorders.* Kalamazoo, MI: Upjohn.

Hartmann, E. (1977). L-tryptophan: A rational hypnotic with clinical potential. *American Journal of Psychiatry, 123*, 366.

Hawkins, D., & Mendels, J. (1966). Sleep disturbance in depressive syndromes. *American Journal of Psychiatry, 123*, 6.

Kahn, E., & Fisher, C. (1969). The sleep characteristics of the normal aged male. *Journal of Nervous and Mental Disease, 148*, 477–494.

Kales, A., Beall, G.N., & Berger, R.J. (1968). Sleep and dreams: Recent research on clinical aspects. *Annals of Internal Medicine, 68*, 1078–1104.

Kales, A., Heuser, G., Jacobson, A., Kales, J.D., Hanley, J., Zweizig, J.R., & Paulson, M.R. (1967). All night sleep studies in hypothyroid patients, before and after treatment. *Journal of Clinical Endocrinology, 27*, 1593–1599.

Kales, A., & Kales, J.D. (1970). Evaluation, diagnosis and treatment of clinical conditions related to sleep. *Journal of the American Medical Association, 213*, 2229–2234.

Kapnick, P.L. (1978). Organic treatment of the elderly. In M. Storandt, I.C. Siegler, & M.F. Elias (Eds.), *The clinical psychology of aging* (pp. 225–251). New York: Plenum Press.

Kay, D.W.K. (1963). Late paraphrenia and its bearing on the etiology of schizophrenia. *Acta Psychiatrica Scandinavica, 39*, 159–169.

Kay, D.W.K., Cooper, A.F., Garside, R.R., & Roth, M. (1976). The differentiation of paranoid from affective psychoses by patients' premorbid characteristics. *British Journal of Psychiatry, 129,* 207–215.

Kinsey, A.C., Pomeroy, W.B., & Martin, C.E. (1948). *Sexual behavior in the human male.* Philadelphia: W.B. Saunders Co.

Kirven, L.E., & Montero, F.F. (1973). Comparison of thioridazine and diazepam in the control of nonpsychotic symptoms associated with senility: Double-blind study. *Journal of the American Geriatrics Society, 21,* 546–551.

Knight, R.P. (1937). The dynamics and treatment of chronic alcohol addiction. *Bulletin of the Menninger Clinic, 1,* 233–250.

Laforet, E.G., Sidd, J.J., & Waterman, W.E. (1974). The relationship of heart rate to mood in patients with heart block: Effects of pacing. *Journal of Gerontology, 29,* 643–644.

Larson, R. (1978). Thirty years of research on the subjective well-being of older Americans. *Journal of Gerontology, 33,* 109–129.

Lehmann, H.E., & Ban, T.A. (1969). Chemotherapy in aged psychiatric patients. *Canadian Psychiatric Association Journal, 14,* 361–369.

Lesse, S. (1967). Apparent remission in depressed suicidal patients. *Journal of Nervous and Mental Disorders, 144,* 291–307.

Litman, R.E., Curphey, T., & Shneidman, E.S. (1963). Investigations of equivocal suicide. *Journal of the American Medical Association, 184,* 924–929.

Litman, R.E., & Wold, C.I. (1974). Masked depression and suicide. In S. Lesse (Ed.), *Masked depression* (pp. 105–117). New York: Jason Aronson.

Lutterotti, A. (1967). De l'aspect social de l'alcoholisme dans la viellesse. *Revue d'Hygiene et Medecine Scolaries et Universitaires, 15,* 751–760.

Maddox, G. (1964). Self-assessment of health status: A longitudinal study of selected elderly subjects. *Journal of Chronic Diseases, 17,* 449–460.

Masters, W.H., & Johnson, V.E. (1966). *Human sexual response.* Boston: Little, Brown & Co.

Masters, W.H., & Johnson, V.E. (1970). *Human sexual inadequacy.* Boston: Little, Brown & Co.

McCrae, R.R., Bartone, P.T., & Costa, P.T. (1976). Age, anxiety and self-reported health. *International Journal of Aging and Human Development, 7,* 49–58.

McNair, D.M., Lorr, M., & Droppleman, L.F. (1971). *Profile of mood states: Manual.* San Diego, CA: Educational and Industrial Testing Service.

Mechanic, D. (1972). Social factors affecting the presentation of bodily complaints. *New England Journal of Medicine, 286,* 1132–1139.

Mendels, J., & Chernik, D.A. (1975). Sleep changes and affective illness. In F.F. Flach & S.C. Draghi (Eds.), *The nature and treatment of depression* (pp. 309–333). New York: John Wiley & Sons.

Mendels, J., & Hawkins, D.R. (1968). Sleep and depression: Further considerations. *Archives of General Psychiatry, 19,* 445.

Mendels, J., Stern, S., & Frazer, A. (1976). A biochemistry of depression. *Diseases of the Nervous System, 37,* 3.

Miller, M. (1978). Geriatric suicide: The Arizona study. *Gerontologist, 18,* 188–195.

Miller, M. (1979). *Suicide after 60—The final alternative.* New York: Springer.

Mintz, R.S. (1968). Psychotherapy of the suicidal patient. In H.L.P. Resnick (Ed.), *Suicidal behaviors: Diagnosis and management* (pp. 271–296). Boston: Little, Brown & Co.

Mishara, B.L., & Kastenbaum, R. (1980). *Alcohol and old age.* New York: Grune & Stratton.

Murphy, G.E., & Robins, E. (1968). The communication of suicidal ideas. In H.L.P. Resnick (Ed.), *Suicidal behaviors: Diagnosis and management* (pp. 163–170). Boston: Little, Brown & Co.

National Council on Alcoholism, Criteria Committee (1972). Criteria for the diagnosis of alcoholism. *American Journal of Psychiatry, 129,* 127–135.

Nowlin, J.B. (1965). The associations of nocturnal angina pectoris with dreaming. *Annals of Internal Medicine, 63,* 1040.

Osgood, N.J. (1982). Suicide in the elderly. *Postgraduate Medicine, 72,* 123–130.

Osgood, N.J. (1985). *Suicide in the elderly: A practitioner's guide to diagnosis and mental health intervention.* Rockville, MD: Aspen Systems Corp.

Pattison, E.M. (1974). Rehabilitation of the chronic alcoholic. In B. Kissin & H. Begleiter (Eds.), *The biology of alcoholism* (Vol. 3, pp. 587–658). New York: Plenum Press.

Pfeiffer, E. (1975). A short mental status questionnaire for the assessment of organic brain deficit in elderly patients. *Journal of American Geriatrics Society, 23,* 433–441.

Pfeiffer, E. (1977). Psychopathology and social pathology. In J.E. Birren & K.W. Schaie (Eds.), *Handbook of psychology and aging* (pp. 650–671). New York: Van Nostrand Reinhold Co.

Pfeiffer, E., & Busse, E.W. (1973). Mental disorders in late-life affective disorders: Paranoid, neurotic and situational reactions. In E.W. Busse and E. Pfeiffer (Eds.), *Mental illness in later life* (pp. 107–144). Washington: American Psychiatric Association.

Pfeiffer, E., Verwoerdt, A., & Davis, G.C. (1972). Sexual behavior in middle life. *American Journal of Psychiatry, 128,* 10.

Pfeiffer, E., Verwoerdt, A., & Wang, H.S. (1968). Sexual behavior in aged men and women. Observations on 254 community volunteers. *Archives of General Psychiatry, 19,* 641–646.

Piland, B. (1979). The aging process and psychoactive drug use in clinical treatment. In *The aging process and psychoactive drug use* (Service Research Monograph Series, DHEW Publication no. 79-813, pp. 1–16). Washington: Government Printing Office.

Pilowsky, I. (1970). Primary and secondary hypochondriasis. *Acta Psychiatrica Scandinavica, 46,* 273–285.

Pokorny, A.D. (1968). Myths about suicide. In H.L.P. Resnick (Ed.), *Suicidal behaviors: Diagnosis and management* (pp. 57–62). Boston: Little, Brown & Co.

Polatin, P. (1975). Psychotic disorders, paranoid states. In A.M. Freedman, H.I. Kaplan, & B.J. Sadock (Eds.), *Comprehensive textbook of psychiatry* (Vol. 1, pp. 992–1002). Baltimore: Williams & Wilkins.

Post, F. (1966). *Persistent persecutory states in the elderly.* New York: Pergamon.

Post, F. (1968). Psychological aspects of geriatrics. *Postgraduate Medicine, 4,* 307–318.

Post, F. (1973). Paranoid disorders in the elderly. *Postgraduate Medicine, 53,* 52–56.

Post, F. (1982). Functional disorders, description, incidence and recognition. In R. Levy & F. Post (Eds.), *The psychiatry of late life* (pp. 176–196). Oxford: Blackwell Scientific Publications.

Powers, R.J., & Kutash, I.L. (1980). Alcohol abuse and anxiety. In I.L. Kutash, L.B. Schlesinger & associates (Eds.), *Handbook of stress and anxiety* (pp. 329–343). San Francisco: Jossey-Bass.

Resnick, H.L.P., & Cantor, J.M. (1970). Suicide and aging. *Journal of American Geriatrics Society, 18,* 152–158.

Retterstol, N. (1968). Paranoid psychoses. *British Journal of Psychiatry, 114,* 553–562.

Rosin, A.J., & Glatt, M.M. (1971). Alcohol excess in the elderly. *Quarterly Journal of Studies on Alcoholism, 32,* 53–59.

Rosow, I. (1973). The social context of the aging self. *Gerontologist, 13,* 82–87.

Roth, M. (1955). The natural history of mental disorder in old age. *Journal of Mental Science, 101,* 281–289.

Sainsbury, P. (1962). Suicide in later life. *Gerontologica Clinica, 4,* 161–170.

Salzman, C., & Shader, R.I. (1972). Response to psychotropic drugs in the normal elderly. In C. Eisdorfer & W.E. Fann (Eds.), *Psychopharmacology and aging* (pp. 159–168). New York: Plenum Press.

Schildkraut, J.J. (1965). Catecholamine hypothesis of affective disorders. *American Journal of Psychiatry, 122,* 509.

Schuckit, M.A. (1977). Geriatric alcoholism and drug abuse. *Gerontologist, 17,* 168–174.

Schuckit, M.A., & Miller, E.L. (1976). Alcoholism in elderly men: A survey of a general medical ward. *Annals of the New York Academy of Science, 273,* 558–571.

Schuckit, M.A., & Pastor, P.A. (1979). Alcohol-related psychopathology in the aged. In H.I. Kaplan (Ed.), *Psychopathology of aging* (pp. 211–227). New York: Academic Press.

Shanas, E. (1969). Living arrangements and housing of old people. In E.W. Busse & E. Pfeiffer (Eds.), *Behavior and adaptation in late life* (pp. 129–149). Boston: Little, Brown & Co.

Shneidman, E.S., & Faberow, N.L. (1968). The suicide prevention center of Los Angeles. In H.L.P. Resnick (Ed.), *Suicidal behaviors: Diagnosis and management* (pp. 367–380). Boston: Little, Brown & Co.

Simon, A., Epstein, L.J., & Reynolds, L. (1968). Alcoholism in the geriatric mentally ill. *Geriatrics, 23,* 125–131.

Strain, J.J., & Grossman, S. (1975). Psychological reactions to medical illness and hospitalization. In J.J. Strain & S. Grossman (Eds.), *Psychological care of the medically ill: A primer in liaison psychiatry* (pp. 23–57). New York: Appleton-Century-Crofts.

Tanna, V. (1974). Paranoid states: A selected review. *Comprehensive Psychiatry, 15,* 453–470.

Taylor, J.A. (1955). A personality scale of manifest anxiety. *Journal of Abnormal and Social Psychology, 48,* 285–290.

Timiras, P.S. (1972). *Developmental physiology and aging.* New York: Macmillan Publishing Co.

U.S. Public Health Service (1974). *Vital statistics of the United States, Volume II, 1970, Mortality Part A.* Rockville, MD: Department of Health, Education, & Welfare, Public Health Service.

Verwoerdt, A. (1976). *Clinical geropsychiatry.* Baltimore: Williams & Wilkins.

Verwoerdt, A. (1980). Anxiety, dissociative and personality disorders in the elderly. In E.W. Busse & D.G. Blazer (Eds.), *Handbook of geriatric psychiatry* (pp. 368–380). New York: Van Nostrand Reinhold Co.

Verwoerdt, A. (1981). *Clinical geropsychiatry* (2nd ed.). Baltimore: Williams & Wilkins.

Verwoerdt, A., Pfeiffer, E., & Wang, H. (1969). Sexual behavior in senescence. I. Changes in sexual activity and interest of aging men and women. *Journal of Geriatric Psychiatry, 24,* 163.

Wax, T. (1975). *Alcohol abuse among the elderly.* Paper presented at the annual scientific meeting of the Gerontological Society, Louisville, Kentucky.

Weinberg, J. (1975). Geriatric psychiatry. In A.M. Freedman, H.I. Kaplan, & B.J. Sadock (Eds.), *Comprehensive textbook of psychiatry* (Vol. 2, pp. 2405–2420). Baltimore: Williams & Wilkins.

Weiss, J.M.A. (1968). Suicide in the aged. In H.L.P. Resnick (Ed.), *Suicidal behaviors: Diagnosis and management* (pp. 255–267). Boston: Little, Brown & Co.

Whitehead, T. (1975). Long-acting phenothiazines. *British Medical Journal, 2,* 502.

Williams, E.P., & Mysak, P. (1973). Alcoholism and problem drinking among older persons. In E.P. Williams & P. Mysak (Eds.), *Alcoholism and problem drinking among older persons* (pp. 10–15). Springfield, VA: National Technical Information Service.

Williams, J.D., Ray, G.G., & Overall, J.E. (1973). Mental aging and organicity in an alcoholic population. *Journal of Consulting and Clinical Psychology, 41,* 392–396.

Wood, J.S. (1975). Drug effects on human sexual behavior. In N.F. Wood (Ed.), *Human sexuality in health and illness* (pp. 201–211). St. Louis: C.V. Mosby Co.

Wood, W.G. (1978). The elderly alcoholic: Some diagnostic problems and considerations. In M. Storandt, I.C. Siegler & M.F. Elias (Eds.), *The clinical psychology of aging* (pp. 97–113). New York: Plenum Press.

Young, J. (1972). Acute psychiatric disturbances in the elderly and their treatment. *Clinical Practice, 25,* 513–516.

Zarit, S.H. (1980). *Aging and mental disorders: Psychological approaches to assessment and treatment.* New York: Free Press.

Zimberg, S. (1975). The elderly alcoholic. *Gerontologist, 14,* 221–224.

Zung, W.W.K. (1971). A rating instrument for anxiety disorders. *Psychosomatics, 12,* 371–379.

Zung, W.W.K., Gianturco, D., Pfeiffer, E., Wang, H.S., Whanger, A., Bridge, T.P., & Potkin, S.G. (1974). Pharmacology of depression in the aged: Evaluation of Gerovital-H3 as an antidepressant drug. *Psychosomatics, 15,* 127–131.

Zung, W.W.K., & Green, R.L. (1973). Detection of affective disorders in the aged. In C. Eisdorfer & W.E. Fann (Eds.), *Psychopharmacology and aging* (pp. 213–224). New York: Plenum Press.

Chapter 7

Special Considerations in Psychotherapy of the Elderly

Developmental psychologists and clinicians have reviewed a number of perspectives for psychotherapy with the elderly. This chapter explores some of the special issues in the psychotherapy of the elderly and proposes that psychotherapy, if properly conceptualized and structured, can be effective in meeting the elderly clients' needs through individual and group work.

RATIONALE FOR PSYCHOTHERAPY OF THE AGED

Psychotherapy of the elderly clients has received little attention in the professional literature, both in terms of a systematic rational approach and in terms of outcome data. Recent years have brought new growth in the awareness of the problems that are faced by older persons and a renewal of interest in the question of whether the aged can benefit from psychotherapy. This interest has included consideration of the role that individual and group psychotherapy, family therapy, and behavior therapy can play in resolving some of the problems of the aged. In particular it is questioned as to whether application of therapy might require a reconsideration of goals and modification of techniques that have been primarily developed and assessed with younger adult clients.

Recent discussion has also focused on the question of whether psychotherapy for the elderly should be more palliative in nature as opposed to insight-oriented and change-oriented. Given the psychodynamics of the aged, another important question is whether psychotherapy should be brief in structure as opposed to long-term therapy. The use of psychotherapy with the aged has long been hampered by pessimism. Pfeiffer (1971) holds psychiatry as largely responsible for the widespread myth that elderly patients are not amenable to psychotherapy. Therefore, attention by psychiatrists has for the most part consisted of gratuitous comments about the desirability of psychotherapeutic involvement with the elderly. Most psychotherapy with the elderly is being conducted experimentally in hospitals for the mentally ill rather than in outpatient clinics or private practice. Pfeiffer (1971) has also commented on the limited clinical involvement of psychotherapists with geriatric outpatients who account for approximately 2 percent of the outpatient clinic populations but for nearly 30 percent of the mental hospital populations.

These demographic data suggest that the elderly in society tend to receive either no therapeutic care at all or total custodial care in institutional contexts (Goldfarb, 1969; Kahn, 1975). Butler's (1975b) overview makes it obvious that little progress has been made in providing psychotherapeutic services to the aged in the communities. He charges that therapeutic nihilism is reflected in the increasing incidence of psychopathology in later life. As noted by several observers (e.g., Butler, 1975b; Redlich & Kellert, 1978), this lack of service to outpatient elderly in the communities also indicates that psychologists and psychiatrists in private practice work primarily with economically advantaged adults rather than the socially and economically deprived, aged persons.

Professionals' Disenchantment with Psychogeriatric Clients

It is fairly clear that the aged population includes about 17 to 20 percent of individuals who are psychologically distressed and in need of mental health services including outpatient psychotherapy (Abrahams & Patterson, 1978–1979). A number of contemporary writers have discussed other social issues regarding treatment of the elderly that have caused professionals to become personally disenchanted with psychogeriatrics. Butler and Lewis (1977) reviewed a variety of therapist-related barriers to psychological treatment in old age, which they subsumed under the rubrics of professional ageism. According to these authors professionals have operated from an unspoken and self-protective belief that it would be a waste of precious professional time to invest on people with limited futurity or to bear witness to the last struggles of the dying. Zinberg (1965) commented on the practitioners' reluctance to treat the older patient. Treatment of the elderly, dealing as it does with loss, incapacity, and finally death, was depressing for full-time geriatric psychiatrists. Kastenbaum (1978) notes that association with the low-status aged clients tends to lower the clinician's self-esteem and standing with colleagues and consequently produces further depression and comparative reluctance to offer treatment.

Another set of attitudes centers around the clinician's own fears and anxieties. First, there is the generalized expectation that interaction with the elderly client will result in much personal distress and fear, and second, there is the anxiety that the elderly may die during treatment. Often the therapists' overidentification with the aged also stimulates the therapists' fears regarding their own eventual old age and death (Butler & Lewis, 1977). Although it is not clear which of the preceding factors may be prepotent, their cumulative negative impact has been confirmed in Ginsberg and Goldstein's report (Ginsberg & Goldstein, 1974) and in Kahn's study (1975, p. 25), which documents a 45 percent reduction in the number of referrals of older persons for psychological consultation from 1966 to 1971.

General aversion of mental health practitioners toward treating the aged may be causally related to the paucity of psychogeriatric training. Pfeiffer (1971) observed that few practitioners have had sufficient formal training in those psychotherapeutic procedures most suitable for the aged, and most practitioners' knowledge of geriatrics is acquired during infrequent contacts with elderly persons (Lawton & Gottesman, 1974).

Kahn (1975) sees the patterns of psychotherapeutic attention to the aged as the product of "reciprocal aversiveness" between the elderly and the mental health establishment. There has been so little basic contact between the vulnerable elderly and the mental health professions that the type of assessment from which treatment choices might be determined has seldom been done (Kastenbaum, 1978).

In general there has been an underuse of mental health services by the aged, suggesting that both the demand and the need for treatment may not be as great among the elderly as among younger adults (Gottesman, Quarterman, & Cohn, 1973). It is plausible to suppose that the elderly have not viewed therapy as a solution to their problems and have consequently avoided it. However, the tendency of the aged to shun psychotherapy may be conceptualized as part of a gestalt in which the aged view psychotherapy as a badge of a weakness and disgrace instead of a sign of urbane sophistication (Sparacino, 1978–1979). Other factors that may contribute to the elderly's low demand and rejection of psychotherapy include their lack of faith in the "clumsy, insensitive or patronizing intervention techniques" (p. 200) often used by the mental health staff.

In part this state of affairs probably reflects cohort effects. The aged are disproportionately composed of the more poorly educated, who have not accumulated enough knowledge about the causes and cures of mental illness. Many elderly firmly believe that mental illness is an inherited condition from which complete recovery is not possible (Riley & Foner, 1968). Kahn (1975) therefore postulates that the current group of cohorts may easily attribute many reversible and correctable psychological conditions to what they consider normal aging process. The general conservatism of the aged with respect to finances, personal worth, and individual rights might also explain why the aged generally reject psychotherapy (Glamser, 1974).

Kahn (1975) and Sarason, Sarason, and Cowden (1975) predict that the next generation of elderly will comprise a better educated segment of the population. The overall prediction is that "the aged of the future will be more psychologically-minded" (Sarason, Sarason, & Cowden, 1975, p. 584) and will increasingly reject the custodial care typically provided to the elderly. Kahn (1975) anticipates that many more elderly will be exposed to a psychogenic model of mental health and will likely insist on improved mental health care, forcing professionals to eschew custodialism and to become increasingly concerned with prevention in all its aspects.

Calls for more extensive therapeutic efforts with the elderly have blamed current prejudices that the elderly cannot be reeducated, that they are too inflexible to learn, and that there is too much life history to deal with in therapy. This pessimism about the inability of the elderly to profit from psychotherapy because of the irreversible disabilities of old age began with Freud (Rechtschaffen, 1959). Even today it is sustained by many nonanalytical therapists, who regard the aged to be too rigid, lacking in insight and motivation, and too uninteresting to attract the attention of practitioners (Dye, 1978).

Current research, however, presents a different picture of the elderly's ability to benefit from psychotherapy. There is evidence that aging can bring increased level of functioning and motivation to older adults. Rechtschaffen (1959) cited evidence that the aged are more open to alternative interpretations in therapy than are younger clients, that they desire intervention and want therapeutic involvement. Numerous case histories reviewed by Rechtschaffen indicated that various therapists had been successful with aged clients using psychoanalysis (in both traditional and modified forms); Jungian analysis; a blend of life review, reassurance, and supportive therapy; and a combination of drug, diet, and environmental therapies. A review by Eisdorfer and Stotsky (1977) described the varied procedures that have been used successfully in the treatment of the aged.

In general, however, reports of outcome studies are fragmentary and infrequent due to several contributing factors. Principal among these determining factors is that psychotherapy seems to be fashioned predominantly for achieving personality change, insight, and self-awareness. McGee and Lakin (1977) postulate that current psychotherapy procedures are designed for the better-educated and more vocal and expressive youth and adults. Because of educational and other cultural differences, today's cohort of aged persons are less expressive and therefore less receptive to predominantly verbal methods used in psychotherapy. Looft (1973) notes that the elderly are often under incredible pressure not to affirm their selfhood and to assume and maintain a childlike dependence in which they ought not to be too expressive. This may explain their widespread acceptance of the notion that aging is an inevitable and irreversible decline that cannot be remediated by psychotherapy.

PSYCHOSOCIAL CONSIDERATIONS IN PLANNING PSYCHOTHERAPY FOR THE AGED

Various issues may be raised in any discussion of psychogeriatrics, including the dimensions of the mental health problem and the potentials of the elderly to gain from intervention. A number of the more useful clinical dimensions are discussed here.

Elderly's Prospects for Benefiting from Psychotherapy

Kastenbaum (1964) notes that the evaluation of the prospects of the elderly to profit from psychotherapy on the basis of age and life expectancy is clearly associated with the attitudes and values of society, which will determine whether the elderly are good or bad risks. In this regard Kastenbaum poses two opposing questions: Should older individuals be described as an unprofitable prospect because they do not have much time to live? Should we evaluate the older individual's life as more valuable because there is so little left of it?

According to Ingebretsen (1977) such a discussion is reminiscent of the insurance companies' evaluation of individuals as good or bad insurance risks. McGee and Lakin (1977) caution that this perspective focuses attention on the market economy aspects of the therapeutic relationship. It suggests that because there is a limited supply of therapists to serve the mental health needs of society as a whole, the elderly must assume a low priority in the allocation of therapeutic resources. Shanas and Hauser (1974) contend that psychotherapy remains a relatively high-priced service for the elderly. It may remain very low on a total list of priorities for an economy that has not yet developed adequate support for even such obvious necessities as nutrition and medical care for the elderly.

This question turns primarily on whether we regard the elderly as a valuable source of sustenance, maturity, and wisdom and are therefore willing to allocate our limited therapeutic resources to them. A central notion pertains to important developmental tasks of aging, which are often overlooked by the psychotherapy establishment. For Erikson (1968), old-age ushers in the culmination of the life cycle with the accumulation of knowledge and mature judgment "freed of temporal relativity." Reisman (1954) views a majority of the aged as being a self-sustaining and autonomous group anxious to accommodate to life in constructive ways. Similarly Grotjahn (1955) believes that the developmental task of the aging person lies in the integration of the past leading from maturity to wisdom. He evaluates the elderly's prospects for achieving integration and mastery in a most positive light.

Thus the question of whether the elderly are a good or bad prospect for therapy cannot use age per se as a definitive criterion. The assessment depends first on the therapist's own values and frame of reference and second on the elderly client's special problems and concerns. Typically the psychotherapist's reluctance to treat the elderly represents the basic discriminatory attitudes in our society, which suggest that the aged have low social status and are therefore not preferred as clients (Ford & Sbordone, 1981). Kastenbaum (1978) thinks that most clinicians have little hope for the elderly clients. Despite growing evidence to the contrary, the stereotypic belief persists that old age is a period of disintegration and decline and that older patients have low conceptual ability, are usually lacking in energy, and are therefore relatively useless and unproductive (Davis & Klopfer, 1977, p. 343) in psychotherapy.

Social and Emotional Dependency of the Elderly

Many writers (e.g., Goldfarb, 1955; Safirstein, 1972) have pointed out that the elderly present certain social problems that set precise limits on the effectiveness of therapy. Many elderly persons, lonely and fearful of isolation, may permanently align themselves with a protective other who will not forsake or abandon them. The increasing dependency need of the elderly persons to find protectors and providers poses a major problem in psychotherapy. For Erikson (1968) and Reisman (1954) the elderly's withdrawal and dependency reflect a state of anomie and despair. These combine to a state of inattention on the part of many elderly to the outside world.

Extreme dependency in the client may often provoke the therapist, who may react with anger and attempts to avoid the client. Goldfarb (1954) and Stern, Smith, and Frank (1953) postulate that the elderly client's dependency relationship arouses in therapists an unconscious mixture of guilt and hostility "stemming essentially from their own relationship with their parents." However, denying the elderly clients their dependency with a significant other can also lead to friction in the therapist-client relationship. Most elderly patients voluntarily elevate the physician or therapist to a parental status. From the therapist's perspective, however, the inability of the inexperienced therapist to use these illusions for the patients' benefit may pose a serious problem in psychotherapy (Goldfarb, 1971).

The key condition of dependency makes it more difficult for the therapist to accomplish anything instrumental in the therapeutic encounter. While most therapists recommend that client dependency be minimized in the therapeutic relationship, in practice it is difficult for the relatively less experienced practitioner to foster autonomy in the elderly client. This represents a serious roadblock to the therapist whose mandate is to promote growth and change in the elderly client.

While differences exist in the psychological picture of old age, manifest data point to the increasing insecurity of the elderly and the resulting decreased mastery, lowered self-esteem, and increasing invalidism and depression (Peck, 1966). Peck notes that old age means serious depression in a culture that emphasizes youth, beauty, and success. The most obvious losses that accompany old age are physical decline and loss of functions, which may threaten the elderly's concept of self and disintegrate the personality. Thus the psychotherapist who knowingly or unknowingly takes on the responsibility of working with the locked-in feelings of the elderly client is faced with a difficult and time-consuming task.

Elderly's Rehabilitation Potentials

Given the poverty of the aged, financial considerations definitely play a role in their acceptance in psychotherapy. The decisive factor, however, is their capability for redirection and rehabilitation through psychotherapy. The answer to this question is not just of significance to the elderly but to society as a whole, which must assess the prognosis and decide whether therapeutic resources should be allocated to the aged. The prejudicial view is that emotional disorders of the elderly are intractable, untreatable, and peculiar to old age. The aged are viewed as being too rigid and uncooperative, and the question turns primarily on whether they have the intellectual capacity for change. However, one of the important factors overlooked is that older patients are not considered for intervention until an emergency state of mental and personality breakdown has developed (Oberleder, 1964, 1970). Butler (1963) observes that older persons must qualify for therapy on the basis of a severe loss of memory, disorientation, or incontinence, at which time paradoxically the feasibility of therapy may be seriously questioned.

Rosenthal (1959) maintains that the idea the elderly are without the emotional flexibility and intellectual capacity for change is a cultural stereotype. He and others (e.g., Butler, 1963; Oberleder, 1964) refute the position that decline in intelligence occurs as a function of age. Clinical data show that when the intelligence of the elderly was tested by means of verbal tasks, as opposed to tasks requiring speed, fine motor control, and coordination, the elderly obtained higher scores than younger subjects (Pressey, 1957). Similarly, when differentiation was made between fluid and crystallized intelligence, the clinical results show that although fluid intelligence, which has a neural base, reduces somewhat with age, crystallized intelligence, which incorporates verbal comprehension and social awareness, may gain from the greater maturity and the richer life experiences of the elderly.

Mental functioning of the elderly when measured by traditional tests of abstraction shows results that reflect negatively on their capability for change. The empirical evidence, however, does not unequivocally support the argument that gross decline in cognitive abilities and verbal expressiveness with old age makes the elderly unsuitable candidates for psychotherapy (McGee & Lakin, 1977, p. 336).

Others who have worked with the elderly (Rosenthal, 1959; Grotjahn, 1951; Butler, 1963) have argued that for many elderly their greater motivation to find better ways of living for the short span of life left to them produces a striving for change that often far outweighs the strivings of younger clients. Ingebretsen (1977) and Butler (1975b) have argued that the elderly client's shortage of time is a distinct advantage. Most elderly, aware of the decline in their psychological functioning and their general slowness, recognize that they must take greater responsibility for their betterment.

Another favorable factor is that the older adult is more likely to have experienced adapting to stressful situations. Even minimal attention from the therapist may assist these clients to reassert their previously learned coping skills. Davis and Klopfer (1977) believe that most elderly have significant inner resilience and potential for living their lives at a better level of functioning. Frequently the existence of survival and coping resources is obscured by the elderly clients' feelings of anxiety stemming from environmental stresses. The therapists' communication of respect and appropriate admiration for the clients' potentialities can be useful in their recovery. If therapeutic help is not provided promptly or is restricted, it has the effect of reducing motivation for change and increasing despondency in the elderly individuals. Treatment by therapists whose basic training is not for work with the aged also has a negative effect on their well-being (Wolff, 1962; Wolk et al., 1965).

Psychological problems of the elderly range from existential concerns, special crises, neurotic anxiety to organic brain syndromes and mental deterioriation (Schmidt, 1974). Some conditions are irreversible. In general, however, most behavioral and emotional problems of the elderly are within the province of psychotherapy, and promising results have been obtained in group and individual psychotherapy.

Type of Available Therapy for the Elderly

There are many opposing views concerning the nature of therapy for the elderly and the extent to which the therapeutic approach should be similar to that adopted with younger adults. Oberleder (1964) maintains that the problems of the aged can be treated with the same methods and conceptualizations used with the nonaged. Rosenthal (1959) advocates the attainment of goals similar to those used with other adults. Bromley (1966), however, warns against generalizing from therapy developed with younger clients to an older population.

Several observers (Butler, 1975a, 1975b; Goldfarb, 1955; Knight, 1978–79; Post, 1965) suggest that the aged are a distinctive subgroup within society and may well have special needs and concerns that must be treated differently. Cohen (1981) notes that not only do many therapists confuse the clinical picture of the elderly with that of the young adults but also many therapists confuse the clinical picture of the minority of elderly who are cognitively impaired and disordered with that of the majority who are intact. Many elderly are functioning satisfactorily in many areas of their lives while others have functional disorders. Developmental considerations and views of the interplay of age, experience, and disorder in later life will therefore determine what form of psychotherapy is appropriate for the aged.

Several questions seem relevant. Muslin and Epstein (1980) suggest that while age per se indicates nothing definite about the needs and motivations of the client, a number of age-specific ambiguities must be considered. For example, it is not clear whether there are emotional syndromes or complaints specific to the aged or whether neurosis of later life represents a distinct similarity to neurotic syndromes found in youth or adults. Several authors (e.g., Cameron, 1956; Muslin & Epstein, 1980) are of the opinion that the neurosis of late life does not represent any change from the psychotherapeutic involvement with nonaged patients. For many elderly, neurotic disorders represent the emergence of anxiety or depression for the first time and may be precipitated by emotionally charged events in old age. Ingebretsen (1977, p. 319) notes parallels between the situation of the elderly and younger adults in role change, in building and terminating careers and relationships, and in the debate over the meaning of life. Thus in the elderly, as with other age groups, stresses and depressions reveal themselves in both phase-specific and age-specific ways.

Therapy modalities will vary depending on the therapist's individual orientation and the preferences of the family members of the elderly clients. Generally speaking, however, directive, supportive, and activity-oriented approaches are advocated (Oberleder, 1964, 1966). Even deep analytic therapy and complete personality reconstruction are possible with the elderly. However, an intense therapeutic relationship may be ill-advised because of the client's sense of personal loss when therapy ends (Da Silva, 1965). Goldfarb (1969) therefore suggests that the therapist must endeavor to substitute a symbolic rather than a real close interpersonal relationship with the client. To renounce deep personality change does not, however, imply that the elderly cannot change or that they must settle for second-best goals for therapy (Hiatt, 1971).

The question of what kind of therapy we offer the elderly must be determined on the basis of the individual's emotional, physical, and intellectual resources. The specific problems of the elderly client (whether existential in nature or crisis-oriented) will also determine the urgency of the therapeutic help. In general, Ingebretsen (1977, p. 330) recommends that the elderly be helped with concrete problems and crises situations, rather than with a proposal of a deep personality change. Hiatt (1971) advises that long-term therapy goals should be relinquished in order to help the elderly client rehabilitate in a modified environment. Other authors (e.g., Peterson, 1973; Spark, 1974; Brody, 1974) have emphasized the value of individual psychotherapy as an adjunct to group and family therapy.

Goals for Therapy with the Aged

In setting treatment goals Yesavage and Karasu (1982, p. 44) observe that the elderly vary considerably with regard to the strength of their internal and external resources. The elderly show wide individual differences with regard to intellectual and emotional capabilities and disabilities. In their life reviews they demonstrate a marked drive to restructure their lives, seek meaning, and achieve emotional gratification. Accordingly, clinicians and therapists should remain open to a variety of possible approaches in therapy with elderly and be geared toward consolidation, that is, mastery of the past as a basis for adapting to the present.

Several areas of concern are obvious in the geriatric literature on goals for psychotherapy. The goals depend very much on the nature of the problem rather than on the age of the client (Schaie, 1973) although it would not be surprising if therapy goals for the functionally disordered aged were different from therapy goals for the functionally disordered younger adults.

In most instances therapy with the aging has two main goals: the alleviation of anxiety, and the maintenance or rehabilitation of psychological functioning (Stotsky, 1972). Other important goals central to the practice of therapy with the aged follow.

Actualizing Client Potentials

Goldfarb (1955) has argued that a central therapeutic goal is to enable elderly clients to actualize their potentials by bringing about changes in feeling, thinking, and acting that will improve the clients' relationships, facilitate relief from culturally determined tensions, and help them attain a sense of satisfaction and completion. Others have argued that the attainment of all these goals in psychotherapy with the elderly may be an unrealistic proposal. It may inevitably lead to anxiety, frustration, or pessimistic efforts in both the therapist and the client, especially if the therapist believes in the value of short-term therapy. One or two intermediate treatment objectives that seek to reinstate the best level of functioning of the client may be appropriate (Sparacino, 1978–79). Even if this goal is achieved only in small part, it will increase the self-esteem and dignity of the elderly.

Pfeiffer (1976) stresses effective interpersonal relationships as a goal for psychotherapy with the elderly. Patterson (1974) believes that much of the depression we see in older persons results from their deprivation of meaningful relationships with significant others. He emphasizes core conditions of empathic understanding, acceptance, and nonpossessive warmth in the therapist-client relationship. It is particularly important, however, that one not shape relationships to fit narrow concepts of how the elderly ought to behave, relate, or think. Patterson notes that too many psychotherapists are seeking for something to do to their clients. By contrast, therapists who see value in waiting, respecting, and attending to the elderly patient's burdens and struggles, and to the persons themselves, are calling attention to the healing value of a caring relationship (Davis & Klopfer, 1977, p. 345). Such therapists are less concerned about structured intervention and specific techniques and more concerned about the therapeutic value of relationships.

Preventing Social and Emotional Deterioration

A number of observers (e.g., Cath, 1965; Kahn, 1965; Dovenmuehle, 1965) share the view that the therapist's primary responsibility is to prevent the emotional deterioration that results from social withdrawal, disuse, and isolation. Often the disoriented state of the elderly person is really unorientation associated with panic periods and is the result of feelings of guilt, anxiety, and social rejection. Oberleder (1966, p. 142) therefore suggests the need for continuing human contacts, social participation, and meaningful work in order to maintain function.

In setting goals for therapy, Rustin and Wolk (1963) advocate the alleviation of anxiety concerning adaptation and death. In order to achieve this goal, it is important to provide elderly clients opportunity for ventilating feelings of anger, fear, isolation, and rejection. Ventilation of pent-up anger and resentment (even if directed toward the therapist) can release the patient's resources for constructive adjustment and prevent further social or emotional deterioration. Thus insight formation, at least in the initial stages of psychotherapy, is less important than the expression and release of deep emotion.

Accepting Aging

Hammer (1972) and Stotsky (1972) note that the therapeutic goal of accepting old age is by its very nature specific to aged clients. Old age to some elderly comes as an unexpected crisis and needs an explanation. This is true in the same sense that an explanation is required by a senior student who has been diligent and conscientious but fails an important examination. When the elderly have had self-perceptions of high productivity and energy, the effects of declining strength in old age are often negative. Conflict in accepting old age arises from the fact that such an acceptance is not just a task for the aged individual but a task for society as a whole. Therefore psychotherapy aimed at increased acceptance of aging and old age must include within its framework the changing of social attitudes and policies as well as the changing of the elderly person's attitudes toward the bodily image.

The goal of psychotherapy then becomes to help the elderly client come to grips with the realities of diminishing physical capacities, personal losses, and unresolved grief feelings that may be causing depression. The clinician's task is twofold: (1) to help the older patients adjust to what has been taken away in later life and (2) to assist them in mobilizing their life experiences such that they are motivated to reach out for what can be added. Zinberg (1964) advocates that therapy should reinforce concrete activity programs that give the elderly a sense of value and esteem.

Goldfarb (1964) stresses the importance of the therapist's involvement in the client. Perhaps the greatest danger to the client-therapist relationship in the later years lies in the therapist assuming a distant or dominating attitude toward the aged client struggling to accept old age. Equally threatening to this relationship would be the therapist's tendency to be guided by sentimentality and pity for the aged client rather than accurate understanding. The therapist's reluctance to accept the client's dependency relationship may also interfere with the elderly client's struggle to accept old age.

On the other hand therapists working with the elderly frequently observe the emergence of a strong transference (Pfeiffer, 1976). According to Ingebretsen (1977, p. 327) *transference* refers to the feelings and attitudes the client manifests toward the therapist. The transference concept, rooted in psychoanalysis, implies that the feelings projected on to the therapist originate from other people significant in the client's life. Goldfarb (1954) places great value on the transference relationship and warns that the therapist may often be required to enter the relationship as a parent surrogate. In his view it is essential that the therapist be able to capitalize on the authority relationship to provide importantly needed support and security for the client. In the relationship with elderly clients the transference phenomenon may assume many different directions. Elderly clients may frequently ascribe to the therapist characteristics of their adult children and express criticism, pride, or jealousy, thus turning the usual dependency relationship upside down (Pfeiffer, 1976).

Therapists accustomed to such transference responses as anger, criticism, or rebellion from their clients can deal with them effectively by making client feelings the main thrust and goal of therapy. Even when elderly clients direct feelings of hostility, resentment, or dependency, support from the therapist can encourage the elderly toward the necessary regression and subsequent resolution of conflicts. When elderly clients experience uncritical acceptance and respect, there is a noticeable increase in their capacity for self-esteem. Goldfarb (1969) cautions that the therapist's involvement may lead to a substantial increase in the client's dependency. Therefore, in accepting the dependency relationship the therapist must be careful not to dominate or overprotect the client nor to set oneself up as the only person concerned about the elderly individual's welfare.

If there is a significant chronological age difference between the elderly client and the therapist, the transference may assume a different direction. It can often lead to a tendency for the elderly client to describe the young therapist as the eldest child in the relationship or for a client to experience strong sexual transference. Such a transference is by definition an unconscious phenomenon. A number of therapists (e.g., Berezin, 1972; Hiatt, 1971; Ingebretsen, 1977) caution that regardless of the therapist's age or sex or the specific interpretation of the transference it is important for the therapist to consider the logic of the transference relationship with the elderly client. The therapist must be prepared to be perceived as a child, sexual partner, or protective parent and be ready to capitalize on the quality of the transference in order to serve best the needs of the elderly client.

SPECIAL PROBLEMS OF PSYCHOTHERAPY WITH THE ELDERLY

Ingebretsen (1977) and Schmidt (1974) emphasize that the term *elderly* covers a wide range of persons not only in age but also in types of people and kinds of problems. These problems can have unexpected similarities to those of younger persons. Similarly the kinds of psychiatric disturbances that concern adults can also be found in geriatric patients. However, certain crises and existential tasks are particularly central in the later years, and therapists must be prepared in terms of skills and training to deal with some of the special crises and problems of old age.

Adaptation to Losses

Psychotherapeutic themes of physical decline, loss of functions, and marked loss of physical capacities leading to dependence and depression in the elderly are situations of such a character that they will emerge as problems of therapy regardless of how normal and creative the elderly individual's earlier life has been. Helping the aged to cope with major losses must therefore be an important theme of therapy (Hammer, 1972). Old-age losses such as death of a spouse, loss of a job, and loss of status may precipitate depressive reactions in the elderly, and many aged persons may need prolonged help in their search for an acceptable identity.

Retirement can also create a crisis for many industrious and diligent elderly whose self-worth and dignity has been locked into their work. According to Butler (1963) and Seligman (1974) the loss of work for many elderly may mean a loss of the meaning of existence resulting from a loss of relationship with coworkers and a loss of economic control.

Butler (1963) observes that as a rule the elderly must deal with greater difficulties than any other age group. However, most of the emotional disturbances of the aged tend to fall into a relatively small cluster of psychiatric syndromes. Among the most common syndromes that may be manifested in old age are depressive reactions, paranoid reactions, hypochondriacal states, acute and chronic anxiety states, and organic brain syndromes. All of these experiential syndromes in one way or another are characterized by feelings of helplessness and dependency and depression. In dealing with these syndromes, it is important for therapists to note that the elderly make use of relatively basic psychological mechanisms, the most prominent of which are withdrawal, denial, projection, and somatization (Pfeiffer, 1976, p. 199).

Similarly therapists need to be aware that about 50 percent of all depressive problems in the elderly are functional (Pfeiffer, 1976). This implies that in 50 percent of the cases depression is associated with situations when there are precipitating circumstances and when there are stern situational deprivations and age-related physical, psychological, and economic losses leading to feelings of despondency and sadness. Meerloo (1955, 1961) emphasizes that in the many instances of depression that develop from loss of relationships and deprivation, the emotional needs should be identified and partially fulfilled before attempting to analyze the person's psychodynamics.

Contact with Reality

Power and McCarron (1975) stress that the therapist's first goal in psychotherapy of the depressed elderly is to help the aged client regain contact with reality. An essential first step in treating depression is for the therapist to make contact with the withdrawn person. Many depressed elderly do not respond to verbal stimuli alone. A complementary interactive-contact method of reaching the depressed elderly is recommended and has been observed to be more effective with the elderly than any other age group (Power & McCarron, 1975). Ronch and Maizler (1977) and Verwoerdt (1976) also agree about the value of physical contact in the context of a warm supportive relationship with the elderly patient. These authors emphasize the importance of limited goals and greater nonverbal immediacy (e.g., more frequently smiling, eye contact, or touch and physical support). Actions such as stroking the individual's arm or shoulder and holding the hand for a while serve not only to gain the withdrawn person's attention, but the described relationship serves primarily to dispel feelings of anxiety, tension, and agitation.

Salzman and Shader (1978) note that the elderly often have problems in verbal communications. Nonverbal behavior may be the only real communication of accurate affective experiences. In this respect the practitioner's observations of the subtle nuances of bodily gestures, facial expressions, and posture may be extremely vital. Therapists who work with aged clients may clearly note the elderly's anger, disappointment, or despondency in such bodily gestures as unfocused staring into space, nervous movements of the fingers, or hanging head. Therapists need to be able to discuss the elderly's nonverbally expressed concerns in a way that benefits the client.

The next question hinges on an assessment of what the reality of the client has to offer. In many cases it can be a difficult problem to offer consolation or compensation for a series of losses. It is then appropriate to try to change the elderly person's milieu through work with the family, neighbors, and other health and social welfare personnel.

Existential Concerns

Another area of common concern among the elderly, although not mutually exclusive from other concerns, relates to existential and developmental problems that the elderly have in integrating their earlier life with present circumstances. According to developmental theorists (e.g., Erikson, 1968) the acceptance of death and the search for meaning in life constitute some of the existential tasks central to the later years. Neugarten (1968, 1974) has argued that in order to achieve ego integrity, the individual must accept life as it has turned out. A critical question that often arises for the elderly is, "How did I use my life?" (Moberg, 1963, p. 8). Acceptance of life also implies an acceptance of death. Thus the essential question in psychotherapy with the elderly is to recognize the elderly's need for not only continuity in their past and present life but also continuity beyond death (Kübler-Ross, 1975).

Available evidence suggests that the aged generally hold more positive attitudes toward death than do many younger persons (Saul & Saul, 1973). However, a number of external factors may negatively affect the elderly's attitudes toward death. Principal among these are the attitudes of family and friends who may consider death a taboo subject and would be reluctant to discuss it (Jeffers & Verwoerdt, 1969). The elderly are likely to be impeded in their preparation for dying by therapists who are not skilled in reflecting meanings and feelings about death. Knight (1978–1979) therefore feels that therapists who work with aged clients need to develop skills for discussing anxiety about death in a way that benefits the client.

Integration of the Past, Present, and Future

The importance of maintaining an intimate connection between the past, present, and approaching death has been emphasized by a number of authors (e.g., Butler, 1969; Kübler-Ross, 1969, 1975; Meerloo, 1961) who have studied how the elderly orient themselves toward the past through a life review and in doing so achieve a reorganization of the personality. According to Butler (1969, p. 7) the awareness of death can lead to a focused awareness of the limited future and can result in an extra strong motivation for therapy. Usually the systematic life review process results in better temporalization along the time line, and for many elderly, psychotherapeutic exploration of the past provides greater self-understanding for the present and the future. Butler (1969) cautions, however, that many practitioners who have worked with the elderly have been concerned with the frequent emergence of bitterness, disappointment, and despondency in remembering the past. In many other elderly there is a regressive preoccupation with the past, which interferes with a realistic acceptance of the present. Advocates of the life review emphasize that the object of reminiscence is to help the elderly find confirmation of present or past identity. Therefore, reminiscence or the life review should take the form of a reinforced structuring of the past rather than a destructuring of the past in which the psychotherapeutic objective is often to free oneself from the bonds of the past.

Kübler-Ross (1969) and Weisman (1972) advocate that psychotherapy with the elderly should be oriented toward providing effective opportunity to talk about death, to discuss feelings about dying and the loss of friends. One important component is giving the person repeated assurance that life has been of great value (Wolff, 1966) especially in the case of the elderly who engage in severe self-criticism. If the therapist can maintain a close relationship with the patient and show high regard, this contributes more to the person's self-respect than does easy assurance.

Unresolved Grief

Unresolved grief is particularly central in the later years and is characterized by feelings of hopelessness and depression. Hypochondriacal symptoms, bodily preoccupations, and withdrawal also characterize the functioning of many depressed elderly. The therapist must be attentive to feelings of unresolved grief, loneliness, and isolation. Such feelings may become especially accentuated in the relationship with the therapist. Zinberg (1965) and Gramlick (1968) alert the therapist to the danger of locked-in feelings of guilt and anger. They emphasize the importance of helping the elderly to work through sorrow and to acknowledge their unresolved grief feelings (Levin, 1964).

Weinberg (1951, 1975a, 1975b) and Kahana (1980) suggest a few helpful points for therapists working with the elderly. These include being empathic listeners, encouraging the elderly persons to talk about themselves, understanding and considering the validity of the elderly persons' feelings, and projecting optimism in order to help clients and their families feel that their sharing of information and personal insights has been of much value.

Organic Problems

Among the late-life disabilities capable of arousing considerable anxiety in the therapist are the organic brain syndromes found in almost half of the geriatric patients (Simon & Cahan, 1963). These can often bring out psychotic conditions and other psychological dysfunctions such as memory loss, orientation problems, and depression.

Simon and Cahan (1963) have attempted to differentiate acute but reversible brain syndrome symptoms from other irreversible symptoms. They have argued that with appropriate adaptation in therapy techniques brain syndrome symptoms of depression are amenable to treatment and reversible through psychotherapy. Symptoms of depression, apathy, helplessness, and insecurity that accompany many forms of organic brain dysfunction can be partially reversed when appropriate reality orientation support is provided (Saul & Saul, 1974).

Psychotherapy as an adjunct to other forms of management (Kahana, 1980) is often useful in reducing symptoms of agitation in brain syndrome patients (Kahana, 1971). Saul and Saul (1974) report positive results with group reconstructive psychotherapy, and Oberleder (1970) recommends various forms of ecologic or milieu therapy in which involvement in concrete activity and recreation is advocated. The teaching of mnemonic techniques can be of assistance in promoting reorientation and contact with reality. A directive approach to therapy is recommended, including direct suggestions for action and self-controls. The fact that one attempts these forms of reconstructive psychotherapy with elderly clients presenting organic brain syndrome symptoms is an expression of optimism that may have an interaction with the family members' treatment of the elderly relative.

SPECIFIC FACTORS OF SESSIONS

Frequency of Sessions

In view of the diminishing emotional and physical energy of the aged as compared to nonaged in the general population, most psychotherapists recommend shorter and more frequent therapy sessions. Ross (1959), for example, reports successful use of brief therapy sessions made more comfortable by serving refreshments and having light music and informal conversation. Bromley (1966) and Stotsky (1972) recommend a much more relaxed and informal relationship with the client than is the case in traditional psychotherapy.

Structure and Direction

Generally speaking, psychotherapy with the elderly requires a more active role on the part of the therapist and a more explicit indication of whether the client should consider psychotherapy or any other form of treatment. The boundaries of the therapist's professional competence should be explicitly stated for the benefit of both the client and the family members of the elderly. Perhaps a more explicit indication should be given of the nature and kinds of psychotherapeutic help the client may expect to receive and eventually to accept. McGee and Lakin (1977) caution that many elderly are not familiar with the scope and sequence of psychotherapy and may therefore make inappropriate requests for legal and medical help and medication for somatic complaints. The aged clients will probably have other needs related to their mental health, including a need for companionship and activity (Hammer, 1972). Cumming and Cumming (1975) suggest that while the therapist is not able to meet these needs directly, referral to appropriate agencies that can help the elderly client is considered essential to therapy. To a limited extent the therapist must be prepared to assume the role of social planner, family consultant, recreational adviser, and good friend. In the initial meeting with the elderly client (or the family members) the therapist's primary task would involve consultation and education concerning the scope, value, and delimitations of psychotherapy.

Psychotherapy with elderly clients will usually require more structure in the form of questioning and probing. As opposed to nondirective counseling more commonly used to elicit ideas and attitudes of younger adults, questioning with the elderly should be more direct and ask for specific information, beliefs, or opinion. Structured questioning and probing are especially recommended in the case of those elderly who are mildly or moderately disoriented and who may therefore be rambling and unfocused in their responses.

Brink (1979) and Butler and Lewis (1977) have noted the inappropriate use of silence on the part of many elderly clients. If silences are of long duration, occur frequently, or cannot be attributed to such known characteristics of the elderly as shyness, fear, or deep emotion, they may frequently be indicative of mild organic impairment. Other behavioral symptoms of the client such as gazing into space, random mumbling, and irrelevant talk may indicate the client's disorientation to place and surroundings or may suggest that the client . experiencing brief seizures of organic origin requiring medical attention. Butler (1975b), however, cautions that the client's silence may also indicate self-preoccupation often characteristic of many elderly who have experienced grief. Butler suggests that it is important to intervene by asking open-ended questions that will bring an elderly person back on track to reality.

The reported benefits of the therapist being more active and structured have been extensively documented. It is argued that most elderly clients feel helpless and anxious and expect the therapist to play a parent surrogate role and to steer them through psychotherapy (Goldfarb, 1954). This form of direct structured support can be particularly helpful in psychotherapy with brain-impaired elderly clients who suffer from lack of impulse control and who need frequent reminders to keep going (Meerloo, 1955).

Medical Referral

A key ingredient in therapy with the elderly is differentiation between symptoms and situations that have medical implications, psychotherapy implications, or both. However, an eclectic orientation calling for a combined approach (including medical treatment, supportive and insight therapy, behavior change techniques, family therapy, and even pharmacology) is advocated with the elderly. The described eclectic approach is useful especially when one therapist is able to act as a reservoir of several external resources.

Medical referral is often indicated when medication can be a supportive adjunct to reduce stress and fatigue. Some other aspects of psychotherapy for the elderly who often require medical consultation or referral are symptoms of organic brain syndrome and somatic symptoms that can be easily confused with symptoms of medical disease. Somatic symptoms are commonly used by the elderly to gain emotional or economic support from family and friends (Peck, 1966). The therapist must tread carefully between acknowledging the person's somatic symptoms as indicators of medical illness or succumbing to overgeneralized devaluation of the patient's somatic symptoms, based on the advanced age. In either case medical referral of the elderly is advisable whenever a clear differentiation of medical and psychological symptoms is not possible.

The Role of Significant Others in Therapy with the Elderly

Supportive psychotherapy for the aged is arousing considerable interest. For best effects such psychotherapy should enlist all available help in the environment. If the elderly person is living in the community, those closest to the person—family, friends, or neighbors—are also seen by the therapist in order to assess their understanding of the psychodynamics of aging (Peck, 1966). The closest family members whose active cooperation will be solicited may merit careful interviews. Davis and Klopfer (1977, p. 347) caution that many times close relatives of the elderly persons may actually scapegoat and harass them. It is important for the therapist not to be seen as taking sides with those relatives who, however well meaning, are perceived by the elderly patient as being unsympathetic or unkind.

Generally speaking, the therapist must use authority and professional position to preserve an orientation of firmness with the elderly person and to avoid the extremes of over- and underinvolvement in the family. Davis and Klopfer (1977) observe that families get upset about their elderly members, often because of guilt. They may tend to be overprotective and treat the elderly person as more fragile than justified. The therapist needs to recognize the power of family members. Sometimes certain family members may present roadblocks to treatment. Family members should be asked for information about patients and to give firsthand observations on the elderly client's functioning. They should be consulted in such practical matters as changes of living quarters, involvement in social groups, and medical treatment for the elderly person (Peck, 1966, p. 750). The status of the psychotherapist is of great importance in the treatment of the elderly client and may often be used to protect the client against well-meaning but rather controlling relatives.

The therapist may be called on to arbitrate in the disputes of the family. Such arbitration may be necessary when the elderly person's problems are actually situational. In these circumstances the therapist serves as a kind of referee who avoids blaming anyone and offers various options for solution (Davis & Klopfer, 1977, p. 347). Family members may have to be called in for direct assistance when the members' own anxiety about death and dying is having negative effects on the elderly client. Adult children or relatives of the elderly person may have to be trained to function as parent surrogates, acting to gratify the elderly's need for protection and reassurance. The therapist's direct power intervention may be useful in those situations when the elderly person is engaging in much self-reproach and guilt.

In short, therapists working with the elderly are advised to be much less territorial than they might be with younger adults and to enlist the auxiliary help of the social support system. It may be profitable for the therapist to space out sessions and then continue to be available on an on-call basis. The social support system can be trained to serve as auxiliary helpers or props. The therapist's main function may be to play the role of a benevolent parent providing empathy, noncritical understanding, permission to ventilate feelings, and token but real help during brief meetings.

Thus a notion is advanced of the generalist in the psychological treatment of geriatric patients. It is suggested that the therapist of the elderly must be conversant with a variety of techniques in psychotherapy, at least with the methodologies of supportive or insight therapies and eclectic medical approaches that take due note of the physical conditions and inner strength of the elderly persons. Certainly it helps if therapists have some personal experiences and background knowledge of geropsychology that enrich their understanding of the critical needs of the aged and their ability to deal with the social, emotional, and biological problems that figure prominently in old age.

Although the aged have been described as a subgroup throughout the discussion, one of the important findings of the therapy literature is that all the aged do not change in the same ways on the same measures of aging (Kastenbaum, 1973). An effective psychotherapeutic approach to the elderly must be based on an unbiased assessment of available data for each client. Each clinical and developmental task must be approached by both therapist and client with a minimum of stereotyping of the aged.

Many therapists are surprised to discover how satisfying psychotherapy with the elderly can be. The elderly are often more realistic in their expectations about treatment and are most grateful to their therapists when they experience clinical progress (Goldfarb, 1971).

SUMMARY

It is fairly clear that the aged population includes a substantial portion (i.e., 17 to 20 percent) of individuals who are psychologically distressed and continue to resist psycho-therapeutic intervention. A number of social factors may explain the underutilization of outpatient facilities by the aged. The prejudiced attitudes of the therapists toward the elderly patients' ability to benefit from therapy have contributed to a marked decline in the number of elderly receiving any form of active therapeutic care.

Older persons can and do respond to psychotherapy, but success in therapy will depend on the skills of the therapists and their ability to assess the elderly clients' special problems and concerns. Clearly there is a need for healthy self-questioning by therapists about possible biases toward the aged. Therapists can function more effectively with the elderly if they could be desensitized to their own fears of working with the elderly. It may also be useful for therapists to evaluate their own tendencies to be too dominant in the relationship with the elderly.

In order to be successful, therapy will also require changes in the therapists' basic assumptions about the goals of therapy and the ability of the elderly to benefit from it. Success depends also on improvement in the general societal position of the elderly. With notable increases predicted in the educational attainment and psychological sophistication of the elderly, it is important to counter the therapists' current lack of interest and training in geropsychotherapy. Given that psychotherapy with the aged may show a considerable increase in the years ahead, simple forms of custodial caregiving will not be sufficient. More attention in training needs to be given to the relative efficacy of different forms of psychotherapeutic approaches with the aged. Most therapists have not received sufficient training for work with the elderly and continue to use therapy procedures designed primarily for younger adults. The therapists of the elderly must become more familiar with the special concerns of the aged including their fears, anxieties, and the need for supportive relationships. Future training of therapists must include some time in settings where the elderly are the focus of treatment.

The chapters which follow will examine the strengths and limitations of individual and group psychotherapeutic approaches that have potentials for being effective with the elderly.

REFERENCES

Abrahams, R.B., & Patterson, R.D. (1978–79). Psychological distress among the community elderly: Prevalence, characteristics and implications for service. *International Journal of Aging and Human Development, 9,* 1–18.

Berezin, M.A. (1972). Psychodynamic considerations of aging and the aged: An overview. *American Journal of Psychiatry, 128,* 1483–1491.

Brink, T.L. (1979). *Geriatric psychotherapy.* New York: Human Sciences Press.

Brody, E.M. (1974). Aging and family personality: A developmental view. *Family Process, 13,* 23–25.

Bromley, D.B. (1966). *The psychology of human ageing.* Baltimore: Penguin.

Butler, R.N. (1963). Psychiatric evaluation of the aged. *Geriatrics, 18,* 220–232.

Butler, R.N. (1969). The life review: An interpretation of reminiscence in the aged. In R. Kastenbaum (Ed.), *New thoughts on old age* (pp. 265–280). New York: Springer.

Butler, R.N. (1975a). Psychotherapy in old age. In S. Arieti (Ed.), *American handbook of psychiatry* (Vol. 5, 2nd ed., pp. 807–828). New York: Basic Books.

Butler, R.N. (1975b). Psychiatry and the elderly: An overview. *American Journal of Psychiatry, 132,* 893–900.

Butler, R.N., & Lewis, M.I. (1973). *Aging and mental health: Positive psychosocial approaches.* St. Louis: CV Mosby Co.

Butler, R.N., & Lewis, M.I. (1977). *Aging and mental health: Positive psychosocial approaches* (2nd ed.). St. Louis: C.V. Mosby Co.

Cameron, N. (1956). Neurosis of later maturity. In O.J. Kaplan (Ed.), *Mental disorders in later life* (2nd ed., pp. 201–243). Stanford, CA: Stanford University Press.

Cath, S.H. (1965). Some dynamics of middle and later years: A study in depletion and restitution. In M.A. Berezin & S.H. Cath (Eds.), *Geriatric psychiatry: Grief, loss and emotional disorders in the aging process* (pp. 21–72). New York: International Universities Press.

Cohen, G.D. (1981). Perspectives on psychotherapy with the elderly. *American Journal of Psychiatry, 138,* 347–350.

Cumming, J., & Cumming, E. (1975). Care in the community. In J.G. Howells (Ed.), *Modern perspective in the psychiatry of old age* (pp. 486–509). New York: Brunner/Mazel.

Da Silva, G. (1965). Loneliness and death of an 81-year-old man. *Geriatric Focus, 4*, 11–14.

Davis, R.W., & Klopfer, W.G. (1977). Issues in psychotherapy with the aged. *Psychotherapy: Theory, Research and Practice, 14*, 343–348.

Dovenmuehle, R.H. (1965). Psychiatry: Implementation. In J.T. Freeman (Ed.), *Clinical features of the older patient* (pp. 266–272). Springfield, IL: Charles C Thomas.

Dye, C.J. (1978). Psychologists' role in the provision of mental health care for the elderly. *Professional Psychology, 9*, 38.

Eisdorfer, C., & Stotsky, B.A. (1977). Intervention, treatment and rehabilitation of psychiatric disorders. In J.E. Birren & K.W. Schaie (Eds.), *The handbook of psychology of aging* (pp. 724–748). New York: Van Nostrand Reinhold Co.

Erikson, E. (1968). The human life cycle. In D.L. Sills (Ed.), *International encyclopedia of the social sciences*. New York: Macmillan Publishing Co.

Ford, C.V., & Sbordone, R.J. (1981). Attitudes of psychiatrists toward elderly patients. *American Journal of Psychiatry, 137*, 571.

Ginsberg, A.B., & Goldstein, S.G. (1974). Age bias in referral for psychological consultation. *Journal of Gerontology, 29*, 410–415.

Glamser, F.D. (1974). The importance of age to conservative opinions: A multivariate analysis. *Journal of Gerontology, 29*, 549–554.

Goldfarb, A.I. (1954). Orientation of staff in a home for the aged. *Mental Hygiene, 37*, 76–83.

Goldfarb, A.I. (1955). Psychotherapy of aged persons. IV. One aspect of the psychodynamics of the therapeutic situation with aged patients. *Psychoanalytic Review, 42*, 180–187.

Goldfarb, A.I. (1964). Patient-doctor relationship in treatment of aged persons. *Geriatrics, 19*, 18–23.

Goldfarb, A.I. (1969). Institutional care of the aged. In E.W. Busse & E. Pfeiffer (Eds.), *Behavior and adaptation in late life* (pp. 289–313). Boston: Little, Brown & Co.

Goldfarb, A.I. (1971). Group therapy with the old and aged. In H.I. Kaplan & B.J. Sadock (Eds.), *Comprehensive group psychotherapy* (pp. 623–642). Baltimore: Williams & Wilkins.

Gottesman, L.E., Quarterman, C.E., & Cohn, G.M. (1973). Psychosocial treatment of the aged. In C. Eisdorfer & M.P. Lawton (Eds.), *The psychology of adult development and aging* (pp. 378–427). Washington: American Psychological Association.

Gramlick, E.P. (1968). Recognition and management of grief in elderly patients. *Geriatrics, 23*, 87–92.

Grotjahn, M. (1951). Some analytic observations about the process of growing old. In G. Rogheim (Ed.), *Psychoanalysis and social science* (Vol. 3, pp. 301–312). New York: International Universities Press.

Grotjahn, M. (1955). Analytic psychotherapy with the elderly. *Psychoanalytic Review, 42*, 419–427.

Hammer, M. (1972). Psychotherapy with the aged. In M. Hammer (Ed.), *The theory and practice of psychotherapy with specific disorders* Springfield, IL: Charles C Thomas.

Hiatt, H. (1971). Dynamic psychotherapy with the aging patient. *American Journal of Psychotherapy, 25*, 591–600.

Ingebretsen, R. (1977). Psychotherapy with the elderly. *Psychotherapy: Theory, Research and Practice, 14*, 319–332.

Jeffers, F.C., & Verwoerdt, A. (1969). How the old face death. In E.W. Busse & E. Pfeiffer (Eds.), *Behavior and adaptation in late life* (pp. 163–182). Boston: Little, Brown & Co.

Kahana, R. (1971). The humane treatment of old people in institutions. *Gerontologist, 11*, 282–289.

Kahana, R. (1980). Psychotherapy: The elderly. In T.B. Karasu & L. Bellak (Eds.), *Specialized techniques in psychotherapy* (pp. 314–336). New York: Brunner/Mazel.

Kahn, R.L. (1965). *Emotional needs of older people*. Paper read at American Psychological Association Meetings, Chicago.

Kahn, R.L. (1975). The mental health system and the future aged. *Gerontologist, 15* (1, pt. 2), 24–31.

Kastenbaum, R. (1964). The reluctant therapist. In R. Kastenbaum (Ed.), *New thoughts on old age* (pp. 139–145). New York: Springer.

Kastenbaum, R. (1973). Loving, dying, and other gerontologic addenda. In C. Eisdorfer & M.P. Lawton (Eds.), *The psychology of adult development and aging* (pp. 699–708). Washington: American Psychological Association.

Kastenbaum, R. (1978). Personality theory, therapeutic approaches, and the elderly client. In M. Storandt, I.C. Siegler, & M.F. Elias (Eds.), *The clinical psychology of aging* (pp. 199–224). New York: Plenum Press.

Knight, R. (1978–79). Psychotherapy and behavior change with the non-institutionalized aged. *International Journal of Aging and Human Development, 9(3),* 221–238.

Kübler-Ross, E. (1969). *On death and dying.* New York: Macmillan Publishing Co.

Kübler-Ross, E. (1975). Facing death. In J.G. Howells (Ed.), *Modern perspectives in the psychiatry of old age* (pp. 531–539). New York: Brunner/Mazel.

Lawton, M.P., & Gottesman, L.E. (1974). Psychological services to the elderly. *American Psychologist, 29,* 689–693.

Levin, S. (1964). Depression and the aged: The importance of external factors. In R. Kastenbaum (Ed.), *New thoughts on old age* (pp. 179–185). New York: Springer.

Looft, W.R. (1973). Reflections on intervention in old age: Motives, goals, and assumptions. *Gerontologist, 13,* 6–9.

McGee, J., & Lakin, M. (1977). Social perspectives on psychotherapy with the aged. *Psychotherapy: Theory, Research and Practice, 14,* 333–342.

Meerloo, J.A.M. (1955). Psychotherapy with elderly people. *Geriatrics, 10,* 583–587.

Meerloo, J.A.M. (1961). Modes of psychotherapy in the aged. *Journal of the American Geriatrics Society, 8,* 225–234.

Moberg, V. (1963). *Din stund pa jorden.* Stockholm: Bokforlaget Aldus/fionnier.

Muslin, H., & Epstein, L.J. (1980). Preliminary remarks on the rationale for psychotherapy of the aged. *Comprehensive Psychiatry, 21,* 1–12.

Neugarten, B.L. (1968). *Middle age and aging.* Chicago: University of Chicago Press.

Neugarten, B.L. (1974). Age in American society and the rise of the young-old. *Annals of the American Academy, September,* 187–198.

Oberleder, M. (1964). Aging: Its importance for clinical psychology. In L.E. Abt & B.F. Riess (Eds.), *Progress in clinical psychology* (pp. 158–171). New York: Grune & Stratton.

Oberleder, M. (1966). Psychotherapy with the aging: An art of the possible? *Psychotherapy: Theory, Research and Practice, 3,* 139–142.

Oberleder, M. (1970). Crisis therapy in mental breakdown of the aging. *Gerontologist, 10,* 111–114.

Patterson, C.H. (1974). *Relationship counseling and psychotherapy.* New York: Harper & Row.

Peck, A. (1966). Psychotherapy of the aged. *Journal of the American Geriatrics Society, 14,* 748–753.

Peterson, J.A. (1973). Marital and family therapy including the aged. *Gerontologist, 13,* 27–31.

Pfeiffer, E. (1971). Psychotherapy with elderly patients. *Postgraduate Medicine, 50,* 254–258.

Pfeiffer, E. (1976). Psychotherapy with elderly patients. In L. Bellak & T.B. Karasu (Eds.), *Geriatric psychiatry* (pp. 191–205). New York: Grune & Stratton.

Post, F. (1965). *The clinical psychiatry of late life.* Oxford: Pergamon.

Power, C.A., & McCarron, L.T. (1975). Treatment of depression in persons residing in homes for the aged. *Gerontologist, 15,* 132–135.

Pressey, S.L. (1957). Tests "indigenous" to the adults and older years. *Journal of Counseling Psychology, 4,* 144–148.

Rechtschaffen, A. (1959). Psychotherapy with geriatric patients: A review of the literature. *Journal of Gerontology, 14,* 73–84.

Redlich, F., & Kellert, S.R. (1978). Trends in American mental health. *American Journal of Psychiatry, 135,* 22–28.

Reisman, D. (1954). Some clinical and cultural aspects of aging. *American Journal of Sociology, 59,* 379–383.

Riley, M.W., & Foner, A. (1968). *Aging and society.* New York: Russell Sage Foundation.

Ronch, J.L., & Maizler, J.S. (1977). Individual psychotherapy with the institutionalized aged. *American Journal of Orthopsychiatry, 47,* 275–283.

Rosenthal, H.R. (1959). Psychotherapy of the aging. *American Journal of Psychotherapy, 17,* 55–65.

Ross, M. (1959). Recent contributions to gerontologic group psychotherapy. *International Journal of Group Psychotherapy, 9,* 442–450.

Rustin, S.L., & Wolk, R.L. (1963). The use of specialized group psychotherapy techniques in a home for the aged. In J.L. Moreno (Ed.), *Group psychotherapy* (Vol. 16, pp. 25–29). Beacon, NY: Beacon House.

Safirstein, S. (1972). Psychotherapy for geriatric patients. *New York State Medical Journal, 72,* 2743–2748.

Salzman, C., & Shader, R.I. (1978). Depression in the elderly: II. Possible drug etiologies. *Journal of American Geriatrics Society, 26,* 303–308.

Sarason, S.B., Sarason, E.K., & Cowden, P. (1975). Aging and the nature of work. *American Psychologist, 30,* 584–592.

Saul, S.R., & Saul, S. (1973). Old people talk about death. *Omega, 4,* 27–35.

Saul, S.R., & Saul, S. (1974). Group psychotherapy in a proprietary nursing home. *Gerontologist, 14,* 446–450.

Schaie, K.W. (1973). Intervention toward an ageless society? *Gerontologist, 13,* 31–35.

Schmidt, C.W. (1974). Psychiatric problems of the aged. *Journal of American Geriatrics Society, 22*(8), 355–359.

Seligman, S. (1974). Submissive death: Giving up on life. *Psychology Today, 7*(12), 80–85.

Shanas, E., & Hauser, P.M. (1974). Zero population growth and the family life of old people. *Journal of the Psychological Study of Social Issues, 30,* 79–92.

Simon, A., & Cahan, R. (1963). The acute brain syndrome in geriatric patients. In W.M. Mendel & L.J. Epstein (Eds.), *Acute psychotic reaction.* Washington: American Psychological Association.

Sparacino, J. (1978–79). Individual psychotherapy with the aged: A selective review. *International Journal of Aging and Human Development, 9*(3), 197–220.

Spark, G.M. (1974). Grandparents and intergenerational family therapy. *Family Process, 13,* 225–239.

Stern, K., Smith, J.M., & Frank, M. (1953). Mechanism of transference and counter transference in psychotherapeutic and social work with the aged. *Journal of Gerontology, 8,* 328–332.

Stotsky, B.A. (1972). Social and clinical issues in geriatric psychiatry. *American Journal of Psychiatry, 129,* 117–126.

Verwoerdt, A. (1976). *Clinical geropsychiatry.* Baltimore: Williams & Wilkins.

Weinberg, J. (1951). Psychiatric techniques in the treatment of older people. In W. Donahue & C. Tibbitts (Eds.), *Growing in the older years.* Ann Arbor: University of Michigan Press.

Weinberg, J. (1975a). Psychopathology. In J.G. Howells (Ed.), *Modern perspectives in the psychiatry of old age* (pp. 234–252). New York: Brunner/Mazel.

Weinberg, J. (1975b). Geriatric psychiatry. In A.M. Freedman, H.I. Kaplan, & B.J. Sadock (Eds.), *Comprehensive textbook of psychiatry* (Vol. 2, pp. 2405–2420). Baltimore: Williams & Wilkins.

Weisman, A. (1972). A psychosocial death. *Psychology Today,* November, 77–78, 83–86.

Wolff, K. (1962). Group psychotherapy. Group psychotherapy with geriatric patients in a psychiatric hospital: Six-year study. *Journal of American Geriatrics Society, 10,* 1077–1080.

Wolff, K. (1966). The emotional rehabilitation of the geriatric patient. II: Therapeutic principles. *Journal of American Geriatrics Society, 14,* 1150–1152.

Wolk, R.L., Reder, E.L., Seiden, R.B., & Solomon, V. (1965). Five-year psychiatric assessment of the patients in an out-patient geriatric guidance clinic. *Journal of American Geriatrics Society, 13,* 222–239.

Yesavage, J.A., & Karasu, T.B. (1982). Psychotherapy with elderly patients. *American Journal of Psychotherapy, 36,* 41–55.

Zinberg, N.E. (1964). Geriatric psychiatry: Need and problems. *Gerontologist, 4,* 130–135.

Zinberg, N.E. (1965). Special problems of gerontologic psychiatry. In M.A. Berezin & S.H. Cath (Eds.), *Geriatric psychiatry: Grief, loss and emotional disorders in the aging process* (pp. 147–159). New York: International Universities Press.

Chapter 8

Individual Psychotherapy for Depression: Supportive, Interpersonal, and Cognitive-Behavioral Approaches

Despite the widespread need for treating depression, there have been few attempts to develop a systematic body of knowledge and information concerning models, strategies, and procedures appropriate for use with depressed elderly. Eisdorfer and Stotsky (1977) reviewed the smorgasbord of techniques that have been employed in psychotherapy with the elderly. Without controlled outcome studies, formulations of effective psychotherapy strategies and techniques are derived from isolated case histories and clinical experience, with clients referred by families of the elderly and social workers to physicians and mental health practitioners. For the most part, therefore, the question of whether psychotherapy for depression is effective with the elderly remains an ideological issue, and empirical formulations are lacking (Zarit, 1980).

This chapter focuses on time-limited brief psychotherapies for treatment of depression in the elderly. Guidelines and recommendations have been developed from three sources: (1) authoritative conceptualizations of depression and theoretical positions discussed in the clinical literature (see Beck, 1967; Brown & Harris, 1978; Ferster, 1973; Lewinsohn, 1974; Rogers, 1951; Seligman, 1975; Small, 1979), (2) recent advances in the use of supportive and cognitive-behavioral interventions designed specifically for the elderly (see Fry, 1984a, 1984b, 1984c; Gallagher & Thompson, 1981, 1982, 1983; Hammen & Cohen, 1980; Steuer & Hammen, 1983; Jarvik et al., 1983; Kastenbaum, 1978), and (3) the experience of the author in supervising psychotherapy research on depression in the elderly (see Fry, 1983–1986). This chapter considers individual psychotherapy modalities (supportive, interpersonal, and cognitive-behavioral) for the treatment of depression. Group psychotherapy and psychopharmacological approaches to intervention with the elderly are considered in Chapters 10 and 12.

SUPPORTIVE THERAPY

Although psychotherapy has been practiced with the elderly to a limited degree, evidence suggests that the supportive mode is the single most innovative and effective approach to the treatment of depressed elderly. The time-honored, face-to-face interaction mode of therapy with the elderly not only has the weight of tradition but provides the maximum flexibility and adaptability to those needs of the elderly person that are age and stage specific. The supportive interpersonal relation that the mental health practitioner establishes is designed to bring about modification of feelings, cognitions, attitudes, and behavior that have proven troublesome or problematic to the elderly. Gutmann (1980) makes strong appeals for a genuinely developmental approach to the supportive therapy of later life, noting that the elderly have a multiplicity of social and affective concerns, and therapy can be sought for many problems. Often there is conflict at this stage in determining which is the core primary concern and distinguishing it from other concerns about the past and future. Many elderly are troubled by the emergence of more agentic problems that will render them helpless victims of circumstance, organic problems, and illness. Thus many elderly may respond to their emerging feelings and desires with depression, physical illness, alcoholism, and suicide attempts (Gutmann, 1980).

From a psychodynamic perspective, stresses and changes associated with later years are typically seen as a process of depletion, with loss of health, fertility, loved ones, and social status being the predictable consequences of aging, and depression, anxiety, and dependency being the inevitable problems of later life. Seen from a developmental perspective, however, the elderly's behavior reflects patterns of strength and vulnerability specific both to their past experiences and to their current life period. Such an approach makes it possible for the therapist to go beyond the simple goal of alleviation and relief to wider goals of restitution and enrichment.

The alleviation function holds that a cathartic expression of grief and depression over loss of persons and objects is the first step toward helping to restore normal functioning in the elderly. Since issues of loss are a common concern in psychotherapy with the elderly, the first step toward the goal of alleviation is often for the therapist to listen in supportive, empathic, and caring ways to the elderly client's expression of grief and through empathic listening to explore with the client the unique meaning of this loss (Rogers, 1951).

Although most of the psychotherapy efforts directed toward the elderly are designed to help them accommodate to their losses and accept their grief, Butler (1977) stresses that at some point the counselor should shift from expressions of reassurance and empathy to a process of restitution and later to one of enrichment. Restitution and enrichment, according to Butler, involve several features. Through supportive therapy the therapist may initially attempt to understand the elderly client's fears, normalize the emergent desires, and eventually turn the potentials into strength. The restitution goal, by contrast, entails strengthening the adaptive capacity of the elderly individual.

As Goldfarb (1956) noted, many elderly persons, despite their pain and depression, seem motivated to improve their level of adaptive behavior. Their ability to benefit from minimal psychotherapeutic contact with the therapist makes it efficient for the therapist to work with them. Rather than become rooted in their grief, clients may be encouraged toward new restitutive adjustments to circumstances for which they may have only limited preparation. The goal of restitution would entail strengthening the adaptive capacities of elderly individuals at risk. Via supportive restitutive therapy there may be an attempt to encourage clients to take more active control of their activities and thus to regain a partial sense of mastery over their lives.

As part of a restitutive program some elderly persons may benefit from learning new behavioral-social skills that will help them to adapt to changed aspects of their environment. Some may need to take over new roles and learn assertive skills. Others may wish to work toward strengthening support systems within their environment. A widow, for example, may be fearful of excessive loneliness and social isolation following the death of the spouse and may need the assistance of the therapist in increasing social participation and social stimulation. A widower may need help in interacting in more effective ways with his children and neighbors. From a restitution perspective, therefore, intervention would be designed to compensate for this elderly person's social deficits. Supportive therapy might involve simplifying the environment so the individual could continue to function at home (as opposed to moving to a custodial home or living with children).

In the supportive role the therapist has a unique opportunity and responsibility to ameliorate the depressive conditions as much as possible, to strengthen the support systems within the environment that can facilitate the process of restitution for losses incurred by the elderly (Gutmann, 1980; Kessler & Albee, 1975), and motivate the client toward enrichment activities. The enrichment perspective implies that every elder has some potentials for growth and fulfillment. Regardless of age, some strengths and capabilities of the elderly, if properly nurtured, can bring their level of functioning beyond the minimal or usual (Gutmann, 1980). The following case illustrates this point. Mrs. A.D., a 76-year-old client confined to a wheelchair, was referred for therapy. She appeared disoriented, anxious, and withdrawn. She had lost her husband a month before and her son died three months preceding her husband's death. Her therapist had little incentive to work with her precisely because he felt little could be done about the losses that Mrs. A.D. had endured. He felt that she must go through a normal grief period and therapy was not indicated.

Mrs. A.D. subsequently went to see a female counselor and sought her assistance in adapting to her changed circumstances. Therapy focused on concrete issues such as legal advice in recovering money from her husband's estate and social services assistance in helping her move to another residential area where she could be closer to friends. The counselor helped Mrs. A.D. in making arrangements for in-home services. Within a matter of weeks Mrs. A.D. looked more alert and communicative. She was visibly relieved after the counselor helped her with the practical concerns that were distressing her and contributing to her depressed mental outlook.

In the course of counseling Mrs. A.D., the therapist noted that the client was uniquely unafraid of death and even when she spoke about her husband and son's deaths, she did not feel she had been singled out by bad fortune. Contrary to what the therapist had assumed, it was not a depressive experience for Mrs. A.D. to explore her grief concerns, and she showed a remarkable degree of philosophical composure in coming to terms with the death of her husband and son. As became obvious later in counseling, problems for which she really needed help were only tangentially related to the death of her husband. Mrs. A.D. recovered from her depression after receiving help with her immediate needs.

As a part of therapeutic intervention Mrs. A.D. was persuaded to help counsel another elderly lady and her sister, both terrified by the thought of approaching death. This latter experience served to enhance Mrs. A.D.'s sense of self-fulfillment and improved her interpersonal adaptiveness. The therapy helped Mrs. A.D. not only to understand her own anxieties better; it also contributed to making her more confident in her interpersonal relations with the other two elderly ladies. The therapist had identified Mrs. A.D.'s potentials for enrichment and turned the potentials into new strengths.

Much of the therapeutic intervention described in Mrs. A.D.'s case goes beyond the narrow conception of the therapist's role as the manager of anxiety, depression, and confusion commonly seen as specific symptoms of mental illness in the elderly. But it is well within the broader conception of the geriatric practitioner's role. As Pfeiffer and Busse (1973) suggest, the geriatric practitioner may often have to assume responsibility for the general psychosocial care of the elderly. In our increasingly specialized society more elderly persons can be expected to turn to mental health practitioners for this broader intervention, advice, and channeling of energies. Social contact is often severely restricted among older persons in terms of daily contacts and visitations, and virtual isolation places many elderly at risk for certain kinds of depressive reactions arising from physical and emotional neglect, insufficient cognitive stimulation, and insufficient opportunity for self-actualization.

Cohen (1976) and Kessler and Albee (1975) therefore make a strong plea for both ameliorative and restitutive psychotherapy to forestall reactive depression in the elderly. Instead of trying to change paranoid and hypochondriacal responses so commonly observed in later life, restitutive therapy recommends action that would reduce the likelihood of old-age isolationism and provide opportunities for social support and friendship. Ultimately a supportive therapy program that combines amelioration, restitution, and enrichment works toward a reduction of pathogenic factors in the environment of the elderly and a strengthening of the social support systems. It supports rapid, prompt, and effective intervention when critical problems become evident, and it demonstrates concern for the immediate consequences of the problems as well as the immediate effect of changed life circumstances. Even minimal supportive contact between an elderly client and a concerned counselor is often sufficient to give the client a sense that the individual can now deal with those situations that had seemed so overwhelming. For many depressed elderly the counseling contacts may be the person's only significant social interactions, and because of their depressed state therapy may indeed be a substitute for friendship. These unusual situations and client needs must be accepted by the practitioner, who must attempt to be both an advocate and a therapist.

Unfortunately a developmental perspective in psychotherapy with the elderly is not the dominant view nor is the focus on goals designed to restore the elderly individual to an improved level of functioning. In most cases the therapist focuses on a more limited goal of providing immediate relief of symptoms through medication or at best providing services for the elderly who are handicapped or have brain damage. With many elderly, depression is not an illness but the product of problems in adaptation to the changed environment. Supportive therapy is successful if it teaches them even one or two coping strategies for dealing with environmental change.

As seen in Chapter 7, goals in psychotherapy for the elderly are generally more narrowly drawn than in treating younger persons. Total reorganization of life style is rarely attempted nor is it desirable. Rarely do elderly persons have such optimistic goals or resources allocated to meet these goals. Generally speaking more short-term and realistic goals are advocated. Principal among these are acceptance of a more dependent status as a natural concomitant of old age, a new adaptation to a changed life situation (e.g., acceptance of a less active role after widowhood), or relearning of practical daily living skills lost through injury.

When working with the elderly, there can be no quarrel with limited objectives, provided that therapists learn to investigate the limits by appropriate consultation with clients and their families. Achieving a focus for brief supportive psychotherapy is an important goal. Short-term supportive therapy provides the therapist an opportunity to assess the ego functions and emotional resources of the elderly person. The need for such an assessment has often been overlooked, and the elderly person's adaptive capacities and ego strengths to cope with the crisis are frequently overrated. The following situation illustrates the point.

Mr. S.K. at age 76 appeared calm and sufficiently alert after his wife's funeral. He admitted that he was quite shaken up but wished to be left alone so that he could get himself in hand. Supportive treatment did not seem indicated as Mr. S.K. sounded composed and told his neighbors he would ask for help if he needed it. No specific measures were taken to give him ego support. Three days later Mr. S.K. took his life through an overdose of sleeping pills.

This case illustrates that certain reactive disorders (e.g., grief and loneliness resulting from the death of a spouse) call for supportive work even when no obvious verbal indication or self-disclosure is given by the client. Certain nonverbal aspects of the elderly client's stance and qualities of the silences constitute the elderly person's indications of an underlying crisis situation (Karpf, 1980). Bellak (1976) recommends that the loss of a loved person be invariably understood in relation to the unique history and current situation of the bereaved individual. For many elderly the loss of a spouse is invariably a precipitating event and always has a certain dynamic effect. The current effect of any loss must be assessed in terms of the client's current social functioning, family networks, and history of depression and anxiety.

A supportive and compensating relationship with the therapist or other professional can often help elderly individuals to continue functioning adaptively even in the face of emotional losses. Even cognitively competent and physically healthy elderly may develop pathological behaviors if overwhelmed by stressful, nonsupportive circumstances. Thus some assessment of the client's ego readiness to deal with a crisis is an important criterion (Karpf, 1980). Decisions concerning long-term therapy will by their nature require time and thought, but short-term interventions aimed at providing subjective relief through supportive therapy are indispensable. Such therapy may take the form of catharsis or release of tension, mild ego-strengthening, and lessening of the superego pressure. Supportive therapy is often denigrated by viewing it as a mindless hand-holding exercise. However, a number of therapists (Herr & Weakland, 1979; Karpf, 1980) believe that it should be the treatment of choice for many elderly whenever the conditions suggest mild psychopathology, depression, bereavement, grief, and loss. It is the indicated treatment at some times for as simple a reason as the therapist's lack of understanding of the client's deeper crisis.

An elderly man who has lost his wife, for example, has lost not only a person with whom he had a strong affectional bond but also the person on whom he depended for physical care. An elderly woman who loses her husband has lost not only his companionship but the financial, legal, and physical support he provided. Lack of such support may in itself be cause for a severe depressive reaction or anxiety (Silverstone, 1976) and comprise the basis for supportive therapy following a crisis. Trained volunteers may be useful in meeting the emotional needs of these individuals. Some recent projects have demonstrated that older persons can acquire the communication skills of empathy, acceptance, and genuineness that enable them to serve in the role of peer counselors (Alpaugh & Hickey-Haney, 1978; Becker & Zarit, 1978). Such trained volunteers can be used effectively with many isolated and lonely older persons.

Professionals trained in the psychoanalytic tradition have attempted to apply more psychoanalytic concepts to supportive therapy with the depressed elderly. Psychoanalytic therapy is not regarded as a treatment for depression but rather as an approach toward strengthening the patient's adaptive capacities. According to Cath (1966) depressive reactions in the elderly are precipitated by loss, the loss being internal as well as external. As people grow older, the ego loses capacity to refuel itself, and the multiple losses deplete the ego's capacity for nourishment, gratification, and nurturance. The person regresses and the total self begins to shrink. Applications of psychodynamic treatment of depression are also aimed at increased nourishment and support, increased activity and socialization, involvement of the elderly client in meaningful intergenerational human interaction, and establishment of the therapist as a caring individual. This formulation of the dynamics of depression links almost directly to the interpersonal treatment approach advocated by other therapists (e.g., Frank, 1974; Rounsaville & Chevron, 1982).

The interpersonal therapists relate the severance of attachment and social bonds, the absence of intimate and confiding relationships, and the impairment of social roles with the onset of depression in the elderly. Although no integrated body of research literature supports the effectiveness of interpersonal therapy for treating depression in the elderly, the available clinical evidence suggests its usefulness. Elderly individuals presenting a history of mild depression, losses, social impoverishment, and difficulty in role transitions can be helped through supportive interpersonal therapy.

The goal for interpersonal therapy of depression in the elderly is similar to other supportive approaches: restoring self-esteem by developing in the client a sense of mastery vis-à-vis the demands of the new role-related situation. Techniques are similar to those used for grief resolution: facilitating a realistic evaluation of what has been lost, encouraging appropriate expression of effect, and helping the elderly individual develop a social support system and a repertoire of new or regained behavioral and social skills necessary for this new phase of life. Detailed description of strategies, techniques and rationale for the interpersonal therapy of depression are considered to be beyond the scope of this chapter. The interested reader is referred to Rounsaville and Chevron (1982) and Klerman, Rounsaville, Chevron, Neu and Weissman's (1979) manual.

Basic Skills and Techniques in Supportive Therapy

The therapist chooses from a variety of intervention techniques to attend to the depressed client. The particular techniques of therapy are advice, guidance, reassurance, assumption of a protective role, permissive attitudes, and catharsis. The same need for proper training and experience is crucial in supportive work as in other clinical work. Herr and Weakland (1979) stress that supportive therapy with the elderly takes sound judgments and astute clinical skills to understand ego functioning, ego defenses, repression, denial, and the extent of other clinical disorders. If defenses are too weak or resistance too characterologically fixed in an older individual, it takes a knowledge of defense mechanisms and an understanding of resistance to realize this (Freud, 1959). One cannot give sound advice to the elderly unless this advice is based on knowledge of gerontology and understanding of reactive disorders of the elderly. Relaxed listening and expressions of care and concern by the therapist constitute an effort to create a special atmosphere that offers the older client a sense of security, safety, and an opportunity to express sadness (Karpf, 1981). The elderly are often quite sensitive to what is left unsaid, and therefore the therapist must be prepared to respond sensitively to nonverbalized feelings as well as verbal expressions. Frequently self-disclosure on the part of the therapist may encourage the client in self-disclosures of blame, guilt, unhappiness, and depression. Respect for the uniqueness of each elderly person's grief and the individuality of each person's need for comfort and encouragement is a key ingredient of supportive therapy.

Status of Supportive Therapy

It is suggested that brief supportive psychotherapy is practical for the elderly in ambulatory care settings. The emphasis is on limited goals, some understanding of the etiology of the depression, some recognition of current contributing factors, and some comprehension of measures that can remedy the difficulties (Karpf, 1981). This concentrated focus of the therapeutic effort on immediately relevant concerns (Small, 1979) often increases the need for activity on the part of the client and aims at helping the client cope with crisis.

Many authors (e.g., Eisdorfer & Cohen, 1976; Herr & Weakland, 1979; Verwoerdt, 1976) observe that supportive treatment for the elderly depends on the resources assigned to psychotherapeutic care of the elderly, on the priorities established by the communities and neighborhoods in which the elderly reside, and on the conspicuousness of the dysfunctioning and impairment reflected in the behaviors at various ages (Eisdorfer & Cohen, 1978). Older persons may, for example, tolerate significant pain and emotional anguish as a normal accompaniment of aging. Verwoerdt (1976) noted that depression in old age is frequently untreated because depressive symptoms such as sad feelings, loss of appetite, self-reproach, and guilt cognitions are much less conspicuous.

The supportive approach is geared to limited goals. Many elderly persons do not need or desire intensive therapy nor are they prepared to invest the effort in working toward it. There is little doubt that what a majority of depressed elderly need is a benign helper willing to assist them in realigning their feelings and behavior in the context of new situations and new human relationships. For many other elders, supportive therapy alone may not be enough. It must remain an open question whether and to what extent therapeutic pressures may be applied to the elderly beyond supportive therapy and to what extent their therapy needs are compatible with the tenets of other modalities such as cognitive-behavioral therapy, insight therapy, and pharmacological or somatic treatment.

BEHAVIORAL APPROACH

A treatment modality that offers an approach for actively dealing with problems of the aged or aging is the behavioral model. This approach focuses primarily on behaviors that are unadaptive and targeted for change and on the environmental variables and persons that are maintaining these behaviors.

Advantages of This Approach

Cautela and Mansfield (1977) suggest several advantages of a behavioral model for treatment of the depressed elderly:

- Time is not unnecessarily spent on assessing the relevance of past experiences and gleaning insights from the past. Present behavior itself is the target for change, and the focus of therapy is present, immediate intervention. This orientation is particularly effective for the elderly, many of whom tend to glorify the past and to assess the present most unfavorably by comparison. Focus on present social problems and management of present interactions and present deficits in coping serve as useful key ingredients of therapy with the elderly.

- The therapist's active role in the behavioral treatment and the therapist's efforts at making intervention structured, precise, and limited help more older clients compared to younger ones (Rechtschaffen, 1959). Most older persons, when compared to the younger persons, profit from approaches in which the therapist plays a more active role. Because of the direct behavioral approach of the behavior therapist, behavior therapy should achieve a greater measure of success with the aged.

- The stress of old age is often accompanied by anxiety for which behavioral techniques are relatively more useful.

- The behavioral model emphasizes self-change and self-reliance, processes emphasized in therapy with the elderly. In old age, more so than in youth, individuals are confronted with feelings of limited capabilities and a sense of helplessness. An intervention model that opens up prospects of teaching the elderly methods of self-control and self-management of their environments is more in keeping with the elderly persons' perceptions of their dignity and self-efficacy. Within this framework the agent of change is the elderly individual. Teaching the elderly person methods of self-control increases feelings of control over the environment and helps to reduce feelings of helplessness and dependency on others.

- In the behavioral model no attempt is made to use negative diagnostic labels such as brain syndrome, senility, cognitive impairment, or dementia to explain the depression. The same shaping or modeling procedures are used with a person whose depression is a result of rejection or cognitive impairment.

Behavioral therapies have been shown to be effective for several problems of the aged. They are especially valuable for changing depressive responses of many elderly whose depression is an outcome of role status changes, social and emotional losses, and severe reduction in the rate of positive reinforcement from other adults in their environment. Behavioral interventions are also useful for treating depression in many elderly who may be unsuitable, unavailable, or unwilling to participate in more dynamic, insight-oriented therapies. Our challenge is to establish and maintain the consistent programs of reinforcement necessary to modify behaviors; when this can be done, it may be a useful substitute for other long-term and expensive interventions of a psychodynamic nature.

The cognitive-behavioral orientation to psychotherapeutic intervention involves three components: (1) behavioral, (2) social, and (3) cognitive. The behavioral component attends only to observable behaviors whereas the cognitive emphasizes the client's internal experiences, such as thoughts, wishes, and attitudes. The social component is an integral part of both the behavioral and cognitive approaches. Neither model was designed specifically for the treatment of depression in the elderly, but several of the behavioral theorists (e.g., Fuchs & Rehm, 1977; Lewinsohn, 1974; Lewinsohn, Youngren, & Grosscup, 1979) and cognitive theorists (Beck, 1967; Beck, Rush, Shaw, & Emery, 1979; Seligman, 1975) have suggested useful departures from traditional therapy techniques, which can be extremely effective in treating depression in many elderly clients. Both behavioral and cognitive theorists have stressed the functional relationship between everyday behaviors and depression and dominant cognitions and depression that have special relevance for the elderly.

A third group of therapists (e.g., Fry, 1984a, 1984b, 1984c; Fry & Grover, 1982; Dessonville, Gallagher, Thompson, & Finnel, 1980; Gallagher & Thompson, 1983; Steuer & Hammen, 1983) have begun to examine the usefulness of cognitive and behavioral strategies in intervention programs for the elderly. These researchers stress the efficacy of a joint cognitive-behavioral position to the treatment of depression. Thus, overall, the expectation for cognitive-behavioral therapy is that it would desensitize the elderly to specific fears and anxieties, alter maladaptive beliefs, enhance self-efficacy, and thereby reduce depression.

Various response modalities that need to be assessed are listed in Table 8–1 (McLean, 1976). McLean stresses cognitive-response modalities such as deficits in concentration and decision-making abilities, and rate and duration of automatic depressive thoughts; behavioral response modalities such as frequency of social activity, frequency of self-initiated tasks, perceptions of work performance, and amount of physical activity; and somatic response modalities such as level of agitation, fatigue, weight loss, bodily pain, etc. The overall assessment of response modalities will facilitate the therapist's decision as to whether behavioral strategies are appropriate with a given elderly client. Behavioral therapy may be designed for deficits or disorders in any one of the response modalities or clusters of responses listed in Table 8–1. It is generally assumed that in the case of depressed elderly clients there will be the overlapping presence of several cognitive, behavioral, and somatic symptoms. For example, there may be complaints of fatigue, weight loss, appetite loss accompanied by complaints of poor memory and concentration, lack of interest in social interaction, and infrequency of pleasant activity. A specific behavioral therapy program may be designed separately for each response modality.

Behavioral Therapies: Modifying Behaviors

This major form of psychotherapeutic intervention systematically applies principles of learning to the modification of functional disorders and reactive disorders related to depression. We frequently assume that all psychotherapy must uncover the roots of a problem in order for meaningful change. Thus most psychodynamic formulations of maladaptive behaviors and affective disorders attempt to give the client insight or awareness. However, in the behavioral intervention the assumption is that insight into one's past is not a necessary condition for behavioral change. Behavioral methods of psychotherapy are based on the assumption that desirable behaviors can be learned by the manipulation of environmental contingencies and that psychiatric disorders such as abnormal depressive reactions are the consequence of specific habits or thoughts of the client and are shaped by the reinforcements or negative responses from significant individuals in the environment.

Reinforcement Therapy for Depression

Behaviorally oriented therapists (e.g., Dessonville et al., 1980; Fry, 1984a, 1984b; Fuchs & Rehm, 1977) note the importance of reinforcement and reward strategies in treating depression. Research with the elderly has shown that two sets of conditions are likely to precede and sustain depressive episodes of clinical and psychiatric proportions: (1) reduced rate of response-contingent positive reinforcement (this occurs primarily through reduction in the number of pleasurable activities and increase in the number of unhappy activities and events including losses, grief, and bereavement) and (2) reduction of instrumental social skills that permit individuals to obtain positive reinforcements or relaxation experiences in their environment (Lewinsohn, 1976).

Ferster (1966) was one of the first to link the state of depression with the reinforcement history of the organism and to call for a functional analysis of depression in which antecedents and consequences related to this state would be investigated. In the elderly especially, depression is directly a consequence of the decreased frequency of positively

Table 8-1 Evaluation Content Areas, by Response Modality

Scaled and operationally defined specific and global (where appropriate) measures are to be attained on the specific areas organized by the following three response modalities:

Cognitive/affective response modality
- rate of suicidal ideation
- decision-making ability
- memory
- concentration
- rate of laughter per day
- rate of crying per day
- rate and duration of automatic depressive thoughts (i.e., worthlessness, hopelessness, helplessness, and worry)

Behavioral response modality

work performance	—interest in work
	—feeling of competence
	—time lost
	—% accomplished compared to average day
eating	—a checklist of the amount of food consumed for each meal and snack
social interaction	—frequency of self-initiated social activity
	—average daily time spent with friends over last 2 weeks
	—frequency of sexual intercourse
	—interest in sexual interaction

if married:
- —average time spent talking to spouse
- —average time in shared activities with spouse per day
- —marital satisfaction over last week

if single:
- —average time spent talking with friends over last week
- —average time spent in shared activity with friends over last week
- —degree of enjoyment experienced interacting with friends during past week

social interaction (cont.)—general	—frequency of attending social events during past 2 weeks
	—satisfaction from attending social events during past 2 weeks
physical exercise	—type and amount of physical exercise

Somatic response modality

sleep	—average number of hours
	—early morning waking
constipation	
presence of aches and pains	
agitation	—pacing
	—tremors
	—handwringing
fatigue	
appetite	
weight lost	

Source: From *The Behavioral Management of Anxiety, Depression and Pain* (p. 90) edited by P.O. Davidson, 1976, Larchmont, NY: Brunner/Mazel. Copyright 1976 by Brunner/Mazel. Reprinted by permission.

reinforced behavior. To the extent to which social behaviors decrease with aging, there is an increasing failure to handle or avoid unpleasant social consequences and a tendency instead to engage in a great deal of self-criticism and self-blame. Ferster (1973) also emphasizes the increased frequency of avoidance and escape behaviors. The elderly, when depressed, will typically avoid reporting medical problems and requesting help and may escape to bed instead of running the risk of social confrontation with family or facing unpleasantness resulting from behavior such as complaints or dissatisfaction with life events.

Factors Maintaining Depression in the Elderly

Depression may be related to a variety of maintaining factors that are unique to the elderly. These are discussed next.

Abrupt Changes in the Environment

Behavior may be weakened by a sudden change in the environment such as when the spouse of an elderly person dies. To the extent the elderly person's repertoire is intimately related to the loss, there will be a total dampening of the behavior (Ferster, 1973). Frequently, therefore, depression will follow the death of a spouse or an old-age injury or illness that deprives the elderly person of an important set of skills such as social interaction or independent functioning (Paykel et al., 1969).

After retirement, many elderly suddenly placed in a free-work environment may become depressed. In the past, work-related behavior was maintained mainly by positive consequences. After retirement, little behavior may result since there is an impoverished repertoire in relation to positive reinforcement. Behavior may also be weakened in many elderly who go to live with their children and perceive themselves vulnerable to their criticisms, directions, or indications of rejection.

Anger in Relation to Depression

The prominence of anger in many elderly persons' repertoire may be related to the low frequency of positive reinforcement. Many elderly persons in their later years feel that their life has been a waste. They suffer frustration and anger toward significant others (living and dead) who denied them praise, encouragement, and recognition and robbed them of a right to status and productive living. Many elderly become paranoid in their later years and harbor resentment and anger. Since one cannot expect people one is angry at to offer positive reinforcement, many elderly unconsciously distort all positive reinforcements offered by friends and family. Insufficient positive reinforcement and aversive control are highlighted by other behavioral writers (e.g., Seligman, 1975) as contributing to an increased sense of helplessness and decrease in the elderly person's behavioral repertoire.

Lack of Social Skills

Lewinsohn and his colleagues (Lewinsohn, Weinstein, & Alper, 1970; Lewinsohn, Biglan, & Zeiss, 1976) focused on possible deficits in social skills among depressed persons. The major difference found between depressed young adults and depressed elderly was a negative social reaction of self-blame. In situations in which the elderly were ignored, criticized, or disagreed with, they expressed more apologies, self-blaming, and self-critical statements (Fry & Grover, 1982; Fry, 1984c). Many depressed elderly in relating to their families expressed more positive reactions of gratitude and appreciation but expected fewer positive reactions in return. Gradually there was a notable reduction in the frequency of social interactions with various members of the family (Fry, 1984c). The following case of an elderly woman demonstrates the influence of the various depression-maintaining factors, for example, loss of reinforcement, repressed anger and hostility, and deficits in social skills that characterize the lives of elderly.

Client 1

Mrs. L. was born in 1909. In the intake interview she reported being depressed, spending large amounts of time in bed, and having no interest in food. She complained about the absence of close friends, blaming the situation on her husband, who professed no need for people. He had allowed no visitors to the house for the last three years. She said that she no longer had any feelings for her husband or her oldest son, Roger, both without capacity to show care or concern for any living person. Her younger son, Jack, whom she described as being a caring and nurturant person, died in a car accident. Jack had taken her on several trips and lavished her with gifts from time to time. Mrs. L. appeared alert and energetic while discussing her positive relations with Jack but made frequent statements of guilt, sorrow, and depression when talking about Roger and her husband. She admitted to feeling much anger toward Roger and Mr. L., both responsible for kicking Jack out of the house.

Two home observations were conducted during the diagnostic phase. On both occasions the two observers went as visitors calling on Mrs. L. at a time of the day when other family members were present. The lack of any positive interaction among the members, and especially between Mrs. L. and other members, was striking. The three conversational interchanges in the family centered around the weather, the dog, and the doorbell, which was not functioning.

Using the Libet and Lewinsohn (1973) coding procedure, the following data were obtained:

- activity level of Mrs. L.: total number of actions = 2
- interpersonal efficiency of Mrs. L.: ratio of number of behaviors directed toward the client divided by the number of behaviors she displayed toward others per hour = 1
- interpersonal range: the number of people with whom the person interacts = 1
- use of positive reactions: the extent to which the person reinforces actions directed toward self by others = 2
- silence: the number of intervals per hour during which the person neither acts nor reacts to others = 10 intervals of 4 minutes each
- initiation level: the number of actions per hour initiated by the client = 2

Mrs. L.'s case supports both a reinforcement model of depression and a social interaction model of depression.

Social Interaction Model

In this model it is proposed that social factors play an important role in causation, maintenance, and treatment of depression (Brown & Harris, 1978; Lewinsohn, 1976). Entries and exits from the individual's social field, the quality and quantity of social interaction, and the rate of social reinforcement are the three important factors influencing the degree of depression in the individual. These variables are considered to reside outside the individual and within the context of the social environment (Lewinsohn, 1974).

Brown and Harris (1978) found four main factors that render individuals vulnerable to depression:

1. low intimacy or lack of valuable confidant
2. unemployment
3. absence of adults in the environment
4. loss of nurturant-reinforcing adults in the environment

This finding supports the argument that loss of interest in the environment so characteristic of depression is related to loss of reinforcer effectiveness. Lewinsohn, Youngren, and Grosscup's (1979) data showed that depressed individuals interact socially at lower rates, receive and offer less social reinforcement, report lower levels of enjoyment for activities in which they engage, are less comfortable in asserting themselves socially, and display fewer skills in social interaction.

Bothwell and Weissman (1977) reported a number of social deficits in the functioning of depressed individuals and argued that this social skills deficit may be an accompaniment to depression rather than a deficit in the social skills repertoire of individuals. Vaughn and Leff (1977) demonstrated that the major difference in depressed and nondepressed people followed a negative social reaction in which they were ignored, criticized, or disagreed with. These authors found that family members and relatives of depressed persons could induce relapse by means of verbal criticism. They suggested that depressed persons are differentially reactive to success and failure and have a tendency to withdraw from situations in which they fear a withdrawal of reinforcers (see Lewinsohn, 1974) or a related loss of control.

Although results may be due to nonspecific treatment effects, as proposed by Zeiss, Lewinsohn, and Munoz (1979), there is little question of a relation between social interaction rates and depression. Pointing to the relationship among depressed mood, pleasant activity level, and quality of social interaction, McLean's (1982) data showed that non-depressed but relatively socially inactive clients compared to active ones became depressed later. The social interaction model of depression therefore suggests the importance of considering the depressed clients' social network and their perceptions of it, as well as their difficulties in social interaction. In terms of treatment potentials of this model, McLean (1982, pp. 35–36) suggests that the challenge lies in identifying antecedent and current conditions for promoting social interactions that could serve the following purposes:

- opportunities for social reinforcement
- potential introduction of new social interactions, people, ideas, etc.
- increased opportunities for self-reinforcement and social interaction performance
- increased opportunity to use others as a sounding board and to redirect unrealistic standards or expectations before they begin to handicap the individual's social and personal functioning

These objectives of behavioral therapy have special applicability value for intervention with the elderly. As seen in Mrs. L.'s case, observation of her social exchanges showed that she exhibited few interpersonal behaviors, had a restricted range of persons with whom she interacted, received little social reinforcement from the individuals in her environment, and had few skills with which to reciprocate reinforcement.

From an operant-learning theory, depression in Mrs. L.'s case may have been a natural consequence of sustained reduction in the amount of personal reinforcement from her husband and son. After the death of her son Jack, who according to Mrs. L. had been an unusually attentive individual, Mrs. L. experienced a grave reduction in the number of pleasant events that characterized her life and she had few opportunities to use her social skills. All these observations about Mrs. L.'s interpersonal reactions supported the notion that she might be a good candidate for behavioral treatment aimed at increasing appropriate sources of positive reinforcement.

Behavioral Treatment Programs for the Elderly

Few studies have examined the effectiveness of behavioral interventions on elderly individuals living in community settings and faced with depression arising from problems of social inattention, lack of reinforcements, and lack of assertion and other self-control skills. Studies have looked at problems of depressed elderly living in nursing home settings (Riedel, 1980). Behavioral treatment modules with core ingredients such as assertion training, relaxation training, self-reinforcement, and social interactional strategies have been suggested in a variety of treatment packages designed especially for the elderly (see Gallagher & Thompson, 1981; Fry, 1983–86). These programs stress a variety of principles, procedures, and techniques.

Once a differential diagnosis of depression has been made, a functional analysis to pinpoint concrete events related to a person's depression should be carried out. Evaluation is ongoing and involves periodic assessments throughout treatment not only of changes in depression level but also of concomitant changes in the events presumed to be related to the patient's depression.

Treatment techniques are aimed at increasing the person's pleasant interactions with the environment and decreasing unpleasant ones. A variety of strategies, techniques, and rating instruments are available. However, only those strategies that have direct relevance to the needs of the elderly are discussed here.

Techniques fall into three general categories:

1. those that focus on changing environmental conditions
2. those that focus on teaching depressed individuals skills that they can use to change problematic patterns of interaction with the environment
3. those that focus on enhancing the pleasantness and decreasing the aversiveness of the person-environment interactions

Environmental interventions are useful if the client's environment is impoverished or aversive. Contingency management is a kind of environmental intervention if, for example, the therapist involves family members to make attention and praise contingent on the adaptive behaviors of the elderly client.

Skill-training techniques teach skills that can be used to change problematic patterns of interaction with the environment. Many standardized programs or procedures can be individually designed. Training usually involves didactic introduction to the skills involved; coaching by the therapist; role playing, rehearsal, and practice by the client in and out of treatment sessions; and finally application of the skills in the real world.

Techniques that are aimed at allowing the client to change the quantity and the quality of interpersonal relationships typically cover three aspects of interpersonal behaviors: (1) assertion, (2) interpersonal style of expressive behavior, and (3) social activity. The instruction format usually consists of modeling, rehearsal, and feedback. Goals are set by client and therapist together. Other techniques that can be used with elderly clients are learning to increase one's social activity; relaxation in situations that may induce dysphoria; and daily planning and time management in order to achieve time for pleasant events.

Since each depressed person is unique, treatment techniques should be flexible. Clients need to be provided with a rationale for what is being done, and this should be acceptable to both client and therapist. The treatment program is presented as task-oriented and educational in its goal, ultimately leading to client self-change and self-reliance.

A behavioral perspective maintains that a person's difficulties in functioning effectively involve how the individual acts, thinks, and feels in particular settings or in response to specific environmental events. In other words the person's problem behaviors are not necessarily symptomatic of underlying conflict or intrapsychic problems as assumed in a psychodynamic orientation. Treatment might involve coaching or teaching the elderly individual how to overcome anxiety and to interact more effectively in new individual relationships. To promote positive change, the treatment program must be carefully tailored to the specific context and situation of each elderly person seeking help. Since the environmental and social context is often far less accommodating for the elderly, older persons rarely experience warm strokes or support and encouragement. Because many elderly fail to reinforce themselves adequately, they become depressed and experience a decline in feelings of self-efficacy (Bandura, 1977). Thus behavioral treatment is necessary for strengthening self-reinforcement strategies in the elderly.

According to Gallagher and Thompson (1981) the aim of the behavioral treatment is to develop a generic set of skills for coping with depression, and this requires that the client interact with the environment to produce concrete changes. Many elderly may concede that strategies that they had used for coping or for manipulating contingencies are no longer effective. This requires that many elderly learn new instrumental behaviors so that they can operate effectively on their changed or restructured environment. The following case illustrates this point.

Client 2

Mr. and Mrs. A. were married more than 55 years and had been active members of the community, well known to their neighbors and to friends who lived outside the neighborhood. When Mr. and Mrs. A. needed any help, neighbors were eager to help. Now things have changed drastically. When they take walks during the morning or afternoon, they walk past the neighbors sitting on their porches. The families appear young to Mr. and Mrs. A. Nobody recognizes them, nobody greets them. When Mr. A. took seriously ill one night, Mrs. A. phoned one of the neighbors whose name she remembered.

Mrs. A.: I'm Mrs. A. I am sorry to bother you but . . .

Neighbor: Mrs. who? I'm sorry, I don't recall meeting you.

Mrs. A. gets upset at not being recognized. She is hurt and confused and hangs up without explaining her reason for phoning.

Mrs. A. had been well known to her neighbors and able to cope with emergencies by phoning the next-door neighbor. The old strategy doesn't work any more. The neighbors aren't as friendly. Mrs. A. feels she is too old to make friends with the new neighbors. They are much younger than she is and she is afraid of rejection and condescension.

Within a behavioral orientation the therapist helps the elderly individuals define the behavior patterns to be changed and establishes a program of external reinforcements and rewards designed to modify the problem behavior rooted in the individuals gradually, to monitor and control their own behaviors, and to use self-reinforcements to shape their own behaviors systematically. The goal is to develop in the client resources that will ultimately prove self-rewarding because the behavior leads to social and intrinsic satisfactions.

Systematic application of such strategies through behaviorally oriented treatment should be valuable in helping the elderly in initial recovery from depression and subsequent prevention of such episodes. Of more immediate significance is an explanation and discussion of the primary steps in treatment.

Primary Steps in Behavioral Treatment

Some of the important mediational steps are summarized as follows.

Step 1 is for the client to understand the relation between mood and activity. This requires that the elderly client be helped in monitoring or observing behavior and moods. More effort has to be made to identify activities that can be changed and also better ways to deal with the unchangeable ones.

Client 3

Mr. O. is a 74-year-old widower living alone. He expressed two major concerns: sadness and loneliness. More specifically he was concerned about his lack of motivation to engage in any activity. He spent the majority of his time in bed resting because of his heart condition and his sore foot. His depression peaked during his first visit when he heard that his son and daughter-in-law were on a trip to Bermuda. They were his only family who came to visit him periodically. He spent a great deal of time attributing his sadness to his inability to move around freely, no money to engage in pleasurable activities, and nothing of interest to do. Early in the therapy sessions it was clear that Mr. O. engaged in few pleasant activities. He had few opportunities for obtaining social reinforcements from others because of a marked reduction in the number of individuals with whom he had daily contacts.

Through discussion three principal goals were set: (1) to monitor activities in his daily life that either created tension or alleviated sad feelings, (2) to increase activity level that would not interfere with his heart condition, and (3) to increase assertive behavior in order to obtain more pleasure from his son's visits and to make new friends. From the first day of the treatment procedure Mr. O. was encouraged to monitor his moods and activities. About one week following the meeting it became apparent that Mr. O. was doing well in terms of monitoring activity and mood ratings. He was encouraged subsequently to increase social activity. Mr. O. reported he felt happier when, at his suggestion, his housekeeper agreed to stay and play cards with him. Mr. O.'s neighbor was urged to watch a television movie with him; the company became more interesting than watching the show alone. Mr. O. quickly recognized the connection between his activities and his moods. Most of the tension-producing situations involved his son and family, who were unable to stretch their visiting time to keep him company. Assertion training was recommended so that other friends could become involved in visiting and increasing his activity level.

Monitoring of moods and activities had a positive impact on this client's depression. Here was a client who preceding treatment saw himself as a passive victim of a heart condition. Through monitoring, Mr. O. observed that he was most depressed at the end of the day when he was alone or on Sunday morning, when he did not expect to be visited.

Two important techniques—time management and positive self-statements—were added to therapy. Time management allowed him to distribute interesting activities and visits from friends evenly through the week so that he had one or two interesting events to look forward to on a daily basis. Positive self-statements, such as "I am well able to be cheerful and enjoy some activities on my own," permitted him to engage in some pleasant activities, such as telephone conversations with family members, crossword puzzles, reading the newspaper, and painting when alone.

Step 2 involves encouraging the client to focus on acquiring new skills needed to increase pleasant activities or to decrease the impact of unpleasant ones (such as being alone) only after the person has been helped to see the relationship between moods and activity level. This is illustrated in Mr. O.'s behavioral treatment. In our experience with the elderly (Fry, 1983–86) as compared to other age groups, several depression-inducing aspects of their lives cannot be changed, for example, chronic illness, reduced income, and social isolation. However, once the skill in recognizing mood-activity relationships has been acquired, even seriously depressed elderly can be helped to modify moods by increasing activity level.

In Mr. O.'s case he recognized that he could not change the fact of his physical illness or improve his economic means. The behavioral treatment approach, however, was most useful in getting him to recognize that one component of his behavior that he could selectively control was his depressive response by substituting that with some pleasurable or constructive activity. In deciding what activities to pursue, both therapist and Mr. O. had to work toward the goal of selecting activities that did not either impose a physical strain or require much additional expense. Once significant activities having potentials for pleasure and enjoyment were identified, increase in the level of pleasurable activities was produced through behavioral practices.

Once a sense of effectiveness develops, the elderly client's motivation to maintain activity level and to monitor sad effects related to certain specific events and activities depends on the extent of social reinforcement and support that the elderly person obtains from the environment. Unfortunately through no fault of their own many elderly who begin to engage in independent activities experience a reduction in the amount and quality of attention and assistance from family members and friends.

Step 3 in behavioral therapy is that positive reinforcement, praise, and encouragement of newly acquired skills are essential to the maintenance of the positive responses. Most elderly individuals' depression is related to a loss of self-confidence. Once improvement in behavior is attained, it is important that a steady supply of social reinforcements be provided to encourage the client in behavioral improvement. The following example illustrates the value of sustained positive reinforcement.

Client 4

Mrs. M., an active 76-year-old widow who had a reduced income, went to live with her well-to-do son-in-law and daughter. After a year or so, treatment began because of an abrupt history of panic attacks. These attacks usually came on suddenly, sometimes as often as three or four a day. During the attacks she suffered shortness of breath, extreme sweating, coldness, and pallor of face.

Although Mrs. M.'s family members knew these attacks were psychological in nature and always subsided in time, an overwhelming concern prompted the daughter and son-in-law to rush home from work and to give Mrs. M. attention and care. Mrs. M., meanwhile, was depressed at her inability to control the panic attacks, and her feelings of helplessness and hopelessness about her future intensified. When the attacks became frequent, Mrs. M.'s family sought psychological help for her.

The goals of Mrs. M.'s treatment, set early, changed relatively little throughout therapy. Early in the treatment sessions it became clear that lack of self-esteem was limiting the pleasure that Mrs. M. could obtain by living in a rich household. Mrs. M. felt unneeded, worthless, and helpless.

The first three sessions focused primarily on teaching her relaxation training. Mrs. M. was encouraged to concentrate on monitoring the situations that caused a reduction in tension or that created tension. Mrs. M. observed that tension was highest for her when her daughter and son-in-law were too busy and preoccupied to give her attention. Conversely tension was reduced whenever Mrs. M. was asked occasionally to help in chores and activities that would normally be done by the family or household help. Through discussion of Mrs. M.'s feelings of uselessness and purposelessness two goals were set: (1) to increase Mrs. M.'s involvement in household activity so that she would feel that she was pulling her own weight and being useful and (2) to increase her relaxation level through relaxation exercises during the day, when her children were away at work.

After six therapy sessions, tremendous improvement could be seen in Mrs. M.'s self-report and through improved Beck Depression Inventory Scores (41 initially, reduced to 19). Mrs. M. monitored the number of household activities in which she helped and the effect on her moods. There was a significant reduction in the number of panic attacks. Following the ninth session, however, Mrs. M. began to call to reschedule, cancel, and reschedule. This pattern covered a few weeks. When she finally returned to therapy, she appeared depressed and most unwilling to continue with treatment.

In retrospect several reasons for Mrs. M.'s regression emerged. Mrs. M. received little or no praise or encouragement from her family once she began to show a decline in panic attacks. The daughter and son-in-law who had habitually phoned home during the day to inquire about her panic attacks became so relieved that they stopped being concerned about her. In the early stages of therapy Mrs. M.'s daughter expressed much gratitude for Mrs. M.'s help in the household work but later became too preoccupied to note the many extra chores her mother had done. Mrs. M. received much less attention from the family after they became used to her improvement.

Mrs. M. was reengaged in therapy. Additional sessions were arranged with Mrs. M.'s daughter and son-in-law to instruct them in the value of positive reinforcement and the possible danger of extinction. It was explained to them how extinction may occur as a result of the removal of reinforcement for a behavior that gradually dies out because it is no longer reinforced with attention. It was pointed out to them that the only time they had paid Mrs. M. a lot of attention was when she displayed panic attacks. When panic attacks subsided, Mrs. M. was relatively ignored by her family. Mrs. M.'s children were subsequently trained to give her lots of praise, support, and encouragement for being active, useful, and a highly contributing member of the family.

This case illustrates an important step necessary to effective treatment: the value of ongoing and sustained positive reinforcement and encouragement. As a sense of effectiveness develops in the client and success is experienced with greater frequency, motivation to continue with changes that will promise increasing benefits is contingent on the client receiving more attention and reinforcement for positive behaviors than the client received for maladaptive and depressive responses.

This case also illustrates the dominant need in most elderly to feel useful contributing members of a given social setting. Many elderly, despite serious physical limitations, desire opportunities to contribute, to give more than they receive, and to be involved in constructive activities that may initially bring praise and reinforcement but eventually motivate them to become more self-sufficient and self-reliant through self-initiated changes.

Step 4 in behavioral therapy is that of the client assuming more self-initiated changes. In Mrs. M.'s case, once she had pinpointed the changes she wanted to accomplish, she was able to initiate additional activities that would increase positive benefits. For example, Mrs. M. felt that attention to concrete activities was beneficial to her when she felt depressed. Mrs. M. worked out an arrangement for phoning her daughter or a neighbor when she felt an anxiety attack coming on. Mrs. M. was visibly relieved by this plan since she was assured that she would always receive some attention when she needed it. Follow-up showed that she had continued with the activities that made her feel useful. Mrs. M. was able to regain her self-confidence with the help of the supportive arrangements worked out with her daughter and son-in-law.

Step 5 in behavioral therapy involves generalization or transfer of skills learned to multiple situations in one's everyday world (Gallagher & Thompson, 1981). For some elderly clients this is the most difficult part of the process, and many elderly need long periods of reinforcement before they are able to function primarily on their own with minimal therapist contact. Many elderly become aware that they have learned the essential social skills for functioning independently but continue to need periodic booster sessions to uphold their self-confidence. According to Gallagher and Thompson (1981, p. 8) the purpose of these booster sessions is to provide opportunities to the client to discuss successful and unsuccessful use of behavior strategies as well as to problem-solve about new situations that may have developed in the interim.

State-dependent learning has also been found to contribute to the need for repetition in behavioral therapy. A client who can function with minimal therapist contact in some situations may regress because of additional stress and be unable to see how a previously learned coping skill applies to a new situation. In order to foster generalization of skills, clients should be forewarned about how state-dependent learning operates so that they do not become too discouraged when it happens. The following case illustrates the point.

Client 5

With the help of the therapist's aide Mr. J., a depressed elderly client, had worked out a plan to visit his daughter once a week. Time had been spent in therapy coaching Mr. J. on which bus route to take, questions to ask at the bus stop, and precautions to take en route to his daughter's home. Mr. J.'s daughter worked out arrangements to meet him at the bus stop, which was just a few blocks from her house. After Mr. J. had made a few successful visits, he was forewarned of the possibility that his daughter might not be at the bus stop to greet him. Mr. J. had rehearsed alternative courses of action in the event of his daughter not showing up at the bus stop or not being at home when he arrived. This practice in how to cope with unforeseen situations was of much value when he actually faced the unexpected situation.

Technical Issues and Concerns for the Behavior Therapist

Gallagher and Thompson (1981) address several general issues that frequently arise for the therapist doing behavioral therapy with depressed elderly clients. These authors stress the following aspects of therapy:

Protocol in the Structure of Therapy and the Client-Therapist Relationship

It is important that the elderly client understand the rationale for behavior therapy. Even after the rationale has been understood and accepted, many elderly clients will show resistance in the implementation stage, and many forget why and what they were supposed to be monitoring and observing.

Beck et al. (1979) stress the significance of scheduling the client's activities. Especially for depressed elderly clients it may be necessary to schedule activities hour by hour in order to counteract loss of motivation, rumination, and hopelessness. The specific technique of scheduling the client's time allows the therapist to collect concrete data concerning the client's functional capacity. This capacity may vary considerably, depending on factors of illness, cognitive impairment, and social support available. Beck et al. (1979, pp. 121–124) suggest a number of basic principles that should be explained to the client before using the schedule technique.

- "No one accomplishes everything he plans, so don't feel bad if you don't realize all your plans."
- "In planning, state what kind of activity you will undertake, not how much you will accomplish."
- "Even if you don't succeed, be sure to remind yourself that trying to carry out plans is the most important step. This step provides useful information for setting the next goal."
- "Set aside some time to plan for the next day; write your plans for each hour."

Botwinick (1978) observed that the older person may need more time to assimilate and try out new ideas than a younger person and may need more concerted help and behavioral practice in translating ideas into concrete everyday realities specific to their living environment. Materials may have to be presented more than once with many illustrations and examples, and the therapist needs to be much more flexible, patient, and persistent.

Homework is an integral part of this therapy, and therefore the therapist must ensure the client knows exactly what must be accomplished between therapy sessions. Efforts to complete homework assignments can be reinforced by encouraging the client to confront difficult issues, develop self-rewards for completion, and always review completed homework at the start of the therapy sessions. If necessary, the client should be helped to set a definite scheduled time each day for completing assignments.

Redefinition of the Therapist's Traditional Role

In order to accomplish the various steps in behavioral therapy, the therapist needs to define the role as primarily that of an educator and collaborator. According to Pfeiffer and

Busse (1973) this involves taking an active rather than a passive stance toward the client. Most aged people respond better to treatment when there are specific goals and the therapist plays a more active role than with the young.

With each elderly client the therapist has to find a unique balance between how much to do for the client and how much independence to encourage in the client. Teaching time management in therapy sessions is important as elderly clients may wish to talk at great length and in great detail about events that are not directly relevant to behavioral therapy but merely provide emotional release. While being direct is essential in early treatment sessions, increasing emphasis on the collaborative nature of therapy is beneficial in the middle and late stages.

Promotion of Self-Reliance in Clients

Often therapists beginning work with older adults feel they should assume the advocacy role and extend themselves in doing a great deal for the elderly. However, the elderly person's increasing dependence on others is a major contributing factor in their depression. Most behaviorally oriented therapists, therefore, feel that promoting self-reliance in older persons is a significant part of the treatment. Thus therapists who believe in the primacy of the therapist's supportive-nurturant role may find it difficult to abandon their advocacy role and to assume a firm and demanding but reinforcing stance with the client.

Considerable interpersonal skill is also needed by the behavioral therapist to assess the comfort level of the depressed client and initially to engage clients in treatment. Successful treatment depends on the therapist's skills to provide a reinforcing atmosphere that encourages clients to continue to do their homework and engage in relevant behavioral practice. With elderly clients especially, frequent eliciting of feedback is necessary to determine if the client has comprehended what was explained or if amplification is necessary. The depressed client's willingness to proceed through the designated steps and to be convinced that this approach will be useful in the reduction of depression is the key ingredient of behavioral therapy.

Attitudes of Client and Therapist

If clients feel they are too old to learn or too set in their ways to change their behaviors, tasks can be reframed in such a way that the therapist uses techniques that are more specifically age and stage appropriate. For example, techniques may have to be modified to suit the needs of the elderly person who may be physically sick and become easily stressed and anxious when any suggestions are made for new responses. Personal values and social-cultural factors may inhibit an older person from adopting effective behavioral interventions such as muscle relaxation, assertiveness training, and group therapy. The therapist's task, therefore, is to modify techniques creatively to suit each elderly client's physical needs, skill levels, and social-cultural background. The following case illustrates modifications necessary in standard intervention procedures.

Client 6

Mrs. T. is a 72-year-old alcoholic who lived with her adult son and daughter. She was agitated, reported herself on the brink of total despair, finding it increasingly difficult to keep going with her arthritis and lack of sleep. She also complained about the aggressive attitudes of her children. The lack of any positive interactions between Mrs. T. and her children on a daily basis was also a contributing factor in her depression.

Through discussion, three principal goals were set to (1) increase muscle relaxation, (2) increase assertiveness behavior in order to deal with her aggressive children, and (3) resume attendance at Alcoholics Anonymous (AA) meetings in order to get help for her alcohol problems. As treatment proceeded, a number of adjustments in behavioral techniques had to be made to suit Mrs. T.'s age-related and family-related needs and in order to motivate her to continue using social skills. Because the client had problems with the relaxation exercises due to arthritis, the program was modified to include relaxation sessions while in the bathtub—much more successful and pleasant for her.

She was encouraged to concentrate on monitoring the specific situations in her daily living that created tension. Almost all these tension-producing situations involved her relationships with her children. Assertion training was started, but it became evident early in the treatment that although Mrs. T. was quite adept in assertive skills in the therapist's presence, from a practical standpoint it was not appropriate to be assertive with her children, who had their own problems of aggression. Because of the enmeshed family situation it was decided that Mrs. T.'s assertive responses in relating to the children would be counterproductive to therapeutic aims. Therefore systematic application of other strategies such as increasing level of pleasant activities outside the home had to be implemented.

Concerning attendance at AA meetings, Mrs. T. knew it was important to overcome her habit of solitary drinking. When she took the final step of going to AA meetings, her son was rough on her since other members of the AA group were known to him through his office. The therapist subsequently decided that a suitable alternative would be to work on Mrs. T.'s negative self-image and negative self-statements, which contributed to her depression and drinking. The treatment plan was changed to focus on the modification of negative self-talk, which proved successful.

Mrs. T. was also encouraged to join another group therapy program in which she was able to discuss her negative self-image and shame at being an alcoholic. Since Mrs. T.'s drinking problem was of recent origin and related to her immediate depressions, therapy efforts to increase personal self-confidence proved successful in alleviating depression.

This case illustrates that a client may find considerable benefit from treatment even if goals and strategies initially selected as most appropriate are not used in the final plan. The behavioral therapist's flexibility in restructuring strategies based on insights developed from discussion of personal and sociocultural concerns of the client are valuable strengths.

When working with elderly clients, many of whom have enmeshed family circumstances and social conditions that cannot be changed too easily, the therapist must bow to the judgments of the client. Therapists must be careful to examine their own attitudes and tendencies to be too directive and dominant throughout the treatment program.

Termination Problems

Premature termination is a problem in all modes of therapy, particularly behavior therapy. Reasons given by clients are usually related to logistical problems such as lack of transportation, shortage of money, and difficulty in completing homework assignments. With older clients these are sometimes realistic issues. To minimize the incidence of dropout due to logistic problems, the therapist needs to play an active problem-solving role and help clients to continue in therapy.

The preceding are some of the more salient points that are necessary conditions when developing behavior therapy programs. The treatment manual developed by Gallagher and Thompson (1981) is the only program analysis that has been designed specifically for the elderly and has detailed explanation and discussion relating to conceptual and technical issues.

Behavioral Programs for the Elderly

Fry (1984a, 1984b, 1984c) has also assembled a series of behavioral programs that have been effective in dealing with certain negative behavioral responses that are the indirect consequences of old-age depressive states, for example, accident proneness, alcohol consumption, loss of appetite, restlessness and trembling, and impulsive behavior. Some of the techniques suggested in these behavioral programs, however, are more cognitive in nature and aimed at enhancing self-esteem and morale, components considerably affected during depression.

Fry's (1984a) behavioral programs are predicated on the assumption that most depressed elderly because of preoccupation and poor concentration have difficulties in carrying out tasks that require successive steps for completion. Therefore a cognitive rehearsal technique is employed to help the depressive to pay attention to specific tasks and to counteract the tendency to wander. The therapist requires the elderly client to imagine each step in the sequence leading to the completion of an assignment that the client may have previously been able to accomplish but now lacks the confidence to pursue. By rehearsing the sequence of steps the client has a preprogrammed system to carry out the task. The rehearsal strategy helps the client to identify roadblocks impeding the completion of the task (Beck et al., 1979). The following example illustrates behavioral components of a program designed to elicit greater behavioral activation in a depressed elderly client who became acutely accident-prone following a depression episode.

Client 7

Mr. H. is a 76-year-old physically healthy individual. Mr. H.'s careful history examination suggested that there might indeed be some triggering or exacerbating factors causing his acute accident-proneness in his daily activities. A successful businessman, on his retirement Mr. H. became the volunteer founder of an organization. His medical examination indicated he was in good health and there was no significant loss of hearing or eyesight. Till recently Mr. H. had driven his car to various places of business. But lately he became afraid. He panicked every time he had to plan a short driving trip. He slipped on the stairs at home, bumped into tables and chairs obviously in sight, and hurt himself several times. In his preoccupied state he broke objects of sentimental value to him and as a result became more depressed.

In the first interview Mr. H. declared that his accident-proneness was evidence that he was losing his mind. He repeatedly wondered why he should be so poor in navigating his way around the house or in walking to various places he had been to many times before.

Discussions of his confusion in the morning and late at night, his loss of appetite, and psychomotor slowness suggested that his accident-proneness was an indirect result of depression triggered by cohorts at work. A few cohorts had commented that Mr. H. was no longer with it and was losing his presence of mind.

A behavioral program was set up for him, requiring the following:

- Mr. H. must practice muscle relaxation exercises before any significant move, for example, going down the steps, stepping in and out of the bathtub, navigating his way through the sunroom, which contained several plants, tables, and boards.
- Before deciding to go downstairs, for example, Mr. H. must remind himself that there were 24 steps downstairs and one landing area after the 15th step. Mr. H. must close his eyes and visualize himself going down the steps, resting on the landing area, and taking a deep breath before descending the last 8 steps.
- Mr. H. must monitor his tension state, for example, being wobbly on his legs, drowsy when stepping into the bath, light-headed after a shower. He must attempt to relate that tension state to the particular task he was performing.
- Mr. H. must monitor the number of accident-free mornings and afternoons, when he was able to walk around firmly and securely, did not bump into objects, and was able to go down the steps without clinging to the rails.
- Mr. H. must reinforce himself every 30 minutes that he was able to have an accident-free period.
- Mr. H. must increase his physical activity level by climbing steps more frequently, walking across the lawn onto the pavement even if covered with snow and ice.
- Mr. H. must increase the frequency of using positive self-instruction and self-reinforcing statements that he had rehearsed in therapy (e.g., I've been climbing these steps all my life, there is no reason I should fall today; I was successful this morning and yesterday evening, there is no reason why I should fall now; I must not allow myself to become anxious by the comments of my colleagues at work; The more self-confidently I behave, the more self-confident I will feel).

Within 2 to 3 weeks of implementing the behavioral program Mr. H. considered himself on the ball again. His tendency to worry about a possible accident, to be miserable over little details, and then to withdraw from potentially fear-inducing activities was substantially reduced. It was several weeks before Mr. H. felt ready to resume driving. After 12 weeks of therapy he felt he had regained control of his mind and his depression. Soon he was ready to cope with his work routine. Therapy on a regular schedule was terminated although Mr. H. came back for many booster sessions.

Another technique that is frequently stressed in Fry's (1984a) behavioral programs is that of systematic desensitization, which is used with many stressed and depressed elderly clients who avoid anxiety by withdrawing from a situation. Developed by Wolpe (1958), systematic desensitization involves training the client to experience a state of deep muscle relaxation through tensing and relaxing various muscle groups. When a state of relaxation has been induced, the person is instructed to imagine the anxiety-producing situation in a series of steps or a hierarchy. An anxiety hierarchy is ordered in terms of how much anxiety is aroused when the client is in various situations, beginning with scenes that evoke little anxiety and progressing to more difficult situations. The goal of this progressive desensitization procedure is for the client to remain relaxed even when imagining—and ultimately experiencing—the situations that aroused the greatest anxiety. To gain maximum benefit from desensitization, the client must be sufficiently relaxed to imagine the scenes associated with even a small amount of the anxiety-producing situation. Feldman and DiScipio (1972) cite the use of desensitization with someone hospitalized with Parkinson's disease to reduce a fear of falling. Once this fear was reduced through desensitization procedures, the patient could participate in physical therapy.

Fry (1984b) notes that desensitization is appropriate as treatment for particular kinds of depressions of the elderly, especially when fear and depression coexist. Fears associated with specific types of situations such as fear of visiting and being alone with the physician, fear of walking on the pavement lest one should slip on the ice, fear of medical procedures such as x-rays, fear of crossing the street at a busy intersection, fear of being rejected in group situations. At times the anxiety can become so dominant that the client ceases to participate in daily activities. Fry's (1984a, 1984b, 1984c) experience with elderly clients suggests that depression is often a contributing factor to loss of self-confidence and the subsequent emergence of irrational fears and phobias.

Desensitization can occur either through the use of imagery or in the actual situation. For some persons, imagery does not produce feelings of anxiety similar to the actual situation, and desensitization can take place only through actual involvement in the real-life situation. Fry (1984a, 1984b, 1984c) recommends the use of imagery first, followed by gradual participation in the actual situation. The following case illustrates the use of desensitization procedures with an elderly woman.

Client 8

Mrs. K. became afraid of visiting her doctor (Dr. S.) and still more afraid of being alone with him in his office. Mrs. K. admitted that her fear was most irrational. She confirmed that Dr. S. was indeed a nice man and had given her a number of useful treatments. She did not have any specific reasons for being afraid of him, but she nevertheless experienced much trembling of the body and fear of passing out whenever she was obliged to be alone with him. On one occasion she broke into a cold sweat, fled from his office, and demanded to be taken home. Subsequently she confined herself to her room for several hours until she was able to control her panic state. Her fears reached a peak during a visit when her doctor suggested that she needed a chest examination.

Since Mrs. K. was a chronic bronchitis patient, regular visits to the doctor's office were important and could not be avoided. An anxiety hierarchy was constructed for Mrs. K. where she began by imagining a scene associated with only a small amount of anxiety, such as thinking about the appointment with the doctor a few days before the actual date. After repeated pairings of each scene with a relaxed state, Mrs. K. was able to envision it with less experience of anxiety. The therapist then presented the next scene in the hierarchy, such as being driven to the doctor's office by her daughter, being accompanied by the doctor's receptionist into the doctor's interior office, and being left there alone with him. These scenes were paired repeatedly with relaxation until they produced minimal anxiety. Mrs. K. was also encouraged to engage in these imagery exercises and cognitive rehearsal exercises as a part of homework assignments. After a few sessions of relaxation and desensitization she felt ready to return to the actual situation of the doctor's office.

Participation in the actual situation was also graduated. Mrs. K. was first driven to the doctor's office. Her daughter accompanied her to the interior office, but no face-to-face visit with the doctor was planned. Subsequently the daughter stayed with the mother during the entire visit and assisted Mrs. K. in undressing and dressing activities for the medical test. Mrs. K.'s doctor, who was notified of the panic attack, also cooperated in the desensitization procedures by initially letting the daughter and the nurse stay in the office for the entire checkup.

After several in vivo practices Mrs. K. was able to control her anxiety and stay relaxed even when alone with the doctor. Anxiety control was finally achieved through muscle relaxation training, graduated exercises in desensitization imagery control, cognitive rehearsals, and in vivo practice. While application of desensitization treatment with the elderly has been limited, increasing use of desensitization procedures is taking place with elderly clients who report depression due to specific fears and anxieties associated with daily functioning. Mr. H., who developed an anxiety about driving his car or stepping into the bathtub, was also treated successfully through desensitization.

Clients who receive training in relaxation and desensitization also report immediate relief in sad mood. Lewinsohn, Munoz, Youngren, and Zeiss (1978) report that depressed persons generally respond favorably to these procedures. Self-induced relaxation and self-management of anxiety procedures are therefore a useful adjunct to other forms of intervention for depressed elderly. Many elderly who become depressed by their own fears in group situations can be taught ways of managing their fears of rejection, criticism, and tension in social and interpersonal contexts. In these cases relaxation and desensitization are successful in shaping more effective interpersonal behaviors (Fedoravicius, 1977).

Status of Behavior Therapy for Depressed Elderly

The decision to use behavior therapy rather than another treatment modality must be based on consideration of several factors: the client's motivation to participate in an active problem-solving program for the treatment of depression, the therapist's commitment to social learning theory as a plausible and feasible way to explain the origin and maintenance of depression, and the presence of specific behavioral excesses or deficits that could become targets for intervention. There are no hard-and-fast guidelines to help the clinician determine which older clients are good candidates for behavioral therapy or when to select the behavioral approach over others in treating depression. In general, good candidates are those depressed elderly who have many unpleasant events and few pleasant events and who come from social environments lacking in reinforcement, positive experiences, and social support.

COGNITIVE THERAPY OF DEPRESSION

Cognitive therapy, the only psychotherapy designed specifically to treat depression, was developed by Beck (Beck, 1967; Beck et al., 1979). According to Beck depression may be viewed as the activation of three major cognitive patterns that lead individuals to see themselves, their surroundings, and their prospects in irrational and idiosyncratic ways. Since the contents of these patterns revolve mainly around themes of loss and deprivation, this makes the cognitive model of depression particularly relevant to the elderly. Thomae (1970, 1980) notes that depression in the elderly is directly related to reminiscences of loss and anticipations of physical, emotional, and cognitive deprivations. This conceptual analysis of the causes of depression is consistent with Beck's Cognitive Triad.

The first component of the cognitive triad (i.e., the self, surroundings, and the future) is the negative view of self as deprived, defective, or defeated. Depressed clients notably believe that they are inadequate or defective and therefore undesirable. Because of their alleged defects depressed clients invariably reject themselves and consequently suffer a severe decline in self-esteem and self-control. This decline takes the form of personal criticism, self-blame, and underestimation of one's abilities and capabilities.

The second component is the negative view of experiences. Depressed clients view interactions with the environment as inordinately demanding, obstructive, or difficult. They therefore interpret most of their interactions with the environment as representation of deprivation and defeat. These interpretations are taken as evidence to support their ideas of personal rejection, deprivation, and increased dependency on others who are always viewed to be more capable. Compared to the nondepressed, depressed persons minimize success experiences and emphasize failures.

Finally, the negative view of the future permeates the ideations of the depressed persons. As they look ahead, they see their future as holding nothing of value; therefore they fear an indefinite continuation of their present hardships and a life of unremitting deprivation, frustration, and further losses.

Beck's (1967) tricomponent theory of depression rejects the view of depression as an affective disorder in which cognitions related to low self-esteem are secondary to the affective disorder. He considers the cognitions the primary cause of depressions. An examination of the thought contents of depressives reveals distortions and unrealistic perceptions in which clients exaggerate their faults and believe therefore that they are social and emotional outcasts and must endure loneliness. As Beck (1974) notes, several other phenomena of depression such as dependency and helplessness may also be considered as consequences of the negative cognitive pattern. Increased dependency may be attributed to negative concepts. As most depressed individuals expect things to turn out badly, many depressed persons yearn for help from other persons whom they consider to be strong.

According to most cognitive theorists (Kovacs, Rush, Beck & Hollan, 1981; Beck et al., 1979) increased depression results from the rekindling or restimulation of major constructs, or depressive schemas, in the sensitized person's repertoire. Although the schemas may be latent or inactive at a given time, they are activated by particular kinds of circumstances and may consequently lead to a full-blown depression. A depressed client's ideation is marked by typically depressive themes going back to earlier stages that render the individual vulnerable to psychological dysfunction. As the depression deepens, the thought contents are increasingly saturated with themes of failure, hardships, and insolvable problems. These conceptualizations of depression proposed by Beck et al. have special relevance to the understanding of depression in the elderly.

Cognitive Distortion Model and Depression in the Elderly

Traditionally depression in the elderly has not been considered a cognitive disorder. However, there is increasing evidence to indicate otherwise. The characteristic manner in which the depressed elderly construe themselves, their environment, and their future invites confrontation on the part of many younger friends and family members in an attempt to dissuade them from their irrational feelings of despair, hopelessness, and worthlessness.

Thomae (1970, 1980) notes that as individuals grow older, they tend to adopt a negative attitude toward aging. Automatic thoughts that precede their anxiety and depression are related to the belief that being old is being inferior. Certain clusters of cognitive distortions and dysfunctional maladaptive beliefs more commonly found among the elderly involve life-style changes, health issues, and relationships with others. Thomae (1970) postulates that a person's perceptions of growing older rather than any external (social) or internal (biological) changes determine their mode of adaptation to aging, and depression arises because many elderly have distorted perceptions, expectations, and concerns about the outcomes of old age. The dominant sentiment experienced by a considerable number of depressed elderly is a sense of loss—irrevocable loss of valued relationships, attributes, and opportunities. Sensitized by unfavorable life circumstances and insidious conditions over a prolonged period, many depressed elderly become prone to misinterpretation or magnification of problems. Such magnification helps to provide a reason or meaning for their depression.

Many elderly faced with problems of adjustment become prone to jumping to negative conclusions, tuning out of positive factors, and presenting the worst picture of their situation. Systematic cognitive distortions work further to engender sadness, low self-esteem, self-criticism, and self-blame. Beck (Beck et al., 1979) and Ellis (1970) have made an important contribution to the understanding of depression in terms of the type of distorted thinking that occurs.

Role of Cognitive Errors

Cognitive errors or irrational thinking in the information-processing system helps the depressed person to maintain and retain the beliefs in negative views despite strong evidence to the contrary. Beck et al. (1979) identified six sets of cognitive errors, which are described here for purposes of clarification. Examples and illustrations of statements representing cognitive errors have been drawn from therapy sessions with a number of depressed elderly clients:

1. Arbitrary inference (response set), that is, drawing incorrect conclusions from existing evidence. For example, "When I phoned to speak with my grandson, my daughter-in-law answered the telephone and said that Jeff was in the middle of doing his homework and that he would have to phone me back later. Obviously, she doesn't want me to make contacts with her children."
2. Selective abstraction (stimulus set), that is, focusing on a single aspect of a situation. For example, "My son and his family come twice a year to visit us from Toronto. As I grow older, I wish they could come more frequently but I get the feeling they are just too busy and not interested enough in us."
3. Overgeneralization (response set), that is, drawing conclusions from single bits of information. For example, "My legs felt wobbly when I got up this morning. I know I'm headed for some serious illness."
4. Magnification and minimization (response set). Similar to overgeneralization but including an evaluative component. "My boss disagreed with me about my decision to buy the apparatus. He and I will never see eye to eye on anything."
5. Personalization (response set). For example, "My husband was late coming home to our anniversary celebration and when he finally did arrive, he didn't apologize. There is something very wrong about our marriage, I know."
6. Absolutist, dichotomous thinking (response set), that is, seeing every experience in opposite terms. "This year everything, and I mean everything, has gone wrong for me. It makes me feel absolutely useless."

Cognitive errors tend to become autonomous as the depression deepens and the person's interactions with others in the environment decrease. A woman whose adult children have stopped communicating with her may feel appropriately sad or disappointed, but if she views this to be the end of the world and feels that her life is meaningless, she will become increasingly inactive or despondent. Clients may reason on the basis of self-defeating assumptions, may incorrectly interpret life stresses, may judge themselves too harshly, may jump to inaccurate conclusions, or may fail to generate adequate plans or strategies to deal with external problems because of their inability to respond rationally and objectively to the social environment. Beck views depressive thoughts as being latent in most persons but coming to the fore during stress.

Kahn, Zarit, Hilbert, and Niederehe (1975) and Kahn and Fink (1958) note that the tendency to view oneself in an exaggerated negative way may increase with age. These authors propose that depressed elderly tend to perceive events in stereotyped and cliched ways. With increasing age, many elderly come to view themselves in terms of negative stereotypes about old age and to be overly despondent about their abilities. Consistent with this view, Fry (1982) observed that depressed elderly condemn themselves in irrational and oversimplified ways, making statements such as "my whole life has been a failure" and "I can't seem to do anything properly." According to Kahn et al. (1975) this tendency to be overly self-critical and to perceive events in oversimplified ways is related to poor adaptation.

Working in a similar vein, Ellis (1970) has identified several patterns of irrational thought that are associated with disturbing emotions and which cause depressive disorders. Ellis proposes that many distressing emotional reactions are the result of not appraising one's actions correctly or rationally and of overgeneralizing the impact of failures or disappointments.

Irrational Beliefs

While not all of the irrational thoughts identified by Ellis (1970) characterize the cognitions of the elderly, a few are notably present in the thinking processes of the elderly and influence their appraisals, attributions, and expectations. A few examples follow:

- One common irrational belief is that the past remains all important and that because something once strongly influenced life, it must continue to determine feelings and behavior today. Many elderly who had influential relationships in the past and acknowledged the strength of their influence feel that they can no longer function effectively in any sphere without the support of those influential individuals or be successful without their mediation. According to Ellis this idea is irrational because in the course of everyday events an individual can accomplish success in many situations and in many activities without assistance from others.

- Older patients frequently have irrational and dysfunctional beliefs about the role their children should play in their lives. Since many elderly cohorts grew up in the period before old-age insurance, when older persons were mainly cared for by their children, they believe that they should be supported by their adult children. Some well-to-do elderly parents believe their children are selfish for not doing more for them. Others believe irrationally that their children should come to visit them frequently and if they do not, then obviously they have failed as parents. The therapist must dispel some of these irrational beliefs by discussing with these patients the changing nature of adult children's responsibilities and their occupational commitments, which keep them busy. The therapist must correct any specific misattributions about their children and their own role as parents.

- Another irrational belief that many elderly cling to is the notion that it is necessary to be loved by all persons and in all situations. Many elderly persons are known to become depressed when even a single member of the family rejects or ignores them. According to Ellis this idea is irrational because it is most unlikely that a person will be appreciated by everyone for all actions. Moreover, the fact that a person is not appreciated by someone should not automatically imply that the person is inferior, worthless, or defective; it only implies that different persons appreciate and value different things.

- The older patients' irrational beliefs about how everyone should treat them with respect (because of their age) often lead to self-defeating behavior patterns. An elderly father becomes angry with his son for not consulting with him about a business deal. An older woman gets angry at her children when they visit because they do not visit frequently enough. These parents cling to an irrational belief that their children should always involve them in decision making and consult with them as in the old days. An elderly man who is financially independent still expects that he is entitled to receive offers of financial help from his children.

- Another irrational belief that many elderly uphold is that one's depression comes from external pressures and that one has little ability to control one's feelings or to rid oneself of depression. The idea is irrational because in the course of everyday events there are many opportunities for both pleasure and depression, and it is important to try to change one's depressive conditions so that they become more pleasurable. It is irrational to believe that one cannot control one's emotions. The consequences of this belief are, first, to make a person feel helpless and, second, to make a person believe that there is no point in attempting to change a situation because the ability to control lies with others and not within oneself.

The overall effect of such longstanding irrational beliefs is that many elderly become dependent on others whom they invariably regard to be superior and much stronger than themselves and whom they must try to please at whatever the cost.

Cognitive therapy is useful in correcting cognitive distortions and irrational beliefs. It is called *cognitive therapy* because it is believed (Beck et al., 1979) that psychological disturbances frequently stem from specific habitual errors or deficits in thinking and from nonspecific faulty information processes. Friends and relatives play an important auxiliary role most frequently when the patient is suffering from dysfunctional beliefs involving family conflicts, family responsibilities, and obligations toward the elderly. In these cases the therapist may choose to have one or more sessions with the children alone so that they can be helped to alleviate guilt feelings toward elderly parents.

Children too frequently have irrational beliefs or dysfunctional attitudes toward the older persons that could interfere with their relationship. Common dysfunctional beliefs are "They are going to die soon; I should be able to do something to stop that." "My parents are old and helpless and completely dependent on me. I must do *everything* I can to help them." Such belief can lead children to wear themselves out in the process of looking after their elderly parents. By spending some time with the elderly parent, an adult son can correct his own erroneous assumptions about the father's inability to care for himself. The latter erroneous belief is counterproductive for the elderly father.

According to both Beck and Ellis the therapeutic task is to pinpoint the depressed client's particular cognitive distortions and maladaptive beliefs that result, first, in communication disturbances and, second, in the individual's maladaptive attempts to manipulate the interpersonal environment. The depressed client may be confronted with reactions of rejection, hostility, or retaliation. Such social reactions may arouse further depression ultimately leading to feelings of despair, powerlessness, and dependency.

This attempt to account for the development of social interaction difficulties in depression has given impetus to the interpersonal disturbance model (Stuart, 1967), the learned helplessness model (Seligman, 1973, 1975), and the life stress model, all deserving some discussion because of their immediate relevance and application to cognitive-behavioral intervention with the elderly. All these models emphasize the need for reinforcement and emotional support during prolonged intervals of stress and depression and are therefore compatible with the basic tenets of supportive therapy.

Interpersonal Disturbance Model of Depression

According to McLean (1976) this model appropriately underscores the position that depression must be understood in terms of the depressed client's interaction with the social environment and must be treated within a social context. The interpersonal disturbance that the depressed elderly person shows is generally the result of reflected appraisal from others in the environment. This external appraisal is seen to influence the self-appraisal of the depression to an extent that the individual believes that the ability has been lost to control the interpersonal environment effectively. Such perceptions of loss of control lead to further cognitions of depression and side effects of depression such as withdrawal, avoidance of communication, or maladaptive attempts at coercive communication.

Within an interpersonal disturbance framework, therapy involves certain behavioral components such as training in social learning principles, verbal interaction, monitoring and feedback, and training in the construction and use of reciprocal behavioral contracts (McLean, Ogston, & Grauer, 1973). The difference between the interpersonal disturbance model of intervention for depression and other cognitive-behavioral models is that the former builds in procedures for including the relevant social network members as an integral component of therapy. Compared to conventionally treated comparison groups, results of interpersonal therapy (McLean, 1974; McLean et al., 1973) indicate a significant improvement in the management of problem behaviors, moods, and communication style, through using behavioral rehearsals, assertion training, and social skills training. The development of cognitive-behavioral skills such as cognitive rehearsal, cognitive restructuring of communication modes, and thought-stopping provides therapeutic vehicles by which negative interpersonal encounters (e.g., control through aggression, coercion, or withdrawal) can be transformed to more socially acceptable forms of control.

Learned Helplessness Model of Depression

This model (Seligman, 1973, 1975) proposes that depression is produced by the belief that responding is useless. Learned helplessness concentrates on those depressions that begin with a reaction to loss of control over gratification and the relief of suffering. The depressed individual is generally slow to initiate responses, believing oneself to be powerless and hopeless in the results or consequences of actions. This model of the development of depression is particularly relevant to many elderly who believe in effect that there is no point in bothering to control or respond since no matter whatever they try to do will be ineffective in bringing about change. Many of the domestic environments in which the elderly reside are insidious combinations of dependency and passivity: self-conscious and unassertive elderly give up trying because they lack a sense of efficacy in achieving the required goals. Many elderly may have exceptional capabilities and competence that they acquired earlier. However they may give up trying because they no longer expect their behavior to have an effect on the unresponsive environment (Bandura, 1977).

The sequence of events in the learned helplessness model of depression is continuous frustrations in goal attainment, learning that one's efforts make no difference, a belief in hopelessness, confirmation of this belief through further experiences of personal ineffectiveness, a generalized feeling of helplessness, and the development of depressive symptomatology. Most depressed elderly have excessively high standards of performance that will not permit self-reinforcement. They also have a tendency to evaluate their present performance against perfectionistic standards of accomplishment that they held in the past. Because of these tendencies, depressed elderly continually evaluate themselves as being a failure (see Fry, 1984a, 1984b, 1984c).

Seligman (1975) suggests, therefore, that therapy must consist of a twofold recovery: recovery of realistic standards of performance and recovery of the belief that responding produces reinforcement. The learned helplessness view of depression emphasizes attainment of client influence over positive consequences through exposure to successful experiences. The induction of mastery, or personal effectiveness, then occurs in the reverse order to which it was originally lost (McLean, 1976).

Successful therapy is said to have occurred when clients believe that they can command acknowledgment, attention, and recognition from others. However, what constitutes a successful response is defined not by the client alone but also by the social environment with which the client is interacting. From a cognitive-behavioral perspective the therapy must consider expectations that the social context has of the client and the expectations that the client has of the self. Therapy consists of changing the client's internal dialogue through reappraisals and restructuring of learned helplessness cognitions. The client is taught to emit thoughts that are incompatible with thoughts of dependency, helplessness, and lack of control. The client engages in imagery rehearsal of stressful events and practices self-statements designed to engender a sense of learned resourcefulness to replace the learned helplessness.

Both the interpersonal disturbance view and the learned helplessness view of geriatric depression complement a life-stress model in which depression is related to stressful conditions. Most individuals, by the time they reach old age, have experienced a number of losses, separations, and concrete hardships. Proponents of the cognitive distortion model propose that in old age depression is directly related to stress conditions such as a multifaceted increase in spousal arguments, family discord, death of spouse or immediate family member, serious personal illness, and change in living conditions. During old age reduced physical and emotional energies combine with excesses of stressful events to produce a formative effect increasing the probability of depression.

PRECEPTS OF COGNITIVE THERAPY WITH THE ELDERLY

Cognitive therapy as a single treatment modality is seldom effective in the treatment of depression and is often combined with other supportive, behavioral, and life-stress concepts of therapy. Ultimately a combination of cognitive-behavioral and interpersonal-supportive therapies (sometimes integrated with pharmacotherapy) are brought to bear on the depressed individual to modify negative cognitions, provide more rational feedback to the client, and help the client regain more objectivity and reasoning. However, before the decision to use cognitive therapy or any other form is made, Beck et al. (1979) point out that the therapist should have a clear understanding of the syndrome of depression. Beck et al. (1979) warn that therapists should limit the use of cognitive therapy to those patients with unipolar nonpsychotic depression differentiated clearly from other forms of affective disorders. A number of fundamental precepts are emphasized, principally the following:

- There must be a collaborative relationship between the client and the therapist. This collaboration takes the form of a therapeutic alliance in which therapist and client work together to fight a common enemy: the client's depression. The collaboration demands that the client and therapist trust each other. Like most forms of supportive therapies, the cognitive technique must be learned and practiced in an atmosphere of concern for the client's special needs. The importance of empathy, warmth, and genuineness in establishing a therapeutic relationship is stressed. The elderly may often show resistance in tasks requiring them to evaluate strengths and deficits in their existing cognitive styles and beliefs and in tasks requiring them to change their ways of looking at themselves and others. Thus more than in any other therapeutic technique, the therapist's interpersonal skills and confidence in the ability of the elderly to succeed will influence treatment.

- A selection of target problems is made for the therapist and client to address during the course of therapy. Throughout each session the therapist tries to find out if the client is responding positively to the therapeutic process and always asks the client for evaluative feedback of each session. Another element of this feedback process is that the therapist explains the rationale for each intervention. This procedure is of special significance when working with the elderly. It demystifies the process of therapy: if the client can see a relationship between a technique or assignment and the solution to a problem, then the client is more likely to participate in the therapy. The therapist has to check that the client has understood the therapist's formulations.

- Once the collaboration between therapist and client has been established, they can begin to work together as a team. In this process of collaborative empiricism each of the client's maladaptive thoughts or underlying assumptions is approached in the same way that a scientist would approach a problem. In the initial sessions the therapist has six major goals (Young & Beck, 1982):

1. Define with the client specific problems to work on.
2. Set priorities regarding the order in which to attack the problems already defined.
3. Select a target problem that can be alleviated quickly to show the client that the individual is not hopeless and thus have empirical evidence to show that the client's problems are not insoluble.
4. Demonstrate to the client the relationship between cognition and emotion, for example, ask what the person was thinking at the time of an apparent mood change.
5. The client has to be socialized into the therapeutic milieu of cognitive therapy in that this is an active and structured therapy.
6. The importance of self-help homework strategies is stressed, especially since the homework is more important than the time during the session.

The structure of cognitive therapy does not change as treatment progresses, only the content. The middle and later sessions are more likely to focus on problems that require more intensive cognitive probing in order to understand and modify the client's negative cognitions.

- Two major cognitive processes comprise the therapeutic approach:

1. Eliciting automatic thoughts. Conscious thoughts often intervene between external events and an individual's emotional reaction to these events. The therapist trains the client to focus on automatic thoughts. Strategies that can be used include inductive questioning, imagery, role playing, noting of mood shifts in the session, and daily record of dysfunctional thoughts.
2. Identifying maladaptive assumptions. General patterns seem to underlie the client's automatic thoughts. Such patterns act as a set of rules that guide the way a client reacts to many different situations. These assumptions are far less accessible, for example, "I cannot live without my husband." When these rules are framed in absolute terms, unrealistic, or used inappropriately or excessively, they often lead to such disturbances as depression, anxiety, and paranoia (Beck et al., 1979). As noted also by Ellis (1970), such rules are maladaptive. The therapist has to identify and challenge these maladaptive beliefs used by the client. Contradictions of problems inherent in the assumptions and beliefs can be identified.

The cognitive therapist also uses a variety of behavioral techniques to help the client cope better with situational or interpersonal problems. In contrast to behavioral techniques, however, cognitive techniques focus more on how to view or interpret events (Shaw, 1977). The behavioral change (for example, engaging in more pleasurable activities) may however be used as evidence to bring about cognitive change.

COGNITIVE-BEHAVIORAL TREATMENT OF DEPRESSION

Therapy consists of three distinct phases: (1) monitoring, (2) cognitive training, and (3) applications.

Monitoring Phase

The first phase of cognitive-behavioral therapy for depression is an educational one in which clients are given a conceptualization of how to view their depressive thoughts in terms of a series of cognitive distortions. In the initial stages the therapist may give assignments to clients to monitor their thoughts in situations where they make negative self-evaluations or engage in an irrational dialogue with the self. Because the concept of inner speech can be readily grasped by most older persons, this procedure for monitoring their private speech appears to have potential in many situations. Another function served by this monitoring is that negative thoughts and negative self-statements that lead to depressive feelings can also be identified.

Although depression in the elderly encompasses a number of specific cognitive-behavioral problems such as social skills deficits, sleep problems, verbal inactivity, and attentional deficits, research (see Fry, 1982, 1983, 1984a; Fry & Grover, 1982) shows that depression in the elderly is largely defined by a number of depressive internal dialogues and negative cognitions concerning their ability to make new friends and feel accepted by neighbors and associates. In a series of interviews conducted as part of a proposed three-year longitudinal study with depressed elderly (Fry, 1983–86), Fry charted the contents of their internal dialogue perceived as contributing to their depression.

Internal Dialogues

MRS. Y: "My next-door neighbor is a young woman about 22-years-old. She saw me walking across her yard and asked me if I would like to come in and have coffee. I was thinking . . . she's just being kind to an old woman. There's nothing very interesting that she and I can talk about anyway . . . so I said, No-thank-you . . . another time perhaps. She's never asked me again. You see, I was right . . . she's not very interested in me. Very few people are interested in us older folks. I keep saying to myself it doesn't matter that she didn't ask me again, but deep down it does matter to me and it makes me sad."

This is an illustration of an internal dialogue of self-disparagement and self-devaluation. The self-statements reflect the subject's sense of low self-worth, not being interesting to others, others not really interested in her.

MRS. P: "When my daughter-in-law comes to visit me, she brings me a lot of fancy clothes. She always wants to know what I think about the clothes she brings. They are really very nice, but I say to myself, 'There is no way I'm going to look good in them. My body is all out of shape and nothing looks good on me anymore. Once upon a time I did look attractive, but not any more.' And these thoughts make me sad. Anyway, my daughter-in-law insists that I try on the clothes. She thinks I look good, but I think she's just being kind to me. I wish she wouldn't keep asking me what I think. I'm afraid to say the wrong thing so I say nothing at all. I know she thinks I'm ungrateful and I get depressed worrying about her opinion of me."

This is an illustration of an internal dialogue of conflict in which positive and negative self-statements compete against one another, interfering with interpersonal behavior and eliciting interpersonal anxiety and depression.

MR. T: "After I retired, Carl, who was my colleague at work, would come around and visit me. The conversation was always about people at work and how well everyone at work is doing. Carl always wants to know what I do with my time and how come the wife and I haven't gone on a trip. I keep thinking to myself, 'It's not your business . . . why do you come around bragging about yourself and showing me down?' I feel I should not let him push me around with all his peculiar questions. He'd probably love to get me really angry and I get upset with myself thinking that I let him get me down.

"Deep inside me I know I'm not really enjoying my retirement. I think Carl senses that. I know that just by the way he looks at me, almost feeling sorry for me. However, I'm not going to give him the satisfaction of knowing that. I get very depressed every time I meet with Carl and I think I must stop seeing him. But when he comes I'm afraid he'll get hurt and insulted if I don't invite him in."

This internal dialogue reflects a sense of personal incompetence in managing provocations and regulation of anger arousal—a phenomenon quite commonly seen in many depressed elderly males. As Novaco (1977) notes, feelings of anger are influenced by the client's thoughts. A basic premise is that this anger is fomented, maintained, and influenced by the negative self-statements that are made in the provocation situations and subsequently lead to depression.

In this case analysis what Mr. T. perceives as a provocation, what he says to himself when provoked, and the contents of his self-statements contribute to the depressive reaction. Mr. T.'s negative self-statements include assumptions about Carl's design to put him down and the necessity for control or retaliation on his part.

MR. R: "I've just lost my wife and she's everything I had. My children won't talk about her and they change the subject whenever I mention her. I know they would like me to forget her and put her out of my mind but that's not fair to her. Makes me wonder whether they really ever cared for their mother.

"Now my children want me to come and live with them. I say to myself, 'No, sir, you won't get me under your control. No, sir . . . I'm not going to go to live with you.' It's true my children gave us a very good time when we visited them last year and no matter what happened they did come to their mother's funeral. But I know things have changed between us. It never will be the same between us and that depresses me."

This is an illustration of an internal dialogue in which rational and irrational belief statements compete against one another interfering with earlier beliefs of positive parent-child relationships. Mr. R. makes arbitrary inferences about his children's lack of feelings for their mother and exaggerates the extent of the problem between him and the children. There appear to be several cognitive errors in the subject's thinking, helping him to retain depressive thoughts. He clings to negative views of the children despite other information suggesting that his children have considerable concern for him. Common to each of the four clients is the notion that it is not the situations per se that provoke depression and engender anxiety and helplessness, but rather the subject's constructions and beliefs about these events.

Cognitive Training Phase

In the second phase of cognitive therapy clients are taught that forced mediation by means of an alternative set of thoughts and cognitions can deautomatize cognitions of dependency, self-criticism, and self-disparagement. In this phase clients are given relaxation and cognitive skills training, the latter in the form of cognitive restructuring (adapted from Kranzler, 1974; Meichenbaum, 1977) and self-instructional rehearsals with a view to helping clients substitute more positive images and positive rational beliefs for negative and irrational belief systems (Meichenbaum, 1974).

Let us return to a case presented earlier in order to illustrate the cognitive techniques of helping clients restructure self-statements and helping clients to view situations and persons more rationally. In Mr. R.'s case depression was, at least in part, a result of the subject's magnification of the fear that his children had lost interest in him and his wife. He harbored the irrational beliefs that his children did not care for him and wanted to control him. Therapy involved labeling the errors in his thinking and identifying the cognitive distortions and faulty beliefs which were maintaining the depression.

Initial sessions were devoted to examining concrete elements. "Let us look at the concrete good things your children have done for you. Let us examine the negative things that they have done. In the balance are there more good or bad things your children have done?" In the later sessions the focus was on the identification of maladaptive assumptions in the client's thinking. Time was spent in analyzing the validity of Mr. R.'s assumption that his children did not care for him and wanted to control him through such questions as Is it possible that your children won't talk about their mother because they think it will upset you? Is it possible they want you to go and live with them because they think you might be lonely? Is it possible that your children are so grieved by their mother's death that they can't talk about her? Is it possible that your children want you to comfort them? Is it possible your children want you to live with them so that they can cheer you up? In what kind of ways do you think your children would want to control you?

As this case illustrates, the therapist teaches the client to recognize the negative automatic thoughts that precede the emotions of anger, anxiety, or helplessness that in turn precede the depression (Meichenbaum & Turk, 1976). Automatic thoughts refer to ideation that interferes with the ability of the client to cope rationally with life experiences.

Application Phase

In the third phase, which is the application phase, clients are asked to imagine various depression-engendering situations and cognitively to rehearse coping with such situations by conjuring positive images and generating positive self-statements. Whereas before treatment, maladaptive thoughts and images would be harbingers or precipitators of depression, in therapy clients are reminded to engage in different internal dialogues, first by restructuring their cognitions of self-criticism, self-disparagement, and dependency and second by emitting more positive statements of self-reinforcement, independence, and self-efficacy. To illustrate these procedures, let us return to the cases discussed earlier in terms of internal dialogues.

Mrs. P. continually conjures up images of an emaciated body and sagging figure. She becomes depressed thinking that no clothes ever look good on her. Mrs. P. is taught imagery manipulation. She is instructed to visualize herself as standing upright and confident and looking smart in her new clothes. Mrs. P. is instructed to adopt the role of an external observer looking at her own body and making positive self-statements (I look nice. There's nothing the matter with my body. I am probably not as attractive as I was 10 years ago, but I'm pretty good for my age. Patricia says I look nice; Mrs. Z. from the church said I look smart. Now why would they lie to me. I must believe them.). Through these cognitive exercises Mrs. P. learns to control her negative imagery and to control her negative thoughts about herself and others.

Mr. T., who is threatened by Carl, is taught how to reconstrue Carl's provocations, to mitigate the sense of personal threat, and to instruct himself to attend to self-cognitions of competence (e.g., Carl has no influence over me. He is not my boss, he is not superior to me in skills or competence. I must not allow him to get me down. Any time Carl attempts to put me down, I must remind myself that I was much more competent than he when we worked together. In the last two years I earned many more bonuses than he. Just because I'm retired doesn't make me incompetent.).

In the preceding examples of negative self-statements and internal dialogue the focus is always on the clients' perceived threat to self-worth, their desire to be in control of the situation, and their cognitions of failure and helplessness, which arouse high levels of depression in these elderly. Provocation-related statements ("Why does he come to make a fool of me?" "He'd probably love to get me really angry." "I don't think she really cares for my opinions but she won't stop asking me what I think.") in combination with helplessness statements define the depression reactions.

In the examples cited, depression reactions consisted of two cognitive components, namely, irrational emotional arousal and negative cognitive activity (i.e., negative appraisals, attributions, self-statements, and imagery). A cognitive-behavioral treatment regimen was therefore suggested for all clients. All clients were typically taught to use relaxation skills to enable them to reduce arousal and acquire cognitive controls over their attentional processes, irrational thoughts, images, and feelings.

In a structured way, each client was taught to conduct a situational analysis of what triggered depression and to reflect on the set of positive cognitions and behavioral alternatives available. For example,

- Mrs. T., who got depressed on receiving lovely clothes from her daughter-in-law, realizes that she becomes depressed because of her constructions and beliefs that she will never look pretty and attractive again. The clothes trigger thoughts of how attractive she once was. The client visualizes herself in these lovely clothes but produces images of poor physical shape and emaciated body. She produces incompatible thoughts of wanting to be attractive again but feeling hopeless about doing so.

- Mrs. Y., who is invited for coffee by her lively young neighbor, produces incompatible thoughts and images of wanting to be interesting and intellectually bright but feeling hopeless and therefore withdrawing from an otherwise pleasant activity. In order to modify her negative cognitions, Mrs. Y. is instructed to remind herself that five years ago she too was an interesting hostess and the life of the party. "If I could be interesting then, surely I can be interesting now. The mere fact that I am older doesn't make me any less skilled. I have the choice of trying out my old skills or withdrawing and being depressed afterward."

Clients are taught to verbalize statements in the context of experimental roles specifically designed to promote self-confidence, self-efficacy, and outgoingness. The following examples illustrate the point (see Fry, 1984a, 1984b, 1984c for details).

- Cognitions of independence (e.g., My daughter-in-law wants to know my opinions so I should express my views. I should not worry about what she thinks of me. So what if I am old; I still have a right to my opinions.)

- Cognitions of self-efficacy (e.g., I must not dwell on things in which I have failed or things that I did not do appropriately. I must concentrate on the many things I accomplished. I can still do a lot if I only give myself a chance. It's stupid to miss a chance for doing something interesting and to get depressed after the opportunity has passed.)

- Cognitions of extroversion (e.g., I want others to take an interest in me, which means I must try to be cheerful, energetic, and pleasant in talking with others. The more I get together with other people and talk with them, the more I will learn to enjoy them and the more they will enjoy me.)

- Cognitions of rational thinking (e.g., I must not worry about how I can repay my daughter-in-law for her gifts. The best repayment is to tell her how I feel about the gifts and what they mean to me. The more I enjoy the gifts and let her know, the more she will enjoy giving them to me.)

Thus, overall, a cognitive-behavioral treatment module is aimed at changing subjects' self-perceptions and negative belief systems. The module is tailored to each client's need and incorporates a convincing rationale for improving mental outlook.

Following Ellis (1970), the cognitive-behavioral treatment program involves identifying the client's self-defeating and irrational thoughts and gradually replacing them with a more adaptive belief system that alleviates the depression. In this way clients begin to control the negative emotional consequences of their negative cognitions. A woman who reports feeling depressed when her husband is late for an anniversary dinner is taught how to express disappointment or even annoyance rather than hopelessness or worthlessness. A man who reports depression after retirement is taught how to express feelings of boredom rather than uselessness and obsolescence; rather than tell himself he is worthless, he substitutes thoughts of more pleasant activity and useful involvement. In a cognitive approach clients remind themselves that they have positive abilities and creative skills.

Current Status of Cognitive-Behavioral Treatment of the Elderly

Cognitive therapy has a number of features that make it a particularly attractive approach for working with the aged who are victims of ageism. Gerontologists have found that the aged in Western societies are involved in a chronic conflict between stereotypes of the elderly as weak and incompetent and their own concepts of themselves as active and competent (Thomae, 1970). Typically the aged resolve this conflict by adopting more negative concepts of themselves or by becoming even more rigid and stereotypic in their expectations of others. Given this situation, cognitive therapy can play an important part in helping the elderly to overcome their negative and depressive attitudes toward their own aging and the excessively restrictive behavioral standards they impose on themselves in how they should act or behave. Elderly cohorts may believe that they are too old to have sex, too old to enjoy themselves, too old to adjust to new experiences, or too old to do anything productive after retirement. Cognitive therapy can be helpful in irrational beliefs about aging and ageism.

Another area in which cognitive therapy can be helpful to the elderly is the domain of physical health problems. The importance of psychological factors has been acknowledged in the successful management of a wide range of physical disorders as contributing to depression. The therapist can use cognitive approaches to help in the management of physical problems (e.g., problems with ambulation, pressure sores, pain and incontinence) by teaching the patient to recognize and modify dysfunctional ruminations, exaggerations, and catastrophic thoughts about the physical ailment. Many elderly have fixed delusional beliefs that their health is irreparably impaired and no medication can help. Cognitive therapy can help the client with the psychological aspects of the ailment by convincing clients of the importance of carrying out prescribed medical recommendations on dietary management, medication, and exercise programs. The emphasis is on encouraging the patient to let go of dysfunctional beliefs about health.

In examining the current status of cognitive-behavioral interventions with the elderly, a number of issues need to be addressed for future therapy work using cognitive approaches.

- Therapists must continue to experiment with a variety of cognitive-behavioral techniques with which they feel comfortable and which have an increasing probability of meeting the individual needs of the elderly client. Techniques may have to be modified in order to accommodate the social-cultural expectations of the family and community.

- In the cognitive-behavioral approach a number of specific strategies such as reinforcement and direct one-to-one contact with the therapist have the effect of improving morale even before intervention begins. Cognitive-behavioral intervention must often be implemented in combination with other supportive and interpersonal forms of therapy, and there is a considerable reliance on a collaborative therapist-client relationship and on other familiar techniques such as reassurance, clarification of internal emotional states, improvement of communication, and reality testing of perceptions and performance.

• Recent studies (e.g., Dessonville, Gallagher, Thompson, Finnell, & Lewinsohn, 1982; Fry, 1984a; Steuer & Hammen, 1983) have noted that the cognitive components of the intervention may be useful only to those elderly clients who are not cognitively impaired and do not have serious emotional disturbance. Clinical experience suggests that elderly clients with impaired reality testing, reasoning abilities, or memory functions (e.g., organic brain syndromes) or those with functional disorders and borderline personality structures will not respond to this treatment. Most of the studies using cognitive approaches with the elderly have been conducted on subclinical samples. Overall, the positive results obtained in initial studies of cognitive-behavioral interventions with elderly clients may serve as preliminary analogue findings whose application to more severely depressed and disturbed samples require further research (Fry, 1982).

• The cognitive-behavioral treatment techniques, while giving tacit acknowledgment to the significance of a variety of psychological problems in the elderly, have been extremely useful with elderly clients having characteristics of unassertiveness, helplessness, and hopelessness. Therefore, one of the problems inherent in cognitive-behavioral interventions with depressed elders is a ceiling effect. No matter how efficacious a procedure or coping strategy may be, at some point or in some situation the hopelessness may become unbearable for a subject. Coping self-statements that work successfully for an elderly person living with the family may be quite unsuccessful in another situation when the client is alone or even in the same situation at a different time when a key environmental support is missing. In short the amount and quality of perceived hopelessness, dependency, and sad effect in any elderly individual are multidetermined by a variety of psychosocial factors as well as the cognitive and sensory input. Thus a combination of cognitive-behavioral and other supportive therapeutic modalities is recommended in intervention programs for depression. Some of these strategies may be used to modify the negative and depressive environments in which the elderly live.

In conclusion it is suggested that many elderly are known to lack in environmental support and reinforcements. A therapy orientation based on behavioral principles of support, encouragement, and reinforcement is bound to be advantageous for the elderly.

Cognitive-behavioral therapy has several possible advantages over more traditional interventions as a treatment for depression in the elderly. It is time limited, and it has a problem-solving orientation with emphasis on present problems and on coping skills (Steuer, 1982). The technique may be more acceptable to geriatric clients whose key concern is with problems of coping and surviving than treatments aimed at insight or personality reconstruction. The behavioral components of this treatment have as their key ingredients reinforcement, increased activity, pleasurable experiences, and increased interpersonal effectiveness. These are valid techniques for affecting social isolation, loneliness, and lack of social response, which commonly characterize depression in the elderly. The cognitive components impact directly on the irrational and dysfunctional beliefs that many elderly tend to develop and indirectly on the loss of self-esteem and morale that is inextricably linked with depression. Behavioral therapies reveal that "change in environmental conditions can change gerontological behaviors and thereby undermine the common opinion that old age with its detrimental behaviors is only due to biological deterioration" (Baltes & Lascomb, 1975, p. 6). This fact underlies the special importance of employing a combination of cognitive-behavioral modalities and integrated therapies in intervention programs for depression.

Frequently caregivers of the elderly are resistant to the use of behavioral therapy on moral or ethical grounds, feeling it is inappropriate to brainwash or control the behaviors of clients who are just as helpless as young children. Although Strupp (1973) has reassuringly pointed out that all psychotherapies involve an element of control, concerns about the ethics of cognitive-behavioral treatment should be foremost in the mind of each therapist for each elderly client seen. Behavioral and cognitive approaches such as those presented in this chapter have immense potentials for manipulation of the client's behaviors and thoughts. The history of psychotherapy with the elderly shows numerous examples of therapists imposing their personal values and preferences on the clients. An elderly person's life style may have many features that the family and therapist find old-fashioned or inappropriate, but these belief systems or behaviors should be made a part of the treatment regimen only when related to the elderly client's problems in functioning. The aged as a group are likely to have values about family life, spousal intimacy, interpersonal relations, and finances that are quite different from those of a younger therapist. These values, although somewhat outmoded, are not necessarily inappropriate and should not be criticized or modified through behavioral or cognitive therapy unless they present problems of interpersonal disturbance for the elderly. For these reasons it is critical for the therapist to develop treatment plans that are reflective of the goals and values of the client.

Those therapists or caregivers who work with severely depressed elderly or chronically ill elderly are frequently the most hesitant to apply cognitive-behavioral treatments. Their concern may be realistic. The increased vulnerability of these elderly clients engendered by enforced activities, drugs and medication contributes to the therapist's misgivings about the application of behavioral therapies. However, behavioral therapies that attempt to restructure the elderly clients' actions and emotions by using techniques of positive reinforcement, positive attention and social-instrumental support, as a rule, are more effective in relieving the elderly client's psychological distress (Baltes & Lascomb, 1975) than are other therapies most of which also involve elements of control by the therapist. This fact underlies the importance of using specific behavioral procedures involving positive reinforcement as opposed to punishment, aversion therapy, or time-out procedures.

CONCLUDING REMARKS

This chapter has introduced a number of rationales, sets of strategies, and tactics for the treatment of depressed elderly. An overview of the basic principles and elements of a supportive and cognitive-behavioral framework for psychotherapy with the elderly has been provided. The aim has been to present each approach in a manner that facilitates its use by therapists of various persuasions working with depressed elderly.

The relationship between depression and supportive and reinforcing interactions is central to all three approaches outlined. Therefore specific tactics aimed at enhancing the quality and quantity of the elderly person's social, emotional, and cognitive interactions have been delineated. Different response modalities of the client—the cognitive/affective modality, behavioral response modality, and the somatic response modality—need to be monitored and evaluated by content areas (see McLean's [1976] suggested breakdown; Table 8–1). The main virtue of this approach is that it provides a structured setting in which a few clear-cut and functional goals for alleviation of depression can be pinpointed and defined as targets for intervention. For example, alleviating the elderly client's sense of helplessness, hopelessness, and dependency through supportive or cognitive-behavioral techniques may be a reasonable therapeutic goal. Generally the focus has been on improving daily behaviors and day-to-day functioning rather than on broad life styles (Table 8–1). This emphasis is recommended as appropriate for short-term intervention procedures that have as their goal the relief of situationally determined anxiety and depression.

Practitioners must note that psychotherapy of whatever description has not proven notably successful in treating severe forms of depression in the elderly. Clinical evidence suggests that a fusion of supportive and cognitive-behavioral approaches promises to alleviate the current unhappiness of many elderly clients and is therefore deserving of serious attention.

The relatively confused results of many recent attempts to provide supportive and cognitive behaviorally oriented therapy to the elderly are instructive in that they suggest two conclusions: first, that the elderly have limited experience with psychotherapy and, second, that no one therapeutic approach (supportive, cognitive, behavioral, or psychodynamic) holds the ultimate answers to the alleviation of their depression. There are effective elements in all approaches, and most therapeutic approaches recommended for use with the elderly are not as divergent as presumed. This chapter has attempted to show how the various approaches are similar and integrated in terms of conceptualization, rationale for treatment, and actual methods.

Because of this situation, which some would regard as a certain maturing of geriatric therapy, the trend to combine supportive and cognitive-behavioral methods allows the practitioner to be both an advocate of the elderly and a therapist. The chapter has addressed several practical concerns. The first of these is that depression in the elderly is a rather complex conceptual phenomenon, a function of many emergent events requiring multimodal attention. Many adaptations and simplifications of procedures will be necessary. The veracity of daily monitoring of behaviors, although typically not a problem, is of occasional concern to elderly clients.

Perhaps the most formidable obstacle for clinicians and therapists centers around the nature of the collaboration between the elderly client and therapist. It is vital for therapists to convey warmth and concern for the client through both verbal and nonverbal behaviors and to be careful that they do not seem to be disapproving or cynical of the client's needs, values, and perspectives. It is also vital for therapists to display a professional manner and to convey a relaxed confidence about their willingness and ability to help the depressed elderly.

We do not know how older adults differ from younger persons with respect to therapy demands to learn new social skills of assertion and self-confidence, and discrimination with respect to their application. Although the evidence is still somewhat unclear, it is thought that older persons may find new social skills and discriminations somewhat harder to learn because of sensory and neurological changes associated with increased age. Motivation to succeed in therapy, as related to age, is an unexplored area. This is especially true of the complex motivations, as compared with the basic needs of the elderly for shelter and safety.

Although the evidence is unclear, there is some suggestion (Lieberman & Gourash, 1979) that older persons have a great desire to relieve psychological distress, and are therefore generally quite cooperative in therapy.

Finally, the therapeutic approaches outlined are probably most suitable for unipolar nonpsychotic depressives, and other treatments (e.g., lithium and other medication) should be considered for other depressive disorders resulting from organic brain disease or psychosis. It must remain an open question whether and to what extent pharmacological treatment is a useful adjunct to psychotherapy. All these approaches are geared to limited goals. In the case of depression any technique—pharmacological or psychological—that promises to alleviate the client's unhappiness and suffering deserves serious attention (Strupp, Sandel, Waterhouse, Malley, & Anderson, 1982). Through the renewed interest in the biologic and genetic bases of depression, progress has been made in developing pharmacological and somatic treatments especially for use with depressed elderly. Thus, it is likely that the present trend toward greater eclecticism among psychotherapists will also accept the amalgamation of pharmacological and psychological treatments for depression. Most practitioners must accept the position that psychoactive medication can play a major part in the treatment of depression in late life and that psychotherapy is an important adjunct to pharmacology.

SUMMARY

This chapter has introduced the reader to supportive and cognitive-behavioral approaches to psychotherapy for depression in the elderly. There has been limited clinical work using the cognitive-behavioral modality with older clients whose basic problem is one of depression. However, whatever preliminary work has been done is encouraging in its findings. The models of psychotherapy for depression have focused on elements of supportive therapy and the use of social, behavioral, and cognitive techniques. Behavioral and cognitive methods are based on the premise that in the absence of physiological disturbances, depression is the result of specific habits or thoughts of the client and depressive reactions are precipitated by particular environmental events. The chapter presents an overview of behavioral methods that can be used to increase the occurrence of desirable behaviors and strengthen self-efficacy through relevant social skills. Cognitive methods are advocated to modify irrational thoughts and distorted cognitions that precipitate depressive emotions.

The behavior therapist must weigh a variety of ethical considerations in the application of treatment procedures, especially to the depressed and chronically ill older clients. The principles of supportive therapy, however, operate in most settings and therapists and caregivers of the elderly should have few misgivings about the application of supportive interpersonal treatment procedures. Older people have a great desire to relieve psychological stress, and respond favorably to most treatment procedures using interpersonally-oriented supportive techniques.

The aim has been to present each approach in a manner that facilitates its use by therapists of varied persuasions who are reasonably familiar with the cognitive-behavioral formulations and other supportive-psychodynamic constructs. A number of case histories and description of techniques have been presented in order to illustrate the modifications in concepts and techniques that are necessary in psychotherapy with the elderly. There are effective elements in all these approaches and no one therapeutic approach holds the ultimate answers. The emphasis is on short-term treatment and the use of supportive procedures that have as their goal the relief of situationally determined depression through active participation of the client.

REFERENCES

Alpaugh, P., & Hickey-Haney, M. (1978). *Counseling older adults: A training manual for beginning counselors and paraprofessionals*. Los Angeles: Andrus Gerontology Center, Southern California University.

Baltes, M.M., & Lascomb, S.L. (1975). Creating a healthy institutional environment for the elderly via behavior management: The nurse as a change agent. *International Journal of Nursing Studies, 12,* 5–12.

Bandura, A. (1977). Self-efficacy: Toward a unifying theory of behavioral change. *Psychological Review, 84,* 191–215.

Beck, A.T. (1967). *The diagnosis and management of depression*. Philadelphia: University of Pennsylvania Press.

Beck, A.T. (1974). The development of depression: A cognitive model. In R.J. Friedman & M.M. Katz (Eds.), *Psychology of depression: Contemporary theory and research* (pp. 3–27). Washington: Winston-Wiley.

Beck, A.T., Rush, A.J., Shaw, B.F., & Emery, G. (1979). *Cognitive therapy of depression*. New York: Guilford Press.

Becker, F., & Zarit, S.H. (1978). Training older adults as peer counselors. *Educational Gerontology, 3,* 241–250.

Bellak, L. (1976). Crisis intervention in geriatric psychiatry. In L. Bellak & T.B. Karasu (Eds.), *Geriatric psychiatry* (pp. 175–189). New York: Grune & Stratton.

Bothwell, S., & Weissman, M. (1977). Social impairment four years after an acute depressive episode. *American Journal of Orthopsychiatry, 47,* 231–237.

Botwinick, J. (1978). *Aging and behavior* (2nd ed.). New York: Springer.

Brown, G.W., & Harris, T. (1978). *Social origins of depression*. New York: Free Press.

Butler, R.N. (1977). Toward a psychiatry of the life cycle: Implications of socio-psychologic studies of the aging process for the psychotherapeutic situation. In S.H. Zarit (Ed.), *Readings in aging and death: Contemporary perspectives* (pp. 213–224). New York: Harper & Row.

Cath, S. (1966). Beyond depression: The depleted state. A study in ego psychology in the aged. *Canadian Psychiatric Association Journal, 11* (special suppl.) S329–S339.

Cautela, J.P., & Mansfield, L. (1977). A behavioral approach to geriatrics. In W.P. Gentry (Ed.), *Geropsychology* (pp. 21–42). Cambridge, MA: Ballinger Publishing Co.

Cohen, E.S. (1976). Comment: Editor's note. *Gerontologist, 16,* 270–275.

Dessonville, C., Gallagher, D., Thompson, L., Finnell, K., & Lewinsohn, P.M. (1982). Relation of age and health status to depressive symptoms in normal and depressed older adults. *Essence, 5,* 90–117.

Eisdorfer, C., & Cohen, D. (1978). The cognitively impaired elderly: Differential diagnosis. In M. Storandt, I.C. Siegler, & M.F. Elias (Eds.), *The clinical psychology of aging* (pp. 7–42). New York: Plenum Press.

Eisdorfer, C., & Stotsky, B.A. (1977). Intervention, treatment and rehabilitation of psychiatric disorders. In J.E. Birren & K.W. Schaie (Eds.), *The handbook of the psychology of aging* (pp. 724–748). New York: Van Nostrand Reinhold Co.

Ellis, A. (1970). *The essence of rational psychotherapy: A comprehensive approach to treatment*. New York: Institute for Rational Living.

Fedoravicius, A.S. (1977). *When relaxation treatment fails. . . .* Paper presented at the meetings of the American Psychological Association, San Francisco.

Feldman, M.G., & DiScipio, W.J. (1972). Integrating physical therapy with behavior therapy. *Physical Therapy, 52,* 1283–1285.

Ferster, C.B. (1966). Animal behavior and mental illness. *Psychological Record, 16,* 345–356.

Ferster, C.B. (1973). A functional analysis of depression. *American Psychologist, 28,* 857–870.

Frank, J.D. (1974). Psychotherapy: The restoration of morale. *American Journal of Psychiatry, 131,* 271–274.

Freud, S. (1959). Mourning and melancholia. In *Collected Papers* Vol. 4 (pp. 152–170). London: Hogarth Press.

Fry, P.S. (1982). *Social, affective and cognitive mediators of depression in the elderly*. Progress report submitted to Department of National Health and Welfare, Canada. Unpublished report.

Fry, P.S. (1983). Structured and unstructured reminiscence training and depression among the elderly. *Clinical Gerontologist, 1,* 15–37.

Fry, P.S. (1983–86). *Psychosocial mediators of depression in the elderly.* Social Sciences and Humanities Research Council of Canada, Research Grant (in progress).

Fry., P.S. (1984a). Cognitive training and cognitive variables in the treatment of depression in the elderly. *Clinical Gerontologist, 3,* 25–45.

Fry, P.S. (1984b). Development of a geriatric scale of hopelessness: Implications for counseling and intervention with the depressed elderly. *Journal of Counseling Psychology, 31,* 322–331.

Fry, P.S. (1984c). Thematic contents of depressive cognitions in the elderly. In R. Schwarzer (Ed.), *The self in anxiety, stress and depression* (pp. 313–327). Amsterdam: North Holland Publishers.

Fry, P.S., & Grover, S.C. (1982). Cognitive appraisals of life stress and depression in the elderly: A cross-cultural comparison of Asians and Caucasians. *International Journal of Psychology, 17,* 437–454.

Fuchs, C.Z., & Rehm, L.P. (1977). A self-control behavior therapy program for depression. *Journal of Consulting and Clinical Psychology, 45,* 206–215.

Gallagher, D., & Thompson, L.W. (1981). *Depression in the elderly: A behavioral treatment manual.* Los Angeles: University of Southern California Press.

Gallagher, D., & Thompson, L.W. (1982). Treatment of major depressive disorders in older adult outpatients with brief psychotherapies. *Psychotherapy: Theory, Research and Practice, 19,* 482–490.

Gallagher, D., & Thompson, L.W. (1983). Cognitive therapy for depression in the elderly. In L.D. Breslau & M.R. Haug (Eds.), *Depression in the elderly: Causes, care and consequences* (pp. 168–192). New York: Springer.

Goldfarb, A.T. (1956). The rationale for psychotherapy with older persons. *American Journal of Medical Science, 232,* 181–185.

Gutmann, D. (1980). Psychoanalysis and aging: A developmental view. In S.I. Greenspan & G.H. Pollack (Eds.), *The course of life: Psychoanalytic contributions toward understanding personality development, Vol. 3: Adulthood and the aging process.* Washington: U.S. Government Printing Office.

Hammen, C., & Cohen, R. (1980). *Cognitive-behavioral therapy for depression in the elderly.* Paper presented at the Western Psychological Association Annual Meeting, Hawaii.

Herr, J.J., & Weakland, J.H. (1979). *Counseling elders and their families.* New York: Springer.

Jarvik, L., Mintz, J., Steuer, J., Gerner, R., Aldrich, J., Hammen, C., Linde, S., McCarley, T., Motoike, P., & Rosen, R. (1983). Comparison of tricyclic antidepressants and group psychotherapies in geriatric depressed patients: An interim analysis. In P.J. Clayton & J.E. Barrett (Eds.), *Treatment of depression: Old controversies and new approaches* (pp. 299–308). New York: Raven Press.

Kahn, R.L., & Fink, M. (1958). Changes in language during electroshock therapy. In P.H. Hoch & J. Zubin (Eds.), *Psychopathology of communication* (pp. 126–139). New York: Grune & Stratton.

Kahn, R.L., Zarit, S.H., Hilbert, N.M., & Niederehe, G. (1975). Memory complaint and impairment in the aged. *Archives of General Psychiatry, 32,* 1569–1573.

Karpf, R.J. (1980). Modalities of psychotherapy with the elderly. *Journal of American Geriatrics Society, 28,* 367–371.

Karpf, R.J. (1981). Individual psychotherapy with the elderly. In A.M. Horton (Ed.), *Mental health interventions for aging* (pp. 21–49). New York: Praeger Scientific-A, J.F. Bergin Publishers.

Kastenbaum, R. (1978). Personality theory, therapeutic approaches and the elderly client. In M. Storandt, I.C. Siegler, & M.F. Elias (Eds.), *The clinical psychology of aging* (pp. 199–224). New Pork: Plenum Press.

Kessler, M., & Albee, G.W. (1975). Primary prevention. *Annual Review of Psychology, 26,* 557–592.

Klerman, G.L., Rounsaville, B.J., Chevron, E.S., Neu, C., & Weissman, M.M. (1979). *Manual for short-term interpersonal psychotherapy (IPT) of depression.* Unpublished manuscript.

Kovacs, M., Rush, A.J., Beck, A.T., & Hollon, S.D. (1981). Depressed outpatients treated with cognitive therapy or pharmacotherapy: A one-year follow-up. *Archives of General Psychiatry, 38,* 33–39.

Kranzler, G. (1974). *You can change how you feel: A rational-emotive approach.* Eugene, OR: RETC Press.

Lewinsohn, P.M. (1974). A behavioral approach to depression. In R.J. Friedman & M.M. Katz (Eds.), *Psychology of depression: Contemporary theory and research* (pp. 157–179). Washington: Winston–Wiley.

Lewinsohn, P.M. (1976). Activity schedules in the treatment of depressed individuals. In J.D. Krumboltz & C.E. Thoresen (Eds.), *Counseling methods* (pp. 74–83). New York: Holt, Rinehart & Winston.

Lewinsohn, P.M., Biglan, A., & Zeiss, A.M. (1976). Behavioral treatment of depression. In P.O. Davidson (Ed.), *The behavioral management of anxiety, depression and pain* (pp. 91–146). New York: Brunner/Mazel.

Lewinsohn, P.M., Munoz, R.F., Youngren, M.A., & Zeiss, A.M. (1978). *Control your depression*. Englewood Cliffs, NJ: Prentice-Hall, Inc.

Lewinsohn, P.M., Weinstein, M.S., & Alper, T. (1970). A behaviorally oriented approach to the group treatment of depressed persons: A methodological contribution. *Journal of Clinical Psychology, 26,* 525–532.

Lewinsohn, P.M., Youngren, M.A., & Grosscup, S.J. (1979). Reinforcement and depression. In R.A. Depue (Ed.), *The psychobiology of the depressive disorders* (pp. 291–361). New York: Academic Press.

Libet, J., & Lewinsohn, P.M. (1973). The concept of social skills with special references to the behavior of depressed persons. *Journal of Consulting and Clinical Psychology, 40,* 304–312.

Lieberman, M.A. & Gourash, N. (1979). Evaluating the effects of change groups on the elderly. *International Journal of Group Psychotherapy, 29,* 283–304.

McLean, P. (1974). Evaluating community-based psychiatric services. In P.O. Davidson, F.W. Chark, & L.A. Hamerlynck (Eds.), *Evaluation of behavioral programs*. Champaign, IL: Research Press.

McLean, P. (1976). Therapeutic decision-making in the behavioral treatment of depression. In P.O. Davidson (Ed.), *The behavioral management of anxiety, depression and pain* (pp. 54–90). New York: Brunner/Mazel.

McLean, P. (1982). Behavioral therapy: Theory and research. In A.J. Rush (Ed.), *Short-term psychotherapies for depression* (pp. 19–49). New York: Guilford Press.

McLean, P., Ogston, K., & Grauer, L. (1973). A behavioral approach to the treatment of depression. *Journal of Behavior Therapy and Experimental Psychiatry, 4,* 323–330.

Meichenbaum, D. (1977). *Cognitive-behavior modification*. New York: Plenum Press.

Meichenbaum, D., & Turk, D. (1976). The cognitive-behavioral management of anxiety, anger, and pain. In P.O. Davidson (Ed.), *The behavioral management of anxiety, depression and pain* (pp. 1–34). New York: Brunner/Mazel.

Novaco, R.W. (1977). Stress inoculation: A cognitive therapy for anger and its application to a case of depression. *Journal of Consulting and Clinical Psychology, 45,* 600–608.

Paykel, E.S., Myers, J.K., Dienelt, M.W., Klerman, G.L., Lindenthal, J.J., & Pepper, M.P. (1969). Life events and depression: A controlled study. *Archives of General Psychiatry, 21,* 753–760.

Pfeiffer, E., & Busse, E.W. (1973). Mental disorders in later life—affective disorders: Paranoid, neurotic and situational reactions. In E.W. Busse & E. Pfeiffer (Eds.), *Mental illness in later life* (pp. 107–144). Washington: American Psychiatric Association.

Rechtschaffen, A. (1959). Psychotherapy with geriatric patients: A review of the literature. *Journal of Gerontology, 14,* 73–84.

Riedel, R.G. (1980). Behavior therapies. In C. Eisdorfer (Ed.), *Annual review of gerontology and geriatrics* (Vol. 2, pp. 160–195). New York: Springer.

Rogers, C.R. (1951). *Client-centered therapy*. Boston: Houghton Mifflin.

Rounsaville, B.J., & Chevron, E.S. (1982). Interpersonal psychotherapy: Clinical applications. In A.J. Rush (Ed.), *Short-term psychotherapies for depression* (pp. 107–142). New York: Guilford Press.

Seligman, M.E.P. (1973, June). Fall into helplessness. *Psychology Today*, pp. 43–48.

Seligman, M.E.P. (1975). *Helplessness: On depression, development, and death*. San Francisco: W.H. Freeman & Co.

Shaw, B.F. (1977). Comparison of cognitive therapy and behavior therapy in the treatment of depression. *Journal of Consulting and Clinical Psychology, 45,* 543–551.

Silverstone, B.M. (1976). Beyond the one-to-one treatment relationship. In L. Bellak & T.B. Karasu (Eds.), *Geriatric psychiatry* (pp. 207–224). New York: Grune & Stratton.

Small, L. (1979). *The briefer psychotherapies*. New York: Brunner/Mazel.

Steuer, J.L. (1982). Psychotherapy for depressed elders. In D.G. Blazer, *Depression in late life* (pp. 195–220). St. Louis: C.V. Mosby Co.

Steuer, J.L., & Hammen, C. (1983). Cognitive-behavioral group therapy for the depressed elderly: Issues and adaptations. *Cognitive Therapy and Research, 7,* 285–296.

Strupp, H.H. (1973). On the basic ingredients of psychotherapy. *Journal of Consulting and Clinical Psychology, 41,* 1–8.

Strupp, H.H., Sandell, J.A., Waterhouse, G.J., Malley, S.S., & Anderson, J.L. (1982). Psychodynamic therapy: Theory and research. In A.J. Rush (Ed.), *Short-term psychotherapies for depression* (pp. 215–248). New York: Guilford Press.

Stuart, R.B. (1967). Casework treatment of depression viewed as an interpersonal disturbance. *Social Work, 12,* 27–36.

Thomae, H. (1970). Cognitive theory of personality and theory of aging. *Human Development, 13,* 1–10.

Thomae, H. (1980). Personality and adjustment to aging. In J.E. Birren & R.B. Sloane (Eds.), *Handbook of mental health and aging* (pp. 285–309). Englewood Cliffs, NJ: Prentice-Hall, Inc.

Vaughn, C.E., & Leff, J.R. (1977). The influence of family and social factors on the course of psychiatric illness. *British Journal of Psychiatry, 129,* 125–137.

Verwoerdt, A. (1976). *Clinical geropsychiatry.* Baltimore: Williams & Wilkins.

Wolpe, J. (1958). *Psychotherapy by reciprocal inhibition.* Stanford, CA: Stanford University Press.

Young, J.E., & Beck, A.T. (1982). Cognitive therapy: Clinical applications. In A.J. Rush (Ed.), *Short-term psychotherapies for depression: Behavioral, interpersonal, cognitive and psychodynamic approaches* (pp. 182–214). New York: Guilford Press.

Zarit, S.H. (1980). *Aging and mental disorders: Psychological approaches to asessment and treatment.* New York: Free Press.

Zeiss, A.M., Lewinsohn, P.M., & Munoz, R.F. (1979). Non-specific improvement effects in depression using interpersonal, cognitive, and pleasant events' focused treatments. *Journal of Consulting and Clinical Psychology, 47,* 427–439.

Chapter 9

Grief, Death, and Dying in the Aged: Assessment and Therapeutic Considerations

While several forms of social and emotional stress may contribute to depressive reactions and disorders in the elderly, bereavement, grief, and mourning constitute by far the most pervasive stress that the elders have to endure. Each day almost 4,000 Americans celebrate their 65th birthday and about 3,000 persons aged 65 or over die. Nearly half of these deaths are linked to prolonged grief, chronic conditions of heart disease, and cerebrovascular disease. There is documented evidence that the presence of physical illness, reduction in cognitive capacity, and prolonged grief resulting from the death of spouse or peers have a profound effect on the elderly's adaptation to late life (Brotman, 1973). Grief also serves in varying degrees to underline increasing feelings of helplessness, anhedonia, dependency, and depression.

Clinical studies and observations suggest that the ability to tolerate grief and bereavement is considerably impaired as a function of physical decline. The decline of the extended family structure and the decrease in social contact aggravates the sense of isolation and grief. Barriers to the therapeutic working through of the grieving process may often alter the natural course of grief and bereavement to an extent that it interferes permanently with the elderly's communications and coping capacities. Insensitive rejection of the elderly's grief and sadness may cause other functional disorders and abnormal behavioral tendencies.

The evaluation of what coping mechanisms are being used by the elderly and an assessment of the psychodynamics of each person's grief by the practitioner are important to an understanding of the long-term effects of the bereavement process and the appropriateness of psychosocial interventions at the time of stress. The purpose of this chapter, therefore, is first to examine the psychodynamics of grief and to discuss implications and applications of the psychosocial processes for practitioners and clinicians working with the elderly. The second purpose is to evaluate the elderly's fears and anxieties concerning death and dying and to discuss diagnostic and assessment procedures and therapeutic approaches commonly used in working with dying elderly clients. The role of primary caregivers with special reference to the function of psychotherapists, families, physicians, nurses, social workers, and clergy is of significance in the management of the dying elderly.

NORMAL AND ABNORMAL GRIEF

In order to understand the nature of the grieving process and its normal and abnormal features, some clinicians have examined its three separate components: (1) bereavement,

(2) grief, and (3) mourning. Kastenbaum and Costa (1977) describe *bereavement* as referring to survivorship status, *grief* as being the survivor's state of distress and response to loss, and *mourning* as being the culturally accepted behaviors that express the survivor's responses to death.

A number of authors (e.g., Jacobs & Douglas, 1979; Wahl, 1979) have described abnormal grief reactions separate from normal grief with normal grief defined as a "self-limited process requiring no medical attention" (Engel, 1961, p. 2). In the case of the elderly, however, there is a greater risk of abnormal grief because of the prolonged period the elders may need in accepting the loss, readjusting to the environmental changes that may occur from the loss, and forming new relationships after surviving the loss (Lindemann, 1944). These are often difficult tasks for older people due to a common reduction in social activity levels. Other researchers (e.g., Bornstein, Clayton, Halikas, Maurice, & Robins, 1973) caution against viewing severe depression in the elderly as abnormal even if it persists for a time. The grieving process in the case of the elderly may be characterized not only by typical grief symptoms (e.g., agitation and crying) but very often by disease symptoms that may produce their own depressive effects.

Skelskie (1975) has examined age differences in the mourning process, and his findings indicate that mourning in aged persons is different from typical adult mourning. Since grief is only one of the many stresses experienced by old people, it is more diffuse and obscured than in younger age groups. The danger is that in older people grief reactions may often be misdiagnosed as symptoms of organic brain syndrome (Burnside, 1969) because the grieving client's clinical picture is characteristic of the cognitive and psychomotor retardation often noted in organic impairment.

DSM III Criteria for Assessing Grief

The elderly person may concentrate on particular themes of grief and may spend considerable time discussing the many losses experienced in late life. According to Clayton (1979) the practitioner needs to assess, both socially and psychologically, whether the themes of grief are normal or pathological in terms of reality distortion, intensity, duration, and frequency and whether the client is at risk for becoming severely depressed. According to DSM III (1980) criteria bereavement is considered uncomplicated unless there is a premorbid preoccupation with worthlessness and prolonged and marked functional impairment and psychomotor retardation. In uncomplicated bereavement, guilt is present but is chiefly about things done or not done at the time of the death. Depressed mood is regarded as normal, but most of the acute reactions about the death rarely occur after the first two or three months of the death.

There will be many individual variations in the grief responses. Therefore, the practitioner needs to evaluate at the individual level the short-term and long-term effects of grief on the elderly person's physical and psychosocial functioning. Major effects of grief reactions, generally observed in the elderly, are summarized in Table 9–1 with suggestions for management of clinically complicated effects.

Grief and Physical Health Effects

Bartrop (1977), who examined the relationship between bereavement and physical illness, notes that most often bereavement causes catastrophic stress for the older person, and often this stress leads to maladaptive body changes in the elderly (Cox & Ford, 1964).

Table 9–1 Effects of Grief Reactions of the Elderly and Their Management

Area Affected	Effects of Grief Reactions	Management of Complicated Grief Reactions
Physical health effects	Disturbances in sleep Lack of strength and physical fatigue Loss of appetite Predisposition to physical symptoms such as dizziness, bodily pain, palpitation, and breathing difficulties	Provide a balanced psychological regimen of diet, activity, and relaxation. Hospitalize elderly with severe and complex grief reactions involving intense depression, severe withdrawal and loss of appetite; electroconvulsive therapy may be indicated for complicated grief reactions.
Psychosocial and emotional effects	Depression, agitation, and lack of concentration Anhedonia Tendency for self-neglect, self-punitiveness, and hostility or punitiveness toward others instrumental in the grieving Expressions of guilt, anger, and self-deprecation Suicidal ideations and psychomotor retardation Intense cognitive preoccupation with person who died	Psychotropic medication for mild depression, agitation, and sleep disturbance. Promote and foster a number of supportive relationships with confidants, friends, and family. Encourage bereaved person to explore feelings of loss and to communicate emotions of helplessness, guilt, self-blame, etc. In cases of bereaved persons denying grief, encourage such persons to mourn, cry, or show distress.
Life-style changes	Increased helplessness and hopelessness in daily functioning Increased isolation Reduced physical activity and inertia Decreased capacity for self-care Decreased ability for carrying out routine functions	Provide assistance in basic self-care tasks and tangible problems of daily living. Encourage social interaction and involvement in pleasant activity. Provide substantial reinforcement and encouragement for reality orientation.

Note: The greater the number of areas affected with respect to physical and emotional health and life-style changes, the more complicated will be the grief reactions.

In interpreting the origins of these bodily changes, Blazer (1982) emphasizes the notion that "the stress of loss and the psychologic responses to this stress are transduced into physical changes that predispose to a variety of illness" (Blazer, 1982, p. 38), often culminating in cardiovascular disease or the broken heart syndrome, a term coined by Parkes (1970). In the elderly, somatic grief reactions including disturbances in sleep, lack of strength, and sometimes physical exhaustion, and loss of appetite may often predispose elderly individuals to serious physical illness. Cognitive distortions and cognitive reactions may give rise to inactivity, difficulty in concentration, and loss of interest in previously preferred activities (Table 9–1). The elderly may need a prolonged phase of restitution and recovery to accept the loss and to return to a state of well-being and health. As noted by Clayton

(1979) and Engel (1961), the expected return to physical well-being and health may be indefinitely impaired for some older individuals.

Grief and Psychosocial Effects

There are variations in the impact and general effects of grief depending on the developmental status of the elderly client and the extent to which the loss of a loved one produces changes (both short- and long-term) in the life style of the client.

Developmental Effects. Psychosocial effects of grief will vary according to the developmental phase of the grief and whether the individual is at the stage of anticipatory or postponed grief.

Blazer (1982) notes that older persons who experience significant losses may overreact to these losses. After one loss is experienced, the individual may feel more easily threatened and may develop a cognitive attitude of anticipating many losses. While these anticipated losses are not realistic, they do represent a psychic reality to the elderly mourner who may generalize easily from specific loss to general loss. Several authors (e.g., Lindemann, 1944; Fulton & Gottesman, 1980; Carey, 1977), in discussing the notion of anticipatory grief and loss, contend that this capacity to experience grief and accept a loss before it occurs may often have a positive effect on the individual's adjustment to loss. In the case of the elderly, however, the assumption that anticipatory grief will facilitate their adjustment to loss may not be valid. Older people, while not obsessed with the anticipation of the death of spouse and elderly friends and neighbors, do agonize over potential loss of spouse, family members, and friends. Thus anticipatory grief is always present for the elderly, and during the period of anticipatory grief potentially hazardous forces (e.g., sensory deprivation, physical illness, social isolation) may mitigate against normal stress reactions to give rise to many other negative emotional reactions such as depression, agitation, repression, and intense identification with the person whose death is anticipated (Parkes, 1970; Switzer, 1970).

Conversely some elderly may deny the terminal illness of their loved ones and may unconsciously postpone the grief until the actual loss. These individuals who omitted the grieving or postponed it may experience even greater agitation and stress than others who anticipated the loss and perhaps went through a phase of partial grieving before the actual loss. Myers, Murphey, and Riker (1981) caution that gerontologists and other health practitioners may find it useful to discuss and subsequently to assess the origins of morbid grief reactions in the elderly and to take stock not only of the number of losses and bereavements the elderly individual has experienced but also the intensity and duration of the grieving with respect to the developmental phases of the grief. The assumption that the severe, prolonged, or morbid grief reactions of the elderly are always abnormal or pathological is not always valid. Fulton and Gottesman (1980) recommend a periodic reconsideration and reassessment of the developmental aspects of grief. Especially in the case of the elderly who live in constant fear of their own death and the death of other elders, it is important to assess whether the elderly person is going through a phase of anticipatory grief or postponed grief.

Life-Style Changes. Jacobs and Ostfeld (1977), who examined the association between bereavement and death, speculate that bereavement may lead to significant life-style changes in the bereaved widow or widower who may choose to live alone and in turn may be subjected to changes in dietary habits, increased social isolation, reduced physical activity, and decreased capacity for self-care (Table 9–1). Cumming and Henry (1961) state that the tendency for social isolation is typical in the elderly and to be expected as a part of the "disengagement process." Maddox (1963), however, refutes this notion and contends that social isolation is imposed on many elderly by circumstances arising from the death of the spouse. It increases feelings of loneliness, boredom, and hopelessness in the grieving elderly, further predisposing them to a variety of illnesses. These observations suggest that bereavement and grief may be important predictors of emotional and physical illness in the elderly. These variables may work through a common intervening variable such as the strength of the social support network and may therefore not intrinsically be the most important predictors.

Generally speaking social isolation, lack of emotional support, or abrupt changes in the environmental support may increase the potential for abnormal grief reactions among older persons. The assumption that the elderly who are bereaved (because of death due to chronic illness or advanced age) will adjust better than those experiencing a sudden loss is not always valid. On the contrary the grieving process in the case of the anticipated death may add to the existing disturbance of the anticipatory grief by intensifying and prolonging the reaction and by generating feelings of self-blame.

In assessing the grief reactions of normally bereaved elderly, a number of factors need to be observed:

- Loss of spouse. Parkes (1970) notes that the most severe form of psychological stress is caused by the loss of a spouse. With the majority of the elderly the spousal bereavement is not only the most significant of the losses experienced (Holmes & Rahe, 1967) but is almost inevitable for many elderly individuals. Stone and Fletcher (1981) note that the possibility of widowhood, especially for elderly women, increases dramatically after the sixth decade. Practitioners and family members of the elderly are therefore cautioned to observe the prolonged pining that many widowed elderly may go through, resulting in increasing feelings of isolation and behavioral withdrawal. Several authors (e.g., Abrahams & Patterson, 1978; Butler & Lewis, 1973; Parkes, 1982) observed that social isolation following the death of a spouse was significantly related to a variety of negative psychological consequences. While recognizing that no one dies of grief per se, research has indicated that the health of recently bereaved elderly widows and widowers is known to deteriorate following bereavement and that a significant number of widowed elderly die within 6 to 12 months following bereavement.

- Significance of anniversary dates. Jacobs and Douglas (1979) postulate that perhaps grief serves as a mediating process or bridge between a conjugal loss and an ensuing illness or death. Barraclough and Shepherd (1976) therefore suggest the significance of noting the psychiatric effects of anniversary dates and the fact that many elderly widowed individuals die close to or at the time of individually significant dates. Gerontologists need to recognize that widowed elderly are at greater risk for serious depressive disorders around anniversary dates, birthdays, and special celebrations.

- Atypical grief reactions. While the criteria for distinguishing normal grief reactions, clinical depression, and atypical grief are not clear, Parkes (1982) suggests a close examination and assessment of the atypical grief reactions in which there is a prolonged stage of feeling sad, helpless, and hopeless. Intense feelings of hopelessness, helplessness, and self-blame may lead to depressive disorders associated with clinical depression (Table 9–1). Symptoms of pining, searching for the lost one, preoccupation with thoughts of worthlessness, marked functional impairment and marked psychomotor retardation suggest that the bereavement is complicated by the development of a major depression (DSM-III, 1980).

There are few empirical data on whether finer distinctions between atypical grief and clinical depression are possible and valid in the case of elderly subjects. Therefore, it may be hard for the average family or professional to distinguish between normal appropriate grief and a clinically significant affective disorder. A number of authors (e.g., Berezin, 1972; Blazer, 1982; Parkes, 1970) suggest that various aspects of grief and bereavement (e.g., anticipatory grief, cf. Lindemann [1976]; partial grief, Berezin [1972]; omitted grief, Deutsch [1937]; preterminal and postponed grief) be monitored and assessed in any overall psychosocial evaluation of the depressed elderly. Special attention should be given to nonverbal behavior and to morbid grief reactions including delayed reactions, distorted reactions, medical diseases, anger against specific persons, absence of emotional expression, self-punitive behavior, and agitated depression accompanied by symptoms such as insomnia and self-accusation (Lindemann, 1944) (Table 9–1).

According to Goldfarb (1974) practitioners need to be cautioned about the bereaved elderly's tendency to use pseudoanhedonia, a mechanism by which patients express apathy and the desire to be left alone and not pushed around. Pseudoanhedonia clients act self-punitive and punitive to other persons and on a short-term basis use self-punitiveness as a mechanism for eliciting support from the social support system. These behavior patterns may overlap the diagnostic criteria of a major depressive episode. Goldfarb (1974) characterizes these bereaved clients as demonstrating an exaggerated show of helplessness, self-neglect, inability to carry out routine functions, and vehement fear of losing their minds. Closely associated with these symptoms are frequent somatic complaints such as inertia, bodily pain, malfunction of organs, and depressive symptoms such as loss of interest, loss of purpose, suicidal cognitions, and preoccupation with their sad state (Table 9–1).

Similarly Blazer (1982) observes that older adults with complicated bereavement frequently exhibit manipulative and coercive behaviors to modify the environment to their dependency needs. He notes that passive aggressive behavior is not uncommon in abnormal bereavement. Symptoms of physical and mental impairment are also easily incorporated into the daily interactional style of the bereaved person, often leading to a diagnosis of significant physical-organic or cognitive deficits. Blazer cautions that individual reactions to death and dying are expected to vary from day to day. Practitioners must be flexible in their orientation and tailor their approaches to the client's unique background, personality attributes and life style, personal needs, and circumstances.

Psychological functioning following bereavement should be assessed and predicated on the basis of interaction among specific coping strengths of the elderly individual, social support networks available, and subsequent stressors in the environment. Thus Parkes's (1982) model would assist practitioners in predicting that clinical depression may result in those elderly individuals with limited coping abilities and limited social support.

Psychosocial Correlates of Grief

Heyman and Gianturco (1973) note that many older people can and do adjust satisfactorily to loss and grief. These authors draw attention to several factors correlating significantly with both positive and negative outcomes of grieving:

- High socioeconomic status and high educational attainment (Glick, Weiss, & Parkes, 1974) are linked with positive outcomes of grieving and satisfactory adjustment. A plausible explanation for this is that the elderly from high socioeconomic status conditions may have relatively more social support at the time of bereavement. These elderly may therefore be less at risk for severe depression than their counterparts with less social backing and support.

- The elderly's reactions to bereavement may vary with other factors such as spousal death and whether the death was due to natural causes. Following Silverman (1972), the elderly who have been bereaved as a result of the spouse's suicide may face additional trauma beyond the immediate loss, including a fruitless search for self-blame. Generally speaking most elderly adjust satisfactorily within a year.

- Seligman (1975) introduced the concept of learned helplessness resulting from death of loved ones. This concept applied to the elderly suggests that when they are exposed to a series of uncontrollable events such as the death of a spouse, loss of finance, and illness, they may learn that active responding is futile and that quiet grieving is more adaptive. Such learning, according to Seligman (1975), undermines the incentive and motivation to adapt to the loss. Grief reactions and helplessness reactions become inextricably linked in the bereavement process. Goldfarb (1974) notes that learned helplessness in bereaved and depressed elderly may cause them to advertise their weaknesses, their ineptitude, or their memory problems, which all may be a part of the mechanism of pseudoanhedonia. Verwoerdt (1976) takes a similar orientation toward the phenomenology of the bereaved elderly. He notes that the depressed elderly may often withdraw as a protection against the potential for uncontrollable events and their own helplessness in the presence of hurt. Verwoerdt speculates that the elderly may seek only partial resolution of grief, and their avoidance of further object relations may lead to somatization.

More positive reinforcement for greater initiative, self-care, and reality orientation of the elderly will gradually draw them out of their detachment and anhedonia (Table 9–1).

THERAPEUTIC CONSIDERATIONS

Given the conflicting nature of available practitioner experiences and the research data, practitioners and clinicians working with bereaved older clients are cautioned to develop their own diagnostic devices for each particular client. Key points to bear in mind include the interrelationship of the bereaved client's current social and emotional conditions including an assessment of the client's past psychological functioning. The interview must first establish what adversities and bereavement the client has experienced and how the client has coped with the loss and grief. As noted by Pfeiffer (1980), it is assumed that persons who have successfully adapted to grief and bereavement are more likely to continue to do so. Such clients are less at risk than persons who have made poor adjustments. Questions to which the clinician or interviewer must seek answers include the following:

- How many family members, close friends, etc., have died recently or awhile ago?
- How distressed were you by these deaths of friends and family?
- How long did it take you to overcome the grief?
- Do you still tend to think of the losses (through death) that you experienced?

Also the magnitude of the distress experienced (short-term and long-term) must be assessed and compared. It is important that the elderly's grief reactions or subsequent depressive disorders be evaluated in the context of the network of rewarding social relationships available to the elderly client. The quality of the social network will often be a strong determinant of whether a bereaved and grieving widow will be temporarily or indefinitely distressed by the loss of a spouse.

Another important point that needs consideration is the differential assessment and diagnosis of normal and abnormal grief reactions (Wahl, 1979). While such differential diagnosis may be hard to accomplish, the practitioner or clinician may solicit the assistance of the elderly client's family in assessing the intensity of depression and whether the grief reaction is approaching clinical depression. An early differential diagnosis of normal aging reactions to loss and grief and neurotic grief reactions is important since prolonged lack of intervention or treatment increases the potential for abnormal grief reactions among older persons, sometimes culminating in suicide attempts.

Parkes (1970), in analyzing the elderly person's expressions of anger toward physicians, clergy, and family members, suggests that intense feelings must be considered as part of the bereavement reaction. Guilt may be expressed over the deceased spouse's illness and the failure of the widow or widower to attend to the needs of the ill person on time. Clayton, Halikas, and Maurice (1971) observe that much anger is directed at the deceased for having abandoned the spouse in old age. Anger may also be directed toward the physician, who may be charged with having neglected the serious nature of the deceased person's illness.

Caregivers should not overlook the fact that although the angry feelings may be grossly out of line, they are for the most part an appropriate cathartic reaction to the circumstances the bereaved elderly widow or widower faces. Expressions of guilt, anger, and suicidal ideations can be prominent during the bereavement period and should be accepted empathically by the caregiver. Lindemann (1976) stresses the key point that grieving is a constructive process and should be encouraged, especially in the elderly whose reactions to grief frequently tend to take the form of depressive withdrawal (Table 9–1).

It is sometimes felt that the best treatment includes helping the widowed person to cry and show distress. The available evidence, although rather limited in nature, indicates that widows who showed less distress in the early phases of widowhood had a poorer adjustment after one year (Parkes, 1970). These data suggest that unexpressed feelings of anger, guilt, or regret tend to linger and to impair the person's subsequent functioning. Generalizations concerning the amount of mourning that is healthy are insufficient, and the caregiver will have to monitor the individual variations in grief reactions.

Overall, counseling of the recently bereaved person can have major cathartic effects. Various clinicians (e.g., Lowenthal & Haven, 1968; Parkes, 1970; Silverman, 1977) have advocated the importance of a supportive relationship with a significant other. Caregivers (especially physicians) who talked with the bereaved, offered reassurance, and made some symbolic or real gestures to indicate their concern were seen as helpful and kind (Clayton, Halikas, & Maurice, 1971) by the bereaved client. The presence of a confidant often reduces feelings of distress and loneliness following the death. An empathic counselor or confidant can also help to place the bereaved person's feelings of anger, guilt, and desertion in a broader perspective by reassuring the client that these feelings are a normal reaction and that expression of these feelings can often be helpful (see management considerations in Table 9–1). Conversely, if a bereaved person wishes not to discuss the loss and desires to readjust to a normal routine as soon as possible, the individual should not be pushed into expressions of grief or distress over the loss.

The professional counselor should be aware that depending on the strength and quality of the relationship with the deceased, and depending also on the adaptation history of the bereaved person, there will be individual variations in the intensity of the need to grieve. Many elderly who lived with the chronic illness of a spouse may have engaged in a long period of anticipatory grief. If their relationship with the deceased was good, they may adjust well to their loss without the need for a prolonged expression of grief. Often they may feel relieved of the burden of caring for a spouse who died after a long debilitating illness. In such cases it is presumed that they were able to reconstruct their feelings of guilt or regret.

Barrett (1978) stresses the predominant need of many elderly widows initially to grieve and subsequently (although slowly) to form new social relationships. Widowed elderly persons may also need help with tangible problems involving finances and housing. Many widows or widowers may indulge in the grieving after the routine problems have been solved. A small but selective group may have little or no desire to grieve and will show little distress. History taking may show these individuals often had unusual adaptive qualities in their younger days.

In all events the counselor or caregiver should tentatively explore the bereaved person's wishes to discuss the loss and to deal with tangible problems of daily functioning. The counselor can point out a willingness and availability to help in whatever way the bereaved person deems important. The desires of the bereaved person must be respected in all aspects.

Most of the therapeutic procedures outlined are beneficial for most of the elderly going through a period of normal grief. However, treatment of bereaved older adults who suffer from a complicated grief reaction may require some ancillary procedures for care that must be used as an adjunct to the usual support and encouragement given to grieving elderly. Where grief reactions are intense (i.e., there is a major depressive disorder), treatment may have to be multidimensional, including a decision to hospitalize those elderly persons unable to care for themselves. Psychotropic medications may be useful for some elderly, with careful monitoring and attention being paid to objective measures of impairment in sleep, appetite, and activity. In some cases electroconvulsive therapy may be indicated.

Whether at home or in the hospital facility, companionship of family members will be important. Materials of interest to the person should be provided, and the emphasis should always be on maintaining a warm, supportive, and familylike atmosphere in which the bereaved person may be more willing to express deep feelings of loss and anger. Psychotherapy by a trained counselor may be an important adjunct in the case of some elderly who show complicated grief reactions. A number of important features stressed in the psychotherapy of the bereaved older adults include verbal and nonverbal expression of pain, sorrow, and the finality of bereavement. Also stressed in the verbal and nonverbal expression are the bereaved person's feelings of love, guilt, and hostility toward the deceased. The bereaved person will need assurance that the suffering and pain are transient. Blazer (1982) advocates that the bereaved elderly person be encouraged to review the relationship with the deceased (i.e., a life-history approach) and to recognize some of the expected alterations in cognition, effect, and behavior secondary to the bereavement (see management considerations in Table 9–1).

The professional counselor must work with the client to find an acceptable balance for the future intrapsychic representation of the deceased. Initially the bereaved person will need a considerable amount of support from the counselor, who must allow a positive, even parental, transference to evolve (Blazer, 1982), but gradually the counselor must attempt to encourage the transfer of dependency on the therapist and the deceased to other sources of gratification, namely, friends and family. There should be a steady decrease in the number of sessions with the elderly bereaved person, but termination should be gradual.

There are many inconsistencies as to the important considerations in assessing and treating the grief of the elderly and in identifying those who are especially at risk for suicide or severe depression. Wass and Myers (1982) suggest that research, theory, and practice should be closely aligned wherever possible and that the concepts of clinical depression, atypical grief, abnormal grief reactions, and interventions necessary for the bereaved elderly should receive more careful formulation and explication.

DEATH AND DYING

Several authors (e.g., Kübler-Ross, 1970; Kastenbaum, 1971; Shneidman, 1970) have commented on the fact that until recently death and dying were rather taboo topics for discussion and research. Consequently psychotherapy for the dying elderly or training programs for the professionals and paraprofessionals providing care to the dying have not been developed adequately. Recently, however, thanatology and related areas of grief and bereavement have attracted much public attention. There are research investigations and writings on varying aspects of grief and death and their effects on the mental health and coping capacities of the elderly. While physical death, its meaning, and scope have always been of interest in the medical world, more recently increasing attention is also being given to the areas of psychological and social death. Partially in response to the increasing needs of the terminally ill population, as well as other factors about the cultural milieu of the elderly, there has been a tremendous growth of interest and rapidly expanding psycho-therapy literature about problems and anxieties of the dying elderly persons, their families, their caregivers, and the cultural milieu in which the care is given. This section presents a discussion of some of the issues involved in evaluating the fears, anxieties, and psycho-social-physical needs of the elderly who are dying and to make suggestions concerning their reconstitution and management. (See Exhibit 9–1 presenting a summary of clinical assessment workup of the dying elderly.)

However, the present state of clinical research, assessment measures, and systematic intervention approaches is still quite poor (Kastenbaum & Aisenberg, 1972; Krant, 1974; Weisman, 1974). Appropriate procedures for dealing with the dying are inadequately explained, and few controlled studies have been conducted. Some of the key issues are summarized in Exhibit 9–1.

Kübler-Ross (1969), Eissler (1955), and Norton (1963) speak eloquently of the consequences of the abandonment that the elderly feel when families avoid recognizing their helplessness. It is suggested that depressions occur in the dying because they have no one with whom to share the experience. Dying alone in a hospital, unable to share one's anxiety about the impending death, is the last abandonment. Suffering the loss of life without the protective umbrella of a recognized grieving status could be the most frequent form of abandonment into old age. Spikes (1980) notes that the dynamics of dying is complicated for the elderly person because in old age there is a diminished social value of life; that is, the elderly person places less value on one's own life, while others in the environment also tend to share this reduced evaluation.

If allowed to occur in a milieu of abandonment, the dying process will inevitably lead to depression and other disorders that will dovetail concerns of rejection, loneliness, and

Exhibit 9–1 Clinical Assessment Workup of the Dying Person and Pretherapy Considerations

1. *Assessment of the Dying Person's Emotional States*

   —Denial, helplessness, and passivity
   —Anger, hostility, and frustration
   —Despondency, anxiety, self-pity, and withdrawal
   —Insightful acceptance and quiet constructive resignation

2. *Assessment of the Dying Person's Coping Capabilities*

   —The capacity for tackling, that is, adopting an active attitude or a tendency to fight the illness (adaptive)
   —Timely seeking of medical advice, compliance with therapeutic regimens, active information seeking (adaptive)
   —A tendency for capitulating, taking a passive stance, and withdrawing from interactions with friends and family (unadaptive)
   —Experience of adversities and magnitude of distress successfully tackled and tolerated in the past

3. *Assessment of the Dying Person's Emotional Needs*

   —Need for nurturance, moral support, and protection
   —Need for privacy and autonomous existence
   —Need for social interactions and companionship

4. *Assessment of the Dying Person's Social Support Networks*

   —Number of friends, confidants, and significant relationships
   —Attitudes of the family members toward death and dying and the quality of the family members' relationship with the dying person

5. *Assessment of the Meaning of Death as Perceived by the Dying Person*

   —Threat to the person's psychic integrity
   —Loss of self-esteem, security, and aspirations for the future
   —Abandonment, violence, and manipulation
   —Immortality and a positive life hereafter
   —Relief from pain or a source of psychosocial and economic gain

6. *Assessment of the Dying Person's Major Fears Related to Dying*

   —Fear of abandonment and isolation
   —Fear of physical suffering and pain
   —Fear of loss of mental and physical capacities
   —Fear of disrespect and indignity during and at the time of dying
   —Fear of obsolescence and deterioration

meaninglessness in the elderly. The end result may be that chronic depression will be superimposed on grief and the illness of old age (Spikes, 1980). Spikes (1980) and Katz and Gardner (1972) suggest that the responsibility for developing a viable support system for the elderly must lie with modern medicine designed along biopsychosocial lines. Within the biopsychosocial framework, treating a dying person as one with a status of privilege has a significant meaning.

STAGES OF DYING

It is important for the therapist and practitioner to recognize the client's stages of dying and to understand the specific needs, emotions, and behaviors of the elderly client at a given stage of development. Weisman (1974) and Kübler-Ross (1969) have outlined various stages through which most terminally ill patients pass. Both generally agree that Stage 1 begins with the onset of symptoms until the diagnosis is made. In this stage most patients go through a period of denial that allows them to assimilate the reality and mobilize other defenses in response to the fact of certain death. Stage 2 is the interval between diagnosis and the onset of terminal decline. The patient's denial is replaced by anger and resentment toward others, including family and health care personnel. Stage 3 starts when active treatment is found to have diminishing value. Anger and resentment are replaced by bargaining in an attempt to postpone pain, disability, and death in return for some promise of good behavior.

Death is generally viewed by the elderly as a slow process beginning long before the conventional signs of a terminal disease process are evident (Karasu & Waltzman, 1976). Karasu and Waltzman (1976) observe that for many elderly, recognition of the dying process may be related to the unmistakable signs of physical decline experienced in late life and the accumulation of physical, social, and emotional losses that frequently occur in old age. Chronic disease and the increasing inability to achieve gratifications and satisfactions increase the sense of loss and depression in many elderly long before the terminal illness stage is reached. Often the predeath syndrome defined as "immobility, incontinence and mental incapacity" sets in and serves to increase the sense of helplessness and despondency (Isaacs, Gunn, McKechan, McMillan, & Neville, 1971, p. 1115).

Kübler-Ross (1970) feels that when help is given in working through the various stages of dying, dying persons achieve a stage of acceptance in which they disengage and await death with a greater measure of peace and calm. Although there is considerable controversy as to whether all dying individuals demonstrate all stages on an equivalent basis (cf. Kastenbaum & Weisman, 1969; Hinton, 1963) there is increasing agreement as to the relative importance of all of these stages merging quickly in the elderly dying persons. Karasu and Waltzman (1976) contend that because many elderly have a history of chronic illness and various sensory and cognitive deficits, they go through a longer stage of depression and anxiety with respect to dying. They are increasingly frightened, perhaps because of difficulty in communications, possibly isolated from families and friends and dependent on whoever is available for the gratification of physical needs and emotional nurturance. Thus slow-dying elderly present more problems than other age groups, and their development through the stages of dying is less clear and less continuous.

Although much of what has been discussed appears valid from a psychosocial perspective, the question of training for unpreparedness for death in both the dying and the living elderly is rarely discussed by practitioners and social gerontologists. Whether one attributes social abandonment of the dying to conscious or unconscious death, fear, denial of death, or a kind of emotional apathy or indifference in society, the questions are important enough to deserve some attention if professionals are to provide intervention and therapy. Indeed, as Baum and Baum (1980) conclude, a good case can be made for the assertion that people in an industrialized society are singularly unprepared to deal with the dying. It is unpreparedness in relating to the dying, not having learned how to feel and share emotion, and what to say to the dying person that seem to be at the root of the caregivers' and practitioners' apprehensions about relating to the dying.

The elderly clients' reactions to death will ultimately depend on what death signifies to them. The meanings they associate with death will have been determined by their assimilation of cultural and family attitudes, personal experiences with death of others, their unresolved conflicts, or their sense of satisfaction with achievements (Karasu & Waltzman, 1976). Geriatric professionals and caregivers must attempt, therefore, to understand the elderly persons' cultural milieu, their fears concerning death, their attitudes toward death, and many other aspects of socioeconomic, educational, and occupational status presumed to be linked with the mental well-being of the elderly (see Exhibit 9–1 for clinical assessment guidelines).

UNDERSTANDING OF THE ELDERLY PERSONS' FEARS ABOUT DEATH: THERAPEUTIC CONSIDERATIONS

Issues of personal death become areas of most immediate and conscious concern in the elderly (Spikes, 1980). Kalish and Reynolds (1976) observe that while it is not known how profoundly the fear or fact of death influences the adaptation to late life, psychological studies have documented that thoughts of death are frequently entertained by the elderly. Some old people may not experience a great deal of fear about death; nevertheless it is important that clinicians assess whether their attitudes toward it are negative, positive, or neutral. Death-related attitudes have been explored in a number of studies (e.g., Preston & Williams, 1971; Wass, 1979) and suggest that the immediacy of the elderly's concern about death or fears about death may serve to inform the clinician about the psychological mechanisms that individuals may employ later to adapt to the fears and facts of death (Spikes, 1980).

To perceive more clearly the full dimensions of the subject of death concerns and death fears, clinicians, physicians, or mental health workers working with the elderly need to consider the question of developing a unifying perspective of some of the meanings which the elderly attach to death. As noted by Sobel (1980), death is essentially an unknown state but has many meanings and images projected onto it. Since in the minds of many elderly one of its meanings is loss, abandonment, and violence directed at the helpless individual, the elderly's anxiety toward such an event is reality based. Kübler-Ross's (1969) stages in the reaction to death and dying (i.e., denial, anger, bargaining, fear, and depression and acceptance) are known to many practitioners and clinicians who are aware of the concomitant stress that death and dying produce in the later years. What practitioners and clinicians need to assess, as early as possible, are the elderly persons' thoughts of their own progressing death. As one examines these meanings, one explores with the elderly the wealth of experience they have acquired, the experiences of human vulnerability, and one gains in understanding of the many dimensions of fear associated with death (Exhibit 9–1).

These issues need to be understood and addressed with special reference to the philosophical and psychological perspectives of the elderly. The need for such perspectives may be understood as the need for substantive responses to three central questions:

1. What is the nature of death for the elderly in the cultural context of a death-denial and death-avoidance society?
2. What are the specific fears and anxieties that the elderly have concerning their death?
3. What do caregivers and practitioners need to know about the variety and intensity of the fears related to death and dying?

Some of the assessment needs described above are summarized in Exhibit 9–1.

Individual Differences in the Fears toward Death and Dying

Individual responses to stress and crises vary according to personality patterns that have made an imprint on almost all of the behavioral patterns including those of coping, regression, or anxiety. This is true of the fear of dying. Weisman and Kastenbaum (1968) observed that some elderly had little anxiety or awareness of impending death and gradually withdrew into inactivity. Others remained actively involved in decision making relevant to their lives.

In order that practitioners be able to assist the elderly in the process of reconstitution or resignation to their illness, it is important that they attempt to understand something about the personality of the elderly and the kind of life that the person has lived. Kastenbaum (1971) noted that some elderly looked forward to dying before their time. Some who had experienced many losses, including the will to keep enduring and persevering in life, approached death with some measure of agitation. Still others who possessed a strong religious faith in the significance of an afterlife approached death with composure. The fewest death fears were reported by both the strongly religious and confirmed atheists while the greatest fears of death were reported by individuals who were undecided about religion or who had inconsistent beliefs (Kalish, 1976). The notions of immortality or afterlife were supported by a sizable majority of elderly (see Cavan, Burgess, Havighurst, & Gold-hammer, 1949).

Attitude toward death was shown to be positively related to both educational level and emotional adjustment (Riley, 1970) and all three variables—educational level, emotional adjustment, and attitude toward death—were associated with the quality of the social support available to the elderly. Fear of death was found more often in those living alone than in those living with relatives or in homes for the aged (Swenson, 1961).

Perhaps a greater measure of fear and anguish is noted in those individuals who may come to view death as a punishment for hostile impulses of earlier days or by others in whom the notion of dying may arouse separation anxiety. Clearly an elderly person will greet the idea of death positively if viewing it as an opportunity for reunion with a lost spouse rather than a separation from a loved one. Thus, often an elderly person's view of death as a cosmic reunion or an indefinite continuation of existence in some type of life hereafter will ameliorate the intensity of the fear of death.

The following is an attempt to encapsule several described views (cf. Attig, 1979) and to develop a specific list of the dominant fears and concerns of the dying elderly (see Attig (1979) for a detailed discussion):

- The perceptions of death and dying and the attitudes toward death for many elderly are grounded in a specific culture. The North American culture is not merely a death-denying but rather a vulnerability-denying culture. Many elderly in their lifetime have survived two depressions and two world wars and have attached high value to concepts of individualism, independence, and self-control and autonomy. In a culture that disparages helplessness and dependence many elderly experience fear, shame, and guilt, which are exacerbated by the prospects of being rendered helpless and unable to cope successfully. Fear of being a burden on others produces in many elderly a sense of special suffering (steeped in an ethic of individualism) when they must finally admit to themselves and others their total reliance on external supports.

- Many elderly confined to the sterile environments of their institutional homes, with limited economic and emotional resources available to them, may suffer fear when they are isolated or abandoned while dying and most in need of the companionship of someone who cares.

- Many elderly, victims of stroke and other forms of declining mental functions and physical debilitation, may suffer considerable fear because their continuing motivation for meaningful interaction with the environment may be denigrated and undermined. Many may suffer emotionally as they lose the physical capacities to interact with the environment. Fear of loss of control over their own body functions and fear of the loss of mental capacities to make decisions for themselves are genuine fears for elderly confined to health care institutions.

- For many elderly, fear of physical suffering (associated with the pain of disease and physical debilitation) may increase considerably by the prospects of surgery, cancer, or other painful terminal illness. After learning about their terminal condition, many elderly who have struggled with the common avoidance and denial of death may experience severe anxiety in confronting the prospects of their own deaths.

- Many elderly with terminal illness may be denied information affecting their case, and this fear of the unknown may profoundly affect their emotional endurance. Persons for whom euthanasia is contemplated are among the most vulnerable of the elderly. They may face a future filled with fear and suspense as to whether their wishes for euthanasia will be accepted or denied. These fears concerning the timing of death must be understood as the responses of persons who are at the mercy of physicians and administrators who may not necessarily share their beliefs concerning death or the right to die. The practitioner's respect and sensitive response to the dying elderly depend on an understanding of their fears and anxieties. Without such awareness on the part of the practitioner, the prospects of according these elderly their inviolable dignity are considerably diminished. For many elderly confined to wheelchairs and life-supporting apparatus, their experience of fear and shame is exacerbated by the prospects of indignity and disrespect at the hands of those who are charged with their care.

- Wass and Sisler's (1979) research findings stress the elderly's concerns about the significance of their images surviving through children, good works and achievement, etc. Those elderly concerned about issues of immortality and survival of their images had significantly higher death concern scores than those who were less interested. As Attig (1979) observes, the need for immortality is expressive also of the fear of incompleteness that many elderly feel, that is, the fear that perhaps they did not avail themselves "of opportunities to accumulate experiences, engage in meaningful projects, grow in relationships, achieve integrity, and the like" (p. 11). In old age, therefore, the desire for immortality may be closely associated with the fear that their lives have no intrinsic value and therefore are not worthy of expression or continuation after their physical death.

- Another area of concern frequently associated with death is the elderly person's obsessive anxious concern over external events. It has been commonly observed that many elderly may become fearful of being suddenly taken off Medicare benefits, old-age pension, and welfare benefits and sudden and precipitous relocation into a poorer neighborhood and dwelling. According to Sobel (1980) this can be understood as a symbolic personification of death, which can come suddenly and snatch one away. Similarly fear of being mugged, robbed, or walking alone in the street exemplifies this concern with death. Other materials such as disability, illness, abandonment, and feelings of being cheated can also be construed as reification of death and its actions on the undefended person (Sobel, 1980). The elderly's fears and concerns about death therefore reflect the basic anxiety about social injustices such as robbery and being cheated.

Life in a complex modern society requires that the elderly live with many threats of uncertainty and a high level of trust that they will be cared for. Practitioners must recognize that caring for the elderly implies convincing them that they will be cared for in old age in a manner that meets the intimate needs of the elderly themselves rather than the needs of their families or caretakers. An essential element in respecting the elderly is, then, the appreciation of their fear and anxiety concerning a dignified death. It is imperative that the clinician or counselor give the fears of the elderly regard and consideration commensurate with the seriousness of the problems they can cause (Weisman & Kastenbaum, 1968).

CONSIDERATIONS IN MANAGEMENT AND TREATMENT OF THE DYING ELDERLY

A number of specific management strategies and procedures for working with the dying elderly are recognized to be generally effective. These are summarized in Exhibit 9–2. Fear of death is not especially intense or pervasive in the elderly under circumstances of moral

---

Exhibit 9–2 The Management of the Dying Elderly Client: Caregivers' Role and Functions

1. Empathic and supportive communication of the terminally ill diagnosis by someone close to the dying elderly.
2. Maintenance in the client of sustained and supportive communication with confidants after the disclosure of diagnosis.
3. Respect of client's need to be informed of the details of illness, timing of death, etc., and measures being taken either to prolong life or avoid prolonged dying.
4. Communication with and support of the dying person's family.
5. Preservation for the client of rewarding relationships with family, friends, clergy, social worker, nurse, and physician.

6. Maintenance in the client of a dignified self-image by providing a pleasant environment including activities and relationships enhancing the elderly person's sense of intrinsic worth.
7. Provide client sustained assurance to the very end, that the individual will be treated with courtesy, dignity, and safe conduct.
8. Psychotherapy with the dying person:
   - Help the person to mourn and to develop a fantasy or belief of immortality.
   - Depending on client's need, offer empathy, and unconditional positive regard.
   - Encourage a life review with a view to helping the dying person to gain strength and significance from achievements and past contributory efforts.

support, reassurance, and empathy (Swenson, 1961). Unfortunately many physicians and practitioners view the elderly from a perspective of obsolescence and deterioration. Only to the extent that practitioners try to gain an understanding of the elderly's dimensions of vulnerability, fears, and despondency, will they acquire a basis for ameliorating their fears and concerns about death. The temptation is too great to treat the dying as if they were already dead and had already forfeited their rights to any human needs. Equally of concern is the caregivers' tendency to withhold information or diagnosis from the dying person.

According to Maier (1979, p. 93) the major problem of dying is how not to die alone. ''It should be axiomatic that even under the most adverse conditions, the patient is not alone,'' and therefore the sound of human voices, the clasp and feeling of a human hand are important needs that should not be denied to the dying elderly. Attig (1979) vigorously deplores the lack of involvement on the part of caretakers. He advocates that active support be given; the dying must not be isolated or abandoned. In order to ameliorate their emotional condition and to alleviate their fears, truth must not be kept from them, especially the truth that would enable them to retain control over decisions affecting their lives. As an advocate of the good death, Attig contends that if the dying remain capable of meaningful interaction with the environment and with others, steps must be taken to ensure that the environment promotes as much social interaction as possible and that the lines of communication between caregiver and the dying person are always open.

All of the foregoing emphasizes the notion that the caregivers' decision to persist in avoidance and denial of death for the client or patient has the consequence of making the elderly's fears all the more dominant. Both the patient's self-reflection and the caregivers' reflection on their own fears and attitudes toward death and dying (i.e., concepts of afterlife, suicide, euthanasia, grief and bereavement, care of the dying) can provide a perspective that allows for the articulation and unification of a program of home and hospital care and treatment of the dying elderly. Contemporary literature on the subject of death and dying is growing, but to date there are no well-considered treatment and care plans. Several important questions and concerns need to be addressed before a circumspect treatment program would be acceptable at a broad cultural level.

One of major current concerns has to do with a unified perspective of euthanasia. Preston and Williams (1971) and Wass (1979) stress the importance of discussing with the elderly their views on the right to die. Old people have definite opinions on the issue of the right to die, and by far the large majority wish to be allowed to die naturally rather than to be maintained by artificial or heroic means (Wass & Myers, 1982). Any clinical assessment workup procedures used with the elderly should endeavor to assess the views of the elderly concerning death: their fears, their frustrations, and their rights. Often this kind of clinical assessment may require that the clinician, mental health worker, or physician seek the assistance of the elders' close family members in soliciting the elderly's views on these matters in an objective but empathic manner. In states that have natural death laws clinicians must inform those elderly who do not know of their right under the law, thus helping to alleviate their anxiety. In states without such legislation it would still be important to find out what the older person's anxieties are concerning death. Such an assessment, even though it appears cold and harsh on the surface, should be useful if it is conducted before the elderly person becomes terminally ill and unable to communicate (Wass & Myers, 1982). The knowledge obtained from the clinical assessment of the elderly's fears of death may be shared with family.

Sociodemographic factors relevant to the counselor include the client's level of educational attainment (Jeffers, Nichols, & Eisdorfer, 1961). For example, low levels of formal education have been found related to negative death attitudes and high degree of fears (Berman & Hays, 1973; Riley, 1968; Wass & Sisler, 1979). Personality factors (in the absence of severe cognitive functioning) are clearly the most important indicators, and the dying elderly person's traits and attitudes should be clearly recognized and respected by the practitioner (Spikes, 1980). For example, to the narcissistic person death and old age are seen simply as weakness, and the realization of death may produce strong reactions of humiliation and rage and a denial of the fears pertaining to death. If denial cannot be maintained by counterphobic measures, serious depression of the ego-centered type or even suicide may result (Spikes, 1980). Compulsive personalities on the other hand may suffer more superego or conscience-related depression when faced with death fears and may view their own deaths as punishment. Some frequently observed symptom complexes are depression, regression with anxiety, and social withdrawal. These complexes may occur alone, in combination, or alternately. In most cases, however, they must be viewed by the clinician as an attempt to deal with or deny the death fears (Spikes, 1980, p. 416).

Assessment of the Dying Client's Needs and Wishes

Karasu and Waltzman (1976) suggest evaluation of the coping mechanisms that are being used by the dying elderly person. These clinicians stress that the evaluation must include a consideration of several aspects. For example:

- proximity of the patient to dying
- specific threats to life: physical illness, mental disorders, financial handicaps
- premorbid adaptive techniques
- accumulated life experiences and relationships: past achievements and social roles, challenges, obstacles, and expectations for success
- expectations of those in the immediate environment and the nature of their transactions with the elderly person, i.e., the degree of unconditional support, nurturance, and protection demonstrated by the family, institutional environment, or the community network

For purposes of assessment, a number of scales to assess death concerns are available. The more well-known ones follow.

Abbreviated and Adapted Form of Shneidman's Questionnaire

This scale (1970) may be of some assistance to clinicians and practitioners in understanding some of the psychodynamics of various aspects of death and dying. The abbreviated Shneidman's questionnaire has 18 items adapted from the original 75 items and yields information concerning four distinct categories of dying:

1. Personal meanings of death (To what extent do you believe in a life after death? Regardless of your belief about life after death, what is your wish about it? What aspect of your death is most distasteful to you? To what extent are you interested in having your image survive after your death?)

2. Physical and mental health status (How do you rate your present mental health? When you think of your own death, how do you feel? What is your own orientation to death?)
3. Thoughts concerning the terminal period (If you were told that you are terminally ill, how would you wish to spend your limited time till you died? How would you like your body disposed of after your death?)
4. Concern for others (What are your thoughts about autopsy done on your body? Would you be willing to donate your organs for transplant?)

In using this kind of questionnaire in an interview with the elderly, the practitioner always has to consider the problem of social acquiescence. While one point of view suggests that the elderly as a group are more acquiescent, a conflicting point of view suggests that the elderly can afford to tell what they think and feel and are far less likely to acquiesce. Nevertheless, it is important that confidentiality of information should be assured.

Dickstein Death Concern Scale

This is another example of a death concern assessment scale with 30 test items of particular relevance to the elderly's attitudes to and concerns relating to death. Dickstein (1975a, 1975b) conceptualizes death concern as conscious contemplation of the reality of death and negative evaluation of that reality.

As explained by Wass and Sisler (1979), who have used this scale extensively, the purpose is to measure individual differences in the degree to which one confronts death and is disturbed by its implications. The scale, particularly if used in a semistructured interview, has capabilities to elicit significant information related to aspects of death that are distasteful (e.g., the process of death might be very painful; I am afraid of what happens to my body after I die), motivation to have the image survive, perceptions of mental and physical health, and concerns about autopsy, transplantation of organs, pain and suffering, and artificial means of prolonging life.

Wass and Sisler (1979) using the 30-item Dickstein scale were able to demonstrate the validity and reliability of the scale in the identification of death concerns. Second, they were able to identify significant differences among elderly subjects' death concerns in a number of areas that may have practical relevance for practitioners who work with geriatric patients.

Assessment must include aspects of the ability of elderly persons to maintain interests, relationships, and involvement in activities. Others who adopted patterns of withdrawal, repression, and constriction much earlier in life may be expected to use mechanisms of denial to a greater degree. Far more careful work must be done to define the relative importance of all of the variables in the total clinical picture of the dying elderly person.

CAREGIVERS' THERAPEUTIC ROLES

Kastenbaum and Aisenberg (1972) point out that reactions of the individuals will depend on a sense of time perspective or a sense of acceleration. Their anxiety will be related to their sense of imminence. Kastenbaum (1966) observed that for many elderly, time was not a concern and therefore death was much less formidable. Lieberman (1966), however, noted that those elderly closest to death showed greater interest in other people and high responsiveness to the environment. For the practitioner this should reaffirm the importance of the elderly person's need to make contact with significant others in the environment, particularly with those caregivers who have some measure of control over their physical and emotional health and well-being. Even others who wrap themselves in counterfeit cloaks and show manifest symptoms of withdrawal, insomnia, and psychosomatic disturbances are similarly expressing a desperate need to seek support and human contact with various caregivers such as the therapist, the physician, nurse, social worker, clergy, and family. Each caregiver has a distinct therapeutic function and role with the dying elderly. Some of the roles overlap and so do the functions, but each can help in the management of the elderly person's adaptations.

Psychotherapist's Function

Eissler (1955) advocates that the major therapeutic task with the dying elderly is to help the person to mourn and to develop a fantasy or belief of immortality. Spikes (1980) notes that the aim of mourning is to help the dying person achieve psychological integration. The therapist must assist the client in becoming consciously aware of an actual or anticipated loss and at the same time to erect a fantasy of immortality. If the patient cannot independently erect such a fantasy, it falls on the clinician to aid in doing so (Becker, 1973). Spikes (1980) observes that this ability to generate a fantasy will be less obvious in persons who are intellectually inclined. On the whole the conviction of some sort of immortality such as living on through children or through accomplishments and creations or possessions may be easily erected in most dying elderly.

Psychotherapy for death may become synonymous with psychotherapy for loss. Helping the dying person to come to terms with death means that the person must both integrate the ideal of the eventual loss of self or the object into one's conscious awareness and simultaneously discharge many painful effects, including sadness and rage. The orderly progression of the mourning process from denial to acceptance will require considerable emotional support, time and effort, and proper observation from all persons in the immediate environment including family, health care personnel, and the psychotherapist. Although this point clearly overlaps with the points about human contact and immortality, it is necessary for the practitioner to note that the particular quality of relations with others strongly influences the way the dying elderly handle death.

Eissler (1955) suggests that the therapist who is working with the elderly patient must maintain a paradoxical attitude. The paradoxical attitude requires that the therapist recognizes the magnitude and gravity of the dying person's situation but still impresses on the dying person the notion of personal indestructibility. Stated another way, the process of helping the dying person to mourn is not possible without at the same time convincing the person of possessing permanence. Depending on the individual's belief systems, some can be helped to maintain a sense of immortality through ideas of reincarnation and of life after death. Others may reject these views.

The most systematic and adaptive technique in response to old age and coping with death has been put forward by Butler (1963), who particularly emphasizes the need for life review. In summing up the value of the life-review procedure, Butler notes that it is a naturally occurring, universal mental process characterized by the progressive return to consciousness of past experiences and particularly the resurgence of unresolved conflicts. The life-review process helps the dying person to gain strength and significance from the adaptations and achievements already experienced. In reviving experiences, conflicts are surveyed and reintegrated but more important there are construction, reconstruction, and integration of meaningful, useful, and contributory efforts. The life review is a last attempt to interpret one's identity and transcendence in terms of a permanent status.

The technique is not without some risks. Jeffers and Verwoerdt (1968a) and Becker (1973) caution against encouraging the life review in depressed patients for fear that they experience a resurgence of guilt and sadness for past mistakes. However, generalizations about the use of the life review with dying elderly persons are insufficient. The therapist must carefully evaluate the specific characteristics of each client to decide whether the kind of stock taking involved in the life review will be useful. The major therapeutic task is to develop some sense of personal immortality. Generally speaking the life review is an adaptive technique and like all patterns of adaptation has significant applications in psychotherapy of the dying elderly. The life review is ill-advised, however, in cases where psychopathology is indicated.

Family's Function

The family is regarded vital to the elderly person's successful adaptation to dying. Spikes (1980) notes that when an elderly member is afflicted by a fatal illness, older couples mourning together have been able to help the dying person achieve a sense of permanence.

Kalish (1976) and Jeffers and Verwoerdt (1968a, 1868b) note that the quality of the family members' relationship with the dying person will strongly influence the way that person handles death. One of the most satisfying adaptations to ending of life is a close and nonambivalent relationship with children and grandchildren. Regardless of the history of family relations or deficiencies in other aspects of living, most elderly are able to mourn successfully or to accept approaching death when family members are available and involved. This relationship with children and grandchildren makes it easier for the person partially to satisfy a need for immortality. Not only is the process of mourning greatly facilitated by the presence of interested listeners (Burnside, 1969; Shands, 1955; Feifel & Jones, 1968), but family members also satisfy the mutual affectional needs and bestow on the older persons the reminder of continuity of life and tangible evidence of their ongoing contributions to mankind (Jeffers & Verwoerdt, 1968b).

The mental health workers (who may also be the primary caregivers for the elderly) should be aware that family members frequently need counseling assistance in order to be supportive to the elderly relatives. Peterson (1980) notes that reactions of family members to the dying elderly will depend, in part, on the way that the person functioned within the social structure. If the dying individual was perceived by the rest of the family to be strong and invulnerable, often the family, and especially the spouse, may avoid facing the issue of the person's impending death. The mental health worker's mediation may be important in families communicating feelings of loss and grief to the dying elderly member. Zarit (1980) notes that there is a critical line between helping family members to know they have done what they can in communicating their feelings to the dying person or in settling old problems, and pushing the person too much, so that there is an unnecessary dwelling on depressive feelings. The major task of the family is to explore the feelings of the dying elderly in a supportive atmosphere, and to allow them the opportunity to talk about their situation at their own pace. This may involve being available to the elderly individual as a confidant, listening in a supportive way, or helping the elderly person to reach closure on psychological concerns, desires or wishes.

As death nears, the elderly person may want the companionship of only one or few confidants, and may feel no special need to talk for long periods of time. The family members may have difficulty in accepting the elderly person's withdrawal and the refusal for further treatment. They may inappropriately try to cheer up the dying elderly and encourage them to hold on to life. Kübler-Ross (1970) points out that rather than encouraging the dying person to cheer up, families can be more helpful by accepting the dying person's response and recognizing that death will be made easier by letting go rather than through continuing struggle.

Medical Caregiver's Function

Any treatment procedures should be discussed in detail with the patient, and the dying person's input in the decision making should always be sought unless it has already been established that the individual is not capable of making a rational judgment. Karasu and Waltzman (1976) stress that the elderly patient should be told the details of the illness and the treatment possibilities in specific but careful terms, without removing hope and without discussing specific time limits of life expectancy. However, if the patient wishes to acknowledge death openly and to discuss practical issues such as life expectancy and time limits, the economic costs in terms of hospitalization and financial problems of short-term or long-term care, these issues must be discussed in specific, realistic, and practical terms.

In particular, patients need to know the risks and odds involved in any further treatment. When the only recourse available is complicated and painful treatment that has little probability for success or will cause considerable disfigurement, the elderly patients should have a choice to determine whether they want further treatment. The patient's decision to keep the diagnosis confidential from the family must be respected. However, families who have not been given adequate information to assess the elderly relative's medical condition should also be supported in their right to obtain the information. It is usually assumed that the elderly patient has the right to decide on major issues of care such as the need for further treatment, and the decision to remain in the hospital, to go home, or to a hospice. They also need the opportunity to resolve any personal conflicts with the family members when they feel the timing is right. By contrast, individuals who do not want to know about their condition should not be pressed with the facts, but in many cases the elderly need to be informed that it is their right to ask legitimate questions concerning diagnosis, the potentials for recovery, and the treatment possibilities.

Weisman (1974) emphasizes the need for doctors and professionals to reassure the elderly patient that the individual will be cared for with courtesy, dignity, and safe conduct. Safe conduct implies that the practitioner will provide the patient with knowledge about the nature and course of the disease or illness; will approach the patient with acceptance, clarity, candor, compassion, and mutual acceptability; and will provide the patient with an emotional, social, and physical environment consistent with the diagnostic status or terminal illness status of the patient. This implies that the physical needs of the individual in terms of medication and control of pain and suffering and psychological needs in terms of moral support, right to privacy, autonomous existence, or companionship will be respected (Exhibit 9–2).

An important aspect of the care of dying elderly is the recognition of the time when active treatment is no longer helping the client. In hospital settings it is usually assumed that patients and their families would want to pursue every possible source of cure for terminal illness, but as the chances of remission dim, it has been observed that many more elderly persons, compared to younger adults, prefer to terminate treatment and life-support systems. Although issues of euthanasia are surrounded by much controversy, and decisions in this regard may not be within the jurisdiction of the physicians or the primary health care team, they do present many social, legal, and ethical concerns to the patient. The elderly person's fears, concerns, and queries as to euthanasia can no longer be ignored by the health care professionals. If the client wishes to discuss the subject, the issues must be discussed in specific, realistic, and practical terms.

Nurses' Functions

The doctors' attitudes toward the elderly and their standards of safe conduct will often influence those of the nurses caring for the patient. Since nurses are generally responsible for the care of the immediate physical needs of their patients, their training prepares them essentially for the physical and technical aspects of the care of the dying. However, some observations (Kastenbaum, 1969) stress that nurses may often be expected to deal with the psychosocial aspects of caring for their dying patients. The nurses' lack of inclination to allow patients to talk about their feelings or to relate with the bereaved families (Kastenbaum, 1967) may stem from their lack of self-confidence and lack of training to respond effectively to the clients' thoughts and feelings. As a result of inadequate amount of training to handle the psychosocial aspects of the dying elderly, nurses have tended to insulate themselves from the emotional impact of their relationship and to maintain a rather cool, objective, and detached stance with the dying person. Discontinuous and piecemeal caregiving in the form of physical health care (Krant, 1974) can be protective for nurses but nevertheless tends to increase guilt feelings.

Significant numbers of nurses, doctors, and educators in the medical field are becoming increasingly aware of the potential therapeutic effects of their emotional relationship with patients. Both in the medical profession and in nursing and health care there have been increasing attempts to include specific training programs and conferences and seminars dealing with issues of patients' grief, bereavement, and dying. There appears to be a growing recognition of the need for medical practitioners and nurses to improve their interpersonal abilities to cope with the intense affective situations of their dying patients and to serve them and their families with compassion and personal care.

Social Workers and Clergy

Other health care personnel who are attempting to reformulate their roles in relation to the dying elderly include the clergy and social workers. Karasu and Waltzman (1976) note that the role of the clergy and social worker has expanded rapidly as a result of the increasing emphasis on bereaved families and the need to relate to their psychological needs. Social workers are recognized more formally as a vital part of the primary health care team playing key roles with dying patients and their bereaved families. They act as advocates for the dying and their families by providing social and moral support and by mediating between dying patients and families and other members of the health care staff. The clergy perform a similar role, especially with those elderly who are experiencing guilt with respect to mistakes and other elderly who have concerns about themselves and their families from the perspective of life after death.

Health Care Team

For some patients and families a team approach with different health care members assuming different functions may be satisfactory. Other patients and their families may wish to have only one primary care provider. These needs must be respected as far as possible, without putting undue strain on individual staff members. In either case, appropriate staff transactions and negotiations will be necessary to the well-being of the dying patient.

It is incumbent on all members of the health team, including psychologists, therapists, nurses, clergy, social workers, and other medical specialists, to communicate openly about the needs of the dying individual. It will be important to share medical and psychological information since each member of the health care team may have views and may relate with the elderly and their families under different circumstances. In formulating specific goals for therapy and treatment there must be mutual sharing among staff and support for the individual staff member at all times. Feelings about the dying person, the family, the dying process, or interaction with previous staff members in the other hospitals and nursing homes where the elderly person lived need to be resolved if optimum care is to be provided.

Insights (both positive and negative) about the elderly person's coping resources must be shared among the staff members on the team. They must decide collectively when and how much information should be imparted to the patient or the family. Decisions as to the person who can relate most effectively with the elderly person must also be made by the health team.

In concluding this chapter, it is important to note that while there is ample study of the medical aspects of death and dying, psychosocial aspects and psychological care of the dying elderly are areas in which limited work has been done. Although much of what has been said about the fears and anxieties of the dying persons would appear valid from a clinical point of view, many questions about the management of the concerns and anxieties of the dying have received little attention in the psychological literature.

Many questions about the specific issues of dying (such as euthanasia, the role of the therapist, the responsibilities of the family, and the functions of the medical team and social work personnel) have been raised. How do we evaluate normal grief? How do we facilitate the mourning process? What characteristics must caregivers have? What happens to the psychosocial needs of the dying? What kinds of training programs will help caregivers to improve their relational and social skills? How much information must be shared with the dying and their families? Many of these significant questions need to be discussed urgently and intensively by practitioners.

Recent endeavors in the development of more sophisticated biopsychosocial approaches to the understanding of the dying elderly show promise. However, our basic concern is still with understanding the unique feelings, meanings, and needs of the grieved or dying elderly and with developing more effective ways to communicate comfort and support to them. More advanced assessment techniques must be developed to evaluate the roles that different members of the family and health care team play in the anticipated management of illness, death, and bereavement of the elderly. More advanced training programs and conferences must be organized to teach health care personnel interpersonal skills for serving the emotional needs of the dying.

Geriatric practitioners need to obtain a clearer understanding of the dynamics of death fear or death concern among the elderly in order to assist them in the adaptation to dying. On the positive side there is considerable evidence available to health professionals that the majority of aged are healthy and capable and their attitudes toward death and dying are rational, stable, and positive. It is particularly important therefore for clinicians and health professionals to assess the facts of preventive mental health in the aged on an ongoing basis and to acquire knowledge about their existing coping skills and adaptive capacities.

SUMMARY

This chapter has attempted to elucidate some of the psychosocial aspects of the phenomena of grief, death, and dying in the elderly, including their fears and anxieties about
death. A major focus has been on therapeutic considerations and the management of the
dying elderly. In this respect the role of primary caregivers has been discussed with special
reference to the function of psychotherapists, families, physicians, nurses, social workers,
and clergy. Significant questions that need to be addressed in clinical practice or future research have been raised.

REFERENCES

Abrahams, R.B., & Patterson, R.D. (1978). Psychological distress among the community elders: Prevalence, characteristics, and implications for service. *International Journal of Aging and Human Development, 9*, 1–18.

Attig, T. (1979). Death, respect and vulnerability. In A. deVries & A. Carmi (Eds.), *The dying human* (pp. 3–15). Tel Aviv: Turtledove Publishing Co.

Barraclough, B.M., & Shepherd, D.M. (1976). Birthday blues: The association of birthday with self-inflicted death in the elderly. *Acta Psychiatrica Scandinavica, 54*, 146–149.

Barrett, C.J. (1978). Effectiveness of widows' groups in facilitating change. *Journal of Consulting and Clinical Psychology, 46*, 20–31.

Bartrop, R.W. (1977). Depressed lymphocyte function after bereavement. *Lancet, 1*(801b), 834–836.

Baum, M., & Baum, R.C. (1980). *Growing old: A societal perspective*. Englewood Cliffs, NJ: Prentice-Hall, Inc.

Becker, E. (1973). *The denial of death*. New York: Free Press.

Berezin, M.A. (1972). Psychotherapy for the aged. *Journal of Geriatric Psychiatry, 4*, 34–45.

Berman, A.L., & Hays, J.E. (1973). Relationship between death anxiety, belief in after life and locus of control. *Journal of Consulting and Clinical Psychology, 41*, 318–326.

Blazer, D.G. (1982). *Depression in late life*. St. Louis: C.V. Mosby Co.

Bornstein, P.E., Clayton, P.J., Halikas, J.A., Maurice, W.L., & Robins, E. (1973). The depression of widowhood after thirteen months. *British Journal of Psychiatry, 122*, 561–566.

Brotman, H. (1973). Who are the aging? In E.W. Busse & E. Pfeiffer (Eds.), *Mental illness in later life* (pp. 19–41). Washington: American Psychiatric Association.

Burnside, I.M. (1969). Grief work in the aged patient. *Nursing Forum, 8*, 416–427.

Butler, R.N. (1963). The life review: An interpretation of reminiscence in the aged. *Psychiatry, 26*, 65–76.

Carey, R.G. (1977). The widowed: A year later. *Journal of Counseling Psychology, 24*, 125–131.

Cavan, R.S., Burgess, E.W., Havighurst, R., & Goldhammer, H. (1949). *Personal adjustment in old age*. Chicago: Science Research Associates.

Clayton, P.J. (1979). The sequelae and nonsequelae of conjugal bereavement. *American Journal of Psychiatry, 136*, 1530–1534.

Clayton, P.J., Halikas, J.A., & Maurice, W.L. (1971). The bereavement of the widowed. *Diseases of the Nervous System, 32*, 597–604.

Cox, P.R., & Ford, J.R. (1964). The mortality of widows shortly after widowhood. *Lancet, 1*, 163.

Cumming, E., & Henry, W.E. (1961). *Growing old: The process of disengagement*. New York: Basic Books.

Deutsch, H. (1937). Absence of grief. *Psychoanalytic Quarterly, 6*, 12–22.

Diagnostic and Statistical Manual of Mental Disorders (DSM-III), (1980). Washington: American Psychiatric Association.

Dickstein, L.S. (1975a). Death concern: Measurement and correlates. *Psychological Reports, 37*, 563–571.

Dickstein, L.S. (1975b). Self-report and fantasy: Correlates of death concern. *Psychological Reports, 37*, 147–158.

Eissler, K.R. (1955). *The psychiatrist and the dying patient*. New York: International Universities Press.

Engel, G.L. (1961). Is grief a disease? A challenge for medical research. *Psychosomatic Medicine, 23*, 18–22.

Feifel, H., & Jones, R. (1968). Perception of death as related to nearness of death. *Proceedings of the 76th Annual Convention of the American Psychological Association, 3*, 545–546.

Fulton, R., & Gottesman, D.J. (1980). A psychosocial concept reconsidered. *British Journal of Psychiatry, 137*, 45–54.

Glick, I.O., Weiss, R.S., & Parkes, C.M. (1974). *The first year of bereavement.* New York: John Wiley & Sons, Inc.

Goldfarb, A.I. (1974). Minor maladjustments of the aged. In S. Arieti (Ed.), *American handbook of psychiatry* (Vol. 3, pp. 820–860). New York: Basic Books.

Heyman, D.K., & Gianturco, D.T. (1973). Long-term adaptation by the elderly to bereavement. *Journal of Gerontology, 28*, 359–362.

Hinton, J. (1963). The physical and mental distress of the dying. *Quarterly Journal of Medicine, 32*, 1–21.

Isaacs, B., Gunn, J., McKechan, A., McMillan, I., & Neville, Y. (1971). The concept of pre-death. *Lancet, 1*, 1115.

Jacobs, S., & Douglas, L. (1979). Grief: A mediating process between a loss and illness. *Comprehensive Psychiatry, 20*, 165–176.

Jacobs, S., & Ostfeld, A. (1977). An epidemiologic review of the mortality of bereavement. *Psychosomatic Medicine, 39*, 344–357.

Jeffers, F.C., Nichols, C.R., & Eisdorfer, C. (1961). Attitudes of older persons toward death: A preliminary study. *Journal of Gerontology, 16*, 53–56.

Jeffers, F.C., & Verwoerdt, A. (1968a). How the old face death. In E.W. Busse & E. Pfeiffer (Eds.), *Behavior and adaptation in late life* (pp. 163–181). Boston: Little, Brown & Co.

Jeffers, F.C., & Verwoerdt, A. (1968b). Factors associated with the frequency of death thoughts in the elderly community volunteers. *Proceedings of the Seventh International Congress of Gerontology, 6*, 149. Vienna.

Kalish, R.A. (1976). Death and dying in a social context. In R. Binstock & E. Shanas (Eds.), *Handbook of aging and the social sciences* (pp. 483–507). New York: Van Nostrand Reinhold Co.

Kalish, R.A., & Reynolds, D.K. (1976). *Death and ethnicity: A psychocultural study.* Los Angeles: University of Southern California Press.

Karasu, T.B., & Waltzman, S.A. (1976). Death and dying in the aged. In L. Bellak & T.B. Karasu (Eds.), *Geriatric psychiatry* (pp. 247–278). New York: Grune & Stratton.

Kastenbaum, R. (1966). As the clock runs out. *Mental Hygiene, 50*, 322–326.

Kastenbaum, R. (1967). The mental life of dying geriatric patients. *Gerontologist, 7*, 97–100.

Kastenbaum, R. (1969). Death and bereavement in later life. In A.H. Kutcher (Ed.), *Death and bereavement* (pp. 163–181). Springfield, IL: Charles C Thomas.

Kastenbaum, R. (1971). Age: Getting there on time. *Psychology Today, 5*, 52–54, 82–84.

Kastenbaum, R., & Aisenberg, R. (1972). *The psychology of death.* New York: Springer-Verlag.

Kastenbaum, R., & Costa, P.T. (1977). Psychological perspectives on death. *Annual Review of Psychology, 28*, 225–249.

Kastenbaum, R., & Weisman, A.D. (1969). The psychological autopsy as a research procedure in gerontology. In D.P. Kent, R. Kastenbaum, & S. Sherwood (Eds.), *Research, planning and action for the aged: The power and potential of the social sciences* (pp. 183–195). New York: Behavioral Publications.

Katz, J.L., & Gardner, R. (1972). The intern's dilemma: The request for autopsy consent. *Psychiatry in Medicine, 31*, 197–203.

Krant, M. (1974). *Dying and dignity: The meaning and control of a personal death.* Springfield, IL: Charles C Thomas.

Kübler-Ross, E. (1969). *On death and dying.* New York: Macmillan.

Kübler-Ross, E. (1970). The dying patient's point-of-view. In O.G. Brim, H.E. Freeman, S. Levine, & N.A. Scotch (Eds.), *The dying patient* (pp. 156–170). New York: Russell Sage Foundation.

Lieberman, M. (1966). Observations on death and dying. *Gerontologist, 2*, 70–72.

Lindemann, E. (1944). Symptomatology and management of acute grief. *American Journal of Psychiatry, 10*, 141–148.

Lindemann, E. (1976). Grief and grief management: Some reflections. *Journal of Pastoral Care, 39*, 198–207.

Lowenthal, M.F., & Haven, C. (1968). Interaction and adaptation: Intimacy as a critical variable. *American Sociological Review, 33*, 20–30.

Maddox, G. (1963). Activity and morale: A longitudinal study of selected elderly subjects. *Social Forces, 42*, 195–212.

Maier, D.M. (1979). The conspiracy of silence and the denial of death: A cross cultural examination. In A. deVries & A. Carmi (Eds.), *The dying human* (pp. 89–95). Tel Aviv: Turtledove Publishing Co.

Myers, J.E., Murphey, M., & Riker, H.C. (1981). Mental health needs of older persons. Identifying at-risk populations. *American Mental Health Counselors Association Journal, 3*, 53–61.

Norton, J. (1963). The treatment of a dying patient. *Psychoanalytic Study of the Child, 18*, 541–560.

Parkes, C.M. (1970). The first year of bereavement. *Psychiatry, 33*, 444–467.

Peterson, J.A. (1980). Social–psychological aspects of death and dying and mental health. In J.R. Birren & R.B. Sloane (Eds.), *Handbook of mental health and aging* (pp. 922–942). Englewood Cliffs, NJ: Prentice-Hall, Inc.

Pfeiffer, E. (1980). The psychosocial evaluation of the elderly patient. In E.W. Busse & D.G. Blazer (Eds.), *Handbook of geriatric psychiatry* (pp. 275–284). New York: Van Nostrand Reinhold Co.

Preston, C.W., & Williams, R.H. (1971). Views of the aged on the timing of death. *Gerontologist, 11*, 300–304.

Riley, J. (1970). What people think about death. In O.G. Brim, H.E. Freeman, S. Levine, & N.A. Scotch (Eds.), *The dying patient* (pp. 30–41). New York: Russell Sage Foundation.

Riley, M.W. (1968). Attitudes toward death. In M.W. Riley, A. Foner & associates (Eds.), *Aging and society, Vol. I: An inventory of research findings* (pp. 332–337). New York: Russell Sage Foundation.

Seligman, M.E.P. (1975). *Helplessness: On depression, development and death*. San Francisco: W.H. Freeman.

Shands, H. (1955). An outline of the process of recovery from severe trauma. *AMA Archives of Neurology and Psychiatry, 13*, 401–409.

Shneidman, E.S. (1970, August). You and death. *Psychology Today*, pp. 67–72.

Silverman, P.R. (1972). Intervention with the widow of a suicide. In A.C. Cain (Ed.), *Survivors of suicide* (pp. 186–214). Springfield, IL: Charles C Thomas.

Silverman, P. (1977). Widowhood and preventive intervention. In S.H. Zarit (Ed.), *Readings in aging and death: Contemporary perspectives* (pp. 175–182). New York: Harper & Row.

Skelskie, B.E. (1975). An exploratory study of grief in old age. *Smith College Studies in Social Work, 45*, 159–182.

Sobel, E.F. (1980). Anxiety and stress in later life. In I.L. Kutash, L.B. Schlesinger & associates (Eds.), *Handbook of stress and anxiety* (pp. 317–328). San Francisco: Jossey-Bass.

Spikes, J. (1980). Grief, death and dying. In E.W. Busse & D.G. Blazer (Eds.), *Handbook of geriatric psychiatry* (pp. 415–426). New York: Van Nostrand Reinhold Co.

Stone, L.O., & Fletcher, S. (1981). *Aspects of population aging in Canada*. Ottawa, Canada: National Advisory Council on Aging.

Swenson, W.M. (1961). Attitudes toward death in an aged population. *Journal of Gerontology, 16*, 49–52.

Switzer, D.K. (1970). *Dynamics of grief: Its sources, pain and healing*. Nashville: Abingdon.

Verwoerdt, A. (1976). *Clinical geropsychiatry*. Baltimore: Williams & Wilkins.

Wahl, C.W. (1979). The differential diagnosis of normal and neurotic grief following bereavement. *Psychosomatics, 10*, 104–106.

Wass, H. (1979). Death and the elderly. In H. Wass (Ed.), *Dying—Facing the Facts* (pp. 182–207). New York: Hemisphere & McGraw-Hill.

Wass, H., & Myers, J.E. (1982). Psychosocial aspects of death among the elderly: A review of the literature. *Personnel and Guidance Journal, 61*(3), 131–137.

Wass, H., & Sisler, H.H. (1979). Death concern and views on various aspects of dying among elderly persons. In A. deVries & A. Carmi (Eds.), *The dying human* (pp. 71–86). Tel Aviv: Turtledove Publishing Co.

Weisman, A.D. (1974). Care and comfort for the dying. In S. Troup & W. Greene (Eds.), *The patient, death and the family* (pp. 97–111). New York: Scribner's.

Weisman, A.D., & Kastenbaum, R. (1968). The psychological autopsy: A study of the terminal phase of life. *Community Mental Health Journal Monograph Series*, Monograph 4, (pp. 1–64).

Zarit, S.H. (1980). *Aging and mental disorders: Psychological approaches to assessment and treatment*. New York: Free Press.

Chapter 10

Group Therapy and Group Intervention with the Elderly

In most approaches to psychotherapy of the aged there is the implicit assumption that by bringing groups and families together the system of communications with elderly members of the community can be improved. Thus, the group and family approach to intervention incorporates important aspects of relationships, family ties, and group cohesiveness. The assumption is that these approaches will effectively counter age-related isolation, loneliness, and feelings of abandonment so frequently experienced in late life. This chapter reviews major approaches to group intervention and discusses fundamental implications and applications for caregivers and practitioners working with the elderly persons.

GROUP THERAPY

The application of theory and research connected with group work with the elderly is not new. Since 1970 the use of group work with elderly populations has increased considerably (Burnside, 1978; Goldfarb, 1971; Lewis & Butler, 1974; Mayadas & Hink, 1974; Petty, Moeller, & Campbell, 1976). Groups having many different goals including remotivation, socialization, psychotherapy, reality orientation, and bereavement, have been described. However, as Zarit (1980) observes, one of the major problems of existing group work studies is the lack of clarity of goals. The helping properties of specific treatment programs are usually not spelled out in detail and not measured. Most groups of elderly described in the literature emphasize the improvement or reinstatement of social skills in institutionalized elderly, but as recognized by practitioners working in community settings, goals of behavior established for group work in institutional settings are quite different from those goals set for community settings. Groups reframed within various conceptual models have been described, including psychoanalytic, interpersonal, behavioral, and cognitive frameworks. Procedures have focused on feelings, social behaviors, interpersonal skills, life review, and reminiscences. The practitioner should be aware that these classification schemes are not entirely satisfactory. In many instances group therapy for the elderly, not unlike individual psychotherapy, is an eclectic combination of theories and successful procedures and strategies.

Although the usefulness of group intervention and group therapy with the elderly is well recognized, counselors and therapists have not been exposed to any systematic training for applying technique and process. Furthermore, work with the elderly has been largely atheoretical and has therefore failed to incorporate important concepts of treatment modalities or to assess the relative efficacy of different theoretical approaches and contrasting paradigms. Current group therapies with the aged encompass a broad theoretical spectrum of approaches ranging from the here-and-now groups to others that stress the past or emphasize prospects of the future.

This chapter reviews major concepts of group therapy approaches including behavioral, cognitive, and psychodynamic approaches. The discussion focuses on group types and methods. Special problems of goals for group work with the aged are considered, and the implications for gerontological counselors and therapists are explored.

Group Work and Aging

Burnside (1970) notes that group therapy has been utilized mainly with patients in hospitals and institutions, but the potential for outpatient treatment of older persons functioning in the communities has not been sufficiently explored through group work. These are the persons who are often overlooked in their struggle to adapt to a number of changes inherent in the transition from an active life to a qualitatively dependent life style (Mayadas & Hink, 1974) and who end up functioning at a minimal level of adequacy. In group work there is a preponderant focus on the elderly's adjustment to institutional life and a dire lack of attention to the adaptation of 95 percent of the elderly population living in communities. As Butler (1976) notes, in our therapeutic programs for the elderly we need to bear in mind a basic standard of community health and not be dominated by stereotypes of old-age psychopathology, disorientation, and institutional living.

In group therapy the dichotomy of task versus growth has long permeated typological classification. While such a dichotomy has been useful in its simplicity, it has been unsuccessful in reflecting or capturing the many subtleties that exist in practice. It has been suggested that the elderly are less capable of growth-oriented activities, but group or individual work that teaches them concrete coping skills and tasks has a wider appeal. Papell and Rothman (1966) have proposed three models of group work that have particular relevance to group therapy and intervention with the elderly. Potential benefits and positive outcomes of group interventions are summarized in Table 10–1.

Social Model

This model assumes a unity between social action and individual psychological health. The assumption is that individuals need opportunity and assistance in revitalizing their energies in order to make a social contribution. Such a model would have a wide appeal for many elderly who believe that they are important citizens and have important citizen roles. The orientation of the social model toward creating skilled citizenry and responsible social consciousness seems most appropriate for developmental work with the elderly. As Lowy (1979) notes, this model implies that the elderly are capable of meaningful activity directed toward social change. The suggestion is that the elderly do not need benign protectors and providers in society or in the social groups and that they are fully capable of achieving group identification around social and community issues. Based on the idea that the elderly are well-functioning individuals with ability to manage their own affairs, the emphasis in group work may be on community interests, community issues, and discussion of leadership roles. Recreational play work in a group would be considered a sinful waste in this model.

Table 10–1 Potential Benefits and Positive Outcomes of Group Work with Elderly Clients

Social Model Groups	Remedial Model Groups	Reciprocal Model Groups
Opportunities for elderly individuals to participate in meaningful activities directed toward social change and enhancing social consciousness	Areas identified in which elderly individuals have deficits and dysfunctions; group activity directed toward redressing problems and remediating deficits	Help of group members to one another in the enhancement of their day-to-day functioning, insight, and reciprocal support and reinforcement
Emphasis on promoting leadership roles by orienting group activity toward community interests and community issues	Greatest benefit to elderly clients in hospital and institutional settings	Greatest benefit to elderly clients in community settings
Greatest benefit to elderly clients in community settings		

Curative Factors and Ameliorative Effects of Group Work on Elderly Clients

1. Usefulness for imparting practical and educational information of relevance to groups of elderly clients

2. Self-esteem enhancement

3. Development and enhancement of resocialization and remotivation through group programs aimed at changing self-attitudes and self-image and enhancing self-controls and independent functioning

4. Opportunity for emotional catharsis (i.e., emotional release of feelings of guilt, self-pity, rejection, or anger generated in day-to-day functioning) through communication with group members

5. Expression of existential concerns (e.g., bereavement, loss of spouse, loss of affiliation)

6. Learning of new social relationships and social skills not in the client's existing behavioral repertoire or relearning of lost social skills through observation of group members and through group feedback

Remedial Model

This model establishes a contract for therapy and treatment. Group members are seen in more unhealthy light and with problems that must be redressed and deficits that must be remediated. The goals of the group are for members to help one another get better, and the role of the therapist is to be the protector and counselor who knows what is the best treatment for the group members. Lowy (1979) notes that the remedial model of group work reinforces the view that aging is a form of decline and illness; it emphasizes pathology rather than health and is more appropriate for institutional settings and hospitals. Lowy cautions that while treatment and therapy may be important for some elderly, the therapist would have to be careful not to impose this model when a great majority of the elderly are in fact able to function autonomously and independently (p. 304).

Reciprocal Model

Like the social model, the reciprocal model assumes a fusion between individual psychological health and group enhancement. It views the individual and group in symbiotic interaction and works from the premise that group interactions invariably have a healthy focus. There are no preconceived therapeutic goals and objectives, and therefore no goals of desired outcomes are specified. Individual members may recognize that they have problems and conflicts and may engage group members in a discussion of these problems and difficulties. The goals of group members therefore become defined during the group process, as individuals raise issues of concern or interest. Group members engage in interpersonal relations for problem resolutions. The therapist, as a member of the group, may share in this group process and offers insights that are complementary. Unique demands may be placed on the group therapist who works with older adults. Feil (1967) reported that before group interaction could be achieved, she had to develop a relationship with each individual in the group. In the early period of therapy, she was often called upon to serve as moderator, encourager of free expression, sympathetic authority, and an integrator. Therefore, the therapist's major function is the creation of conditions that allow for reciprocity, mutual trust, and acceptance.

This model advances programs for the aged that go beyond the leader playing the role of physician and clinician. These programs attempt to fill the general goals of searching out common ground between needs of members. Members are seen in a healthy light: they are seen as able to function autonomously and independently. The model allows the elderly to exercise a sense of control and mastery. Such a model, when implemented, has a wide appeal for community elders who formulate their own goals in an existential desire to fulfill their needs for self-esteem.

In choosing a group work model, the nature of the setting (whether institutional, community, or residential) and the preponderant needs of the people will determine which model is most appropriate. The current practice is for institutional settings to focus on the remedial model and for community settings to focus on the reciprocal or social model. Groups of older adults are found in different settings and at different stages of personal control and functioning. The fundamental needs of the members for remedial skills or creative social activity will determine how the group moves along and how the needs of the individual person can be best met in the group. Since the group processes used in the various types of groups are not mutually exclusive, groups may use different models at different stages. One model may be used as a beneficial adjunct to another. As a group member advances from the remedial group, the person may proceed to develop and integrate into a group with a reciprocal and social focus (Lowy, 1979).

Loneliness, isolation, and rejection are conditions often associated with the process of aging. These conditions, stemming from a myriad of sources, give rise to a high incidence of depression and suicide among the community elderly (Capuzzi & Gross, 1980). Apathy, withdrawal, and paranoid tendencies are also likely to be found in the community elderly obscurely hidden away in their private lodgings. Although little empirical knowledge exists about the adaptation patterns of this category of the aged, there is general evidence to indicate that group treatment of older persons has great potential for offering supportive and socializing experiences and for leading to new learning to overcome specific difficulties (Zarit, 1980). Mayadas and Hink (1974) postulate that group therapy can benefit the elderly in adjusting to an entire range of life styles regardless of whether intervention is instituted at the time of a particular crisis or when concerns about aging and adaptation first begin to develop.

GOALS FOR GROUP WORK WITH THE ELDERLY

According to Goldfarb (1971) group therapy is the use of group methods and activities to encourage personal activity, sociability, and social integration of the individual member. The range of group approaches used with old persons goes from motivational through recreational and vocational to physiotherapeutic. Thus one view is that group therapy is the provision of a "beneficial controlled life experience within a group setting by the establishment of relationships with the leader or interaction with group members, or both, together with some clarification of one's motives and those of others in the interaction" (Goldfarb, 1971, p. 624). Group therapy, because of its diversity, can do many things for many people but not necessarily the same things for all the people helped. In this regard the treatment properties are similar for both individuals and groups. The one critical difference between individual psychotherapy and group treatment, however, is that the latter uses specific properties of the group experience to mediate and effect changes (Yalom, 1975; Hartford, 1978).

According to Zarit (1980) an appropriate objective of psychotherapy groups (as differentiated from general groups) is to effect some change in behavior, feelings, or attitudes of group members. Zarit suggests that these groups will not only provide the stimulation or socialized experiences of unfocused groups but will also intervene in specific problems of clients in the group.

Curative Factors and Ameliorative Effects through Group Work

Yalom (1975) has identified a number of curative factors or treatment properties of groups, most of which are reviewed here. Some of these treatment properties have greater applicability to goals of group therapy in institutional settings while others would be more appropriate for outpatient settings (see Table 10–1 for a summary of the ameliorative effects of group activity on the elderly).

Imparting of Information

At a minimal therapeutic level the first curative factor of the group is its usefulness for imparting information (Yalom, 1975). In both hospital settings and outpatient settings groups can be used for the dissemination of information concerning medications, social policy, recreational benefits, and occupational services available to the elderly. This type of information can be imparted both from the therapist to group members and among the group members themselves. At a maximal therapeutic level Yalom considers the two most important curative factors in groups to be the opportunity for interpersonal learning and the instillation of hope. Both these curative features of groups have special implications for group psychotherapy with the elderly. These features provide a framework within which a redefinition of social identity of the elderly is more easily possible. Unger and Kramer (1968) note that the elderly, more than any other age group, have a greater tendency to overemphasize their faults and to make more limited appraisals of their strengths. Hence groups can provide the opportunity to observe other peers and receive feedback about one's interpersonal behaviors.

Lowy (1961) has commented that the elderly attain a state of high anxiety because of society's lack of involvement in them and because of subjection to many losses, role discontinuities, and role reversals. The old suffer self-depreciation and depreciation by others, and they have few opportunities to increase their awareness about their interpersonal behaviors. This problem can be summarized as limited opportunity for role performance (Unger & Kramer, 1968, p. 52).

Self-Esteem Enhancement

Thus in terms of general treatment goals for group therapy, a number of authors (e.g., Brudno & Seltzer, 1968; Unger & Kramer, 1968; Toepfer, Bicknell, & Shaw, 1974) advocate the planning of group programs that would increase the elderly's self-esteem and convictions about their contributive value to others and emphasize replacement of the roleless status by teaching new modes of functioning. A treatment model that stresses the significance of learning new social skills or relearning lost skills through observing and modifying the communications of the elderly members is most valuable to both community centers, housing for the aged, and other residential centers. It is possible to create a climate of trust and acceptance in a group setting in which both inpatient and outpatient elderly can learn more about their own interpersonal behaviors. In order to accomplish this goal, Toepfer, Bicknell, and Shaw (1974) stress the use of remotivation behavioral therapy groups. Brudno and Seltzer (1968) advocate group programs of resocialization therapy for effecting change in the elderly's attitudes toward themselves, toward their own passivity, their self-image, and familial relationships.

Both in outpatient and inpatient elderly the planning of such programs for individuals who function as isolates and who accept inactivity as they grow older or decline in physical strength, lends itself to creative proposals and therapeutic goals. Yalom (1975) notes that one of the curative features of such groups is that they can lead to a sense of universality. Participants discover that they are not unique in their situations. Elderly individuals having psychological problems of enforced dependency often change life patterns of handling interactions with others. Frequently resistance or fighting puts a great strain on already depleted strengths and results in the paralysis of the will. There is little or no attempt at voluntary interchange among the elderly themselves. While they seem to be responding to similar stress and in a similar fashion, there is limited spontaneous formation of groups in the community where attitudes, feelings, and fears can be shared. Thus the provision of group experiences serves to establish ties to other persons and counters the phenomenon of parallel adjustment or maladjustment among the elderly with similar but individual difficulties.

Remotivation and Resocialization Enhancement

Techniques of using remotivation and resocialization group psychotherapy with the elderly can include group discussion and recreation as reinforcers of self-worth and role identity. The curative factor in such group psychotherapy is that the experience can instill hope in clients (Yalom, 1975). Seeing other elderly coping well with similar problems or observing them improve in familial relationships or self-management over the course of sessions can instill hope, self-confidence, and assurance that change is possible. In old age there can also exist other subtle problems in self-definition such as a general feeling of lack of purpose or direction. The group therapist must be alert to the elderly individuals' behavioral cues that suggest role ambiguity and thus help them in enhancing self-esteem through group experiences providing new but relevant and purposive role behaviors. Mayadas and Hink (1974) suggest purposive roles such as foster grandparents, friendly visitors and companions, and volunteer workers. Remotivation, resocialization, and personal identity enhancement groups all have their place and value. However, we need to recognize that the way these group experiences are organized will depend on the style of the therapist's leadership and theoretical preferences. The therapist's theoretical preferences will determine whether the focus will be on behavioral change, cognitive change, or both. Some therapists may stress the here-and-now interactions (Rose, 1977) while others may focus on the there-and-then interactions (Butler, 1976).

Emotional Catharsis

Yalom (1975) considers two other curative dimensions that may have value and significance in some groups of elderly. One is the opportunity for emotional catharsis or the expression of emotions. The fact that many elderly are basically alone in encountering the difficulties in their day-to-day functioning suggests a gradual degeneration into long-term feelings of self-pity, guilt, and failure. Feil (1967), for example, noted suppressed feelings of hostility, submissiveness, and passivity toward family members and institutional staff in many elderly clients. Fearful of deteriorating and full of feelings of rejection and utter loss, many elderly resigned themselves to being dependent, yet felt guilty, angry, and ambivalent.

Yalom (1975) considers emotional release the most vital ingredient to change and successful adaptation of such group members. Viewing group therapy as an opportunity for emotional catharsis, Lieberman, Yalom, and Miles (1973) advocate emotional expression of fears and anxieties and negative feelings about family members through communications among group members. Because of the emphasis on the body as well as the mind, emotional catharsis groups make use of a wide variety of sensory and nonverbal exercises (attention to posture, facial expressions, movement of hands and feet) emphasizing body awareness and synchronization of body and emotions. The purpose of these catharsis groups is to remove mental blocks and depression caused by physical illness, emotional trauma, or crisis. The emphasis is on the integration of the physical, psychological and emotional aspects of the person. Luce (1979) compares these groups to the modern encounter groups especially designed for the elderly (senior actualization and growth experience (SAGE)) which are predicated on the premise that "there is a definite purpose to old age," "that many of the ailments of old age are reversible," "emancipation is necessary from the inhibitions and habits learned in childhood," "old age should be a time of truth" (Luce, 1979, pp. 7–8). One unique component of the SAGE program intended to provide emotional catharsis is its consideration of topics related to grief, bereavement, death and dying. Rather than denying grief and death, elderly participants are encouraged to express their emotions and feelings. Because the SAGE program is new, only one study (Lieberman & Gourash, 1979) evaluating its effectiveness has been reported. Elderly outpatients who participated in these groups were significantly less depressed and had greater self-esteem after the group experience.

Few gerontologists are unequivocally optimistic about this focus on emotional encounter in the face of old-age retrenchment, loss and regression. While such communications are generally therapeutic, Zarit (1980) cautions that leaders who overemphasize confrontation, encounter, and emotional release of hostility and bitterness in elderly group members are likely to cause harm to some participants whose social milieu is fixed and unadaptive. However, groups with the most positive changes were those with both emotional expression and learning of new social relationships and interactions (Lieberman, Yalom, & Miles, 1973).

Expression of Existential Concerns

Another curative factor that may have important significance for group therapy with the elderly pertains to their existential concerns. These include dealing with bereavement, loss of spouse, loss of home, and loss of work and affiliations. Other existential concerns include dealing with the inevitability of death and the elderly persons' sense of futility about their present, past, and future prospects. Empirical studies (e.g., Fry, 1983; Pincus, 1970) found reminiscing a viable tool in helping the elderly cope with feelings of hopelessness and anomie by revitalizing their past sense of esteem. A number of therapists (e.g., Butler, 1976; Lewis & Butler, 1974; Pincus, 1970) have discussed the value of life review and reminiscence as a group psychotherapy procedure for putting memories to work. The opportunity to interact freely with other elderly cohorts and to share memories in a supportive environment may be a crucial element in strengthening the older person's abilities to accept the present (Ingersoll & Silverman, 1978).

Studies in small group research with the elderly report several successful attempts in psychotherapy groups that have incorporated curative dimensions. Finkel and Fillmore (1971) observed that a group of older persons served as a socializing and motivating agent for other elders who had been socially isolated. Other group procedures such as role playing enhanced self-esteem of some elderly (Rose, 1977).

Group treatment programs concentrating on helping older persons to become more communicative and less agitated have been quite successful with elderly clients (see Petty, Moeller, & Campbell, 1976). Such groups have been successful in utilizing problem-solving skills training and rational discussion with the elderly. However, many of these programs showing rehabilitation potential have been tried and tested among institutionalized elderly only. In these settings, group therapy has been offered to old persons whose psychiatric, physical, and social problems cover a wide range of psychopathology. Therefore goals and leadership styles have varied considerably. Treatment procedures may proceed quite differently among community elderly, where group structure and group techniques must be adapted to well-functioning elderly clients with a wide range of psychosocial characteristics. Group processes and outreach strategies may have to be adapted to elderly persons who have had little experience in reaching out to obtain supportive services. Groups with specific goals that meet immediate emotional or activity needs have potentially wide appeal to the community elderly and can have beneficial effects in both community and institutional settings.

GROUP TYPES AND METHODS

In assessing various types of groups that have been successful or shown potential with the elderly, Ingersoll and Silverman (1978) have reviewed group modalities in terms of two basic paradigms: the here-and-now paradigm and the there-and-then paradigm. While they overlap in several respects, for purposes of simplicity the two paradigms are discussed separately in terms of their objectives and the types of group processes which are emphasized. Table 10–2 presents an overview of the major types of groups of immediate and long-term relevance to the improvement and growth of the elderly.

Here-and-Now Paradigm

This paradigm takes the position that the immediate present of the client is the most important component in therapy. Focusing on the past or on future issues and concerns is avoidance of the present and therefore antitherapeutic (Harper, Bauer, & Kommarkat, 1976). The here-and-now model, when applied to the elderly, postulates that by focusing on present problems and offering specific pragmatic help, therapy can decrease anxiety, enhance self-esteem, and alleviate somatic complaints (Ingersoll & Silverman, 1978). This model is based on principles of learning theory and advocates behavioral techniques and behavioral methodology. The focus is twofold: (1) helping the client to cope with anxiety stemming from recent life changes and life events and (2) helping the client to achieve behavioral change and new skills necessary to the performance of concrete activities and developmental tasks of old age.

In order to accomplish these two goals, the here-and-now model stresses a number of therapy components, some with wider applicability for clients in the community and others for clients in institutional settings. While this typology has been useful in its simplicity, it has not always captured existing subtleties and differentiation that exist in practice. However, some of the major characteristics, principal group processes, and strategies of the here-and-now paradigm are reflected in the workings of the following types of groups.

Behaviorally Oriented Management Groups

As opposed to reconstructive psychotherapy and insight-oriented groups, which are concerned with bringing about changes in feeling and thinking, the behaviorally oriented management groups are primarily concerned with the acquisition of behavioral skills and coping strategies. Some of these strategies follow.

Relaxation Training. Quite frequently, behaviorally oriented management groups will attract members who are simultaneously involved in other groups or individual psychotherapy and who have personal anxieties about aging and are depressed to varying degrees (Ingersoll & Silverman, 1978). Thus concepts of deep muscle relaxation and some practice in relaxation exercises are encouraged at the beginning of group work and at the start of each session. Berger and Berger (1972; 1973) noted that some elderly who were experiencing

Table 10–2 Major Types of Groups and Group Approaches

Here-and-Now Groups	There-and-Then Groups
Behaviorally oriented management groups designed to provide Relaxation training Assertion training Self-reinforcement and self-instructional training	Reminiscing groups that encourage elderly to review past accomplishments, past relationships, and past experiences with a view to developing group appreciation and group integration of the richness of the members' lives
Relationship building and communications training groups designed to develop Relationship skills and coping skills Interpersonal effectiveness Effective communications in an atmosphere of group support, acceptance, and regard	Group therapy for depression, groups focusing on Expressive therapy Age-related life-crisis therapy Cognitive therapy for depression (group feedback in cognitive restructuring, cognitive appraisals, self-instructional strategies, self-management of depression)
Reality orientation training groups designed to Assist elderly who are partially disoriented with respect to time, place, people, and objects to regain contact with reality Assist elderly who are isolated and withdrawn to regain social and personal contacts with group members	
Remotivation groups designed to Stimulate and revitalize individuals who have lost interest, motivation, and involvement in their surroundings	
Socialization groups designed to Help shy and timid elderly to practice their social skills through group discussion with members of similar interest, educational attainment, and social background	

insomnia, hypertension, and tension headaches found satisfaction and release in tension by merely participating in relaxation therapy. Relaxation has also been used as a part of a program in treating chronic pain (Beers & Karoly, 1979).

The major emphasis is on developing awareness of body tension and on training in progressive relaxation (Bernstein & Borkovec, 1973). Ingersoll and Silverman (1978) identified 16 muscle groups in different parts of the body (e.g., hands, biceps, triceps, shoulders, neck, head, chest, abdomen, back, mouth, eyes, buttocks, etc.) that are important to body relaxation. Exercises were designed for relaxing each of the muscle groups. Their group therapy clients were trained to relax these muscle groups using a tension-release sequence.

To facilitate individual home practice, members practice relaxation as a group, discuss their difficulties in relaxing certain muscle groups, and then follow a standard listing of the sequence of relaxation steps. One way of explaining differences in the tension level of individual members is to demonstrate that individuals tend to feel tension in different parts of the body. Some persons may feel tension in their abdomen, while others experience it in their shoulders, neck, or back. A particular client may then be asked to monitor tension and to identify the part of the body where tension is felt.

In training clients for relaxation techniques, the group format may be used. The therapist or counselor should ensure that the subjects are in comfortable chairs, have loosened their clothing, with no distracting sounds or glaring lights. The therapist can then instruct the group members to close their eyes and to relax each set of muscles identified in the progressive relaxation program. To gain maximum benefit, each given muscle is tensed for periods of about 10 seconds followed by a relaxation period of 15 seconds. Subjects are urged to concentrate on tensing a given muscle and as far as possible to keep all other muscles relaxed. At the end of an exercise the therapist can instruct clients to focus on a pleasant scene or image while maintaining relaxation in their muscles.

Subjects are taught to monitor feelings of tension and relaxation, and through relaxation exercises they are taught to discriminate better between feelings of anxiety and relaxation. In this way the training helps individuals to identify those situations in which they feel the tension coming on. A particular client may be able to identify where tension is felt and can be taught to modify the relaxation procedure to focus more on the muscle groups that are most tense.

Clients in the group can be taught to bring the feelings of relaxation under voluntary control by pairing relaxation with cue words such as *calm* and *relax* (Paul & Bernstein, 1976) and they can subvocally instruct themselves to be calm or relaxed when they begin to feel anxious. The clients are instructed to take a deep breath, exhale, and say the cue word *relax* or *be calm*. Whenever the client experiences tension in the group setting either in talking or responding, the use of the cue word would help relieve the tension. This self-induced relaxation procedure can be used as an adjunct to other forms of treatment such as assertion training, memory training, or coping skills training.

Although a number of gerontologists have commented on the usefulness of relaxation training in assisting elderly cope with the anxieties of their day-to-day functioning, a number of cautions are necessary in the implementation of relaxation training. As Ingersoll and Silverman (1978) note, compared to middle-aged adults a longer period of training may be necessary to teach elderly people the entire relaxation procedures for the 16 sets of muscles. Due to the time-limited nature of the therapy programs generally advocated for the elderly, there is a risk that some elderly clients may become sensitized to their body tensions without being allowed sufficient time to learn and practice relaxation sequences that may gradually alleviate anxiety.

Most of the relaxation exercises have a calming effect similar to tranquilizers. For some elderly who have arthritis or back pains that would make the tensing of certain muscle groups painful, a medically supervised program of aerobic exercises would be a useful alternative to deep muscle relaxation. Training can be combined with biofeedback equipment, especially if elderly subjects are unable to differentiate between a state of relaxation and tension.

Commercial tapes of relaxation exercises are available and can be used during group sessions. The therapist can then be free to attend to clients' responses and to check whether clients look relaxed and are benefiting from the training. Specific forms of relaxation sequences may be inappropriate for certain elderly clients having specific physical disabilities or handicaps or certain medical and organic impairments or frailties. A medical clearance is advisable, especially for the elderly who have multiple medical problems.

Behavioral Contracts. Problems of some elderly can be dealt with through contracts whereby they undertake to increase their level of independent functioning and the frequency of satisfying activities in which they participated during the week. Members contract to review and record their charts of daily activities and discuss ways in which they could increase the frequency of highly satisfying activities.

Assertion Training. Petty, Moeller, and Campbell (1976) have reported that a majority of elderly experience difficulty in having their needs met because of their inability to assert themselves and to communicate their needs effectively. Thus the difficulty that many older persons experience in asking others for help when help is needed or in handling difficult demands made on them from adult children, relatives, and friends constitutes an increasingly important issue in group therapy. Unsatisfactory personal relationships, often of a longstanding nature, are not resolved because of the elderly's inability for behavioral confrontation. Assertive training can provide ways for aging individuals to express their feelings as they come up. This is a way to prevent depression because when put-downs or slights are countered, they are not internalized and do not eat away at the self-image (Wheeler, 1980). One health-related issue that is often of concern to many elderly clients is their relationship with their physician, specifically in terms of their difficulty in asking doctors questions about diseases and medication. Schwartz (1977) points out that all too often older persons feel they are treated in a patronizing manner in the physicians' offices, demeaned, or treated with indifference. While some old people will fight back, many others tend to lapse into senile or passive-dependent behaviors. In this connection Butler and Lewis (1977) describe the sense of helplessness that can occur in the elderly when they are ill or incapacitated. There is often inadequate emotional energy to be assertive and to deal with put-downs in an effective manner.

Thus a number of gerontologists (e.g., Tournier, 1972; Schwartz, 1977; Wheeler, 1980) believe that assertion training can be useful with a wide variety of target groups of the elderly. It is suggested that the elderly lack effective coping skills in many areas of their functioning such as in developing new friendships, in making their wishes and preferences known to others, and in refusing unreasonable requests. As a consequence, many elderly persons may harbor feelings of anger or resentment toward others or may feel self-pity over their inability to function competently.

Wheeler (1980) enumerates a number of reasons why the assertiveness training approach would have special appeal and relevance to older persons. First, group assertiveness training can be presented as the learning of new skills—a goal that is far less threatening than trying to achieve a change in one's basic personality. Assertiveness training does not carry the implication that the participant is sick or maladjusted, rather it suggests that one has to be firm and personally effective in order to get what one wants. Second, the approach sounds like common sense to many older people who are reluctant to join therapy groups or to articulate their feelings but who may have less difficulty in receiving training that helps them to deal in practical ways with day-to-day situations.

The focus of assertion training with the elderly is the development of behavioral responses that increase personal competency and involve the open and direct expression of feelings and preferences. Assertiveness is differentiated from unassertive behavior, whereby the person inhibits statements about feelings or preferences (Rimm & Masters, 1974) and is also distinguished from aggressive behavior that involves attempts to control and dominate others. Explaining these distinctions between aggressive and assertive behaviors is particularly important when working with groups of elderly, many of whom have had little experience in being assertive. Many individuals of today's cohort of aged persons have grown up with the beliefs that it is improper and impolite to be direct with others about one's feelings, preferences, or rights. Many older persons having stereotypic notions about old age may also believe that it is appropriate to be assertive only when one is young, energetic, and productive but that old age is a time for dependency and relative submissiveness to those in positions of authority and control. Such outmoded beliefs and values may often lead many older persons who once may have acted in assertive ways to behave passively after retirement or loss of role.

Unassertive beliefs are not a problem in and of themselves. However, in the case of many elderly, unassertive beliefs are accompanied by feelings of powerlessness and frustration with regard to several domains of daily functioning. These feelings are reflected in the complaints of many older persons that their doctors and physicians do not listen to them or do not treat them with enough respect. Similarly many elderly persons complain that their adult children ignore them or make excessive demands. When their relationship with the adult children is a problematic one, training in assertive skills may help them to recognize that they do not have to accede to the unreasonable demands of others, including demands made by friends and family members.

Older persons may hold other unassertive beliefs similar to those involving their relationship with authority. Many may feel that it is wrong or even disloyal to the family to reject the requests or needs of their children and relatives. Today's cohort of older persons were socialized to believe that it is important, at whatever the cost, to be useful, if not indispensable, to the family. Generally speaking they feel that if they are loyal and giving to their children, they can expect reciprocity. However, in the adult children's ideas about intergenerational relationships, reciprocity may not be necessary. Hence many older persons feel hurt or neglected because their children let them down and were not sufficiently conscientious in their efforts to help the elderly parents. Thus, assertion training when applied to the elderly has come to acquire two components of almost equal importance: (1) training and practice in assertive behaviors and (2) discussion of assertive rights of the elderly in the context of intergenerational relationships.

With regard to the first component of training, attention is focused on identifying situations and life circumstances of the elderly in which assertive behavior is appropriate. Since many elderly have histories of being unassertive in relationships with authority figures such as physicians, lawyers, or the police, assertion training may be appropriate for groups of elderly who feel uncomfortable, threatened, or anxious in interactions with authority. In assertion training they could be taught ways, for example, of preparing all the questions they want the physicians, lawyers, landlords, bureaucrats, or business people to answer. Clients may be encouraged to rehearse the questions and be persistent in getting the precise information they desire. Such training, when received with the help of other elderly cohorts, is associated with increased positive feelings and increased sense of competence.

Another area of functioning in which most elderly have histories of never having acted assertively is in asking direct requests or favors and making precisely clear what kind of assistance they would like from others. In assertion training sessions groups of elderly can be encouraged to articulate their needs and their preferences.

Assertion training requires the learning of new behaviors. In group sessions attention is given by the group first to the verbal and nonverbal aspects of the unassertive behavior and later to the verbal and nonverbal aspects of the newly acquired assertive behavior. Learning new assertive behaviors will often require behavioral rehearsal in the group setting and further practice through the use of homework assignments.

Other techniques that are often used to shape new behavioral patterns are modeling, whereby the therapist or other group members demonstrate the assertive role. Group reinforcement, praise, and encouragement for successive approximations of appropriate assertive responses is important to the successful shaping of assertive behaviors. Although many older persons are initially uncomfortable in role-playing assertive responses, particularly when these involve relationships with family members and close associates, they gradually begin to acknowledge the positive feelings that result from their assertive performance.

The following case is an example of how assertion training was used with an older client. Mrs. T. was a 75-year-old lady whose husband was confined to a wheelchair. She did most things for him and was reluctant to leave him alone even for brief intervals. Her daughters tended to dominate her and would bring their four young children over to be fed and taken care of. Mrs. T. had trouble expressing her feelings about the impositions that her daughters made on her time. She was also most concerned about her relationship with her husband, who demanded a lot of assistance.

The treatment plan involved the group members teaching Mrs. T. what to say to her daughters and her husband and how to express in assertive ways her personal needs for privacy. Mrs. T. practiced new behavioral and verbal responses until she felt confident that she would be able to reenact these behaviors in strong and assertive ways. The group members and group facilitator helped her to clarify some of the reasons and arguments she could use.

A second important component of assertion training and treatment involves a discussion and clarification of assertive rights (Smith, 1975; Lange & Jakubowski, 1976). More than any other age group, the elderly have difficulty in accepting that they are entitled to any rights in the institutions and settings in which they function. Lange and Jakubowski (1976) stress the importance of convincing unassertive elderly individuals that they have a number of fundamental personal rights, principally the right to respect from other people, the right to have personal needs, and the right to decide the extent to which they may articulate their own needs and respond to others' needs. Elderly persons, especially, need to be convinced that they have a right to their feelings (e.g., feeling tired, happy, angry, insulted) and the right to make their feelings known. Particularly in relationship to authority figures, elderly people need to believe that they have a right to form their own opinions and to act on them assertively.

In group settings, discussions of assertive rights are a stimulating way of reinforcing assertive belief systems in the elderly. Discussion of assertive beliefs involves a clarification of the importance of being assertive as differentiated from being polite and self-defeating. It is important also for the elderly to be convinced that assertive training is not intended to teach them to be manipulative, controlling, or aggressively persistent but to make them more confident about their personal beliefs and rights. Additionally it is important to emphasize that when first learning assertion techniques, most elderly will feel that they are behaving in ways that are self-centered, selfish, and impolite to others, but that ultimately assertion techniques will assist them in feeling more comfortable and competent in a variety of family and social relationships.

Assertiveness training groups for elders are different from those for younger adults in that they are structured to be only mildly confrontative. On the whole they do not attack defenses and are conducive to feelings of confidence, accomplishment, and growth (Wheeler, 1980, p. 17). Assertiveness can be taught in a number of ways. Initially elderly persons are encouarged to be assertive in limited ways with other equally unassertive partners. Sometimes group members are encouraged to talk about their accomplishments and achievements of the past or the immediate present. Members may be encouraged to share the put-downs that they may have experienced or are anticipating, and then the group models ways and means of countering them.

In clinical cases, assertion training (often labeled personal effectiveness training or self-enhancement training) can help older people counter put-downs and paranoid feelings, to stand up for their rights, and to accept aging without being forced to accept ageism. Assertion training appears to be a treatment of choice for aging people suffering losses and depression. If the depression is the result of a drop in reinforcers, a group for assertion training can be a transitional step from emotional withdrawal to building a new social network. Wheeler (1980) notes that when depression is interpreted as anger turned inward, assertion training can help the elderly person to direct the anger more appropriately toward the people in the social milieu who are blocking the creative energies of the individual. On the basis of techniques such as self-report, modeling, role playing, and leader observations, assertion training exercises, combined with self-awareness and self-esteem exercises, become a viable means of helping the elderly to counter internalized stereotypes, clinical syndromes of paranoid states, anhedonia, and hypochondriasis (Comfort, 1976; Butler & Lewis, 1977; Wheeler, 1980). By practicing more assertive roles in a group situation, the elderly learn to recognize more easily their masked depression and to alleviate their depressed and distressed feelings through assertive expression of their needs.

Reinforcement, Shaping, or Modeling Procedures. Persons can obtain reinforcements from other group members or can administer reinforcements to themselves by setting contingency contracts to receive something desirable when they reach a goal, or they may learn to provide self-reinforcements by appraising their own actions favorably when they move toward a goal (Rose, 1977). Sallis (1981) attested to the impact of behaviorally oriented management techniques on community elders who rated high on depression and anxiety. Sallis concluded that while on the whole the elderly respond less favorably to behavioral programs than do younger subjects, still the behaviorally oriented group (compared to other treatment groups) reported more success in anxiety and depression reduction.

Hussian and Lawrence (1981) note that the probability of adaptation behavior in the elderly can be maximized by teaching the elderly appropriate problem-attack behavioral or cognitive-behavioral skills. These authors recommend that when the natural contingencies cannot be easily manipulated by the moderately timid elderly, the perceived control can be cognitively enhanced. When the multiplicity of problematic situations is complex, the teaching of generalized skills might be an alternative tactic to contingency management. Among the more generalized skills that can be taught, relaxation training, goal setting, desensitization training for coping with fears and anxieties, and cognitive intervention have shown most promise with the elderly.

Describing a behaviorally oriented group, Rose (1977) stresses a number of extra measures that have specific relevance to the elderly. Principal among these are goal identification and formulation. The elderly client may need extra help from the therapist or group members in formulating specific goals especially in the initial stages of behavioral goal-setting and programming. Carefully designed homework assignments are useful in order for clients to generalize new behaviors from the therapy session to everyday situations. Success in completing homework assignments or monitoring behaviors may need more frequent reinforcement both by the therapist and participants in the group, as evidence of the person's improvement. Rose (1977) stresses the significance of heavy reinforcement of the initial small steps in implementing a behavioral program particularly when many elderly clients may not see the relationship between specific actions and their presenting problems. For example, a woman who is depressed because she has difficulty in refusing her daughter's requests for baby-sitting or other similar demands from her family may not understand the need for role playing in effectively refusing requests.

Several authors (e.g., Lowy, 1967; Rose, 1977) have emphasized the significance of planning behaviorally oriented assignments and interventions that deal with the immediate issues and immediate concerns of group members. Lowy (1967) notes that the reality needs of older members revolve around such basic concerns as income, health, family relationships, and social interactions. A behavioral focus on these actual situations and group attention to techniques and skills for coping with these problematic issues is important to older persons. Hoyer, Kafer, Simpson and Hoyer (1974) demonstrated that by using contingent reinforcement to increase verbalization several noncommunicative elderly schizophrenics became more reality oriented. Using a stimulus control procedure older insomniacs reduced the time taken to fall asleep (Puder, Lacks, Bertelson, & Storandt, 1982). The leader's major task is to reformulate these general concerns of group participants into specific behaviors and set goals for the learning and mastery of these behaviors.

Relationship Building and Communications Training

After achieving a certain amount of skill in relaxation training and assertion training, the clients' attention may be directed to group interaction through communication and socialization skills. Dyads or triads are encouraged to participate in reflective listening exercises. Subsequently there is encouragement to self-disclose feelings and to provide positive feedback to and from other group members. Members who contribute to individual or group communications are verbally reinforced for their growing awareness. A variety of behavioral techniques—for example, modeling, reinforcing, and role playing—may be introduced to help clients learn new social skills. The opportunity to interact freely with peers in a supportive and accepting environment may be a crucial element in strengthening the elderly person's relationship skills and coping abilities.

Hence it is important that in all communications training the group facilitator work to create a comfortable group climate, define group goals, clarify expectations, and encourage clients to explore common bonds. The importance of unconditional acceptance, confidentiality, and participation needs to be particularly stressed in group work with the elderly. It is generally expected that themes of death, depression, social isolation, and adjustment to sensory and health losses will emerge (Petty, Moeller, & Campbell, 1976). The therapist or the facilitator of the group must have the skills to deal with these entry themes in a here-and-now perspective, emphasizing concrete ways of reducing social isolation and improving the social milieu and the physical environment so that it is more conducive to physical and emotional well-being.

Reality Orientation (RO) Groups

Reality orientation (RO) has gained popularity in the treatment of disoriented or mentally impaired elderly. RO groups were developed to assist individuals experiencing disorientation with respect to time, people, places, or things (Burnside, 1970, 1978). Initially group sessions emphasize basic information covering time, date, next mail, daily activities, etc. As members progress, the level of instruction can be raised to make the classroom activities somewhat more stimulating by including sessions on better grooming, self-care, sensory training, self-control, and management. The ultimate objective is to increase the potentials of members to become more self-sufficient and to establish and maintain contact with the people and events in their immediate environment (Capuzzi & Gross, 1980). According to Taulbee (1978) the most effective RO groups were those that were structured on a 24-hour basis and in which basic principles of individual attention, patience, perseverence, social reinforcement, and positive acceptance were used. Individuals were called by name; told the time, day, and schedule as often as necessary; asked questions; and encouraged to engage in conversation.

The families of elderly clients are also trained in reality orientation techniques (Lee, 1976) and help to use the material when the patients go home so progress can be sustained. The groups are educational rather than counseling or psychotherapy oriented. A variety of reality devices, such as bulletin boards, flashcards with words and pictures, clocks, calendars, scrap books, real objects, and illustrated dictionaries with large print and pictures, are effective stimulus materials that are important to orienting procedures. These groups are along remedial lines and are planned for individuals who are cognitively impaired.

In the more advanced group with fewer orientation difficulties, the most significant problems seem to be remembering dates, medical instructions, and new names as well as forgetting the names of long-time friends. Members frequently interpret memory impairments as a sign of losing one's mind. However, group discussions of the relevant research on memory changes (Meyers, 1974) can greatly help to diminish this fear particularly as members begin to recognize that with varying degrees everyone is experiencing these memory changes. In addition mnemonic techniques and association games are helpful classroom activities. Observation exercises that can help to absorb information and facilitate retention are also useful. Aids suggested by group members and the leaders include writing down information; associating the names of new acquaintances with familiar objects, characteristics, and faces of old friends; repeating new names out loud as well as writing them down; and using large calendars for recording appointments.

Memory training may consist of the use of well-known techniques for improving memory, such as organizing strategies and visual imagery to facilitate learning and recall (see Cermak, 1976; Lorayne & Lucas, 1974 for discussion of various memory strategies).

Zarit, Gallagher, and Kramer (1980) demonstrated that memory training resulted in improved memory and fewer complaints about memory loss.

Zarit (1980) advocates reality orientation therapy for groups of elderly who have concerns about loss of memory. The combination of assurances and positive group interactions can diminish anxiety concerning absent-mindedness and intense anxiety about approaching senility. Actual memory performance, however, is less important for most elderly persons with no apparent signs of senility than is restoring feelings of confidence in their ability to remember and to stay oriented. Zarit, Gallagher, and Kramer (1980) believe that a majority of elderly who show memory loss or poor memory functioning or who complain about inability to recall are often individuals experiencing much depression. In such cases treatment for depression clears up the concerns about memory. Clinicians caution that persons with evidence of severe cognitive deficits associated with senile dementia should not be mixed with other group members who are mildly disoriented, absent-minded, or confused.

Citrin and Dixon (1977), reporting results of one of the few controlled studies of reality orientation training, noted significant improvement of institutionalized elderly on measures of behavior functioning, confusion, and disorientation following 24 hours of classroom instruction. Brook, Degun, and Mather (1975) suggest that reality orientation reverses the process of withdrawal and isolation in the elderly in two ways: first, by stimulating the patient through group attention and repeated orientation to the environment and second, by providing structured interaction with others. Commenting on the significance of structured interaction, Zeplin, Wolfe, and Kleinplatz (1981) noted that it was a useful approach to organizing attention in disoriented elderly clients. Clinical effectiveness of reality orientation may be limited by the severity of the degree of disorientation in elderly persons. Raskind and Storrie (1980) noted no positive change accruing from reality orientation therapy but advocated that best results can be achieved when the specific content of therapy is tailored to the needs of group participants who are selected on the basis of homogeneity in the severity of disorientation.

Reality orientation classes should offer enough choices for the elderly members so that they are not bored but not so many choices that the confusion is increased. Group facilitators, therapists, and cotherapists must consider individual rights and dignity for the confused as basic to any therapeutic plan. Programs should be evaluated regularly and as frequently as possible so that patients' progress through the basic classes can be monitored and patients be moved up to more advanced orientation groups or remotivation groups (Birkett & Boltuch, 1973).

The effectiveness of reality orientation as a treatment for confused older persons has been difficult to demonstrate. Improvement, when observed, has been relatively small and limited to measures of cognitive status (Citrin & Dixon, 1977; Woods, 1979). The procedure does not appear to improve the individual's ability to function with respect to activities of daily living (e.g., personal hygiene, self-control, or locomotion), or diminish behaviors such as anxiety, belligerence or paranoid tendencies (Zeplin, Wolfe, & Kleinplatz, 1981). Reality orientation may be effective for certain types of elderly with a recent onset of organic dysfunction or minimal cognitive impairment (Brook, Degun, & Mather, 1975).

Remotivation Groups

Remotivation therapy is a group technique for stimulating and revitalizing individuals no longer interested and involved in either the present or the future (Dennis, 1978). Remotivation therapy was originally designed to remotivate mentally ill patients and is based on the clinical notion that there are certain parts of the patient's original personality that remain relatively intact and healthy and that group psychotherapy can be used to maintain the intact personality and to protect it from deterioration. The goal of remotivation is to provide a stimulating and supportive environment and continual opportunity to activate the untouched part. Such a goal appears quite consistent not only with current rehabilitation and occupational therapy but also with the goal of psychotherapy for depression for a vast number of elderly who are both unmotivated and inactive.

As described by Dennis (1978), members in remotivation and resocialization therapy groups are strengthened by group encouragement and reinforcement to describe themselves concretely, to speak accurately about past and present experiences, and to participate in various forms of physical therapy, group or individual counseling. The individual also learns to play new roles that do not cause anxiety or create problems. Dennis (1978) advocates that remotivation therapy groups be conducted at least three times a week. Toepfer, Bicknell, and Shaw (1974) suggest a number of therapeutic steps. Principal among these are that the group facilitator attempt to create a climate of appreciation and acceptance. The facilitator then structures each session around nonpathological interests and behaviors (including discussions of holidays, sports, pets, hobbies, etc.) that appeal to a majority of the members. If individual and family problems are brought up by the members, these may be referred to individual counseling sessions, which are a necessary and useful adjunct to group remotivation and resocialization therapy. Controversial subjects such as religion, prejudices, etc., are avoided.

Each remotivation therapy session is based on a different theme selected from a number of topics geared to appeal to diverse backgrounds, experiences, and interests. As far as possible, an attempt should be made to link the topic to previous occupations, hobbies, or interests of the members. The group leader can encourage the elderly clients to rediscover some of their previous interests. Carefully planned questions foster discussion as well as prevent the group members from straying from the topic. The behavioral goal is to encourage the elderly persons to engage in spontaneous verbalizations about the topic and to respond in a relevant manner to the questions of the group facilitator. If the responses are irrelevant and not minimally rational, the leader does not reinforce the individual member; a new question that can be viewed as a restatement of the goal behavior of the group is asked. The leader positively reinforces successive approximations of relevant and rational verbal responses while extinguishing inappropriate ones.

Toepfer, Bicknell, and Shaw (1974) stress that remotivation deals with the crucial behavior of attention. The leader promotes generalization of attention to social cues by promptly and continually reinforcing group members' responses. Thus similarities between remotivation and behavioral therapy are obvious. It is suggested that remotivation be made more systematic by specifying operationally desired behaviors for individuals and group members. The group leader monitors and obtains direct quantitative measures of clients' responses and focuses on differential reinforcement of goal behaviors for the group members. Dennis (1978) advocates the use of interesting audiovisual materials and other sensory items in order to motivate clients. The leader should encourage the expression of pleasure in group discussion and should insist on rational and relevant communications.

In respect to group composition, members should be selected on the basis of ability to interact with others and ability to hear and speak. Unlike members in reality orientation groups, participants in remotivation and resocialization are not severely disoriented or cognitively confused although they may often lack behaviors of attentiveness and prolonged concentration and initially show little interest in the persons and objects in the immediate environment. In respect to skills of the group leader, a number of prerequisites have been suggested. Principal among these are the leader's skills in operationally specifying the behaviors to be promoted in the group. The leaders need to know what behaviors to reinforce and how to do so (Whitney & Barnard, 1966) and what reinforcers are effective with the elderly. Adequately trained leaders should be furnished with precise guidelines for reinforcing desirable responses and extinguishing inappropriate and irrelevant responses. Leaders need also to be skilled at making behavioral observations as opposed to personal interpretations (Watson & Tharp, 1972).

Remotivation and resocialization therapy groups are a step beyond the reality orientation group method. However, in terms of structure, stimulus aids, and the prerequisite social and emotional climate, the two groups are similar. Bovey (1971) has demonstrated that remotivation groups produced changes in the self-concept. However, Birkett and Boltuch (1973) found no significant differences between remotivation and control subjects. Dennis (1976) noted that subjects who received remotivation therapy became initially more depressed than the control subjects. Commenting on this surprising finding of depression, Dennis postulated that the stimulating contents of the remotivation therapy sessions may have presented a sharp and painful contrast to the bleak existence the elderly had in the institutionalized setting. In order to avoid the potentials for any negative outcomes, Dennis (1978) stresses that facilitators need enough training and supervision to be able to identify the emergence of any affective disorders. Despite some potential drawbacks of rigid structure, remotivation therapy offers participants the opportunity to increase their sense of reality, practice healthy roles, and realize a more objective self-image.

Toepfer et al. (1974) stress that remotivation is a promising technique that permits utilization of nonprofessionals more therapeutically, making it possible to reach more clients in groups. However, it remains empirically untested.

The following case is an example of how positive changes were brought about in a hopelessly confused, disoriented, and unmotivated elderly client. Mrs. L., an 86-year-old woman, formerly a highly functioning client, returned home from a long stay at the hospital. She was quite disoriented and withdrawn and showed all the symptoms of acute OBS (organic brain syndrome). She refused to communicate with her spouse and her daughters and for the most part sat slumped over, her eyes fixed on the floor. The family members and elderly friends recognized her as being a highly functioning, alert person and were unwilling to believe that Mrs. L. had an irreversible condition. They asked a therapist and social worker to intervene, and after evaluation an ad hoc group of elderly friends, neighbors, and relatives was formed. The therapist, recognizing that for many elderly past events are easier to recall, began by asking her questions about herself. The group, taking his lead, did the same. At first Mrs. L. refused to acknowledge her husband's presence and protested that she could neither recall who he was nor speak with him or her daughters. The daughters prompted her: "Tell us about the cake you made for Cindy's birthday. How many eggs did you use?" "Tell us about the anniversary present dad gave you." "Do you remember the time that we went to Montreal?" Within half an hour Mrs. L. was sitting up in her chair, attending to the German conversation of an elderly cousin. In the third group session she was able to talk about her recent surgery and her long stay at the hospital. Mrs. L. returned to functioning quite well in the household. However, she was not motivated to interact with her husband and would withdraw to her room and sit alone as soon as the group left. In one group session she confided to her German cousin that she was annoyed with Mr. L. because he had not visited her during her hospital stay. When this erroneous perception was corrected, she returned to interacting with Mr. L.

In a sense this clinical case description encapsulates the ongoing process of evaluation, group treatment, and integration of therapy procedures that are involved in any effectively organized reality orientation and remotivation groups. These positive developments are, of course, individual growth, which results from the combined and coordinated efforts of group treatment, home treatment, and family intervention modalities.

Although remotivation group therapy has been widely used, controlled studies have been few and have not demonstrated its effectiveness.

Socialization Groups

As noted in the implications of abandonment theory and role theory of aging, many elderly do not know how to cope with their loneliness and desire increasing contact with others. It is assumed that people who are drawn into some sort of discussion or socializing groups do not necessarily need psychotherapy, although some implicit or explicit psychotherapy goals are usually included (Zarit, 1980, p. 334). It is understood by socialization group members that they may wish to join a group for socialization and discussion rather than for behavioral or emotional change.

Although originally designed to improve social skills and interpersonal relationships and interactions, socialization groups have advanced to a stage where the objective is to promote self-confidence and self-esteem. By and large such groups are most difficult to conceptualize in terms of goals and procedures. Hanssen et al. (1978) observed that the elderly who join such socialization groups are often among the best-functioning persons in the community. Because of the supportive and cohesive atmosphere encouraged in the groups, such groups principally become a stimulating setting in which to get together with others. Issues that have been considered in such groups include relationship with friends and children; topics of self-esteem, dignity, and privacy for the elderly; problems of insomnia; health and vigor; and assertiveness with family and health care practitioners.

The discussions are lively, although not intensively confrontative, and a lot of mutual support is given by group members. Overall, such groups have a nonspecific impact on the individual member. Petty et al. (1976) report that the supportive groups helped participants reach new insights and develop new patterns of interactions. Toseland (1977) found that problem-solving abilities were improved and there was a significant increase in social skills and assertion behaviors after six sessions. Similarly Weiner and Weinstock (1979) found that interactionally oriented socialization groups produced more change in participants' active problem-solving when compared to two talk groups.

Socialization groups may often have a beneficial impact on a person with major problems or may teach useful problem-solving strategies. However, these goals can be accomplished in a socialization group without a hidden agenda for turning it into a psychotherapy group. For ethical reasons it is important to represent the goals and objectives of the socialization group as accurately as possible to potential participants so that individuals whose primary need may be to work through major conflicts or to acquire specialized problem-solving skills are dissuaded from joining or, having joined, do not dominate the sessions (Zarit, 1980).

There-and-Then Paradigm

The there-and-then model is based on an insight approach that utilizes memory as a tool for therapeutic intervention. The there-and-then model hypothesizes that by reorganizing and understanding past events, feelings of self-esteem will increase and somatic complaints will diminish (Ingersoll & Silverman, 1978). The approach is aimed at bringing about changes in clients' feelings, thinking, and acting, all of which may improve clients' social relationships, enhance personal satisfaction with respect to past productivity, and provide relief from socially determined anxiety and distress.

Through utilizing group and individual intervention the model focuses on helping clients to establish a bridge between the past and the present. A number of group therapeutic approaches and processes fall within the framework of this paradigm.

Reminiscing Groups

These groups are considered by many to represent a third level of group work with the elderly (Dennis, 1978). Originally initiated by Ebersole (1976), these groups use Butler's (1963) work on life review as the theoretical framework. Butler believes that reminiscence is part of a complex developmental process among the aged which is a "naturally occurring universal mental process characterized by the progressive return to consciousness of past experiences, and particularly, the resurgence of unresolved conflicts" (p. 66).

Reminiscence, as a self-reflective process involving the recollection of past events, experiences, and feelings, has an adaptive value for the elderly to the extent that it allows them to work through and mediate personal losses and conflicts of the past (McMahon & Rhudick, 1967). Ebersole (1978) enumerates a number of therapeutic reasons for using reminiscing groups with the elderly. A principal reason proposed is that reminiscing groups enhance a cohort effect. Often the elderly have little desire to spend time with their own age group, especially if they perceive such association to have a social stigma or to be out of step with the mainstream of life. Group participation in reminiscence helps members identify accomplishments and identities in a way that adds to self-esteem and dispels the belief of some cohorts that advanced age is a social disgrace. The point is repeated that a reminiscing life review is not a garrulous storytelling or passive reproduction of past events but an active response to a need for a reorganization of attitudes toward the contents of one's life (Birren, 1964). While the forms of reminiscing and life review may vary from a mild nostalgic recall to severe depression with anxiety, guilt, and suicidal tendencies, Birren (1964) stresses that reminiscing should not be viewed as a psychopathological phenomenon but as a common, normal experience.

More than many younger adults, the older individuals are under greater time pressure to integrate views of the past and to reconcile their past with the world of present relationships. With the likelihood of death in the near future, futurity may no longer be a useful mechanism for maintaining psychological equilibrium (Birren, 1964). As noted by many authors (see Butler, 1963; Birren, 1964; Ebersole, 1978), the essential meaning of life appears to need clarification, and the stewardship of one's life has to be reconciled. There is thus a need for a sophisticated listening audience with a group of other elderly cohorts, or younger adults, who feel the obligations of an interpersonal relationship with the reminiscing elderly individual. Thus, briefly stated, reminiscence has a constructive effect in that it helps the reminiscer not only to recall facts but to weave them into a perspective that is acceptable to the self and to cohorts.

A second major reason for using reminiscing groups is to enhance the individuality of the person by capitalizing on the group exchange of earlier memories (Ebersole, 1978). Reminiscing groups have a therapeutic value in that gradually group participants begin to appreciate the richness of one another's lives through the re-creation of moments of pleasure and accomplishments of satisfaction. Often the individuality of the elderly has been restricted by living conditions and social isolation. Through memory stimulation, through re-creation of joyous events, and through positive reinterpretation, the members learn to come to terms with the totality of life experience and to achieve ego integrity (Erikson, 1963). Ego integrity, according to Erikson, is achieved by using old age as a time to look back, to recount life experiences with a sense of wholeness and sincerity. Without a chance to reminisce and reinterpret life events creatively an individual may view life's efforts as a series of missed opportunities, leading to states of despair and self-disdain (Erikson, 1963).

Formation of Reminiscing Groups. In selecting members for these groups, Ebersole (1978) suggests that potential members should be interviewed individually so that understanding of the aims and objectives of the group can be established. First to be confirmed is the degree of personal commitment that the individual member is prepared to make in terms of the degree of self-disclosure and social interaction involved. Second, in the case of the elderly living at home with family or adult children or in the case of congregate living situations, assurance of confidentiality of information shared may be important. If possible, reminiscing groups should attempt to obtain participants from both community and institutional settings in order to acquire a range of members' past experiences. Third, it is often helpful to place members in reminiscing groups because of their special attributes or deficits (Capuzzi & Gross, 1980). For example, including one or two members who are socially outgoing and one or two members who seem withdrawn may encourage the development of latent strengths in individual group members.

Contents of Reminiscence. The content areas are largely determined by the group members although selection can be guided and reinforced by the group facilitators. Fry (1983) advocates the use of structure in developing reminiscence themes. In Fry's (1983) study, participants in the structured reminiscence groups experienced greater reduction in depression scores than participants in the more unstructured or laissez-faire reminiscence groups in which the life reviewing was quite unselective.

Fry advocates gentle questioning and probing for details. Subjects in Fry's study were asked to give a series of details concerning life events and situations described in the reminiscing. For example, subjects were asked to describe how they felt in a given situation (Did you feel happy, sad, irritated, frustrated, threatened, anxious, in danger?). They were asked to relate hopes and fears associated with an event (Did you wish certain things would happen that would make you feel better? Were there persons that made you feel anxious or happy?) and to describe specific images and thoughts that frequently flooded their minds at the time a particular event was reviewed (Were there thoughts that came into your mind over and over again? Were there persons whose memory you could not dispel from your mind? Were there images that were very strong or images that were vague?). Subjects were asked to describe the kinds of interpersonal interactions they wanted at the time of a particular event (Did you wish people would leave you alone? Did you wish people would stay around and talk with you? Did you want people to give you special attention or special love?). Subjects were encouraged, also, to describe their unresolved feelings associated with a particular life event (Did you feel guilty, responsible, ashamed, lost, confused, embarassed?).

Fry (1983) advocates an attempt by the group members or group facilitator to offer constructive interpretation or reinterpretation of the significance of past events. The therapist may, for example, help participants to recognize patterns in their lives and to develop parallels between their own upbringing, their values and beliefs, and those of their children. The group members should also be urged to reinforce one another, to offer empathy, support, and understanding.

Reminiscing may first be encouraged in dyads and later exchanged in the larger groups. In an effort to enrich their sense of identity and rootedness, clients may be encouraged to keep journals and make genograms (see Guerin & Pendagast, 1976). Hartman (1976) believes that the genogram helps elderly individuals gain an understanding of their family patterns and relationships and thus aids in self-understanding. Deaths, which are often represented visually by the genogram, may generate discussion of feelings of guilt, anger, depression, and conflict. Scrapbooks, photo albums, old letters, and other memorabilia are rich sources of information and can be used in group sessions to stimulate the memory of persons who have resisted participation.

Life review need not be ruled out for brain-damaged elderly. Even persons with moderate brain damage can remember many details through pictures and souvenirs that have emotional meaning for them. While brain damage cannot be reversed through reminiscence therapy, the overlying and underlying depression may be alleviated and adaptation may be facilitated (Lewis & Butler, 1974).

Clinical Evaluation of Reminiscing Groups. In terms of clinical evaluation of the reminiscing procedure, Butler (1963, 1976) notes that a life review can serve to reintegrate the personality, give new meaning to one's life, and help mitigate one's fear of death. The group members can help the individual member to overcome anxieties about the uncertainty of death by reinforcing the elderly member's acceptable image of the self and the positive influences that the individual will leave behind.

McMahon and Rhudick (1967) maintain that participants may often use reminiscing as a means to justify their lives. These authors observed that the reminiscence of many elderly reflected negative themes such as guilt, unrealized goals, and wished-for opportunities to make up for failures. Therapists are therefore cautioned about reminiscing clients who may engage in in-depth breakdown of repression or reminiscence that has too much of the dynamics of despair or life crisis. Similarly, Pincus (1970) notes that reminiscence in relation to situational factors such as stress and emotional factors such as depression may be a valuable source of data for planning appropriate psychological intervention. Harris and Harris (1980) recommend that reminiscence in a group setting be considered as a free-floating oral history interview technique that can provide valuable information concerning psychological factors underlying health and adaptation in the elderly.

At the same time several clinicians (e.g., McMahon & Rhudick, 1967; Pincus, 1970) caution that for some depressed elderly a focus on the past may be highly aversive and should not be encouraged. Many practitioners who have worked with the elderly have been concerned with the frequent emergence of bitterness, disappointment, and despondency in remembering the past.

Grotjahn (1978) advocates that therapists must seriously consider the emotional price sometimes paid when an elderly client reviews, in the presence of cohorts, perceived failures. It can be exceedingly painful for an elderly person to reminisce and reflect on a life that has been characterized by maladjustment, conflict, or neurotic struggles. This clinical consideration has led advocates of the life review and reminiscing group therapy approaches to emphasize the significance of narrating life experiences as they have been lived, not as they might have been lived (Grotjahn, 1955, 1978).

Butler (1963) suggests that reminiscence and life review should take the form of a reinforcing structuring of the past in which the psychotherapeutic objective is to find confirmation of present and past identity. Butler cautions that in the hands of an inexperienced therapist or unstructured group review, reminiscence may take the form of a destructuring of the past in which the goal becomes to free oneself from the past. When reminiscing becomes excessive, morbid, and disorganized for an individual member, the therapist or group facilitator can seek to increase opportunities for gratification in the client's current life situation.

Birren (1964) stresses that sudden emergence of longstanding memories need not be indicative of psychopathology but simply of the fact that the individual has a strong purpose for integrating the past. The controls and inhibitions of previous years are often less important, and many elderly may be willing to speak with new candor. Although the life-review process is intended to be a normative process, group therapists should be prepared to encounter some strong manifestations of effect such as anger and hysterical crying and be ready to deal with this in the group situation.

Lewis and Butler (1974) caution that by its nature reminiscence and life review evoke a sense of regret and sadness at the brevity of life, the missed opportunities, and the chosen paths that turned out badly. In extreme cases old persons may become terror-stricken and panicked if they have privately decided that their life was a total waste. However, Lewis and Butler confirm that these potential risks can be avoided by ensuring that individual reminiscers receive support, positive reinforcement, and unconditional acceptance from the group members and group therapist. Most elderly people, despite their physical frailty, are psychologically capable of reconciling their lives and confronting painful forces in the presence of acceptance and support from others.

On the more positive side Boylin, Gordon, and Nehrke's (1976) findings showed higher levels of ego integrity associated with the frequency of reminiscence in the elderly. Kramer, Kramer, and Dunlop (1966) postulate that reminiscence is a necessary step in the resolution of grief. These authors cite the example of a woman whose husband has died and who recalls and repeats reminiscing until memories lose their painfulness.

Although reminiscence has not been studied widely in respect of its relationship to depression, Fallot's (1980) research reported both positive and negative effects of reminiscing. In terms of positive effects elderly persons categorized as reminiscers were significantly less depressed, made fewer self-blaming attributions about their past experiences, and were less anxious and fatigued than nonreminiscers. However, reminiscers also focused on comparisons between the past and the present and future and showed significantly higher levels of depression and futility concerning the present and future. Thus Fallot (1980) speaks against the advisability of allowing reminiscing members to engage in comparisons of the past and present.

Butler (1963) alerts the therapist or group facilitators to the presence of silent reminiscers in the group whose thinking may be filled with intrusive, negative, and conflictual memories too painful or overwhelming to share with other members of the group. When societal norms have inhibited reminiscing in persons from certain cultural backgrounds or there is conscious avoidance by some members, the group can be led by the group facilitator to discuss and comprehend the adaptational value of reminiscing.

In the opinion of Lewis and Butler (1974) the life review of the elderly in age-integrated and intergenerational groups can be a rich, active reexperiencing of the past through the eyes and judgments of different age groups. In such age-integrated groups all the generations can participate in clarifying past conflicts of the elderly and work at offering solutions for the older persons. This kind of recapitulation of the family members can make a unique contribution to the self-esteem and pride of the elderly members and help to break down some of the stereotyped negative views that the young have of the old and vice versa. Members of all ages may succeed in becoming less conscious of age.

For the therapist and group facilitator, the extent and content of the elderly clients' reminiscences can provide important diagnostic information about self-image, the amount of stress being experienced, and the types of relationships that need to be fostered in the group. On an interpersonal level, reminiscing may have substantial adaptational significance in relation to maintenance of self-concept and self-esteem, resolution of grief, and reaction to specific stressful experiences such as institutionalization or abandonment by family members.

Group Therapy for Depressed Elders

Because of the widespread prevalence of depression among the aged, it is probable that group treatment programs will relate to many participants who are depressed. Different kinds of groups (e.g., reminiscence groups, remotivation groups, socialization groups, and relaxation training groups) may have relevance to the group treatment of depression and may impact nonspecifically in alleviating depression. The discussion here is restricted to those group procedures that relate more specifically to the goals of group treatment of depression. Many of the group procedures suggested are essentially psychodynamic and cognitive in nature.

Expressive Group Therapy. Berland and Poggi (1979) and Lo Gerfo (1980) describe their expressive group therapy program with the very advanced age group of the elderly (72 to 99 years) who were not organically impaired and did not have severe sensory deficits or losses. Through an adaptational use of reminiscing procedures, role modeling, reenactment, and reliving of emotions these elderly individuals were helped to achieve understanding of their thoughts and feelings about current and past experiences and were able to work with themes of loss and death.

Butler (1975) notes that depression-related features most often seen in the elderly include grief, anger, loss of self-esteem, anhedonia, guilt, and anxiety over impending death. Butler notes that in many ways the psychotherapy of depression in old age is the psychotherapy of grief and accommodation, restitution and reconciliation. He advocates the use of group expressive therapy in helping the elderly to achieve the integration and transcendence over bereavement and loss. The role of the group therapist and the participants in expressive therapy is to help the group members to articulate their feelings, to be more expressive about the hurt, the grief, and sorrow, and to use the group media to siphon off some of the deepseated emotions of anger, resentment, and self-pity. The role of the group facilitator is twofold: (1) to assist in providing interpretation, construction, and reconstruction after pent-up emotions are expressed and (2) to provide realistic insight and substitutions for some of the negative thoughts and feelings. Unlike procedures used in individual therapy, the therapist assumes a more passive role but encourages group support, group reinforcement, and group nurturance in the individual member's expression of emotions. The group approach has many advantages for expressive therapy in setting an up tone and providing balance, coverage, training, and richer feedback. Its philosophy is a positive one, emphasizing positive self-concepts—a welcome change from problem-oriented techniques used in other groups.

The preparation that should be given to the group members before expressive therapy should include ground rules of confidentiality, support, and acceptable feedback. The individual member's ability to listen and to hear, as well as to talk, should be generally verified before acceptance into the group.

Contrary to the widely prevailing notion that many elderly are inflexible and lack ability to change, the advocates of expressive group therapy have been able to demonstrate that personality growth and reconstruction continue well into late life and that this kind of therapy should not be excluded as unproductive for the elderly. However, as with a more dynamically oriented group, the level of psychopathology, social and educational status, and other biological handicaps and illnesses of the elderly clients should be considered in introducing them to expressive therapy.

Age-Integrated Life-Crisis Group Therapy. Such a group therapy approach to treatment of depression is based on the notion that increasing age-segregation and social isolation that characterize our society leaves little opportunity for rich exchange of feelings, experiences, and mutual support between the aged and the nonaged. Butler and Lewis (1977) postulate that much of the elderly's depression, including somatic complaints and hypochondriasis, is a reflection of the elderly's need for social interaction and identification with others outside their own cohort groups. Butler and Lewis, therefore, advocate the setting up of age-integrated, intergenerational groups with ages ranging from 15 to 80 years. These groups are set up for the purpose of sharing existential concerns and difficulties in coping as one goes through the life cycle and encounters life crises. Life crisis in this context refers to various critical developmental tasks associated with adolescence, parenthood, occupation, retirement, widowhood, illness, and impending death.

The underlying assumption in this group therapy approach is that alleviation of depression accrues from the opportunity for participants of various ages to share and help one another. The unique contribution of the elderly includes serving as a model for coping and growing older, providing solutions based on experiences related to loss and grief, and sharing insights in the form of creative reminiscences. An age-integrated life crisis group can help the elderly come to terms with many of the issues of loss and bereavement that affect at least 50 percent of the individuals in this age group (Berland & Poggi, 1979). Contrary to the stereotyped view of aging, the elderly have the wish and ability to combat the depression and crises of their life stage and to do so with energy and insight. Through the medium of the intergenerational group the elderly can benefit themselves and other young group participants.

With a view to helping the elderly achieve these goals, Butler recommends the use of cotherapists (both male and female) from different disciplines so as to provide the intergenerational group both a psychodynamic and sociological orientation, as well as the opportunity for useful transference to take place. Group processes involve the use of reminiscence and expressive therapy. The goal is to relieve depression by providing opportunity for new interactions and new interpersonal relations. Advocates of this group approach (e.g., Butler & Lewis, 1977; Berland & Poggi, 1979) stress that interactions of the group should revolve around reality issues, past histories, individual problems of the members, and hopes for the future. Emphasis is, and should be, on the verbalizations of emotions. The expressions of both anger and positive feelings that one generational group feels toward other generational members are encouraged as a step toward constructive resolution of problems.

Butler's criteria for group membership suggest the exclusion of individuals showing active psychosis and suicidal tendencies. Diagnostic categories reflecting reaction to life crisis include depression, anxiety states, hypochondriasis, alcoholism, and mild drug use.

Cognitive-Therapy Groups. Cognitive therapy has long been an effective individual treatment of adult outpatients with moderately severe unipolar depressions (Rush, Hollan, Beck, & Kovacs, 1978). Its application to groups has also been reported (see Jarvik et al., 1983; Morris, 1975; Rush & Watkins, 1981; Shaw, 1977). The usefulness of this treatment to the elderly is in a rather experimental stage. In enumerating several features of the treatment that seem especially promising for use with aged adults, Steuer and Hammen (1983) point out some of the key elements in cognitive therapy that can counter hopelessness. Specifically cognitive psychotherapy attempts to challenge stereotypic beliefs that the elderly have of themselves that they are useless, helpless, and unattractive, incapable of changing their attitudes and rigid in their thinking. These beliefs may be key determinants in much of the elderly's depressions. Cognitive therapy, using the group media, attempts to teach elderly members how to restructure their cognitions of hopelessness, uselessness, and self-devaluation. A number of techniques are used, principally the following.

Group members are taught procedures for thought stopping of negative cognitions, thought catching, and covert self-instruction in order to block dysfunctional and automatic thoughts. Cognitive restructuring procedures require group members to reinforce individuals in challenging and confronting irrational beliefs or distorted cognitions. An elderly woman, for example, may hold on to the irrational belief that other members would not be interested in her problems. Many elderly persons may have the explicit belief that they are too old to change. A retired man may have the distorted perception that his family regards him as useless because he no longer holds a job.

Steuer and Hammen (1983) note a number of adaptations necessary in cognitive-behavioral group therapy with depressed elderly. The elderly have many stereotypic beliefs (exacerbated by depressive distortion), are slow to change, and must be countered both by individual cognitive restructuring and by social pressure from other group members. Group pressure may be necessary to urge members to try new ways of thinking about a situation.

Clients will vary in the degree of cognitive restructuring or positive self-talk that they are able to do. Some elderly clients may be less capable of monitoring or catching dysfunctional and automatic thoughts but may be able to make use of the concept in a therapeutic fashion by giving themselves encouraging pep talks. Steuer and Hammen (1983, p. 293) believe that variability in cognitive restructuring skills is to be expected in the elderly. Variability is accentuated in a group therapy format, which capitalizes on shared or commonly understood experiences. Group members elicit therapeutic participation in cognitive restructuring and induce vicarious learning of related therapeutic strategies. Steuer and Hammen (1983) suggest that cognitive group therapy is especially promising for use with depressed elderly since its focus is not on changing personality structure but on current concerns such as developing problem-solving skills and staying rational.

Case studies drawn from cognitive therapy groups suggest that if such therapy is to be successful with the elderly, certain age-related changes in technique will be necessary. First, age changes in neurological and intellectual functioning may cause the cognitive therapy to proceed more slowly than expected and may make the behavioral components (such as assertion training, increased activity, exploration) useful prerequisites of the cognitive therapy treatment, especially for those elderly who have difficulties in abstract thinking. Second, the physical health status of elderly clients may affect the cognitions and impede the progress in therapy.

Group members must offer support and remind individuals that they may not be able to think clearly on days when they are not feeling well or have not had sufficient sleep. The therapist must monitor the effects of medication on the individual member's ability to think clearly and rationally. Third, group effort to encourage rational responsiveness on the part of the older individuals is important and needs to be discussed. Whenever an individual elderly commences to talk irrationally or to have distorted expectations of self and others, the irrational overgeneralizing and catastrophizing spread easily to other members. A great deal of work on the part of both therapist (or group facilitator) and other group members is required in order to ensure that the members both individually and collectively examine the evidence for and against specific negative automatic thoughts and learn to identify and alter dysfunctional beliefs (schemes) that predispose them to develop these negative cognitions. The process of accomplishing such preventive trends in the group setting may sound deceptively simple but requires that the group facilitator have special skills to work with the group so as to develop more rational, reasonable, and adaptive responses.

As a last point, practitioners caution that often it may be difficult for the therapist or group facilitator to change depressive distortions in elderly who have been exposed to serious real-life hardships. As cognitive therapy is based in part on helping clients distinguish between accurate and distorted cognitions, the therapist is particularly taxed to help elderly clients differentiate between the hopelessness and helplessness characteristic of depression and a realistic recognition of their intellectual, social, and physical limitations.

Continuing research is recommended on the effects of cognitive therapy with depressed elderly. Increasing consideration needs to be given to the adaptations necessary for elderly clients in the standard way that cognitive therapy is done with younger clients. Steuer and Hammen (1983) advocate the use of cognitive group therapy for elderly individuals who understand the relationship between thoughts and feelings and are willing to monitor their cognitions and effects.

CONCLUSIONS

Many types of group therapy have been used with older adults beginning with modified programs of traditional psychodynamic group therapy in the 1950s. Most group therapy has been conducted in institutional settings. However, group therapy is more helpful to older adults living in the community. Group therapy seems quite appropriate for older persons whose problems involve interpersonal relationships or whose social identity may be obscured by factors such as role loss, retirement, or the inaccessibility to friends and family who have provided support and identity confirmation. Problems that can be helped through reinforcement or positive feedback from others are probably dealt with best in a group setting, and sharing experiences and insights with peers provides a sense of emotional security. To a large extent the elderly's needs to belong, be rooted, and be accepted are based on their relationship with those they love most intimately—family and friends. Old-age losses of friends and family necessitate an emotional reorientation, for which many older persons do not have as great a capacity, and also a new role adaptation after, say, retirement or widowhood. Group associations provide opportunities for love and affirmation, to substitute family ties with peer ties, and to give new status and hence new relevance to the existence of many elderly.

If structured well, groups become ego-supportive and can provide what the ego needs—satisfaction from past productivity and a sense of hope for the future. Because older people have rich experiences, well-designed group programs are able to tap their experiences and ability as learners. A concept of considerable significance in androgological and gerontological practice of group therapy is the "unfreezing experience" whereby learners are helped to look at themselves more objectively and to free their minds from the preconceptions (Lowy, 1979, p. 308) and stereotypes of ageism. Group therapy programs can enthuse older people to learn collaboratively, not competitively, and to engage in self-directed inquiry by learning to analyze their life experiences.

Though group approaches have been widely used with the elderly in the past, outcome criteria and measures have not been sufficiently defined to distinguish specific treatment-linked response from general nonspecific symptomatic change. On the one hand there is a need to redefine goals of group work more narrowly and specifically in terms of social, reciprocal, and developmental functions. On the other hand there is a need to propose an expansion in the scope of group work, especially for remedial and psychotherapy functions.

In terms of clinical function old people who are under the stress of declining emotional resources may often be helped through group therapy to clarify and resolve intrapsychic and interpersonal conflict (Lazarus & Weinberg, 1980). In evaluating the psychodynamic processes of group therapy that affect intrapsychic functioning, there is a decrease in guilt and fear because of permissive or reassuring activities on the part of the group facilitator. There is also self-propulsion toward best behavior on the basis of exposure to group consensus. Group therapy cannot and should not be regarded as a specific isolated endeavor since its success depends partly on individual psychotherapy and on social services for achieving changes in the total milieu of the elderly.

SUMMARY

This chapter has examined several perspectives, goals, and intervention approaches in group work. Groups of older persons can have several different objectives including socializing, remotivation, reeducation, communications, and psychotherapy for dealing with specific problems such as cognitive disorders or caring for cognitively impaired or physically ill elderly relatives. Group facilitators need to assess the strengths and limitations of individual elderly members in terms of their being able to profit from group participation. Problems that involve interpersonal relationships, communications, and absence of positive feedback and encouragement can be most appropriately handled through the elderly person's involvement in groups. Though groups have been widely used with the aged, they have been planned mostly along remedial lines and have served the needs of impaired elderly in institutional settings. The scope of group work can be usefully expanded by considering preventive approaches to problems of communications, low self-esteem, and dependency so common among elderly persons. The extent to which older persons can benefit from group therapy has not been evaluated to date. There is sufficient hearsay evidence, however, to indicate that group work with the elderly encourages the development of positive behaviors and adds to the elderly members' sense of well-being. It is suggested that group therapy requires multiple efforts for its support, many of which must come from the community and, most important of all, from family involvement and family intervention.

REFERENCES

Beers, T.M., & Karoly, P. (1979). Cognitive strategies, expectancy and coping style in the control of pain. *Journal of Consulting and Clinical Psychology, 47,* 179–182.

Berger, L.F., & Berger, M.M. (1973). A holistic group approach to psychogeriatric outpatients. *International Journal of Group Psychotherapy, 23,* 432–445.

Berger, M.M., & Berger, L.F. (1972). Psychogeriatric group approaches. In C. Sager & H. Kaplan (Eds.), *Progress in group and family therapy* (pp. 726–736). New York: Brunner/Mazel.

Berland, D.I., & Poggi, R. (1979). Expressive group psychotherapy with the aging. *International Journal of Group Psychotherapy, 29,* 87–108.

Bernstein, D., & Borkovec, T. (1973). *Progressive relaxation training.* Champaign, IL: Research Press.

Birkett, D.P., & Boltuch, B. (1973). Remotivation therapy. *Journal of American Geriatrics Society, 21,* 368–371.

Birren, J.E. (1964). *The psychology of aging.* Englewood Cliffs, NJ: Prentice-Hall, Inc.

Bovey, J.S. (1971). The effect of intensive remotivation techniques on institutionalized geriatric mental patients. *Dissertation Abstracts International, 32,* 4201B–4202B. (University Microfilms No. 72–4064).

Boylin, W., Gordon, S.K., & Nehrke, M.F. (1976). Reminiscing and ego integrity in institutionalized males. *Gerontologist, 16,* 118–124.

Brook, P., Degun, G., & Mather, M. (1975). Reality orientation: A therapy for psychogeriatric patients: A controlled study. *British Journal of Psychiatry, 117,* 42–45.

Brudno, J.J., & Seltzer, H. (1968). Re-socialization therapy through group process with senile patients in a geriatric hospital. *Gerontologist, 8,* 211–214.

Burnside, I.M. (1970). Group work with the aged: Selected literature. *Gerontologist, 10,* 241–246.

Burnside, I.M. (1978). *Working with the elderly: Group process and techniques.* North Scituate, MA: Duxbury Press.

Butler, R.N. (1963). The life review: An interpretation of reminiscence in the aged. *Psychiatry, 26,* 65–76.

Butler, R.N. (1975). Psychiatry and the elderly: An overview. *American Journal of Psychiatry, 132,* 79–84.

Butler, R.N. (1976). Successful aging and the role of the life review. *Journal of American Geriatrics Society, 22,* 529–535.

Butler, R.N., & Lewis, M.I. (1977). *Aging and mental health: Positive psychological approaches* (2nd ed.). St. Louis: C.V. Mosby Co.

Capuzzi, D., & Gross, D. (1980, December). Group work with the elderly: An overview for counselors. *Personnel and Guidance Journal,* pp. 206–210.

Cermak, L.S. (1976). *Improving your memory.* New York: W.W. Norton & Co., Inc.

Citrin, R.S., & Dixon, D.N. (1977). Reality orientation: A milieu therapy used in an institution for the aged. *Gerontologist, 17,* 39–43.

Comfort, A. (1976). *A good age.* New York: Simon & Schuster.

Dennis, H. (1976). *Remotivation therapy for the elderly: A surprising outcome.* Unpublished manuscript.

Dennis, H. (1978). Remotivation therapy groups. In I.M. Burnside (Ed.), *Working with the elderly: Group process and techniques* (pp. 219–235). North Scituate, MA: Duxbury Press.

Ebersole, P.P. (1976). Problems of group reminiscing with the institutionalized aged. *Journal of Gerontological Nursing, 2,* 23–27.

Ebersole, P.P. (1978). Establishing reminiscing groups. In I.M. Burnside (Ed.), *Working with the elderly: Group process and techniques* (pp. 236–254). North Scituate, MA: Duxbury Press.

Erikson, E. (1963). *Childhood and society* (2nd ed.). New York: W.W. Norton & Co., Inc.

Fallot, R.D. (1980). The impact on mood of verbal reminiscing in later adulthood. *International Journal of Aging and Human Development, 10,* 385–400.

Feil, N.W. (1967). Group therapy in a home for the aged. *Gerontologist, 7,* 192–195.

Finkel, S., & Fillmore, W. (1971). Experiences with an older adult group at a private psychiatric hospital. *Journal of Geriatric Psychiatry, 4,* 188–199.

Fry, P.S. (1983). Structured and unstructured reminiscence training and depression in the elderly. *Clinical Gerontologist, 1,* 15–37.

Goldfarb, A.I. (1971). Group therapy with the old and aged. In H.I. Kaplan & B.J. Sadock (Eds.), *Comprehensive group psychotherapy* (pp. 623–642). Baltimore: Williams & Wilkins.

Grotjahn, M. (1955). Analytic psychotherapy with the elderly. *Psychoanalytic Review, 42,* 419–427.

Grotjahn, M. (1978). Group communication and group therapy with the aged: A promising project. In L.F. Jarvik (Ed.), *Aging into the twenty-first century* (pp. 113–122). New York: Gardner Press.

Guerin, P., & Pendagast, E. (1976). Evaluation of family system and genogram. In P. Guerin (Ed.), *Family therapy: Theory and practice* (pp. 450–464). New York: Gardner Press.

Hanssen, A., Meima, N., Buckspan, L., Helbig, T., Henderson, B., & Zarit, S.H. (1978). Correlates of senior center participation. *Gerontologist, 18,* 193–200.

Harper, R., Bauer, R., & Kommarkat, J. (1976). Learning theory and gestalt. *American Journal of Psychotherapy, 30,* 55–71.

Harris, R., & Harris, S. (1980). Therapeutic uses of oral history techniques in medicine. *International Journal of Aging and Human Development, 12,* 27–34.

Hartford, M.E. (1978). Groups in the human services: Some facts and fancies. *Social Work with Groups, 1,* 7–13.

Hartman, A. (1976). *The genogram in the family system through time.* Ann Arbor, Michigan. Unpublished manuscript.

Hoyer, W.J., Kafer, R.A., Simpson, S.C., & Hoyer, F.W. (1974). Reinstatement of verbal behavior in elderly mental patients using operant procedures. *Gerontologist, 14,* 149–152.

Hussian, R.A., & Lawrence, P.S. (1981). Social reinforcement of activity and problem-solving training in the treatment of depressed institutionalized elderly patients. *Cognitive Therapy and Research, 5,* 57–69.

Ingersoll, B., & Silverman, A. (1978). Comparative group psychotherapy for the aged. *Gerontologist, 18,* 201–206.

Jarvik, L., Mintz, J., Steuer, J., Gerner, R., Aldrich, J., Hammen, C., Linde, S., McCarley, T., Motoike, P., & Rosen, R. (1983). Comparison of tricyclic antidepressants and group psychotherapies in geriatric depressed patients: An interim analysis. In P.J. Clayton & J.E. Barrett (Eds.), *Treatment of depression: Old controversies and new approaches* (pp. 299–308). New York: Raven Press.

Kramer, C.H., Kramer, J., & Dunlop, H.E. (1966, July-August). Resolving grief. *Geriatric Nursing,* pp. 14–17.

Lange, A.J., & Jakubowski, P. (1976). *Responsible assertive behavior.* Champaign, IL.: Research Press.

Lazarus, L.W., & Weinberg, J. (1980). Treatment in the ambulatory care setting. In E.W. Busse & D.G. Blazer (Eds.), *Handbook of geriatric psychiatry* (pp. 427–452). New York: Van Nostrand Reinhold Co.

Lee, R.I. (1976). Reality orientation: Restoring the senile to life: Part 1. *Journal of Practical Nursing, 26,* 30–31.

Lewis, M.I., & Butler, R.N. (1974). Life review therapy: Putting memories to work in individual and group psychotherapy. *Geriatrics, 29,* 165–173.

Lieberman, M.A., & Gourash, N. (1979). Evaluating the effects of change groups on the elderly. *International Journal of Group Psychotherapy, 29,* 283–304.

Lieberman, M.A., Yalom, I.D., & Miles, M.B. (1973). *Encounter groups: First facts.* New York: Basic Books.

Lo Gerfo, M. (1980). Three ways of reminiscence in theory and practice. *International Journal of Aging and Human Development, 12,* 39–48.

Lorayne, H., & Lucas, J. (1974). *The memory book.* New York: Ballantine Books.

Lowy, L. (1961, June). Meeting the needs of older people on a differential basis. *Social Group Work with Older People: Proceedings of the Seminar, Lake Mohonk, New Paltz, New York* (pp. 43–67).

Lowy, L. (1967). Roadblocks in group work practice with older people: A framework for analysis. *Gerontologist, 2,* 109–113.

Lowy, L. (1979). *Social work with the aging: The challenge and promise of the later years.* New York: Harper & Row.

Luce, G.G. (1979). *Your second life.* Lawrence, NY: Delacorte Press/Seymour.

Mayadas, N.S., & Hink, D.L. (1974). Group work with the aging. *Gerontologist, 14,* 440–445.

McMahon, A.W., & Rhudick, P.J. (1967). Reminiscing in the aged: An adaptational response. In S. Levin & R.J. Kahana (Eds.), *Psychodynamic studies on aging, creativity, reminiscing, and dying* (pp. 64–78). New York: International Universities Press.

Meyers, R. (1974). *Is my mind slipping?* Los Angeles: Andrus Gerontology Center, University of Southern California.

Morris, N.E. (1975). *A group self-instruction method for the treatment of depressed out patients.* Unpublished doctoral dissertation, University of Toronto.

Papell, C., & Rothman, B. (1966). Social group work models: Possession and heritage. *Journal of Education for Social Work, 2,* 66–77.

Paul, G.L., & Bernstein, D.A. (1976). Anxiety and clinical problems. In J.T. Spence, R.C. Carson, & J.W. Thibaut (Eds.), *Behavioral approaches to therapy* (pp. 167–183). Morristown, NJ: General Learning Press.

Petty, B.J., Moeller, T.P., & Campbell, R.Z. (1976). Support groups for elderly persons in the community. *Gerontologist, 16,* 522–528.

Pincus, A. (1970). Reminiscence in aging and its implications for social work practice. *Social Work, 15,* 47–53.

Puder, R.S., Lacks, P., Bertelson, A., & Storandt, M. (November 1982). Short-term stimulus control treatment of insomnia in older adults. Paper presented at the meeting of the Gerontology Society of America, Boston.

Raskind, M.A., & Storrie, M.C. (1980). The organic mental disorders. In E.W. Busse & D.G. Blazer (Eds.), *Handbook of geriatric psychiatry* (pp. 305–328). New York: Van Nostrand Reinhold Co.

Rimm, D.C., & Masters, J.C. (1974). *Behavior therapy: Techniques and empirical findings.* New York: Academic Press.

Rose, S.D. (1977). *Group therapy: A behavioral approach.* Englewood Cliffs, NJ: Prentice-Hall, Inc.

Rush, A.J., & Watkins, J.T. (1981). Group versus individual cognitive therapy: A pilot study. *Cognitive Therapy and Research, 5,* 95–104.

Rush, A.J., Hollan, S.D., Beck, A.T., & Kovacs, M. (1978). Depression: Must pharmacotherapy fail for cognitive therapy to succeed. *Cognitive Therapy and Research, 2,* 199–206.

Sallis, J.F., Jr. (1981). *Altering arousal level in the elderly: Effects on anxiety and depression.* Unpublished doctoral dissertation, Memphis State University.

Schwartz, A.N. (1977). *Survival handbook for children of aging parents.* Chicago: Follet.

Shaw, B.F. (1977). Comparison of cognitive therapy and behavior therapy in the treatment of depression. *Journal of Consulting and Clinical Psychology, 45,* 543–551.

Smith, M.J. (1975). *When I say no, I feel guilty.* New York: Bantam Books.

Steuer, J.L., & Hammen, C. (1983). Cognitive-behavioral group therapy for the depressed elderly: Issues and adaptations. *Cognitive Therapy and Research, 7,* 285–296.

Taulbee, L.R. (1978). Reality orientation: A therapeutic group activity for elderly persons. In I.M. Burnside (Ed.), *Working with the elderly: Group processes and techniques* (pp. 206–218). North Scituate, MA: Duxbury Press.

Toepfer, C.T., Bicknell, A.T., & Shaw, D.O. (1974). Remotivation as behavior therapy. *Gerontologist, 14,* 451–453.

Toseland, R. (1977). A problem-solving group workshop for older persons. *Social Work, 22,* 325–326.

Tournier, P. (1972). *Learning to grow old.* New York: Harper & Row.

Unger, J., & Kramer, E. (1968). Applying frames of reference in group work with the aged. *Gerontologist, 8,* 51–53.

Watson, D.L., & Tharp, R.G. (1972). *Self-directed behavior: Self-modification for personal adjustment.* Monterey, CA: Brooks/Cole.

Weiner, M.B., & Weinstock, C.S. (1978–1979). Group progress of community elderly as measured by tape recordings, group tempo and group evaluation. *International Journal of Aging and Human Development, 10,* 177–185.

Wheeler, E.G. (1980). Assertive training groups for the elderly. In S.S. Sargent (Ed.), *Nontraditional therapy and counseling with the aged* (pp. 15–29). New York: Springer.

Whitney, L.R., & Barnard, K.E. (1966). Implications of operant learning theory for nursing care of the retarded child. *Mental Retardation, 4,* 26–29.

Woods, R.T. (1979). Reality orientation and staff attention: A controlled study. *British Journal of Psychiatry, 134,* 502–507.

Yalom, I.D. (1975). *The theory and practice of group psychotherapy* (2nd ed.). New York: Basic Books.

Zarit, S.H. (1980). *Aging and mental disorders: Psychological approaches to assessment and treatment.* New York: Free Press.

Zarit, S.H., Gallagher, D., & Kramer, N. (1980). Memory training in the community aged: Effects on depression, memory complaint and memory performance. *Educational Gerontology, 5,* 122–137.

Zeplin, H., Wolfe, C.S., & Kleinplatz, F. (1981). Evaluation of a year-long reality-orientation program. *Journal of Gerontology, 36,* 70–77.

Chapter 11

Family Intervention and Family Therapy with the Elderly

While some of the fears, anxieties, problems of daily functioning, and cognitive-perceptual distortions of the elderly can best be ameliorated through group intervention and group therapy, family factors and home relationships have an equally critical influence on the lives of many elderly and to a large measure determine successful adjustments to old age. If the elders are able to receive adequate help from family members and have a collaborative relationship with them, their whole mental outlook, behavioral functioning, and life adaptations can be significantly improved. As age assaults the individuals and the social support networks are less available, elderly individuals come to rely even more heavily than usual on supportive relationships within the family. From the limited number of empirical studies on the effects of family intervention and family therapy on the mental health of elderly individuals, it is apparent that family ties do not diminish with aging. Many older adults are not isolated from their families but maintain integral ties with their relatives. It is often necessary to consider the entire family system when providing care for an elderly client. When family ties become problematic and conflict-ridden in old age, the fear of abandonment and isolation causes sheer desperation in many elderly who must find solutions to emotional problems in the context of family relations and family therapy. The answer lies in determining how family intervention and family therapy should be reorganized and reconstructed so that it can provide maximum satisfaction to elderly individuals.

This chapter looks at some of the fundamental goals of family intervention for the elderly and discusses some of the components of the elderly individual's family dynamics that need to be evaluated before family therapy. One of the questions that has not been addressed adequately in the family therapy literature is the way in which family therapy for the elderly differs in goals, objectives, and procedures from family therapy with younger adults. These and other related questions are addressed in this chapter.

THE FAMILY OF THE ELDERLY

The classical extended family is not common in our society, and never has been. According to Litwak (1961) the *modified extended family* provides a more appropriate description of family relations in modern American culture. Ties in the modified extended family generally are of an emotional rather than economic nature and are characterized by frequent interactions and common activities between the elders and the adult children. The economic support provided by the modified extended family is in the direction of aged parent to adult child, as well as from adult child to aged family members (Shanas, 1967). From this perspective the family is a unit of persons with emotional ties and sometimes with emotional and behavioral problems.

For purposes of therapy Miller and Miller (1979) believe that the family consists of individuals who are genetically related, who have developed relationships, or who are living together as if they were related. In working with younger families, a number of family therapists (e.g., Berger & Berger, 1972; Haley, 1963; Hops, 1976) agree that the focus should usually be on the so-called nuclear family as opposed to the extended family. Working with the elderly, however, would more frequently entail working with the extended family in which all kin of the elderly couple, such as grandchildren, adult children, or siblings and cousins living outside the family are included.

Depending on the particular emotional or physical problems for which families of the elderly require counseling or therapy, the family therapist will have to decide whether intervention is called for beyond the absolute number of individuals in the family with whom the elderly person comes in frequent contact. Generally speaking Mendlewicz (1975) advocates the use of the modified extended family. He suggests that in the case of depressed elderly the most effective evaluation of family dynamics, family history, and the causes and consequences of depressive disorders can be done when family members from more than one generation are interviewed. On the other hand, in working with the aged there are circumstances in which the family therapist may work with the husband and wife alone. Therapy could easily overwhelm an elderly couple by stressing that they must undertake tasks involving interactions with the extended family. There is considerable awareness of this problem, and a treatment plan for a family that requires a great deal of coordination in assembling various members of the family will interfere markedly with their functioning and may possibly generate conflict and resentment among the family members. Thus, as far as possible the family unit must be defined in such a way as to work out a solution to the problem of the elderly members within the limited structure of individuals with whom the elderly person comes in frequent contact.

An important first step in most cases is to determine which members, if any, of the extended family or the social support system should become involved in family therapy and intervention. In order to accomplish this task, a number of clinicians suggest an assessment of the family interaction. Such an assessment takes into account the frequency of contacts with adult children, visits by the adult children and their families, and telephone contacts. The proximity of family members within 30 minutes' driving distance is also an important consideration.

Involving only relevant family members at each point in the treatment is especially essential for older persons. In some situations the treatment of psychological problems in the elderly may require that only the adult children be present so that they can be trained to understand changed ways of responding to the older person's functioning. In other cases the adult children of the older person's family may bring to the family therapy situation concerns about an elderly parent's functioning. In such cases the presence of both mother and father may not be necessary. The aged person rarely if ever is referred for family therapy as the designated client. According to Brody and Spark (1966) and Brody (1974) experience and practical necessity confirm that the family as a whole feels the crisis of aging. Spark and Brody (1970) stress that the family as a whole should be viewed as a client and all members need to be made aware of the potential consequences of their action or lack of action in the resolution of the crisis of aging.

Miller and Miller (1979) view the family as a system analogous to an organ system, such as the cardiovascular system, and contend that difficulty with one part of the system may have potential or real consequences for other parts of the system. Thus the onset of depression in an older member of the family may place stress on other members, and all members may be forced to play a role in the resolution of the problem of depression in the older member. Family therapy may be necessary to determine the way in which the elderly person's depression or depressive disorder has disrupted the family system.

Evaluation of the Family: Assessing the Strengths and Limitations

In order to understand the nature of the crisis of the family, a systematic evaluation based on various sets of information may be required. First, the family therapist may need to acquire specific information about the general level of stability, compatibility, and flexibility of the family system. Second, the clinician or therapist must assess the degree to which the family functioning has been directly disrupted by the recent sickness, disability, or depression of the elderly member, as opposed to longstanding disruption that has characterized the family functioning. Third, the therapist must identify the specific ways in which the elderly member perceives oneself as disrupting the functioning of various members of the family system.

Blazer (1982) enumerates several other aspects and components of the elderly person's family dynamics that warrant evaluation and assessment before involving the family in a long-term therapeutic endeavor. Among the primary factors that should be considered are quality of family interaction, family atmosphere, family values, family support and tolerance, and family stress (see Blazer, 1982, pp. 222–233, for a detailed discussion of these aspects).

In studying family interaction, Blazer suggests an assessment of the psychological equilibrium of each family in terms of various criteria, principally compatibility in values, beliefs, and viewpoints; cohesiveness and loyalty; ability to be a productive family unit; and the fluidity and flexibility in the roles of various members of the family. Based on clinical experience and research, Blazer concludes that the greater the degree of compatibility in values, beliefs, and viewpoints among various members of the family, the more therapeutic and cooperative will be the relationship that such a family will have with the depressed elderly member.

As in many family relationships, roles within the family may shift, and individuals may assume more than one role at a time. This may cause problems in the relationship between aged parents and adult children. The most obvious is when an elderly parent develops a mental or physical incapacity or becomes severely depressed. Simos (1973) reports that in such circumstances adult children may become involved in managing the consequences of their parents' unadaptive or depressive functioning, monitoring their care, and assuming responsibility for caring for other members of the family who were dependent on the elderly member. When faced with these demands, those adult children who have communicated well with their parents and have had few earlier conflicts with the family may be quite willing to be supportive, helpful, and caring. On the other hand in families with many old unresolved conflicts between the older parents and their middle-aged children, the development of a significant health problem in the elderly parent may increase the anxiety of the individual family members. Angry outbursts may ensue, and conflict and competition may arise among the adult children as to responsibility for the elderly parent. When this conflict among the adult children is coupled with the need to take some responsibility for caring for the incapacitated or depressed elder, the problem of family therapy is considerably magnified.

In families with longstanding problems between the spouses or among the older parents and their middle-aged children, any shift in roles for the elderly members may cause additional problems of interpersonal relationships to surface after many years of latency. Unless the adult children have what Blazer (1982) terms "filial maturity" and are prepared to resolve their conflicts with the depressed or incapacitated elderly parent, the family will experience a life crisis that may have negative outcomes not only for the health of the elderly parents but also for the psychological well-being of the adult children and their families. Because of the difficulties in dealing with the depression or incapacity of an elderly relative, the scope of the family therapy may be considerably enhanced by the need to teach members skills for protecting their own emotional health as well as communicating among themselves. Often family therapy can easily overwhelm the adult children by stressing that tension is building up in their marital and interpersonal relationship.

In conflictual families, where the dominance and control of one or more elderly person has held the family together, the onset of a depression reaction in the previously dominant elder may quickly precipitate further family conflict. Zarit (1980) notes a common conflict when children must assume responsibility for a parent is that the parent resists their attempts to monitor the care. This may result in a powerful resentment between the adult child and the elderly parent or it may lead to overprotectiveness and excessive concern for keeping the family together no matter what the price or sacrifice. Verwoerdt (1981) notes that for some families stress and crises is a way of life. The family members may complain about the burden caused by the presence of an elderly parent in their home, but in fact it is precisely this kind of stress that may hold the family intact. Many conflictual families may welcome the stressful circumstances of providing generous support to the elderly relative because the external crises save them from having to face their own inner conflicts or marital concerns. Thus when such families complain about their elderly relatives but continue beyond the call of duty to support and nurture them, it is important for the family therapist to ascertain the extent to which the family may be crisis prone. If their past is a succession of crises, then the family therapist may assess that the external turmoil serves a defensive purpose for the whole family of the elderly parent.

Certain family members may be less tolerant of the incapacitation, dependency, or sick-role of the elderly member and may refuse to become involved in the treatment and care of this member. These are often individuals who in terms of their upbringing and values do not have a sense of filial maturity, responsibility, or psychological-mindedness toward the specific mental health needs of the elderly relative. The focus of treatment subsequently is on helping the elderly adapt to the idea that their adult children are unable to help. The possibilities of moving to nursing homes, segregated homes for the elderly, or hospital settings should be discussed. For purposes of family assessment only those families relatively free of tension, past conflicts, and internal competitiveness would rate highly on the continuum of family atmosphere and supportive care.

Troll, Miller, and Atchley (1979) suggest that the clinician should assess the older person's perceptions of support that can be expected from the family members. Perceptions of such support as emotional caring, shopping, housework, financial help, and administrative help would rate high on the continuum of family support and tolerance. If the elderly member fears that incapacitation will place a tremendous strain on the time and economic resources of other members of the family (for example, the spouse or other adult children) or if the elderly relative fears reactions of anger and resentment from the adult children, such perceptions are likely to have negative health outcomes for the older person. Through periodic assessment of the quality of family interactions and the level of family support and tolerance, clinicians can increase their own awareness of the level of family stress and the nature of the help, support, and intervention that the family members will be able to provide the elderly relative. These assessments of the family dynamics will in turn help the clinician to make judgments about extrafamilial services that a family will need in caring for the incapacitated or depressed elderly member.

If a family is judged to be unmotivated in caring for the elderly relative, the clinician must attempt to balance the responsibilities that the willing or resisting members may take in the treatment plan for the depressed or incapacitated elderly member. Blazer (1982) cautions that elaborate plans presented by a health care team to an unmotivated family may frequently be a waste of time. Even in unmotivated families considerable stress may occur at the time of institutionalization of an aged family member. The family therapist must impress upon the family members that their attitudes toward nursing-home placement will be most influential in the adjustment of the elderly person to the nursing-home setting (Linn & Gurel, 1972). Nursing home personnel frequently experience family members of the elderly, especially the wives, presenting management problems, or alternatively, avoiding contacts with their elderly spouses, perhaps because of unresolved guilt associated with the act of placement (Linn & Gurel, 1969). According to Brudno (1964), the family therapist's task is to counsel the family and to address problems and conflicts arising from the placement of the elderly member, and to open avenues of communication between the family members and the elderly relative, and between the family members and staff of the nursing home.

Conversely certain other families may be highly motivated to care for their elderly because of a strong tradition of filial responsibility. Seelback (1978) notes that expectations for filial responsibility may vary from family to family depending on the psychological equilibrium of the family. In many cases there are families that have withstood both internal and external stress with a remarkable degree of cohesiveness. By and large families that have a dependable social network system and an ongoing system of communication between the older and younger members maintain a positive outlook toward the life and health of all its members, both young and old. Families having ties of intimacy and belongingness that freely permit all members, young or old, to share emotions and to have a role within the family will remain relatively stable, both in its members and its interactions, over a relatively extended time. Such families will be an excellent means of long-term support in the older person's adaptation to chronic illness regardless of whether this illness is physical, mental, or emotional in nature. The probability of effective family intervention is greatly increased when a family with the desired psychological equilibrium and the clinician can work as a team. The family that has a sense of moral obligation for caring for the senior members could be of great assistance to the clinician in providing a beneficial adjunct to medical treatment.

TYPES OF PROBLEMS IN FAMILIES OF THE ELDERLY

The case for including families of the elderly in the search for solutions to problems of aging is clear and unchallenged. But more frequently the question is how to identify problems within the family and how to deal with the conflicts (Herr & Weakland, 1978).

The overview of general cautions and precautions presented is not meant to be inclusive. Family therapists and researchers may undertake different approaches to the degree of home care desirable or possible by the family of the depressed or incapacitated elderly. Time restraints placed both on the family members and the clinician are recognized, and therefore several strategies presented here may be unrealistic for individual families. The family therapist must choose the diagnostic procedures, goals for treatment, and treatment techniques that are most useful and efficient for the family unit. It must be understood both by the family unit and the therapist that family therapy principles offer some potentially beneficial ways of intervening in various problem situations that arise in families of the elderly. Rather than being an end in themselves, however, these interventions need to be used in the service of specific goals that have been identified jointly by the therapist and the family. While the exact degree to which elderly persons are helped by family therapy remains to be determined, most family therapy interventions, even in unfavorable circumstances, have as their goal the personal happiness and well-being of as many members of the family as possible.

In terms of general problem areas, family therapy in families with elderly members is concerned with examining various conflicts. Principal among these are conflicts between the elderly spouses, conflicts between the elderly parents and their adult children, and conflicts in communications and expectations.

Conflict between the Elderly Spouses

Steuer (1982) notes that changes in the life circumstances of the elderly, for example, retirement, loss of income or old-age illness and incapacitation, may reactivate earlier problems in the marital relationship. Despite unsatisfactory relations many elderly couples may continue together because of a fear of change, or economic necessity. When an elderly member becomes depressed, disabled, or both, this may create dependency on the spouse for physical care, activity, and entertainment. Conflict between the spouses may be precipitated for a number of reasons. Most important, with increasing age many elderly may become both resistant to change and be physically unable to accommodate to the spouse's new needs and disabilities. An incapacitating illness in one spouse may upset the whole balance in the marital relationship. Fengler and Goodrich (1979) have called wives of elderly disabled men "the hidden patients" and urge support for these women who often care singlehandedly for their stricken spouses. The focus of family treatment will then be to help both partners in adapting to the changed capacities of the impaired person and to help the spouse who has become impaired to deal with emotions of despair, anger, self-pity, or resentment (Grauer, Betts, & Birnbom, 1973).

Regressive behavior is often precipitated by the vicissitudes of the aging process. The aged person may react by becoming unduly helpless and turning to the spouse for assistance in almost all life activities. The regressed person may frequently act so angry and hostile in this childlike dependency that it may become impossible to do anything that satisfies that individual. In many cases an aged person's regressive and depressed behavior may take the form of a hostile clinging to the spouse. The following case illustrates this point.

Client 1

A 70-year-old chronically disabled man was so depressed and dependent that he would become seriously upset any time that his wife's friends or the family came to visit or stay.

He had several hypochondriacal concerns that became immensely exacerbated whenever the wife declared that she wanted to go away to visit her friends. This pattern of vicarious dependency gratifications had begun after the children left and he retired from work. In marital therapy, management consisted in allowing him to understand that his wife would indeed abandon him if he insisted on being so physically ill and depressed all the time.

Townsend's (1957) study of intergenerational relationships shows that when aged women become ill or disabled, they tend to depend on their daughters first, then on close female relatives, and last on their husbands. By contrast, when an aged man is ill, the most common source of support, reliance, and aid is his wife. According to several authorities (e.g., Birren, 1964) the role of the elderly man in the multigenerational family is a more difficult one compared to the role of the elderly female. Family therapy may therefore have to stress the significance and importance of the wife vis-à-vis the aged man in times of life crisis and illness.

While Spark and Brody (1970) confirm that physical abandonment of a spouse occurs rarely, there are various ways in which the communication patterns of the elderly spouses begin to change as if from a sense of abandonment. Hinchcliffe, Hooper, and Roberts (1978) note the depressive rule in the communication patterns. According to Hinchcliffe et al. the marital relationship in which one member is depressed shows many unusual signs of hopelessness and apathy. The depressed spouse desperately communicates a need to be cared for by the partner but simultaneously rejects the care. Since little or no appreciation is expressed for the care given, this elicits a distancing response from the caregiving partner, which in time confirms the original sense of despondency.

In family therapy, therefore, it is important that the elderly partner who provides service and care for the depressed spouse be made aware of the psychological difficulty that the depressed spouse may encounter in expressing gratitude or appreciation for the help received. Family and marital therapy will need to focus on the symptoms of anhedonia and masked depression and to teach the partners mutually to recognize symptoms of depression and stress. The caregiving spouse should also be taught techniques for self-care and self-protection. The depressed spouse should be encouraged to express more specifically the need for the particular kinds of help, advice, and attention sought from the caregiving partner.

Blazer and Siegler (1981) enumerate the emotional problems that develop in the marital relationship when an elderly spouse has to care for a disabled, incapacitated, or depressed partner. Principal among these are low morale and strong needs for social support and concerns about social isolation, economic hardship, and role overload (Simos, 1973).

Although marital discord may decrease slightly with age (Hudson & Murphy, 1980), marital problems previously ignored or glossed over may become magnified as a function of the other accompanying hassles and stresses of old age. The readjustment of the house-wife's daily schedule to accommodate a full-time husband, and especially a disabled husband, may present a major difficulty in the relationship of the elderly couple. The elderly spouses may experience stress as the unit strives to adjust after retirement to the impact of the loss of work role and its concomitant rewards for the members of the family unit, including the adult children and grandchildren (Palmore, Cleveland, Nowlin, Ramm, & Siegler, 1979).

The sexual components of the marital relationship may also require therapeutic intervention in later life. Rowland and Haynes (1978) noted that both the family therapist and the elderly couple may avoid the sexual aspect of the relationship because of negative attitudes about sexuality in later life. Murphy, Hudson and Cheung (1980) suggest that family counselors and marital therapists of the aged should discuss the physiological changes that accompany the sexual aging process. How traditional methods of achieving sexual pleasure may be modified (so that sexuality remains a meaningful component of the relationship) should also be examined in therapy. A disabled elderly woman may undergo considerable stress if she perceives her failing health to be a factor in the couple's decline in sexual behavior. Rowland and Haynes (1978) described a two-phase successful program of sexual enhancement for older couples. The initial education phase provided elderly couples with information on sexual functioning in later life, including a discussion of attitudes. In the second phase treatment consisted of exercises designed to improve communication between the spouses, and training in sexual techniques.

It is important for the practitioner to note that at a general level the treatment issues in the marital therapy cases of older couples may not differ from cases of younger couples. Sometimes, however, the difficulties can be longstanding, and the long duration of marital problems may increase feelings of hopelessness. Further problems of distancing and emotional withdrawal in the marital relationship may also become magnified. The pattern of withdrawal may lead to isolation with its risks of absorption, hypochondriasis, disuse atrophy of social skills, or progressive loss of contact with reality (Verwoerdt, 1981). In these situations the practitioner is well advised to stress that marital and family therapy should focus on the dynamics of the relationships and communications rather than on the alleviation of somatic symptoms.

Conflicts between Adult Children and Elderly Parents

Romaniuk (1981) notes the key role that adult children and the elderly spouse play in the home care of the elderly depressed or ailing client. Many adult children assume increasing responsibility for the management of an elderly person, sometimes at a great emotional and financial cost to themselves (Berezin, 1972). Among spouses, caretaking responsibilities may come at a time when physical energies and economic resources are declining.

The family may undergo great stress if living arrangements are changed or if an older adult experiences failing health and joins the nuclear family of an adult child. Considerable conflict and stress can also develop between elderly parents and children when parent-child dependency relationships are reversed.

One type of aggressive reaction often used by elderly parents is the attempt to control their children. Many elderly may feel dependent on their adult children to provide satisfaction, but they may be uncertain that their family members are willing to provide such gratifications. They may attempt to gain control over adult children by using their invalidism, dependency, and depression to make them feel guilty. They may attain a dominating position by making themselves completely dependent on an adult child and becoming permanently sick and incompetent. If this control is directed at a submissive adult child, this may create a number of conflicts and upheavals for the submissive person who resents the manipulation but is unable to discuss the resentment with the dominant elderly parent. As a result, family members may spend tremendous amounts of time and energy in resolving their guilt and resentment. The effects of such controlling maneuvers can be harmful not only to the aging parent but also to the adult children. The following case illustrates the elderly parent's attempt at controlling.

Client 2

Mr. C., a 46-year-old man, was hospitalized for severe headaches and a stomach ulcer. He had been working under high pressure, one reason being that every evening he had to spend time with his elderly father, who was depressed and frequently threatened suicide. The aged father had no other family or friends and counted on his son visiting him every evening. The son was also in chronic conflict with his wife, who had been hospitalized because of recurrent depression. The wife announced her intentions to separate if she did not get more attention from her husband. The wife's physician put more pressure on Mr. C. to spend less time with his father and more time with his wife. Mr. C. revealed in family therapy that he felt controlled by both his father and his wife but tried his best to keep them happy. Management consisted in allowing him to understand that he was being manipulated by both persons. Assertion training helped him to express his resentment and anger toward the father and to assert himself with his wife. Eventually an arrangement evolved with the aged father residing in a rest home. Mr. C. went to visit him once a week and therefore had more time to spend with his wife.

This case illustrates how the family therapist must address the question of the placement of the elderly in long-term care facilities. Such a move is often advisable and may relieve many families. The presence of an aggressive and controlling elderly person in the family of an adult child may create much tension in the family system; however, the family therapist may have to study the delicate balance between the needs of the elderly parent and the needs of the adult child's family. Practical subjects that must be addressed in family therapy include the extent of the obligations that adult children must bear toward the elderly relative, especially in families of cognitively confused and depressed elders.

A number of authors (e.g., Berezin, 1972; Blazer, 1982; Zarit, 1980) observe that potentials for conflict between elderly parents and adult children are greater today because of the absence of cultural norms in the area of intergenerational relationships. Many of the problems encountered seem to be nested within the psychologically larger issues surrounding the management of the role shifts and reversals between parent and child across the life span (Butler & Lewis, 1977). With few exceptions (see Schwartz, 1977; Silverstone & Hyman, 1976) these problems have not been studied in depth by family therapists who must often counsel adult children to cope with the needs of aging parents.

Blazer and Siegler (1981) stress the need for clinicians to become more involved in the roles and interactions of the family. Such role-taking, if planned as a structured intervention, may be useful. Therapists, however, must recognize that such involvement is time-consuming. Families make persistent demands on the therapist in the role as family manager but may simultaneously resent the therapist for taking control of family problems and decisions.

Hausman (1979) advocates the use of support groups designed to assist adult children who are caring for elderly parents. Such groups promote the notion that an important developmental task for the adult child is to view the parents as individuals who both give and receive support. Similarly the developmental task for the elderly parent is to accept the maturity of the children and to enter into a new relationship with them (Brody, 1974). These support groups provide an opportunity for adult children to discuss family issues, air feelings and concerns, and discuss concrete plans for action. Support groups have been instrumental in improving parent-child relationships and have taught families to provide assistance to elderly parents in a constructive manner. They can be a useful adjunct to the therapeutic assistance and counseling provided by a family therapist (Hausman, 1979).

Problems of Communications and Roles

Not all families have sufficient strength to achieve optimal goals of communication with the elderly members and not all families can withstand open conflict within the family system. Families with sufficient strengths in terms of sincerity, empathy and generosity can, however, be helped to achieve improved communications and closeness with the elderly members with respect to new roles and goals.

While there is considerable awareness of the problems faced by middle-aged children in caring for their depressed or chronically ill parent, one problem of family therapy that is often overlooked is the help that elderly parents may give to their adult children. In families of the elderly a number of circumstances develop in which elderly parents may provide comfort and nurturance. For example, an adult child may need emotional support for dealing with midlife crises. In other cases adult children in caring for the ailing elderly parent may become so intensely involved that they may suffer considerable anguish over the thought of losing the "parental child." In many cases adult children may fear death and dying. Various forms of depressive reactions may emerge in adult children caring for an elderly parent. In such cases the family therapist may utilize the help of the elderly parent to offer encouragement and support to the anguished children.

There are cases when the elderly parents are possessive and overinvolved in the family interactions of their adult children. They may make excessive demands on their adult children, thus causing significant disruption in their family life. The source of the problem may originate with the aging parent who tenaciously adheres to an outdated set of roles or obsolete functions. An elderly father may continue to see himself as head of the family or somebody who should have the final word in family decisions. In most cases the difficulties involved in the process of role reversal are due to psychological factors in both the aging parent and the adult child (Verwoerdt, 1981) and may cause considerable upheaval in the day-to-day functioning of the aged parent and adult child (Savitsky & Sharkey, 1972). Such psychological issues surrounding the management of elderly parent and adult child relationships deserve greater attention in family therapy.

Many adult children who have regarded their parents as strong and omnipotent have considerable difficulty in assuming a parental role to their own parents. The filial crisis of this stage occurs when the adult children realize that the aging parents are no longer the pillars of strength and support. This transition involves a reversal of roles, which to many individuals may cause considerable problems. The new filial role involves being depended on and being dependable. In such situations the function of family therapy would be to provide clarification of the adult child's filial role and the delineation of the obligations toward an aging parent.

Spark and Brody (1970) have also referred to problems of abuse of the elderly parent and excessive demands placed on the elderly parents by their adult children. Family therapy sessions have demonstrated how the elderly parent can be extruded, dyadic alliances can occur, and unhealthy symbiotic relationships may develop between adult children and parents. Such problems should also be viewed as legitimate concerns of family therapy for the elderly (Spark & Brody, 1970).

FAMILY AND MARITAL THERAPY WITH THE DEPRESSED ELDERLY

Haley (1963, 1971) maintains that family treatment refers to several different kinds of therapy situations, each having different goals and requiring perhaps somewhat different approaches. However, one common thread in all of the family therapy problems is the recognition that the family as a whole (as opposed to the individual) has a problem. Also the depressions of one person in the family can represent a way of dealing with the depressions of other family members and may also be related to problems of depression shared by the whole family. For example, in the case of families with an elderly relative the elderly person's depression may be a part of sequences of actions, attitudes, and treatment of other family members. An adult son's inability to communicate with the elderly father on certain issues of values, self-esteem, and autonomy may contribute to the depressions of both father and son.

Few advances in therapy can be accomplished if the therapist decides to work with the elderly member alone since the latter's esteem or self-worth may be undermined by other family members. In a majority of cases family members' treatment of the elderly relative needs to be changed before any of the family distress can be reduced. In contrast to individual therapy the persons involved in the family problems interact with one another in front of the family therapist, who can then intervene to change the sequences of behavior in the adult children, which may be leading to depressive and dysfunctional behavior in the elderly parent.

Grolnick (1981) contends that the social context within which a family manages or mismanages its sadness or elation provides a key to the evaluation and treatment of depression in that family. The emotional lability of a depressed family member has a centralizing effect on the whole family's emotional system. When other members are also vulnerable, a contagion of depression and mental dissatisfaction may lead to divorce, recurrent crises, or impaired family organization (Grolnick, 1981). This notion has special relevance for family therapy with the depressed elderly for whom family factors play an extremely important part in symptom formation and maintenance of depression. In the case of the elderly the family therapist can find out what other family members are doing to maintain the depression in the elderly relative; for example, are they uninvolved and indifferent, or are they overly sympathetic and overfunctioning? By taking a familywide view of the depression of the elderly member, the problem is taken from one person and distributed throughout the family system. This can lead to a sense of relief in the identified elderly client who worries about personal responsibility for the depression. It may also bring relief to the adult children, who often feel guilty that they may not be doing enough to care for the elderly parent. Thus each member can gain some awareness of the part each plays in the family process. While the elderly member who is depressed would be viewed as the symptom bearer (Bowen, 1978), those disturbances of effect reflect the disturbances of the family system.

Bowen describes the depressed person as assuming the adaptive position in the family. If this position is adaptive for long periods, the individual can gradually lose self-confidence, and the ability to function independently is markedly impaired. Such a depressed adaptive position is seen often in elderly persons who initially become depressed because of a physical or intellectual incapacitation. Their depression is often exacerbated by the fact that other members of the family, say the spouse or the adult children, may become the overfunctioners or the dominant ones while the elderly persons themselves are compelled into taking the position of underfunctioners or the adaptive ones. Neither position enhances growth for the elderly persons, and such a process can lead to chronic depression or dysfunction. In working with such a family the goal should be to try to get other family members of the elderly (e.g., the spouse or the adult children) to do less and the dysfunctional member (the elderly person) to do more and be more autonomous.

An appropriate treatment plan for a family that must assume responsibility for an invalid elderly parent includes helping them decide what type of care and involvement is necessary or desirable. The therapist must provide a professional judgment of how much self-care the elderly person is capable of and how much help and care is needed from the family. Because of the difficulties in accurately understanding and estimating the amount of care that the elderly person needs, family members may become overprotective, overcaring, and overinvolved. The therapist or clinician must attempt to balance the responsibility that the elderly person takes in self-care and the responsibility delegated to other family members. The family therapist's intervention in assigning tasks to various members will reduce the risk of overprotection of the elderly member or underinvolvement by the family.

It is generally recognized that family members or other caregivers who foster the sick role or promote unnecessary dependence in the elderly relative should be alerted to the negative long-term consequences of their action for the functioning of the elderly person. Families may require counseling in order to learn how to reinforce the aged member to take responsibility for self-care activities and how to deal with the controlling behavior of the elderly relative.

In the case of elderly persons with organic brain dysfunction, family members can learn to contribute to the resocialization, remotivation, or reality orientation of elderly relatives who are confused and disoriented. With a system of comprehensive home care family intervention can significantly increase the number of elderly clients who can be cared for in the community and would otherwise be sent to long-term hospital care for physical disabilities and for behavior problems associated with depression and organic brain syndrome, including senile dementia (Glasscote, Gudeman, & Miles, 1977).

Early intervention and open discussion with all parties involved, including the elderly client, can prevent many potential problems of some family members feeling guilty that they are not doing enough and other members feeling resentful and angry because of the endless demands placed on their time and energies. In this respect Kahn (1975) advises that the most important step in family intervention is to help the adult children and the spouse of the elderly person to realize that they must not neglect their personal needs or make too many sacrifices on their own mental well-being in caring for the elderly person. Alternatives for caring for the elderly, such as nursing homes and institutions for the elderly, should be explored with both the elderly patient and the family members so that the family as a whole is involved in the decision making.

Emotional isolation is an important component of depression in the elderly. Bowen (1978), who introduced the concept of emotional cutoff, contends that the depressed person feels emotionally cut off from other members and therefore increases emotional investment in and preoccupation with the self. This decreases the personal connectedness with others in the family and perpetuates the depression.

When one or both members of an elderly couple become depressed or incapacitated, they tend to become increasingly inactive and feel emotionally cut off from other members of the family. The most frequent situation is when elderly parents have moved in with their adult children or when the adult children were involved in activities with their parents. Although some elderly persons are able to maintain their own set of social activities, others find it hard to live an independent life and expect the adult children to provide some kind of stimulating social life for them. Adult children who react by feeling angry because their parents do so little to keep themselves active or to develop an independent social life may precipitate the elderly members' depressive feelings by emotionally cutting them off (Simos, 1973).

In family therapy sessions it may be possible for younger adults in the family or the therapist to explain to the elders that it is unrealistic of them to expect to be included in the social activities of their adult children. Zarit (1980) notes that it is the expectation of such a responsibility that leads to arguments and guilt feelings in the family members. The family as a system can then be utilized to help various members of the elderly person's family to understand what expectations are fair and possible and others that are unreasonable and to be discouraged. Family therapy must endeavor to teach all members, including the elderly member, how to respond appropriately to their own needs and others' needs without anger or resentment. Perhaps the most important step in family therapy is for various members of the family to communicate more clearly what it is they want from one another and to help one another in responding in new ways to the symptom bearers of the family problem.

When the elderly person is a symptom bearer of depression and anxiety, distancing or withdrawal becomes the initial but major mechanism for handling tension and stress. Depression of one member can often be reduced by increasing the family members' interactions with the depressed person. The key factor in family therapy is for the family to understand that family nurturance and support or family neglect and rejection play an important part in symptom formation and the maintenance of depression in the elderly person. Briefly stated, the goals of family treatment are to open up communications among various members, to bridge the emotional cutoffs between the young and the elderly, and to encourage the elderly members to express their anxieties.

TECHNIQUES FOR FAMILY INTERVENTION

Family treatment techniques offer some direct and potentially beneficial ways of intervening in various problem situations of the families of elderly. These techniques discussed in detail by Herr andWeakland (1978, 1979) and Jackson and Weakland (1971) are summarized in this section.

Communication Skills Training

All families can benefit from simple instructions about communications with elderly persons who are depressed, lonely, or alienated. Learning methods of responding to the elderly person's expressions of low self-esteem and pessimism, such as paraphrase, reflection, and expression of empathic understanding, can be most effective. Paraphrase is a technique for responding to the thoughts and feelings of another person. "I hear what you're saying . . . I understand." The adult talking with a parent might be trained to echo as follows: "Let me check this out with you, Dad, to see that I got it right; you are saying that you are embarrassed because I did not introduce you properly?" "Let me check this out with you, Mom, in case I did not get this right . . . you are saying that you're not sure how much longer you want to stay with us."

In these examples the content of each response is slightly different. They point out the importance of reflective listening as a method to ensure that the message sent by the elderly person is accurately received. Family members must be encouraged to correct one another's perceptions if they are inaccurate.

Determination of the Problem and Relabeling It

Early in the first session it is important to determine the problem through goal clarification and operational specification of the problematic behavior. If necessary, each family member should be asked to state the goals and problems individually. The following case demonstrates this point.

Client 3

Mr. Z. is an elderly man of 86 who is living with his oldest daughter and her family. Mr. Z.'s wife is in an institution. The point of family conflict is that Mr. Z. frequently runs away from home and wishes to return to his farm. He insists he was brought to his daughter's home for a temporary visit. The other members of the family agree that Mr. Z. knew the visit was permanent. When each member of the family was asked to specify the effects of the problem, Mr. Z.'s elder daughter said the whole thing was affecting her work; her husband said it was affecting their marital relationship; the older grandson said he could not bring home any friends because of grandad acting crazy; the older granddaughter complained that her university life was disrupted by constant telephone calls from mom over the new family crisis. Mr. Z.'s son-in-law (Mr. T.) said he did not like to come home from work with his wife (Mrs. T.) always looking and feeling tired. Mr. Z. said he was tired of everyone telling him what to do. He wanted to return to the farm and be left in peace to have his seizures and his spells. Mr. T. maintained that he could not understand why Mr. Z. did not enjoy his easy chair and the leisure of nothing to do. Mr. T. said he could not concentrate on work at the office and worried about Mr. Z. having a seizure and scaring the children. Mrs. T. said she felt responsible for the family upset since it was her father who was brought to stay with them. Mr. Z. said everyone was on his back and he could stand it no more.

During the initial contact the counselor or therapist gives the family members "permission" to talk about feelings and personal problems, in addition to the immediate and objective difficulty that brought the family to therapy. The therapist, in other words, tries to determine the hidden agendas in the family (Herr & Weakland, 1979).

The next step involves the setting of minimal realistic goals. Each family member should be asked to specify the smallest amount of change that could help to solve the problem. Minimizing goals also subdivides the family's problems into smaller, manageable units. By discussing the goals and problems, all the family members can be helped to make clear what is happening in the family and how the events (problems) affect them personally and how they would know if the situation were improving (goals). Although discussions of what the problem is, who is causing it, and how a solution can be negotiated may have fairly free rein during the early part of the session, it is important to secure some final statement of goals and problems from each person, including the elderly member. It is important for the family therapist or counselor to judge whether the goals are realistic, or whether families are setting themselves up for certain failure by aiming too high. Thus the therapist must not only try to determine the problem through role clarification but also try to make sense of the family system. This stage of counseling allows the therapist to observe the various members of the family and their interactions in order to obtain a better idea of how the family system operates.

It is important to note such factors as how people interact with one another, their predominant moods, and what kinds of dyads or alliances they seem to be developing. Haley (1963) suggests a number of important components of how the problems must be relabeled and presented in ways to facilitate their solution. First, he stresses that the family problem should be relabeled only in terms of positive aspects of the existing family relationships and the potential strengths and positive attributes of the family members, including the elderly member, to solve the problem. As an example, when an elderly person becomes depressed, it can be said that the person feels dejected because of declining capacities to contribute to family happiness but the person goes about it the wrong way.

When an elderly mother is demanding in a relationship, it can be said that it is her attempt to communicate with the children. Haley stresses that it is unproductive to focus on negative emotions of anger, resentment, or self-pity in the family relationships.

Second, in relabeling the problem Haley emphasizes the significance of the therapist identifying how all members are contributing to the problem, rather than designating one person (for example, the depressed elderly parent or the detached and rejecting adult son) as the sole contributor. Thus, when a problem is rephrased or relabeled in terms of two or more persons' relationship, the implicit suggestion is that relationships need to be altered and strengthened rather than persons being expected to change.

Determination of Previous Family Solutions

It is important to determine what the family did on previous occasions to solve the problems and to identify the specific techniques, actions, or attitudes that have improved the situation. To elicit this information, it is often useful to ask each family member directly what action was taken and what seemed to work or not to work for the individual person.

Often the family will list all of the things they did, and all of the things that went wrong. At this stage it is important for the therapist to suggest that it is pointless to continue with previous family solutions and that perhaps a new approach should be considered. The therapist must also be attentive to what solutions were not tried as these may reflect actions that are taboo or threatening to the family. For example, a family may not have considered a nursing home for an ailing elderly parent. Another family may have required a cognitively impaired and demented elderly member to stay in a secluded part of the house where the person could not be seen by the neighbors. Such actions reflect family taboo or threat and should be viewed as legitimate concerns of family therapy.

Herr and Weakland (1979) note that most of the problems encountered in counseling elders and their families are "problems created and perpetuated by inappropriate solutions" (p. 102). These authors cite an example that is frequently experienced in families of the elderly. A well-intentioned adult child decides that an elderly parent can no longer live alone and convinces the rest of the family that the parent should move in with one of the adult children. When pressure is put on the aged parent to conform to the new living arrangements the elderly person becomes depressed, hostile, or aggressive thus triggering other family conflicts. Previous appropriate and inappropriate solutions that were attempted by the family must be discussed for their merits and demerits.

After the list of attempted solutions is carefully considered, the therapist must not fall into the trap of offering quick and easy solutions for remediation of the family's problems vis-à-vis the elderly member (Herr & Weakland, 1979). The major responsibility for solving the problems rests with various members of the family. Herr and Weakland (1979) postulate that families undergo considerable stress and suffering in exploring solutions for family problems, and the therapist who quickly assumes the advice-giver's role devalues the suffering experienced by the family and sets the stage for a successful sabotaging, face-saving effort by family members.

Understanding of Family Rules

It is helpful for the counselor to ask, "Are there any family rules?" Herr and Weakland (1978) define the family rule as an unwritten and unspoken agreement among the family members about how the family is to function. Family rules may include such guidelines as "grandfather always makes the decision," "we never allow ourselves to express disappointment," "it is important to be loyal to our elderly parents no matter what is happening." Often, when circumstances force the family to abandon the rules (for example, when the father is incapacitated and must be institutionalized or when the mother is upset and threatens suicide), one family member or another may act in a way to distract the family from dealing with the fact that the family rules must be changed.

Family rules may often have to be dramatically violated when a dominant elderly parent dies, is depressed, or is incapacitated. Haley (1963) suggests that the therapist must intervene in the changes necessary in the family rules by identifying for the family first the rules that must be changed and second the disagreements over who sets the new rules. When an elder who was dominant at one time is no longer capable of making decisions, the therapist must assume the parent role and give specific directives to resolve the conflict over the rules governing the new family relationships.

Also important to consider is how each member of the family system expresses personal power. Some members may exercise power through bankbooks and inheritance, others through psychological intimidation (e.g., the elderly parent who withdraws, refuses to communicate with spouse and children), and still others by becoming weak and helpless or taking on a sick role. Information gained in the analysis is not something openly shared in the family but must be elicited by asking questions about how the family sought solutions to problems in the past. Questions concerning distribution of expenses when an elderly parent moves in with an adult child and expectations of inheritance from an elderly parent must be discussed in the open. Often it is important for the family unit to recognize that resentments may arise because the elderly parent has too much or too little personal power.

Mobilization of Energy of the Family and Specific Directives to Change Behavior

Often families may understand the problems and the conflict but may have difficulties in changing their responses. They may be stuck because through long years of conditioning in one given style they have become resistant to change. Families may also be afraid to change. In such a case Haley's approach is to give directives to families to change certain behaviors. If, for example, an elderly father and adult son always fight over the father not taking his medications or nagging the elderly mother for not giving him enough attention, the therapist might direct someone else in the family to administer the medication or have the mother keep an hourly record of time spent with the spouse.

The use of giving specific directives to family members is not a simple process. In such situations Herr and Weakland (1978) and Jackson and Weakland (1971) suggest that it is often more feasible to ease the family's risk in a behavior transition by reframing a suggested change of behavior into an information-gathering assignment. For example, in the case of an adult son who receives a dozen phone calls from his father every day, it may be advisable to reframe the suggested change in behavior by asking the son to monitor the father's reactions if the son's wife arranges to answer the father's calls.

As in other therapeutic techniques there is always the potential for harm and negative reactions when the therapist attempts to exercise control in giving directives to families to change certain behaviors. Generally speaking, however, the therapist has to assume a substantial measure of control over relationships, especially in those families of the elderly that have a longstanding history of disagreements over rules governing family relationships. In some families, for example, there are conflictual tendencies for scapegoating and victimizing some members, placing others in a permanently sick role and still others in which the elderly members are criticized and made to feel dysfunctional, underfunctioning, and emotionally cut off.

Termination of Family Therapy

After the family has been through a period of exploration, behavioral change, and therapeutic integration the responsibility for terminating therapy rests essentially with the family therapist. The family therapist, in consultation with professional colleagues and the family, must address some of the following questions: Does the family still need counseling? What is the extent of behavioral change accomplished? Where is the therapist in the family system? If the family problem has not been solved, why has it not been solved? Is there an identified member who is sabotaging the therapy process?

The therapist must discuss with the family the specific interventions attempted and their therapeutic effects on family relationships, especially those with the elderly members. The therapist must give family members credit for finding their own solutions and for investing time and effort in therapy. The family members should be urged to resume responsibility for continuation of family relationships, and for both positive and negative events that may occur in the future. Herr and Weakland (1979) suggest that future problems and conflicts should be anticipated so that pitfalls can be avoided and potential saboteurs be identified and discouraged. The termination phase requires that the counselor be restrained in optimism and should convey this sense of restrained optimism to the family.

SUMMARY AND CONCLUSIONS

This chapter has examined family intervention approaches. The special problems and conflicts encountered by families with elderly members were discussed, and assessment and therapy considerations were delineated.

Family therapy and family treatment techniques offer some beneficial ways of intervening in various problem situations of the aged persons. However, as in the case of group therapy, family treatment involves more than applying techniques of individual psychotherapy with all family members present. More important, it involves assessment of the family dynamics and evaluation of the elderly members' contribution to the family conflict.

There are many different approaches to family therapy, that is, psychoanalytic, intergenerational, behavioral, and systems approaches. Few of these approaches have addressed the problems of the elderly. Unique aspects of the family situation of many elderly persons and the therapist's relationship with elderly lend themselves well to a systems approach to family therapy. Herr and Weakland (1978) note that the systems approach to family therapy is the only one to have developed and field-tested programs specifically designed for families with elderly members. Their approach is the strategic approach developed by the Palo Alto Group (Stanton, 1981).

The intergenerational approaches by their very title imply that they have something useful to offer the elderly and their families. Such approaches are predicated on the notion that the struggles and problems of several preceding generations live on in the structure of the nuclear and extended family. Thus, invisible power struggles, family loyalties, and family ties with elderly parents are an important key to understanding guilt feelings, hostilities, and resentments that create a vicious cycle in many extended families (Boszor-menyi-Nagy & Ulrich, 1981).

Bowen's (1978) approach has been mentioned with respect to depression in families of the elderly. The goals in this approach would be to differentiate the elderly individual within the multigenerational family context. Whitaker and Keith (1981) also advocate the multi-generational approach. Others who agree with them suggest that the interests of the elderly persons in family therapy are best served only when generational boundaries are identified and family intervention is confined to three generations: grandparents, adult children, and grandchildren.

Family therapy is a relatively new therapeutic technique. Its use with families of the elderly should not be taken lightly. It is a demanding and complex helping technique often involving the services of more than one therapist or mental health worker. Frequently the management of the elderly and their family members, as compared with the individual treatment of the elders, is the more difficult task (Berezin & Stotsky, 1970).

The success of the family therapy (especially one using a family systems approach) in alleviating problems faced by older adults may depend considerably on the particular type of problem. Baer, Morin and Gaitz (1970) noted that families held negative attitudes toward family therapy for elderly relatives having problems of depression and alcoholism but their attitudes were more positive toward other adults receiving therapy and help for chronic brain syndrome problems. Family attitudes toward older members having hypochondriacal complaints were positive. Thus family therapy was more feasible and effective in the treatment of elders with hypochondriasis (Goldstein & Birnbom, 1976).

Further research, building on an intergenerational approach and a family systems approach to intervention in the families of the elderly, is advocated. The scope of family therapy can be usefully expanded by considering preventive approaches to problems of family communications, fixed hierarchical roles, and fixed family rules that produce conflict in the relationship between elderly members and their adult children.

REFERENCES

Baer, P.E., Morin, L, & Gaitz, C.M. (1970). Family resources of elderly psychiatric patients. *Archives of General Psychiatry, 22,* 343–350.

Berezin, M.A. (1972). Psychodynamic considerations of aging and the aged: An overview. *American Journal of Psychiatry, 128,* 1483–1491.

Berezin, M.A., & Stotsky, B.A. (1970). The geriatric patient. In H. Grunebaum (Ed.), *The practice of community mental health* (pp. 219–244). Boston: Little, Brown & Co.

Berger, M.M., & Berger, L.F. (1972). Psychogeriatric group approaches. In C.J. Sager & H.S. Kaplan (Eds.), *Progress in group and family therapy* (pp. 726–757). New York: Brunner/Mazel.

Birren, J.E. (1964). *The psychology of aging.* Englewood Cliffs, NJ: Prentice-Hall, Inc.

Blazer, D.G. (1982). *Depression in late life.* St. Louis: C.V. Mosby Co.

Blazer, D.G. & Siegler, I.C. (1981). Evaluating the family of the elderly patient. In D.G. Blazer & I.C. Siegler (Eds.), *Working with the family of the older adult.* Menlo Park, CA: Addison Wesley.

Boszormenyi-Nagy, I., & Ulrich, D.N. (1981). Contextual family therapy. In G.S. Gurman & D.P. Kniskern (Eds.), *Handbook of Family Therapy* (pp. 159–186). New York: Brunner/Mazel.

Bowen, M. (1978). *Family therapy in clinical practice.* New York: Jason Aronson.

Brody, E.M. (1974). Aging and family perspective: A developmental view. *Family Process, 13,* 23–38.

Brody, E.M., & Spark, G.M. (1966). Institutionalization of the elderly: A family crisis. *Family Process, 5,* 76–90.

Brudno, J.J. (1964). Group programs with adult offsprings of newly admitted residents in geriatric settings. *Journal of American Geriatrics Society, 12,* 385–394.

Butler, R.N., & Lewis, M.I. (1977). *Aging and mental health: Positive psychological approaches* (2nd ed.). St. Louis: C.V. Mosby Co.

Fengler, A.P., & Goodrich, N. (1979). Wives of elderly disabled men: The hidden victims. *Gerontologist, 19,* 175–183.

Glasscote, R., Gudeman, J.E., & Miles, C.D. (1977). *Creative mental health services for the elderly.* Washington: American Psychiatric Association.

Goldstein, S.W., & Birnbom, F. (1976). Hypochondriasis and the elderly. *Journal of American Geriatrics Society, 24,* 150–154.

Grauer, H., Betts, D., & Birnbom, F. (1973). Welfare emotions and family therapy in geriatrics. *Journal of the American Geriatrics Society, 21,* 21–24.

Grolnick, L. (1981). Evaluation and treatment of affect disturbances within a family context. In A.S. Gurman (Ed.), *Questions and answers in the practice of family therapy* (pp. 244–250). New York: Brunner/Mazel.

Haley, J. (1963). *Strategies of psychotherapy.* New York: Grune & Stratton.

Haley, J. (1971). A review of the family therapy field. In J. Haley (Ed.), *Changing families: A family therapy reader* (pp. 1–12). New York: Grune & Stratton.

Hausman, C. (1979). Short-term counseling groups for people with elderly parents. *Gerontologist, 19,* 102–107.

Herr, J.H., & Weakland, J.H. (1978). The family as a group. In I.M. Burnside (Ed.), *Working with the elderly: Group processes and techniques* (pp. 320–343). Belmont, CA: Duxbury Press.

Herr, J.H., & Weakland, J.H. (1979). *Counseling elders and their families: Practical techniques for applied gerontologists.* New York: Springer.

Hinchcliffe, M.K., Hooper, D., & Roberts, F.J. (1978). *The melancholy marriage.* New York: John Wiley & Sons, Inc.

Hops, H. (1976). Behavioral treatment of marital problems. In W.E. Craighead, A.E. Kazdin, & M.J. Mahoney (Eds.), *Behavior modification* (pp. 431–446). Boston: Houghton Mifflin.

Hudson, W.W., & Murphy, G.J. (1980). The nonlinear relationship between marital satisfaction and stages of the family life cycle: An artifact of Type 1 error. *Journal of Marriage and the Family, 42,* 263–267.

Jackson, D.D., & Weakland, J.H. (1971). Conjoint family therapy: Some considerations on theory, technique and results. In J. Haley (Ed.), *Changing families: A family therapy reader* (pp. 13–35). New York: Grune & Stratton.

Kahn, R.L. (1975). The mental health system and the future aged. *Gerontologist, 15*(1, pt. 2), 24–31.

Linn, M.W., & Gurel, L. (1969). Wives' attitudes in nursing home placement. *Journal of Gerontology, 29,* 368–372.

Linn, M.W., & Gurel, L. (1972). Family attitudes in nursing home placements. *Gerontologist, 12,* 220–224.

Litwak, E. (1961). Geographical mobility and family cohesion. *American Sociological Review, 26,* 258–271.

Mendlewicz, J. (1975). Accuracy of family history method in affective illness. *Archives of General Psychiatry, 32,* 309.

Miller, K.T., & Miller, J.L. (1979, February). *The family as a system.* Paper presented at the annual meeting of the American College of Psychiatrists, Costa Mesta, CA.

Murphy, G.J., Hudson, W.W., & Cheung, P.P.L. (1980). Marital and sexual discord among older couples. *Social Work Research and Abstracts, 16,* 11–16.

Palmore, E., Cleveland, W.P., Nowlin, J.B., Ramm, D., & Siegler, I.C. (1979). Stress and adaptation in later life. *Journal of Gerontology, 34,* 841–851.

Romaniuk, M. (1981). Community mental health practice and the elderly. *Professional Psychology, 8,* 210–217.

Rowland, K.F., & Haynes, S.N. (1978). A sexual enhancement program for elderly couples. *Journal of Sex and Marital Therapy, 4,* 91–113.

Savitsky, E., & Sharkey, H. (1972). The geriatric patient and his family—study of family interaction in the aged. *Journal of Geriatric Psychiatry, 5,* 3–24.

Schwartz, A.N. (1977). *Survival handbook for children of aging parents.* Chicago: Follet.

Seelback, W.C. (1978). Correlates of aged parents and filial responsibility: Expectations and realizations. *Family Coordinator, 27,* 341.

Shanas, E. (1967). Family help patterns and social class in three countries. *Journal of Marriage and the Family, 29,* 257–266.

Silverstone, B., & Hyman, H.K. (1976). *You and your aging parent: The modern family's guide to emotional, physical and financial problems.* New York: Pantheon.

Simos, B.G. (1973). Adult children and their aging parents. *Social Work, 18,* 78–85.

Spark, G.M., & Brody, E.M. (1970). The aged are family members. *Family Process, 9,* 195–210.

Stanton, M.D. (1981). Strategic approaches to family therapy. In A.S. Gurman & D.P. Kniskern (Eds.), *Handbook of family therapy* (pp. 361–402). New York: Brunner/Mazel.

Steuer, J.L. (1982). Psychotherapy for depressed elders. In D.G. Blazer (Ed.), *Depression in late life* (pp. 195–220). St. Louis: C.V. Mosby Co.

Townsend, P. (1957). *The family life of the old people.* London: Penguin Books.

Troll, L.E., Miller, S.J., & Atchley, R.C. (1979). *Families and later life.* Belmont, CA: Wadsworth.

Verwoerdt, A. (1981). *Clinical geropsychiatry* (2nd ed.). Baltimore: Williams & Wilkins.

Whitaker, C.A., & Keith, D.V. (1981). Symbolic-experiential family therapy. In G.S. Gurman & D.P. Kniskern (Eds.), *Handbook of family therapy* (pp. 187–225). New York: Brunner/Mazel.

Zarit, S.H. (1980). *Aging and mental disorders: Psychological approaches to assessment and treatment.* New York: Free Press.

Chapter 12

Psychopharmacology of the Elderly

Advanced age often presents a complex interaction of physical illness, reduced cognitive functioning, and psychopathology. Characteristically a high proportion of the elderly in the sixth and seventh decades of life present with problems of disordered sleep, depressive mood, anxiety, and other affective disorders that necessitate intervention with psychopharmacology and somatic therapy. An appreciation of multiple interactions between age and altered physiologic functioning and the interaction between medical and psychopharmacological drug treatment is a prerequisite to effective mental health intervention for the elderly.

Almost one-third of the elderly over the age of 60 receive psychotropic medication during a year. Prentice (1979) documented the disproportionately high use of tranquilizers, sedatives, hypnotics, and antidepressants in the elderly, especially phenothiazines, which rank among the leading drugs utilized by older adults.

Psychopharmacology is gradually but surely moving into the mainstream of mental health intervention with the elderly. Advances in psychopharmacology have brought about changes in the care of the emotionally disordered and a reexamination of the nosology of depression, anxiety, functional psychoses, and paranoia. Disorders of mood and mental functioning in the elderly generally include depression that accompanies losses, anxiety over present and future health, agitation, and impaired cognitive abilities stemming from a wide range of organic brain dysfunction. Till recently, both physicians and their elderly clients have shared a sense of futility about the ultimate resolution of symptoms present in varying degrees in many elderly persons. With the advancement of psychopharmacology "there seems to be a pharmacological adventurousness that encourages the trial of all sorts of medications for the relief of symptoms which may accompany advancing age" (Salzman & Shader, 1973, p. 159).

Pharmacologic therapy has significantly improved the prognosis and treatment of mental illness in older adults. In our medicated society more and more elderly patients and doctors may agree that psychotropic drugs may be useful. Depression, for example, is now a treatable illness in the elderly, and tricyclic antidepressants are able to shorten the duration of depressive episodes and disorders in all age groups, including the elderly. As a result the issues facing the psychologist, mental health practitioner, social worker, or nursing practitioner involved with geriatric care require a better than usual understanding of the physiological handling of drugs by the elderly. There is a high probability that a geriatric client presenting for psychological and psychotherapeutic intervention will simultaneously or subsequently be subjected to some kind of polypharmacological handling. Thus it is important that mental health workers at all levels and other caregivers, for example, members of the family, who relate with the elderly become familiar with the basic issues relevant to the psychopharmacological treatment of the elderly.

Numerous considerations relevant to dynamics of the aging process and the possibility of single or multiple drug use by the elderly and their particular toxic consequences must enter into an accurate diagnostic understanding by professionals, paraprofessionals, and laypersons involved in providing care to the elderly. There is no doubt that psychopharmacology will play an increasingly important role in psychogeriatric care.

Thus the main concern of this chapter is to alert professionals and paraprofessionals to the pharmacological action and physiological effects of psychotropic drugs and the important psychological and biological issues in drug management. This chapter offers nonmedical paraprofessionals and caregivers an overview of the contemporary pharmacokinetic and pharmacodynamic considerations. The main emphasis is on providing sufficient practically relevant knowledge about the pharmacologic and dynamic interactional properties of specific drugs and the way the elderly generally respond to these drugs. Almost without exception, caregivers involved with elderly individuals are likely to observe the general course of untreated disease states. They will be expected to observe side effects of medication and understand the influence of other medical factors that may contribute to the improvement or deterioration of an elderly person's condition.

Thus this chapter has a twofold purpose. The first purpose is to review some of the iatrogenic illnesses so common in the elderly and the special hazards associated with the use of psychotropic drugs. The second purpose is to draw the attention of practitioners and geriatric caregivers to the cautions necessary in using psychotropic drugs in specific physical and psychological geriatric conditions including indications, contraindications, and therapeutic outcomes. General guidelines for monitoring side effects of psychotropic drugs are discussed, especially for the benefit of nonmedical paraprofessionals involved in caring for the elderly in community-based and nonclinical settings. Only broad generalizations about the usage of psychotropic drugs with the elderly are discussed.

Differential diagnosis of psychiatric syndromes and the selection and dosage of psychotropic drugs for elderly presenting psychological and behavioral symptoms are regarded as the domain of the medical personnel. Physicians and clinicians must necessarily formulate some specific notions concerning the etiology, pathogenesis, and psychodynamics of the disturbed behavior. Nonmedical personnel, however, need to have a good practical understanding of the adverse reactions to drugs that are especially enhanced in the elderly and of the elderly's unique biological processes that are responsible for the adverse reactions. Perhaps the most important skill for nonmedical personnel is to be good observers of elderly patients after medications are introduced or changed in order to identify any adverse consequences. The potential benefits of psychotropic drugs in the management of affective problems of the aged can be increased if nonmedical caregivers, including family members, can be trained to be more attentive to potential adverse effects. Such an approach does not preclude psychotherapeutic and social assistance that nonmedical caregivers can provide to the elderly but only complements them.

GENERAL PRINCIPLES OF PHARMACOLOGY IN THE AGED

With age the body undergoes a wide range of physiological changes that alter the disposition and effects of drugs (Ramsay & Tucker, 1981). These can be discussed under two headings: (1) pharmacokinetics, that is, the effect of the body on drugs, and (2) pharmacodynamics, that is, the effect of drugs on the body. A summary of major pharmacokinetic and pharmacodynamic effects is presented in Table 12–1.

Pharmacokinetics

All four main aspects of pharmacokinetics are altered in old age (Crooks, O'Malley, & Stevenson, 1976; Friedel, 1978, 1980). Physiologic changes with aging alter the activity of psychotropic medication considerably. This is related to specific factors such as absorption and distribution patterns of the drug. A number of clinicians (e.g., Beattie & Sellers, 1979; Burgen & Mitchell, 1978; Friedel, 1978) use the term *pharmacokinetics* to refer to this process of the distribution of drugs in the body and the related processes of absorption, excretion, and metabolism. According to Friedel (1978) knowledge of pharmacokinetics is especially relevant to all personnel concerned with the health care of geriatric persons since it provides understanding of the processes that determine the concentration of different drug agents at their site of action (Blazer, 1982; Burgen & Mitchell, 1978). In other words in addition to specific decreases in capacities (e.g., decrease in the liver's capacity to detoxify, decreased renal capacity to excrete), there is a decrease in the range and resilience of the elderly person's overall capacity for homeostasis and biological stability.

Animal studies suggest a normal tendency toward diminished capacity for metabolic handling of drugs as the aging process ensues. Aging is associated with reduced number of hepatic cells, and therefore enzymatic activity in elderly persons is reduced (Rossman, 1980). Since most psychotropic drugs administered in late life are metabolized by the liver, the biotransformation is predictably slower because the kidney and liver experience a decrease in their efficacy in excreting and metabolizing. Drugs remain in the body longer. Consequently there may be an unexpected increase in the drug level if standard amounts of

---

Table 12–1 General Effects of Drugs in the Aged

Pharmacokinetics (Effects of the Body on Drugs)	Pharmacodynamics (Effects of Drugs on the Body)
Absorption of drugs in the body is slowed because of a decrease in gastrointestinal blood flow that occurs with aging.	Symptoms of withdrawal, lethargy, somnolence, confusion, and agitation caused by long-term use of psychotropic drugs.
Drug distribution in the body is slowed because of the decreased cerebral blood flow that occurs with aging.	Spectrum of symptoms of bodily discomfort, that is, pain, thirst, rectal and vesical distention.
Excretion of the drugs is slowed because of reduced renal blood flow and cardiac output and increased circulation time that occurs with aging.	Disturbed metabolism, that is, dizziness, toxemia, fever, urinary retention, excessively high blood pressure or low blood pressure.
The pharmacologic effects of drugs are heightened because of the altered receptor sensitivity and dramatic loss of neuronal tissue that occur with aging.	Functional disorders, for example, insomnia, hallucinations, weight loss, weight problems.
Prolongation of drug effects because of the body's reduced capacity to excrete drug-drug toxicity selectively.	

drugs are used. It is particularly important, therefore, to be concerned about age-related factors in metabolism and the potential overdosing of elderly patients.

Absorption

The absorption of drugs may be slowed or reduced in aged persons because of a decrease in gastrointestinal blood flow and a reduced gastrointestinal motility associated with a decreased secretion of hydrochloric acid and a secondary elevation of gastric pH (Rossman, 1980). Liver enzyme induction is delayed and renal function is reduced. Thus there is an overall reduction in drug solubility.

Drug Distribution

As the human organism ages, there is a general trend for drugs to stay longer in the body and to have a more prolonged biological activity, and hence generally to have more powerful clinical and toxic effects on the organism (Salzman, Van der Kolk, & Shader, 1975). Most agents prescribed for the treatment of depression in the aged are lipid-soluble. Because blood triglycerides increase with age, lipid-soluble drugs tend to be retained in the lipid compartment for a longer time and tend to accumulate in the fatty tissues and be stored in body fat. Psychotropic drugs typically prescribed for older persons therefore tend to be found in higher concentrations in body fat and to have a longer duration of action secondary to their fat solubility. Since body fat increases with age and protein decreases, highly lipid-soluble drugs are reabsorbed by the renal system and remain longer in the circulation system.

Elderly people have less body mass in general than younger people. Consequently a standard dose in absolute terms will be a high dose in the elderly in terms of dose per kg body weight—and even more so in terms of dose per kg metabolically active mass (Ritschel, 1976).

Cerebral blood flow is decreased in the elderly, and grossly so in patients with cerebral arteriosclerosis. This tends to lessen the effects of drugs as brain perfusion is poor and distribution impaired (Lader, 1982).

The distribution of the drug depends also on the extent to which the drug is bound to the plasma proteins, especially albumin. Protein fractions and plasma albumin may also be reduced with advancing age, which can have prominent effects on metabolism and produce a higher proportion of free drug and a potential for increased storage and increased duration of action of fat-soluble drugs (Vestal, 1978). All these natural and drug-induced effects on metabolic functions point in the direction of cautioning elderly regarding the dangers of overmedication.

Excretion

Once a drug is in circulation, its concentration in the bloodstream is associated with reduced renal blood flow. Renal blood flow and tubular secretion diminish considerably with old age. A decrease in cardiac output and an increase in circulation time delay the circulation and distribution of drugs in the elderly (Salzman et al., 1975) and increase the concentration of the active drug (Holloway, 1974).

Pharmacologic Effects

Aging is associated with altered receptor sensitivity. In the aged there is a gradual but dramatic loss of neurons that are replaced by glial cells. The loss of functional neuronal tissue may be responsible for an increased sensitivity of the brain to the pharmacological action of drugs (Domino, Dren, & Giardina, 1978). This sensitivity may be due to the decreased number of receptor cells coupled with reduced binding of these cells (Roth, 1975). Drugs with central nervous system effects, for example, show changed activity with advancing age and increased variation in the therapeutic response of an older person to a standard dose. Thus, for example, the action of stimulants is reduced with age, while the action of depressants is enhanced. Adverse drug reactions are more common because of the erratic and paradoxical effects of barbiturates and antidepressants on older persons. The specific effects of benzodiazepines or phenothiazines on the older person are almost always difficult to predict because the effect varies with the rate at which these drugs are metabolized and eliminated by given individuals (Verzar, 1961). Therefore close monitoring of the effects of stimulants and antidepressants is important.

Drug Interactions

This category pertains to the interaction between drugs and drug-drug toxicity. Nonmedical personnel in a caregiving relationship to the elderly must be familiar with some of the problems that can result from prescribed or nonprescribed multiple drugs. Hale, Marks, and Stewart (1979) looked at a large cohort of more than 1,700 elderly patients visiting a hypertension screening program over a three-year period and found a consistent increase in the mean number of drug categories with increased age.

Therapeutic effects can be compounded by chemicals interfering with the absorption of drugs and increasing the rate of its metabolism. The potential for drug interactions includes the elderly person's self-medications in ways that are potentially harmful. According to Larson, Whanger, and Busse (1982) two common problems for the caregiver to be aware of are (1) the medicine cabinet, where there may be an increasingly large collection of old drugs that might be indiscriminately taken by an elderly person in an attempt to treat the discomforts of the body or mind, and (2) the interactions of over-the-counter drugs, which include histamines, sleep medications, tricyclic antidepressants, and monoamine oxidase inhibitors (MAO). Many of these nonprescription drugs have anticholinergic effects and interfere with absorption. Antacids, for example, interfere with the gastrointestinal absorption. Many antidepressants may interact with certain types of foods, caffeine, and alcohol to produce symptoms such as confusion, delirium, and psychosis as a result of the interactions between the drugs or between the drug and the medical status of the person (Salzman & Shader, 1978).

In elderly patients on MAO inhibitors, hypertensive crises may result from ingesting certain foods that contain tyramine or other medications such as cold remedies that contain presseramines. The clinical signs of such hypertensive crises consist of severe headache, nausea, sweating, palpitations, rapid pulse, and constricting chest pains. Immediate medical attention is necessary so that an appropriate adrenergic blocking agent can be prescribed. Among the prescription drugs that can lead to significant interactions are diuretics, which cause sodium depletion when combined with lithium carbonate therapy, for the treatment of depression in late life. Selective excretion of sodium leads to an increased reabsorption of lithium, which in turn increases the potential for toxic effects secondary to lithium (Blazer & Friedman, 1979).

Overall, aging is associated with a definite prolongation of the action of most but not all psychotrophic drugs. As a general rule, therefore, the action of a dose of a drug will be longer, sometimes severalfold, in an aged person than in a young or middle-aged adult (Lader, 1982).

Pharmacodynamics

Much less is known of the mechanisms whereby elderly people respond differently than younger people to the same tissue concentration of drugs (Bender, 1974). The responsivity of tissue systems to drugs in general declines with old age (Reidenberg, 1980). According to Bender, however, it is still not clear whether the decline in responsivity is related to a change in the number of receptors, in their affinity for the drug, or in the coupling between surface receptors and intracellular processes. It is generally postulated that several mechanisms operate in interaction. Therefore, in dealing with aged patients the clinicians often find that they have much more than they bargained for. Many of the physical and psychological adaptive systems of older persons are operating near the edge of their reserve capacity. Any additional burdens placed on these diminishing systems will result, more readily in old age than in younger years, in exaggerated symptom formations.

Many of the disequilibrating medical or pharmacological interventions have been attributed to physicians and psychiatric health professionals who have excessive trouble coping with patients who present psychological complaints in the guise of physical complaints and who resist all attempts to retranslate these back into psychological language (Pfeiffer, 1973). Pfeiffer observes that treatment of one symptom or disease process not uncommonly releases or exaggerates other symptoms. A mental health practitioner working with a purely psychological complaint such as depression or anxiety may be unaware of other clinicians who may be treating the same patient for hypertension (say, with reserpine or some combination of a diuretic plus another antihypertensive drug) and may suddenly recognize a suicidal client. A lack of precise definitions and inadequate nosology of symptoms may force clinicians and pharmacotherapists to take a shotgun approach to the prescription of medication and psychotropic drugs. This practice of indiscriminately blanketing the target physical, emotional, and metabolic symptoms with a barrage of drugs is often done by practitioners (who are overwhelmed by the number of symptoms presented) in the hope that at least one of the drugs would be effective.

However, with advancement in our knowledge of psychopharmacology and the risk of drug-drug toxicity in patients with multiple illnesses being treated with multiple drugs, the hazards of a "shotgun" approach are eminently obvious: it may become impossible to distinguish among the intended effect of the drugs, their side effects, and the manifestation of the patient's initial symptoms. Since aged patients frequently have several chronic conditions under simultaneous treatment, overmedication is a constant danger. Learoyd (1972) makes the point about the possible hazards of polypharmacy based on his study in Australia, where 16 percent of a group of psychogeriatric admissions were directly due to the ill effects of questionable drugs and precipitated by adverse effects of psychotropic drugs. Dramatic improvements were observed when the drugs were stopped after geriatric evaluation.

Thus a necessary first step in proper prescription should be a pretreatment evaluation. In addition to assessing the elderly client's social support systems, adequate diagnostic assessment of physical status, medical status, and psychological health is crucial for optimal psychotropic drug use. Since depression in an older person is often multidetermined and presents a variety of physical, medical, and emotional symptoms, the primary health care practitioner (whether this is a psychologist, physician, or psychiatrist) may often have to initiate more than one treatment method. According to Hollister (1974, 1979) and Ayd (1980) pharmacologic therapy is an essential component of this multitherapeutic approach to treatment. Because of high bodily concerns and complicated depressive disorders associated with suicidal tendencies, there is a rapid onset and progression of depressive symptoms in the elderly. Hence, pharmacologic intervention is advised for expeditious treatment of psychological illness. However, much of drug therapy is toward symptomatic relief and there are enormous variations in the responsiveness of the elderly to medications, causing side effects to be frequent and severe. Some general guidelines in the use of drug therapy are in order (see Exhibit 12–1 for brief review).

First, it is important to establish a drug-free baseline by discontinuing all psychotropic medications that are not necessary or essential. Verwoerdt (1981) notes that the discontinuance of all current psychotropic medication to get a drug-free baseline is useful to obtaining an accurate assessment of the efficacy of a prospective drug. Lamy and Kitler (1971) emphasized that care should be exercised in the elderly so that the most important disease is given primary consideration in terms of drug use. When possible, the clinician should treat the primary problem first and evaluate the potential use of other drugs in reference to whether the treatment of the secondary problems will make the primary problem worse or better (Larson et al., 1982).

Since many elderly patients are inadequate in presenting an accurate history of their drug intake, Blazer and Friedman (1979) and Salzman, Van der Kolk, and Shader (1975) suggest that a thorough evaluation of an elderly person should include a careful personal history from the patient and family or friends. In addition to obtaining detailed psychosocial data from which the health professional can derive an impression of the elderly patient's adaptation, the quality of the interpersonal relations, and the general level of mental and emotional strength, there should be a detailed review of the elderly person's present and past

---

Exhibit 12–1 Guidelines for Practitioners and Caregivers in the Use of Drug Therapy with the Elderly

1. Establish a drug-free baseline by discontinuing all nonessential psychotropic medications.
2. Establish a thorough evaluation of the elderly person's history of somatic therapy and drug medication for different psychological ailments and functional and medical disorders.
3. Establish a thorough evaluation of the elderly person's blood pressure and blood count, total protein, albumin ratios, urinalysis, and cardiac and respiratory conditions.
4. Evaluate drug intake and its adverse or positive effects on the elderly person.
5. Starting doses and maintenance doses of drugs for elderly persons should be one-third to one-half of those for younger persons.
6. Administration of drug medication to the elderly person should be the responsibility of an adult who lives permanently with the elderly person and can therefore monitor adverse effects, if any, of the drug.
7. Elderly patients maintained on psychotropic drugs should be observed regularly by caregivers. Their psychological and mental status should be closely monitored for signs of fatigue, withdrawal, cognitive confusion, etc. Close vigilance of the elderly patient is essential.
8. Elderly patients maintained on drugs should be reviewed regularly by their physicians in order to avoid the risk of progressive and often dangerous side effects.

medical history. Especially in the case of those elderly who have had neuroses or psychoses and where somatic therapy or drug medication was prescribed or is anticipated, pretreatment assessment should accurately determine blood pressure and blood count, total protein and albumin ratios, and urinalysis.

A complete evaluation should be made of the pharmaceutical agents used by the elderly person currently and in the past. Frequent offenders are bromides, opiates, and anticholinergic agents. Symptoms of withdrawal, lethargy, somnolence, confusion, and agitation, especially in the evening, may often be an indication that the elderly patient is or has been on long-term use of psychotropic drugs. The natural drop in blood pressure toward evening combined with drug-induced hypotension may cause cerebral anoxia (Salzman et al., 1975). The health care professional, with the assistance of a medical or nonmedical paraprofessional, should go over in detail with the elderly patient as to when the medication was prescribed and whether the medication has been taken regularly, intermittently, or sporadically and describe the effects the patient perceives from the use of the drugs, that is, the spectrum of symptoms of bodily discomfort (e.g., pain, thirst, overheating, or rectal and vesical distention), disturbed metabolism (e.g., fever, dizziness, toxemia), and other functional disorders (e.g., insomnia, hallucinations, appetite loss, weight problems).

After the patient's psychological and physical health status is evaluated, the judgment can be made as to whether the drugs the elderly person is taking are necessary for the emotional or physical discomforts or disorders the person is reporting. Few drugs, if any, should be prescribed unless the clinician is able to formulate some explicit psychodynamic notions or medical hypotheses as to why certain behaviors are occurring. Such a conservative stance based on causal decisions will prevent problems of undermedication, overmedication, or the shotgun approach used by some physicians (Kenny, 1979). Lamy and Kitler (1971) recommend that in order to avoid the risk of many elderly patients using borrowed and outdated preparations and medications, it is generally a good idea to have the family members help the elderly person to get rid of all previous medications stored in the medicine cabinet.

Second, in view of the enormous variations in the responsiveness of the elderly to medication, dosage of psychotropic medication is virtually always started at a potentially therapeutic but probably low level and increased in dosage gradually. As a rule of thumb, starting doses and maintenance doses should be one-third to one-half of those for younger adults. As far as possible, it is useful to follow an individualized approach, particularly in the case of debilitated patients who have multiple ailments; the dosage may be increased according to tolerance (Fann, Wheless, & Richman, 1976).

Tricyclic antidepressants so commonly prescribed for adults often begin with an initial dose of 150 mg, usually given at bedtime, but may be started at 50 mg for an elderly patient and increased from 25 percent to 50 percent of the initial dose every three to five days. The slower metabolism of the tricyclic antidepressants may lead to a toxic reaction from these medications approximately one week after a given dose level is achieved, but at the same time many psychotropic drugs begin to exert their maximum therapeutic effect only two to three weeks following the initial doses. Despite the adverse reactions, to stop treatment before that time, or to fail to increase the dosage to optimal levels, may be worse than no treatment at all. Therefore, periodical review and readjustment of dosage levels are required.

Both the risks of overmedication and undertreatment need to be considered. If the choice of the agent is correct, the dosage should be increased cautiously until the desired effect is achieved. Conversely a side effect (such as urinary retention or severe confusion) may necessitate dose reduction or discontinuation. Friedel (1978) suggests an individualized approach in which a balance is struck between a certain blood level at which there is little therapeutic effect and other higher blood levels at which toxic effects predominate.

The clinician should also question a close family member to determine how well the elderly patient's perceptions of drug intake and its adverse or positive effects correspond with the family member's perceptions. At reevaluations careful questioning about the drug doses actually taken, not the doses prescribed, is necessary.

In most elderly, particularly older adults exhibiting memory disturbance, instructions concerning dosage and regimen have to be given to the relatives or other caregivers who may initially assume the responsibility for the client. Compliance to instructions can be enhanced by the use of a medication calendar, diary, or pill-dispenser.

To avoid potential errors in under- or overmedication, a simple therapeutic regimen should be established to reduce the number of times the medication should be prescribed. Due to the fact that the half-lives of many psychotropic drugs are potent enough, many drugs (particularly neuroleptics and tricyclic antidepressants) can be administered on a once-a-day basis, close to bedtime. Some agents also act as sedatives, thus eliminating or reducing the need for hypnotics or sedatives (Karasu & Murkofsky, 1976).

However, there is no general agreement about the practice of spreading the dosage of psychotropic drugs versus taking the entire amount at bedtime. There is a risk with aged persons, especially those who are in a debilitated condition, that they may be less able to tolerate the sudden absorption of a relatively large drug dosage into their bloodstream and the potential for side effects the following morning. Therefore, some clinicians suggest that the dosage should be divided, usually into halves, with one half given during the day and the other half before bedtime.

Because of possibly impaired disintegration and absorption of tablets, liquid preparations (such as elixirs) are often preferred. Care should be taken in switching from one formulation to another lest the bioavailabilities differ significantly (Lader, 1982).

Third, patients maintained on psychotropic drugs should be reviewed regularly in order to avoid the risk of progressive and sometimes dangerous side effects. According to Whanger and Busse (1975) variations in the responsiveness of elderly patients to drugs may involve a treatment period of several months with subsequent increased risk of debilitating physical effects. Hence the necessity of triannual checkups is emphasized (Whanger & Busse, 1975).

PSYCHOPHARMACOLOGICAL INTERVENTION IN DEPRESSION AND DEPRESSIVE DISORDERS

Depression of varying severity is common in advanced age. Salzman, Van der Kolk, and Shader (1975) note that the development of symptoms may be insidious with no clear precipitants, and increasing social isolation and deterioration of mental and physical capacities may aggravate the mood disturbance. Observable symptoms may include withdrawal and isolation, early morning insomnia, loss of appetite and loss of weight, and general confusion.

There are many different clinical manifestations of depression in the elderly, determining to some extent the type of drugs or treatment approaches to take to a particular patient. Depression in the elderly is easily confused with organic brain syndrome (dementia). Depressions may cause the elderly to become so perplexed or withdrawn that they may be misdiagnosed as having organic brain syndrome. Hence proper diagnosis of the deteriorating mental functioning or cognitive impairment is necessary before embarking on drug therapy. If depression is suspected, a therapeutic trial of antidepressants is indicated and may reverse cognitive deficiencies (Hollister, 1975).

Tricyclic Antidepressants

Since their development in the late 1950s, the tricyclic antidepressants have become the treatment of first choice for patients with biological signs of depression. Six tricyclic compounds are commonly prescribed in the United States and Canada: amitriptyline (Elavil, Endep),[1] imipramine (Trofranil, Presamine),[2] doxepin (Sinequan, Adapin)[3] and its demethylated metabolites nortriptyline (Aventyl, Pamelor),[4] protriptyline (Vivactyl),[5] and desipramine (Norpramin, Pertofrane).[6] The tricyclics can be further grouped according to their nonsedating properties (Trofranil, Pamelor, Aventyl, and Vivactyl). Sedating tricyclics include Elavil and Sinequan. Amitriptyline, doxepin, imipramine, and desipramine can also relieve anxiety in the context of depression. Protriptyline by contrast is a stimulating drug (Prange, 1973).

What distinguishes certain of the newer tricyclics is first their sedative qualities and second their anxiolytic properties (i.e., their beneficial effects on anxiety) (Prange, 1973). Yet it is well known that older patients tolerate the tricyclic antidepressants poorly. As specified earlier there is a high incidence of hypotension, urinary retention, confusion, and blurring of vision in older adults. The goal, of course, is to strike the most favorable balance for each patient between the good and bad aspects of the drugs such as amitriptyline, nortriptyline, and doxepin. These tricyclic drugs have the potential dangers of the anticholinergic effects but also have substances that produce both antidepressant and anxiolytic effects in elderly patients whose depression is coextensive with anxiety (Prange, 1973). For important side effects of tricyclic antidepressants see Table 12–2, adapted from Verwoerdt (1981).

Although the two compounds have significant anticholinergic side effects and a tendency to produce electrocardiographic changes and agitation, imipramine and amitriptyline have been used most extensively in the treatment of the depressed elderly. However, as Nies et al. (1977) point out, older patients often benefit from tricyclic antidepressant therapy in a dose range of approximately 1 mg per kilogram of body weight. In effect this range is less than one-third of that generally administered to younger adults.

Doxepin hydrochloride, according to Ayd (1971a), is the least offensive tricyclic agent with respect to anticholinergic effects. It has a number of advantages when used with the elderly and has become more popular for treating depression in the elderly. The cardiovascular toxicity of doxepin is low (Ayd, 1971b) and the property of blocking the mechanism by which guanethidine is taken into the nerve end is weak. Hence, long-term administration of doxepin (Sinequan) is safe provided a dose can be determined that is

---

[1]cf. Nies, Robinson, & Friedman (1977)

[2]cf. Nies et al. (1977)

[3]cf. Friedel and Raskin (1975)

[4]cf. Reed, Smith, Schoolar, Hu, Leelavathi, Mann, and Lippman (1980)

[5]No studies reported

[6]No studies reported

Table 12–2 Important Side Effects of Tricyclic Antidepressants

Clinical Signs	Causative Factors	Prevention and Treatment
Behavioral		
Excitement, "manic shift"	Stimulating effect	Lower dose or change drug
Exacerbation of psychotic symptoms	Underlying paranoid or schizophrenic disorder	Use antipsychotics in combination or alone
CNS		
Electroencephalogram changes	Large doses; parenteral administration	Lower dose; avoid parenteral administration
Seizures	Family history of epilepsy; history of CNS injury	Don't combine with MAOI
	Combination with MAOI	Wait 2 weeks after one drug before starting another
Parkinsonism; tremors	Unclear; rare	Lower dose or change drug; don't use antiparkinson drugs
Central anticholinergic syndrome	Anticholinergic effects Combination with antipsychotics or antiparkinson drugs	*Differential diagnosis:* Korsakoff; transient ischemic attacks; etc.
Acute confusion		Check peripheral anticholinergic signs
Hallucinations		
Agitation		*Treatment:* physostigmine; stop drugs
Short-term memory loss		
Neurological		
Hypertonus	Anticholinergic or adrenergic effects; combination with MAOI	Lower dose or stop drug
Hyperreflexia		
Ataxia		Avoid polypharmacy
Neuropathies		
Tremors, fasciculations	Old age; vitamin deficiencies	Give vitamins
Cardiovascular		
EKG changes	Preexisting CVD	Do pretreatment EKG
Hypotension		
Myocardial infarcts (CVA)	Adrenergic & anticholinergic effects	Monitor cardiovascular indexes
Increased blood pressure in hypertensive patients	Blocking of guanethidine	Stop drug or use other antihypertensive, e.g., hydralazine
Eyes		
Glaucoma	Anticholinergic effects	Lower dose or stop drug; treat glaucoma
Blurred vision		
Accommodation paralysis		
Genitourinary		
Urinary retention	Prostate hypertrophy	Lower dose or stop drug
Delayed ejaculation		
Gastrointestinal		
Dry mouth, constipation		Lower dose or stop drug; stool softeners
Fecal impaction		Stop drug

Source: From *Clinical Geropsychiatry*, 2nd edition (p. 205) by A. Verwoerdt, 1981, Baltimore: Williams & Wilkins Company. Copyright 1981 by Williams & Wilkins Company. Adapted by permission.

therapeutically antidepressant and has a weak blocking property. Burrows, Vorah, Hunt, Sloman, Scoggins, and Davies (1976) have argued that the increased antianxiety activity, the low anticholinergic properties, and the weak electrocardiac changes make this drug a most acceptable alternative for treating depression in the elderly. Doxepin also has a sedative-tranquilizing action, and "when used with the depressed elderly who also have problems of insomnia, the antidepressant and sedation properties may be a boon" (Prange, 1973, p. 232). Despite the lower anticholinergic properties doxepin may not be as effective on a milligram per milligram basis as other tricyclic antidepressants, and when given in equivalent or full doses, the cardiovascular toxicity of doxepin may become a debatable question. Also, it is a new drug, and clinical testing will be needed to document both the drug efficacy and the severity of side effects that with time tend more and more to resemble those of other members of their class (Ayd, 1979, 1980).

The dosage of the tricyclics is similar in potency of action except for nortriptyline (Aventyl, Pamelor) and protriptyline (Vivactyl), which are both more potent. Nortriptyline has not been used extensively with the elderly, but Reed et al. (1980) found it safe with respect to cardiovascular toxicity and anticholinergic effect when given in a standard dose to geriatric patients. Montgomery, Braithwaite, and Crammer (1977) have argued that optimum benefit from this drug can be derived because of the availability of a therapeutic window for its steady-state plasma levels and therapeutic response levels. This clinical evidence suggests that nortriptyline may be a reasonable alternative to other tricyclic agents mentioned.

Feighner (1980) has discussed the development of tetracyclic compounds, which have been shown to be effective tricyclic antidepressants with a reduced side effect. One hypothesis to explain the reduced side effects is the presence in the tetracyclic compound of maprotiline, which is a specific inhibitor of the norepinephrine uptake.

Tricyclic antidepressants prescribed for bipolar or unipolar depressive disorders have sometimes had the effect of inducing hyperactivity in elderly patients. Also, they have induced seizures and manic episodes (van Scheyen & van Kammen, 1979). Another new class of drugs, however, which has become available in the 1980s, is Trazodone, a triazolopyridine derivative that has proven to be an effective antidepressant for depression and the coexistence of bipolar affective disorders. Triazolopyridine derivatives (Trazodone, Zimeldine) are effective serotonin reuptake inhibitors and blood spectrum antidepressants. Their potential beneficial use with the elderly is indicated in the fact that the drugs are well tolerated, have a faster onset, and show relatively few anticholinergic effects. Specific clinical studies of the elderly are essential for each of these tetracyclic compounds. Clinicians are hopeful that this new class of tricyclic antidepressants may be useful in treating depressed elderly with multiple symptoms of depression, anxiety, insomnia, and agitation.

Tricyclic drugs are most effective in primary affective disease (whether circular or unipolar) and are less effective in the reactive depressions, in which there are clearer precipitants of the depression (Karasu & Murkofsky, 1976). However, in actual clinical practice the distinction between primary depressions and reactive depressions is harder to maintain because reactive etiologies in depression associated with grief, loss, and physical disabilities are almost always present in the elderly. For clinical purposes, therefore, tricyclic antidepressant therapy is frequently used with most depressive syndromes of the elderly, and maintenance of antidepressant therapy is regarded safe and desirable for episodic and recurrent depression in the elderly. With close management and awareness of potential difficulties, tricyclics can be used in significant doses and with most gratifying results. Since all tricyclics have some antidepressant effects, the choice of a tricyclic antidepressant should be determined less by the antidepressant effect itself and more by the properties that induce adverse side effects of beneficial secondary effects. When we consider tricyclic drugs for the elderly, we are most concerned about a lowered threshold for toxic confusion, for glaucoma, for urinary retention, for constipation, for cardiovascular embarrassment, and for Parkinson's disease (Prange, 1973) (Table 12–1).

If tricyclic antidepressants are ineffective in clinical trials, they should be withdrawn. This withdrawal, however, should be effected gradually over a five- to six-day period, with the dose being decreased about 20 percent each day. An abrupt withdrawal of the drug can often produce an overwhelming cholinergic rebound increasing the potential for symptoms such as uncontrolled anxiety, agitation, constipation, stomach cramps, nausea and diarrhea, and insomnia.

Tricyclic drug therapy, if successful, is generally maintained for several months after response. Some patients seem prone to relapse whenever drug therapy is withdrawn, especially those patients who suffer fairly regular cyclical illnesses. Their drug dosage should be increased at the expected time. Lippincourt (1968) advises that as depression lifts, appropriate social measures such as more social activity should be instituted in order to reduce social isolation of the elderly client. It is worth trying to persuade the elderly person to join an interest group or social group that brings the elderly into interaction with other age groups rather than an elderly age group.

MAO (Monoamine Oxidase) Inhibitors

These inhibitors frequently interact adversely with many medical drugs and may cause serious side effects so as to make their routine use in the elderly too hazardous when weighed against their potential benefits (Salzman et al., 1975). These drugs inhibit the breakdown of catecholamines resulting in increased amounts of the neurotransmitters dopamine, serotonin, and norepinephrine at the central receptor sites in the brain. A number of drugs with MAO inhibitors are available in England. The MAO activity that accompanies the aging process suggests that these agents may be useful. However, in the United States and Canada the two chemical groups—the hydrazides (phenelzine sulfate) and non-hydrazides (tranylcypromine sulfate)—are most commonly used (Quitkin, Rifkin, & Klein, 1979). Epstein (1978) advises against the use of MAO inhibitors in the elderly since these drugs may interact adversely with psychomotor stimulants, such as ephedrine, to cause increased agitation, confusion, and disorientation. Although therapeutic for depression, adverse reactions, including the risk of hypertensive crisis, may result if MAO inhibitors are used with the tricyclic antidepressants (Spiker & Pugh, 1976) or sometimes by the ingestion of foods that contain tyramine. Because of the incompatibility of the MAO inhibitors with drugs and foods, these should not be prescribed unless the elderly patient can be relied on to follow a rigid regimen of health care.

Both minor and serious side effects can be anticipated with MAO inhibitors. Hypotension may become serious in the elderly who are at high risk for stroke or myocardial infarction (Walker & Brodie, 1980). They are contraindicated for elderly with liver disease and in interaction with other drugs can potentiate a hypertensive crisis that on occasion may be fatal, cause hallucinations, and hyperreflexia.

Hollister (1979) notes that in low doses they may have some positive effect on mild states of apathy and low energy but recommends they should be used only as a last resort when the response to other antidepressants has been poor or when a particular elderly patient has had a history of responding well to MAO inhibitors. These inhibitors have been proposed as a treatment of atypical depression that has concomitant symptoms of hysteric disorder or somatization disorders (Quitkin, Rifkin, & Klein, 1979). However, since complex depressive disorders are seen fairly frequently in old age, treatment of such depressed aged persons (who are resistant to tricyclic depressants) through MAO inhibitors may be beneficial. The one of the few MAO inhibitors (tranylcypromine) available for clinical use causes severe adverse effects. Improvement in depression should be seen in 48 hours. If no response occurs after three days, the dose may be increased from the initial 10 mg to 30 mg daily. If after a week no improvement occurs, the medication is not expected to be beneficial (Walker & Brodie, 1980).

Goldstein (1977, 1979) suggests a number of precautions that the clinician should impress on the elderly patient or the family concerning the use of MAO inhibitors, principally warning the patient about the potentials for headache and the grave importance of avoiding self-medication (including over-the-counter drugs). The patient should be instructed to report any unusual symptoms immediately.

For the clinician it is important to be aware that tricyclics should not be combined with MAO inhibitors in treating the depressed elderly. Such a combination may lead to synergistic effects manifested by intense CNS sympathetic stimulation, restlessness, muscle twitching, hypertension, and hyperpyrexia (Verwoerdt, 1981).

Gerovital H3

MacFarlane (1973) and Cohen and Ditman (1974) investigated the antidepressant effects of Gerovital H3, first introduced in European clinical studies. Their evidence suggests that it can be safe and effective in treating depression in the elderly. No evidence exists, as rumored, that the medication reverses the process of aging, but a number of double-blind studies (Ostfeld, Smith, & Stotsky, 1977; Zung et al., 1974) have suggested a potential therapeutic benefit of this agent. The drug has been found to have mild antidepressant qualities and is a weak, reversible, and competitive inhibitor of MAO, which selectively inhibits the deamination of certain important brain monoamines. Although there is no risk of the hypertensive crisis so typical of other MAO inhibitors, geriatricians and clinicians in the United States are quite skeptical of the benefits reported from this drug, which has procaine hydrochloride as its basic active ingredient and must be administered intramuscularly.

Table 12–3 presents a list of generic drugs commonly used in treatment of the elderly and their commonly used trade names. Such a description can be useful in examining key ingredients of prescribed and nonprescribed drug medications.

MONITORING OF SIDE EFFECTS AND ASSISTANCE TO THE ELDERLY IN DRUG MANAGEMENT

To what extent will medications used to treat depression, anxiety, and sleep disorders in the elderly produce side effects? (See Table 12–4 for summary review of major side effects.) For the pharmacotherapist the answer is straightforward. In the elderly client the margin for error in expecting and predicting side effects is greatly reduced. Whether or not the elderly patient has frank organic disease of the brain, the cardiovascular system, or the endocrine systems, the compensatory capacities of these systems are sure to be reduced, and

Table 12–3 Generic Drugs with Their Most Commonly Used Trade Names

Generic	Trade	Generic	Trade
Major Tranquilizers		*Antidepressants* (cont.)	
Chlorpromazine	Thorazine	*MAO inhibitors*	
Fluphenazine	Prolixin		
Haloperidol	Haldol	Isocarboxazid	Marplan
Loxapine	Loxitane	Phenelzine	Nardil
Mesoridazine	Serentil	Tranylcypromine	Parnate
Molindone	Moban		
Perphenazine	Trilafon	*Antimanics*	
Prochlorperazine	Compazine	Lithium Carbonate	Eskalith
Thioridazine	Mellaril		
Thiothixene	Navane	*Stimulants*	
Trifluoperazine	Stelazine	Amphetamine	Benzedrine
		Dextroamphetamine	Dexedrine
Minor Tranquilizers		Methylphenidate	Ritalin
Benzodiazepines (Antianxiety)		*Sedatives and Hypnotics*	
		Nonbarbiturate	
Chlordiazepoxide	Librium		
Clorazepate	Tranxene	Chloral Hydrate	Noctec
Diazepam	Valium	Ethchlorvynol	Placidyl
Oxazepam	Serax	Flurazepam	Dalmane
		Glutethimide	Doriden
Mephesine-like compounds		Methaqualone	Quaalude
Meprobamate	Equanil		Sopor
	Miltown	Methyprylon	Noludar
Sedating Antihistamines		*Barbiturate*	
Hydroxyzine	Atarax	Amobarbital	Amytal
	Vistaril	Amobarbital and	Tuinal
Promethazine	Phenergan	Secobarbital	
		Pentobarbital	Nembutal
Antidepressants		Phenobarbital	Luminal
Tricyclics		Secobarbital	Seconal
		Anti-Parkinsonism Agents	
Amitriptyline	Elavil		
Desipramine	Norpramin	Amantadine	Symmetrel
Doxepin	Adapin	Benztropine	Cogentin
	Sinequan	Carbidopa and	Sinemet
Imipramine	Tofranil	Levodopa	
Nortriptyline	Aventyl	Levodopa	Dopar
Perphenazine and	Triavil		Larodopa
Amitriptyline	Etrafon	Trihexyphenidyl	Artane
Protriptyline	Vivactil		

Source: From *Clinical Psychology of Aging* (p. 249) edited by M. Storandt et al., 1978, New York: Plenum Publishing Corporation. Copyright 1978 by Plenum Publishing Corporation. Reprinted by permission.

Table 12–4 Monitoring for Side Effects of Drugs and Guidelines for Management

Major Side Effects	Guidelines for Management
Anticholinergic effects of tricyclic drugs (e.g., toxic confusion, withdrawal, constipation, urinary retention, blurred vision).	Report side effects promptly to pharmacotherapist or physician.
Gastrointestinal effects of lithium treatment (e.g., muscular weakness, nausea, vomiting, toxicity, diarrhea, polyuria, polydipsia).	Report side effects promptly to physician; elderly patient may respond well to propanolol.
Functional disorder effects of antidepressant medication (e.g., sleep disturbances, hypertension, agitation, hand tremors, anxiety disorders, appetite disorders).	Report side effects promptly to physician; elderly patient may respond well to diuretics used with tricyclic antidepressants for the treatment of hypertension.
Behavioral disorder effects of antianxiety agents (e.g., excessive sedation, drowsiness, ataxia, headache, and paradoxical reactions including aggression, anger, and hostility).	Report side effects promptly to physician; elderly patient may not be responding well to barbiturates and may need a change in antianxiety agent.

both potent and nonpotent drugs will produce toxic reactions and other adverse side effects much more readily (Dovenmuehle, 1965).

The most common side effects of medication used to treat depression are the anticholinergic effects. In other words, when we consider tricyclic drugs for the elderly, we are concerned about a lowered threshold for toxic confusion, constipation, urinary retention, cardiovascular embarrassment, blurred vision, inhibition of sweating, and severe mouth dryness.

These matters should be discussed at length between the physician and the elderly patients, but the point to be stressed is the importance of the caregivers recognizing these side effects in their elderly clients. The elderly clients' toxic reactions may readily mimic an aspect of the syndrome for which they may be receiving treatment. For example, depression in the elderly is often accompanied by an element of confusion and withdrawal. This may lead to the prescription of more drug unless side effects produced by the medication are being carefully monitored. The sooner these side effects are reported to the pharmacotherapist or physician, a quick reversal via injectable physostigmine may be achieved.

Many patients receiving treatment within the therapeutic range of lithium may experience side effects. Initial side effects include gastrointestinal symptoms of nausea, vomiting, diarrhea, muscular weakness, polyuria and polydipsia, hand tremor, and tired or dazed feeling (Karasu & Murkofsky, 1976). Some of these late side effects of lithium such as confusion, flushing, and dryness of the skin may persist but, if reported in good time to the physician, may respond well to propanolol.

The contraindications to use lithium are relative and are reflected in the presence of kidney or cardiovascular disease. In the average adult half the lithium is cleared in 24 hours, but the clearance in the elderly is much slower, requiring more careful monitoring of blood level and renal functioning. Normal salt intake is generally adequate to protect against lithium toxic crises, and elderly patients on lithium medication should be encouraged to eat well. Elderly patients having cardiovascular disease are also on a low-salt diet, which increases the potential hazards of toxicity from lithium treatment and low-salt diets.

Cautious vigilance to prevent toxicity is the necessary ingredient of safe treatment. Lithium toxicity may assume various symptomatic forms and affect numerous organ systems. Nonmedical personnel caring for geriatric clients on lithium treatment should monitor for vomiting and diarrhea (GI symptoms), tremor, agitation, and other neuromuscular symptoms. They may observe mental symptoms such as confusion, somnolence and a comalike state, and cardiovascular symptoms such as arrhythmias, hypotension, or even shock. Lithium toxicity is a potential emergency and may require immediate withdrawal of the drug until safe levels of plasma lithium can be achieved (Karasu & Murkofsky, 1976).

Whenever a drug is prescribed for treating depression, the physician should inform the elderly client or the relative of the dose schedule for the medication, the potentials for side effects, and the symptoms likely to be reversed following the administration of the medication. At least initially most antidepressant medications are likely to correct sleep disturbances, agitation, and anxiety disorders and to reverse depressed effect and appetite disorders. The task of making these observations can be delegated to family members as persons in charge of administering the medication. Caregivers should follow up on these patterns and report to the physician if central symptoms of depressed effect do not show signs of improvement.

Because the elderly have a propensity for taking large numbers of prescription and nonprescription drugs for various types of discomforts, it is important to delineate drug-drug interactions between tricyclic antidepressants and other drugs (e.g., alcohol and barbiturates) consumed by the elderly. Tricyclics prolong central nervous system depression associated with alcohol, barbiturates, and antipsychotics and produce more depression and affective withdrawal (Walker & Brodie, 1980). Caregivers need to recognize the dangerous drug-drug interaction, particularly that stemming from the use of alcohol compounds, which should be avoided.

Diuretics can be safely used with the tricyclic antidepressants for the treatment of hypertension. As a rule, however, the use of diuretics must be avoided in the case of the elderly on lithium therapy. Propanolol in combination with hydralazine is also safe to use with antidepressants. High doses of propanolol, however, may cause enough sedation to exacerbate depressive symptomatology (Baldessarini, 1977).

Strain (1975, 1978) summarizes the hazards associated with the use of antidepressants:

- Severe toxicity may often occur at ordinary doses, that is, 75 to 150 mg a day.
- Aged persons are more vulnerable than younger adults to hypersensitivity reactions to psychopharmacological agents. Thus they may more easily develop skin reactions, anemias, and allergies following drug treatment.
- Aged persons are more susceptible than younger adults to cardiovascular and cerebrovascular insufficiencies and hypertensive and hypotensive episodes.
- Paradoxical reactions to drugs (such as barbiturates causing agitation, disorientation, and aggressive behavior; stimulants having a depressive reaction; and sedatives causing agitation) are frequent in late life.
- There is an increased danger of multiple drug or drug-drug interaction or risk of synergistic effects.

ELECTROCONVULSIVE THERAPY

Serious depression in the elderly has uncontrollable potential, either from suicide attempts or as a consequence or cause of severe anorexia and insomnia leading to exhaustion and lethal physical debilitation. For these reasons, rapid treatment of severe depression may be a life-saving procedure for many elderly whose treatment response to antidepressant medication may require several weeks. Tricyclic antidepressants, for example, which are generally given to the elderly at a much reduced dose, produce clinical relief at a much slower pace and may also produce severe cholinergic effects. A faster-acting alternative treatment is often needed. The electroconvulsive treatment (ECT), despite the earlier vilifications, is an important and sometimes life-saving psychiatric and muscle-relaxing procedure that may offer quick and substantial symptomatic relief, particularly for the elderly who are suicidal or severely depressed.

Kopell (1977) points out that the incidence of suicide among those over 65 is nearly twice the national average. In the case of suicidal elderly in particular, it may be inadvisable to proceed on a three- to four-week trial-and-error treatment using tricyclic antidepressants. Instead, one should commence with ECT as soon as possible, especially in the case of elderly with an endogenous depression with psychological and physical symptoms that are concomitant with the onset of depression (Kral, 1976). Anorexia nervosa has been relieved by ECT, which may be a boon in the case of depressed and debilitated elderly. In short, serious depression constitutes the outstanding indication for ECT. Symptoms that predict a good response to ECT are similar in the aged to those in younger adults, that is, low self-esteem, sense of hopelessness, anorexia, weight loss, early morning awakening, and thoughts or acts of destruction (Salzman, 1975). Prout, Allen, and Hamilton (1956) reviewed the early reluctance to use ECT in the aged. Today it is generally conceded that this treatment procedure, when properly administered, is safe and remarkably effective in alleviating the symptoms of severe depression (Salzman, 1975; Salzman et al., 1975; Larson et al., 1982; Walker & Brodie, 1980). Several studies (e.g., Kalinowsky & Hippius, 1969; Goldstein, 1979) have demonstrated that the elderly respond well to ECT. Few secondary problems or problems of mortality have been recorded. Practitioners, therefore, need to be reassured that the ECT procedures are relatively safe. Practitioners should also be able to offer more reassurance and support to depressed elderly clients and their families as to the remarkable effectiveness of ECT on depression.

Kral (1976) has suggested a number of cautions that should be taken in the administration of ECT, and signs and symptoms that definitely contraindicate ECT: signs of recent coronary thrombosis and decompensated heart failure. As a part of the thorough physical examination and diagnostic workup, Kral (1976) emphasizes that there should be no space-occupying lesions in the brain or other problems that might cause increased intracranial pressure with ECT.

Cardiac arrhythmias are another example of ECT problems in the elderly. With adequate muscle relaxation and oxygenation the risk to the elderly is only mildly greater than that of a younger adult. With a pretreatment ECG and cardiac rhythm during treatment, the danger of arrhythmias is greatly reduced and the use of a high-dose pretreatment atropine may protect the elderly patient against poststimulus arrhythmias. Of course, in the case of augmentation of hypertension, the elimination or reduction in the dose of pretreatment atropine should be considered. Pretreatment with 5 mg of diazepam within an hour of treatment may protect against a large increase in blood pressure. When the person is at risk due to respiratory problems, a barbiturate anesthesia is avoided.

Most elderly depressed individuals may show noticeable improvement with two to four ECTs. Salzman (1975) and Salzman, Van der Kolk, and Shader (1975) suggest that after an elderly patient shows some marked improvement from ECT two more treatments should be administered for consolidation of gains. On an average, this comes to five to seven ECTs (Larson et al., 1982).

As the convulsive threshold of the aged brain is higher than for younger adults a number of clinicians (e.g., Lowenbach, 1973; Squire, 1977; Weiner, 1979) suggest additional cautions when ECTs are administered to the elderly. Principal among these are the initial application of 150 volts to induce the full cerebral seizure and the spacing of treatments, allowing three or four days between treatments as opposed to the usual two days used with younger adults. Close monitoring of apnea symptoms, acute memory loss, or confusion is extremely important for at least four hours following treatment. Physical changes in neurologic, cardiovascular, endocrine systems, and autonomic nervous system (ANS) resulting from ECT should be closely observed, and the supervision of a responsible person, often a family member or friend, must be enlisted in the case of outpatient elderly persons receiving ECT treatment. When there is a noticeable increase in confusion following ECT treatment, the use of unilateral treatment to the nondominant hemisphere of the brain should be considered (Salzman et al., 1975; Squire, 1977).

The development of interest in and techniques for ECT has been slow. In fact until the 1950s its use had been regarded to be a form of psychiatric torture. Increasingly, however, it is recognized that when ECT is used properly, it is rapid, safe, and effective in relieving the symptoms of severe depression. The incidence of death in ECT is approximately 1 per 10,000 patients treated, with the major cause of death being cardiac complication, yet ECT is safer in elderly patients with heart disease than is tricyclic antidepressant therapy (Salzman, 1975). Compared to 66 percent of the general population of depressed patients who respond to the tricyclics, 78 percent respond to ECT (Greenblatt, Grosser, & Wechsler, 1964). Nevertheless, it is not sound clinical practice to treat most depressions with ECT. ECT is indicated and can be life saving when it is obvious that delay for trial of drugs is leading to a marked loss in weight, greater risk of suicide, chronicity, and more expense and family disruption.

Nonmedical practitioners are unlikely to become involved in decision making concerning ECT treatment; nevertheless they need to acquire a better understanding of both the risks and hazards and the safety and effectiveness of ECT in the 1980s so that they can support and reinforce the depressed patients and their families when critical decisions concerning certain treatment modalities, including ECT therapy, have to be made.

The physician's mandatory compliance with legal and ethical practices in medicine and therapy ensures that no clinician may use ECT out of frustration in dealing with a difficult client. "ECT is indicated in cases of severe depression only when it is determined unequivocally that drug therapy will take an unacceptably long period to manifest a therapeutic response" (Walker & Brodie, 1980, p. 116). While clinical and research evidence indicates that ECT offers substantial symptomatic relief from depression, it should be used for the maximum benefit of the depressed client in conjunction with psychotherapy and milieu therapy. In many cases of severe depression, mute, withdrawn, and severely agitated elderly who could not communicate verbally have been able to enter into effective psychotherapy after ECT (Salzman, 1975).

ANXIETY

Neurotic disturbances in the elderly typically arise at a greater rate. Loss of important persons, feelings of uselessness, and the experience of physical and intellectual deterioration may often serve to aggravate preexisting neurotic anxiety and helplessness anxiety in many elders. McCrae, Bartone, and Costa (1976) have explained the presence of anxiety in many elderly to be associated with a denial of physical problems, while others (Sathananthan, Gershon, & Ferris, 1976) have documented premorbid personality characteristics that occur with aging and often have hypochondriasis, lethargy, or restlessness and agitation as accompanying symptoms. Psychotherapy with the patients as well as intervention in their social environment and in the family is of great value in the treatment of acute traumatic anxiety in the elderly. Psychotherapy aimed at uncovering and articulating underlying issues of loss, disappointment, or defeat can be quite beneficial; getting patients in touch with their anger and resentment is helpful since anxiety-bound guilt and shame may be prominent features (Shader & Greenblatt, 1975). However, since 1970 it has been seen that antianxiety agents may be of considerable assistance in managing anxiety and agitation in the elderly. The traditional use of benzodiazepines is helpful to some elderly, particularly when the sedating properties of these drugs assist patients in achieving adequate sleep. More commonly barbiturates, propanediols, glycerol derivatives, and some antihistamines have been used to treat anxiety and sleep disturbances in the elderly.

Although barbiturates have been widely used in the general population, they are not recommended in elderly patients "because of the potential for intoxication, lethal overdose, and their propensity to produce paradoxical agitation" (Walker & Brodie, 1980, p. 120). Excessive sedation and resulting motor incoordination can have unwanted consequences such as falls and accidents. Moreover, the barbiturates increase liver enzyme activity, resulting in increased metabolism of steroids. Nevertheless, when antianxiety agents are used appropriately, they will decrease both psychological anxiety and muscle tension.

The benzodiazepines (Table 12–3), the most commonly used antianxiety drugs, include many ancillary drugs (also used to treat depressive disorders) such as diazepam (Valium), chlordiazepoxide (Librium), oxazepam (Serax), and lorazepam (Ativan). They are similar in their muscle-relaxant and sedative properties. Chlordiazepoxide is effective with anxiety in the elderly, and doses need to be much lower than for younger adults (about one-third of the adult dose), but it is moderately sedative and has a potential for habituation and physical illness. Diazepam causes less sedation and has skeletal muscle-relaxant properties, but because of its extended half-life in the aged, prolonged use of it may lead to problems. Oxazepam and lorazepam have the advantage of a lowered half-life when compared to most other benzodiazepines. While these drugs may be frequently prescribed as first-line therapeutic agents for the treatment of anxiety coextensive with depression and agitation, they may produce a complicated therapeutic picture as they also have depressant agents and tend with prolonged use to exacerbate the depressive symptoms.

The major side effects of the benzodiazepines are drowsiness, ataxia, headache, and reduced levels of spontaneous activity and decreased cognitive functioning. Thus the potential for pseudodementia is increased. Paradoxical reactions common in the elderly include agitation, hallucinations, insomnia, and aggression (Walker & Brodie, 1980). The benzodiazepines have been found of some benefit in patients diagnosed as anxious neurotic depressives (Rosenthal & Bowden, 1973). However, they should be cautiously administered as the development of tolerance to the euphorant and antianxiety drugs makes them questionable as effective long-term antidepressants or antianxiety agents (Fann & Wheless, 1975), especially in the elderly.

Benzodiazepines are helpful to elderly clients who have anxious depression. This is an anxiety that encompasses a mixed group of patients in whom anxiety, tension, and agitation are accompanied by overt depressive effect. Many of these elderly are chronically depressed, with intermittent exacerbations of anxiety symptoms, and they frequently complain of difficulty in falling asleep (Shader & Greenblatt, 1975). The sedating qualities of benzodiazepine assist patients in falling asleep. Some anxious depression elderly respond to tricyclic antidepressants such as doxepin or amitriptyline. Combinations of antipsychotic drugs (neuroleptics) and tricyclic antidepressants (perphenazine and amitriptyline) are also used, but this is not at all advisable unless there are psychotic elements in the clinical picture of anxiety and depression.

Caution in treating elderly patients with anxious depression is urged. Excessive sedation and the resulting motor incoordination can have potentials for falls and accidents, as can the anticholinergic, hypotensive, and arrhythmia-producing properties of the antidepressants. Muscle relaxation can be excessive (Linnoila & Vinkari, 1976). Benzodiazepines, even in reduced doses, can produce dependence in the elderly with abstinence symptoms of the barbiturate type on withdrawal (Lader, 1982).

Barbiturates are not generally recommended in the elderly because of their potential for physical addiction and depression of cortical functions but have been tried successfully in low doses with elderly who did not respond well to benzodiazepines (Stotsky & Borozne, 1972). With all these antianxiety agents, patients should be warned about driving and operating dangerous machinery. Interactions with alcohol are often marked.

INSOMNIA

One problem accompanying most forms of anxiety and depression in the elderly is sleep disturbance. Prolonged sleeplessness may often quickly exhaust the elderly person along with the caregivers and support persons. Chemotherapeutic treatment, as opposed to psychotherapy, may be necessary to combat these symptoms before agitation is exacerbated.

The aged, as compared to younger adults, often take longer to go to sleep, have less REM sleep, have less deep sleep, wake faster, and have less total sleep (Kahn & Fisher, 1969; Verwoerdt, 1981). The elderly require less sleep and may regularly awaken once or twice at night. This pattern does not constitute insomnia. However, even when clinically significant insomnia occurs in the elderly, it is rarely an isolated entity and is more frequently a manifestation of other disorders such as anxiety, agitation, or depression. Thus it is advisable that before a hypnotic agent is prescribed, the elderly person should be checked for depression, and psychosis, and physical conditions. Indeed, as Larson, Whanger, and Busse (1982) note, the central cause of fitful sleep may be problems requiring physical and medical attention, such as congestive heart failure, pain, and metabolic abnormalities; drug problems such as habituation to other drugs frequently administered for physical discomforts; and psychological problems such as acute grief, depression, or anxiety. Karasu and Murkofsky (1976) suggest that the safest chemotherapeutic approach to insomnia is to employ the sedative effects of neuroleptics and tricyclic antidepressants in lieu of sedative-hypnotic agents, which are initially quite effective but eventually their withdrawal leads to further deterioration in the sleep. In other words in treating the elderly and recalling their difficulty with metabolizing and excreting drugs, hypnotics should be prescribed for the treatment of simple insomnia, not the insomnia so frequently associated with depression or physical problems.

Taking into consideration the available hypnotics and the rapid habituation they can cause in a matter of two or three weeks, the best present hypnotic for the elderly is chloral hydrate (Noctec) and flurazepam (Dalmane), both of which have a lower risk of habituation and hangover effects. According to Piland (1979), however, these drugs have a long half-life in the elderly, and accumulation can lead to a CNS depressant activity. If the drug is used, it should be tried in 15-mg doses (which is almost half the dose prescribed for adult starters) and taken no more than a couple of times a week for sleep.

Other hypnotic agents such as Seconal, Nembutol, Noludar, and Placidyl (Table 12–3) are habit-forming in the aged. They are potentially toxic and should be avoided. The elderly (especially those living on their own and potentially or actually depressed) should be cautioned about the adverse effects of bromides that can be purchased over-the-counter, without assistance from caregivers. An increasing abuse of bromides may result in subacute or acute organic brain syndrome. Chronic administration of hypnotics to induce sleep can lead to insomnia. Whenever attempts are made to discontinue or merely to reduce the dose of the hypnotic, rebound insomnia may ensue with disturbing effects on the old person (Lader, 1982).

Sedative-hypnotic addiction and opioid abuse are not rare in the elderly. Many elderly may show withdrawal symptoms when the physician or pharmacotherapist attempts to discourage the use of these drugs. The fear of sleepless nights of the depressed person who has lost reserve to cope with physical discomfort or psychological anguish of lonely nights makes it difficult to withdraw these agents. Any attempt at withdrawal should not be encouraged in the absence of considerable social support and control on the part of the family.

In cases of insomnia associated with anxiety, several clinicians (e.g., Chien, 1971; Kastenbaum & Slater, 1964; Mishara & Kastenbaum, 1974) demonstrated that ethyl alcohol or a couple of ounces of wine or beer in the late afternoon improved the elderly person's sleep and anxiety problems. Many elderly do have a decreased tolerance for alcohol and if they are on other medication, the alcohol may potentiate or alter synergistic effects of other psychoactive or psychotropic drugs and produce toxicity.

Alcoholism is also a potential risk for elderly who initially take to alcohol for sleeping purposes. The ratio of elderly who become dependent on larger quantities of alcohol to help them through the day and night has increased considerably and poses many biological, social, and economic problems for elderly males in particular and in elderly women to a lesser degree.

FUNCTIONAL PSYCHOSES

Manic-Depressive Disorders

In the elderly a variety of functional disorders are somewhat common. Some of these such as manic states and schizophrenia may be a carryover from earlier years whereas others such as paranoia may develop for the first time in late life. The outlook for treating the elderly with such disorders has vastly improved with the advancement in a group of drugs called the major tranquilizers. A significant breakthrough in the treatment of manic-depressive illnesses has occurred with the entrance of lithium carbonate into the clinician's regimen. Klein and Davis (1969) have presented evidence to suggest that lithium may be more effective than the tricyclics in preventing the circular mood swings of the manic-depressive disease and possibly in preventing recurrent attacks of unipolar depressive disorders.

The clinician's inability to distinguish manic from depressive attacks in late life and to separate these from confusional states and agitated depressive states has made the outlook for accurate diagnosis and precise selection of psychotropic drugs difficult. Lithium, however, has become a rather popular drug for the effective therapeutic management of those elderly whose recurrent agitated depressive episodes or manic attacks are obscured symptomatically and therefore hard to diagnose. In such a mixed and obscured situation therapeutic trial of lithium carbonate frequently leads to improvement in symptoms and less frequent attacks. Its best indication for use is with milder manic states and the chronic hypomanic states. The drug of choice in the treatment of acute manic state is a sedating phenothiazine such as Thorazine.

Lithium is usually administered in three equally divided daily doses, and for older patients the blood level of lithium required for a therapeutic response is usually in the range of 0.5 to 1 mEq per milliliter. Acute or subacute manic excitement generally responds to lithium within 7 to 10 days.

Many patients receiving treatment within the therapeutic range of lithium experience severe side effects such as nausea, diarrhea, stomach pains, hand tremors, and fatigue. Long-term ingestion of lithium produces a diabetes-insipidus-like syndrome. Polyuria and polydipsia occur with considerable potency and frequency. There are elevation of blood sugar and elevated white blood cell counts. Gattozzi (1970) has reported on thyroid dysfunctioning effects of lithium, which frequently reduces thyroxine secretion. The potential for lithium carbonate to be goitrogenic and to cause renal damage has discouraged the Food and Drug Administration from approving its use for the treatment of recurrent depression. Therefore, the clinician's judgment as to whether the patient's abnormal mood swings are disturbing enough to warrant long-term treatment risks with lithium therapy must be respected. Extreme hyperactivity or talkativeness is rarely a problem in the elderly, but many patients begun on lithium earlier in their lives will need to be maintained on the medication for decades to prevent recurrent attacks in old age.

Lithium is contraindicated in elderly patients with heart disease or on treatment programs that require diuretics or sodium restriction. Since sodium and lithium compete for reabsorption in the renal system, a deficit in sodium results in an increase in lithium reabsorption and lithium retention. The difficulty with cardiovascular diseases is with the low-salt diets that often accompany them. Lithium toxicity is a potential emergency and warrants immediate discontinuance of the drug until safe levels of plasma lithium can be attained. Forced diuresis should aid significantly in the elimination of lithium. Thus close monitoring and vigilance are necessary to prevent toxicity.

Hormone Therapy in the Aged

Aging leads to changes in the endocrine system. The relationship between the biogenic amines and the release of the hormones from the arteriopituitary gland has led to the speculation that hormones may play a major role in depressive illness. Sachar, Finkelstein, and Hellman (1971) demonstrated that depressive illness is associated with an inadequate growth hormone response. Growth hormone is noted to be elevated in stress responses in humans (Brown & Reichlin, 1972), especially in later years.

Concerning the endocrine hypothesis of depressive disorders, clinicians have noted that persons who have an increased secretion of cortisone are more prone to depression. Other endocrine disturbances such as hypothyroidism have also underscored the relationship between endocrine activity and depressive symptoms in the elderly. Thus several different types of endocrine treatments have been considered in the management of depressive disorders in the elderly, including steroids and thyroid medications.

Estrogen, Progestogen, and Testosterone

Although there is continuing controversy concerning the use of sex hormones such as steroids in improving depressive disorders in late life, Greenblatt, Nexhat, Roesel, and Natrajan (1979) feel that androgens are helpful for the climacteric male. Their evidence leads them to believe that androgen replacement therapy in the adult years and late life often lessens fatigue, depression, and headaches in the male. In the experience of some clinicians, testosterone or androgen hormones may be useful in improving appetite and weight loss in climacteric depression. A number of researchers (e.g., Kaplan, 1974; Lehmann, 1972; Jakobovits, 1970) have conceded that while androgen doses of 10 mg orally, stretched over a 12-week period, have been generally helpful in the psychiatric depressions of elderly men, a combination of androgen and other steroid agents is more efficacious. It is suggested that a combination of androgen with either nicotinic acid or thioridazine gave better results than androgen alone.

In the case of female depressed patients gynecological problems and surgery including hysterectomy and the removal of ovaries led to endocrinologically related depression. According to a number of observers about a 50 percent increase was noted in the frequency of elderly women patients experiencing depression, irritability, and nervousness. Estrogen secretion is reduced dramatically in postmenopausal women (Kaplan & Herschyshen, 1971). Deficiencies occur in the reproductive organs with aging, the primary cause of these changes being in the hypothalamus, which becomes less responsive to stimuli that control the release of hormones (Dilman, 1971), and the subsequent imbalance between prolactin and estrogen may be potentially related to depressive symptoms in many elderly women. Estrogen medication has been known to improve anxiety, nervousness, headaches, and depression in the postmenopausal females (Greenblatt et al., 1979) although estrogen causes depression in some women.

Estrogen replacement therapy should be considered for possible inclusion in the management of postmenopausal depression (Wilson & Wilson, 1972; Rhoads, 1974). The use of oral or topical estrogens may be indirectly helpful in the potential depression of women by preserving the tone of the vaginal structures and thereby maintaining the functional genital capacity.

With regard to estrogen replacement therapy there has been some concern about estrogens contributing to the increasing incidence of endometrial carcinoma in postmenopausal women. However, Greenblatt et al. (1979) suggest that this potential problem can be combated especially if regular cyclic causes of oral progestogen are added to the medication regimen. Estrogen has been demonstrated to reduce the availability of serotonin and other amines. Estrogenic steroids may be expected to produce functional vitamin deficiencies, although it is not clear whether such deficiencies are directly linked to the depression or to any other adverse reactions.

Hypothyroidism and Thyroid Preparations

Pituitary thyroid-stimulating hormone (TSH) secretion is under the control of the hypothalamic thyroid-releasing hormone (TRH). Prange, Wilson, Knox, McClane, and Lipton (1970), who reviewed a number of laboratory studies of TRH, concluded that there is a significant connection between thyroid function and catecholamines in the hypothalamus. Finch (1973) has suggested that thyroid function does change with age. Catecholamine-neurons in the hypothalamus may serve as pacemakers of aging by controlling the interaction of pituitary hormones and target cells and may cause an imbalance of the serum thyroid level. These physiologic connections make hypothyroidism a diagnosis that should not be forgotten in old age. Lloyd (1967) found that hypothyroidism is not a rare condition in late life and was found in approximately 2 to 5 percent of all admissions to a geriatric unit. Evidence from Hollister (1973) and Whybrow, Prange, and Treadway (1969) suggests that depression, anxiety, and cognitive disturbances in the elderly with hypothyroidism often show up along with other psychiatric disorders. On occasion the symptoms of hypothyroidism may resemble senile dementia and, if untreated, can lead to states of confusion, cognitive disorientation, and impairment in the aged individuals.

Thyroid has not been considered a major therapeutic agent for depressed elderly patients. However, reversing a low serum thyroid level may alleviate depressive symptoms. It is wise to check routinely the T3 and T4 levels in the elderly with recent development of depression, anxiety, and organic brain changes to examine whether thyroid secretion might possibly be aggravating or even attenuating depressive states. Clinical studies by Prange et al. (1970) and Lloyd (1967) have indicated that the thyroid-stimulating hormone (TSH) and thyroid-releasing hormone (TRH) may be therapeutically responsive agents in the treatment of depression in the elderly. The TSH secretion is generally under the control of the TRH, where suppression may commonly occur and cause a subsequent suppression in the TSH (Loosen, Prange, Wilson, Lara, & Pettus, 1977).

Thyroid preparations, however, should not be administered without rigorous laboratory tests warranting the use of TRH and TSH with the elderly. Many elderly are quite sensitive to thyroid preparations, and indiscriminate use of these may lead to cardiac arrhythmias.

Verwoerdt (1981) strongly advises against the use of estrogen, testosterone, and thyroid preparation with elderly patients diagnosed as having potentials for dementia. Improper administration of thyroid medication in the elderly can commonly lead to apathetic hyperthyroidism, characterized by apathy and depression.

Schizophrenia, Functional Paranoid Disorders, and Antipsychotic Agents

Schizophrenia

Schizophrenia is a disease entity that can continue in a person's later life. Several studies have shown that whenever schizophrenia persists into old age, the clinical picture may change considerably: hallucinations often become less frequent, delusions are modified, and the elderly schizophrenic generally becomes more withdrawn and isolated (Verwoerdt, 1981). When certain personality abnormalities are stabilized, there is a decreased level of social adaptation (Sukhovskiy, 1976; Dvorim, 1977). Kay (1972) believes that the prodromal signs of schizophrenia in the elderly usually occur in the form of seclusion, isolation, and social disengagement but may not have a well-defined symptomatology until many years later, when mild-to-moderate suspiciousness, irritability, and expansive or aggressive behaviors may make the schizophrenia symptoms more detectable (Post, 1973). The mode of actions of the antipsychotic agents in the treatment of schizophrenia is believed to be related to the blockade of dopaminergic receptor sites, suggesting that old-age schizophrenia is associated with the decrease in the brain concentrations of dopamine and the relative increase of dopamine at the postsynaptic receptor sites.

According to Walker and Brodie (1980, p. 104) the selection of an antipsychotic drug from the five major classes of antipsychotic medications (i.e., phenothiazines, butyrophenones, thioxanthenes, dibenzoxazepines, and indoles) depends on the drug's pharmacological properties and side effects. The high-potency drugs used in the elderly—piperazine phenothiazine (Navane) and haloperidol (Haldol), a butyrophene compound—are powerful blockers of dopamine receptors and require a much lower dose to produce the same effects as the low-potency antipsychotics, which are weak blockers of the dopamine receptors—chlorpromazine (Thorazine) or thioridazine (Mellaril).

The low-potency antipsychotics most frequently used in the elderly have the disadvantages of a marked sedative effect and strong anticholinergic effects but the advantage of a low incidence of extrapyramidal symptoms that decidedly ought to be avoided. It is postulated that drug-related extrapyramidal movement disorders are caused by blockade of dopamine receptors in the basal ganglia.

Most of the antipsychotic drugs are equally effective, but individual patients respond differently to each of the three types of phenothiazines, two thioxanthenes, and one butyrophenone. Generally, it is recommended (Hollister, 1972a, 1972b; Branchey, Lee, Amin, & Simpson, 1978) that a start be made with one of the high-potency drugs that have less sedative and less hypotensive effects (e.g., Haldol, Navane). If extrapyramidal signs develop, a reduction in the dose or a change over to thioridazine (Mellaril) or chlorpromazine (Thorazine) is recommended.

Low dosage is particularly important for the elderly in order to avoid the risk of long-term toxicity. Other side effects such as postural hypotension, which contributes to strokes, heart attacks, and dizziness, can be prevented by avoiding the less-potent antipsychotics that have strong sedative and anticholinergic effects (Hollister, 1974, 1979; Jeste & Wyatt, 1981).

For more specific prescriptions for the elderly, antipsychotic agents are available in liquid preparation, which is more easily ingested, and for intramuscular injection. The latter is more potent in its effects than the oral preparations (tablets or liquid) and has the potential for stronger side effects such as hypotensive reactions. Closer vigilance and monitoring of effects are extremely important. Fann and Lake (1972) recommend that in order to prevent hypotensive reactions, the clinician should arrange for drug-free intervals and the prompt cessation of antipsychotic medication when no longer needed. Although extrapyramidal side effects are less common at low doses, they may still occur in the elderly. Prophylactic use of antiparkinsonian drugs is not recommended.

Paranoid Syndromes

Paranoid manifestations can range from suspiciousness to elaborate systematized delusions, both auditory and visual, and hallucinations. Such symptoms and states are quite common in the elderly (Whanger, 1973). Some of these symptoms, however, can be manifestations of other drugs such as amphetamines, which the elderly person may be self-medicating. Thus the need to monitor the person's medication and other psychosocial and biological deficits (e.g., social hearing loss, visual loss), which may be contributing to paranoid thinking in the secluded and isolated elderly person, is important.

Eisdorfer (1980) emphasizes that mildly suspicious elderly may need little or no psychotropic treatment. Antianxiety agents may be sufficient to reduce the anxiety state that may be contributing to the elderly person's paranoid thinking. Antipsychotic agents may be necessary to treat the psychotically paranoid individual. Both hospitalization and drugs will be necessary so as not to increase the existing paranoia.

Both in the moderately or mildly paranoid and the psychotically paranoid individual, the comprehensive treatment plan of drugs and therapy is indicated. The therapist and the family of the elderly can be of value in helping to reduce the suspiciousness of the elderly patient by uncovering the range of situations that are causing anxiety. The therapist's investigative-supportive relationship with the client can elicit the patient's history of fears, anxieties, and suspicious thinking. Antianxiety agents, such as benzodiazepines, may be useful in alleviating paranoid symptoms, but a supportive relationship with family and therapist alone can help to maintain the improvement. The restoration of a supportive social relation with a few friends or relatives is extremely important (Busse & Pfeiffer, 1973).

Behavioral Disorders

Behavioral disturbances in the elderly may result from psychotic, organic, or affective disorders, and it may be difficult to distinguish the variety of functional or psychotic disorders that may be contributing to behavioral disorders. In geriatric patients many of the disorders may be a carryover from early life or may arise for the first time. Hence behavioral disturbances such as psychotic outbursts, acute agitation, and severe anxiety attacks provide a delicate treatment challenge for which a satisfactory solution cannot always be found (Salzman et al., 1975).

Psychosis that begins after 65 is almost always of the paranoid variety and is characterized by symptoms of agitation, paranoid delusions, emotional distress, grandiosity, and thought disorders. According to Salzman et al. (1975) psychotic reactions are often characterized by depression, guilt feelings, self-deprecation, and hypochondriasis; the most frequent behavioral symptoms include agitation, assaultiveness, noisiness, and wandering. These symptoms can be especially distressing since they almost always involve the family and neighbors of the elderly patient, and hence disorders must be treated promptly. In summarizing the various somatic treatments possible for behavioral disturbances, Salzman, Van der Kolk, and Shader (1975) recommend the following. Neuroleptic agents are usually the treatment of choice for geriatric patients. Most neuroleptics (e.g., trademark names [Table 12–3], Thorazine, Mellaril, Tindal, Stelazine, and Haldol) have an equivalent degree of therapeutic usefulness, but selection of drugs must depend more on the unwanted side effects that are produced.

Aliphatic compounds such as chlorpromazine, thioridazine, and butyrophene produce rapid control over psychotic behaviors. The goal is to select an agent that produces minimal sedation or hypotension and the least number of extrapyramidal symptoms that cause difficulties in the motor coordination of elderly patients (Davis, Fann, & El-Yousef, 1973). Acute agitation, severe psychotic outbursts, and anxiety attacks often necessitate parenteral medication as follows: diazepam (5 mg IM) or chlorpromazine (10 to 25 mg IM).

In summary, the following side effects of antipsychotic agents should be carefully monitored. Blood pressure should be monitored. Symptoms of hypotension, agitation, assaultiveness, and confusion may fluctuate in intensity and often appear worse at night. Barbiturates generally should be avoided in the control of nonspecific agitation and confusion in the elderly, and so should routine antiparkinsonian drug administration in the control of extrapyramidal symptoms.

Drug Management of the Elderly's Mental Functioning

CNS Stimulants

Caffeine is a mild cerebral stimulant although excessive use of it in the elderly produces symptoms of anxiety. More powerful CNS stimulants include methylphenidate, which is a sympathomimetic stimulant widely used in the United States to treat the elderly. Crook's (1979) observations led him to conclude that the number of controlled studies that have used amphetamines have been so few that the possible value of these drugs remains controversial. Even where the short-lived, pick-me-up effect is marked, there are serious side effects such as decreased appetite, increased irritability, and perhaps psychotic manifestations. Thus stimulant drugs such as methylphenidate or magnesium pemoline may make some elderly more mentally alert, but overall the drawbacks outweigh the advantages.

Vasodilators

Regli, Yamaguchi, and Waltz (1971) have questioned the use of vasodilators in the treatment of dementia type symptoms in the elderly, especially in the treatment of arteriosclerotic dementia. These authors contend that the rationale for using vasodilators is that they increase the cerebral blood flow, which is normally diminished under conditions of Alzheimer's dementia. However, Obrist, Chivian, Cronqvist, and Ingvar (1970) have argued that vasodilators are incapable of dilating the arteriosclerotic blood vessels, and the general bodily vasodilation results in a lowering of blood pressure, which subsequently produces a diminution rather than an increase in cerebral perfusion (Regli et al., 1971). Furthermore, the diminution is a consequence, not a cause of the dementia, so an increase in blood flow is not likely to exert any useful effect.

However, a certain amount of experimentation continues with the use of vasodilators such as papaverine, isoxsuprine, and cyclandelate, and the results of some studies (e.g., Bazo, 1973; Smith, Lowrey, & Davis, 1968) have provided some encouraging data concerning improvement in mental functioning. While most studies using vasodilators in the treatment of dementia are uncontrolled and do not reach adequate criteria of design, execution, and matched sampling, several of them report positive effects of the drugs on mental functioning, principally less anxiety, more alertness and interest in the surroundings, lighter mood, and more stable mood (Ball & Taylor, 1967; Smith et al., 1968). More recent studies (e.g., Westreich, Alter, & Lundgren, 1975), however, have reported negative effects on mental functioning and adverse side effects such as hypotension, flushing, and tremor. Overall, there is little conclusive evidence of beneficial effects of vasodilators on mental functions.

Cerebral Activators

Meclofenoxate is a drug that modifies cerebral neuronal metabolism without producing vasodilation. Some earlier clinicians (e.g., Oliver & Restell, 1967) had challenged the clinical effectiveness of drugs such as meclofenoxate, which reduces the need of the brain for oxygen and thereby claims to improve memory function. On the whole the area of intellectual and mental deterioration in old age is poorly understood or researched. More attention is being directed to the study of old age dementias and Alzheimer's disease. It is generally hypothesized that decreasing brain acetylcholine levels are the cause of memory impairments in old age. Although the etiology of intellectual degeneration is unclear, some compounds increasing brain acetylcholine levels such as L-dopa have been suggested in the treatment of Alzheimer's disease in order to improve memory functions. Another way to increase acetylcholine concentrations in the brain is to administer lecithin. Overall results of studies that have examined the effects of lecithin have not been encouraging (Glen, 1980). Some improvements in memory have been reported in patients with Alzheimer's disease using physostigmine, which supposedly blocks the breakdown of acetylcholine (which is so important in memory functions) with a cholinesterase inhibitor. Further studies are needed to confirm the benefits of cholinomimetic drugs. Tentatively it is claimed that an approach that does not rely on acetylcholine synthesis for its therapeutic effects is the most promising one to pursue for the treatment of mental deterioration symptoms in the elderly.

Other similar claims are made that Gerovital drugs (deanol, propanolol) and various vitamin supplements can stall cerebral deterioration in aging. Some promising results of dietary prescriptions, vitamin supplements, etc., have been reported (e.g., Zung et al., 1974; Cohen & Ditman, 1974).

PRACTICAL DIETARY CONSIDERATIONS

With many individuals in the seventh and eighth decade of life, suboptimal nutrition and nutritional deficiencies are a common problem among the elderly. These problems are generally associated with depression, grief, and bereavement, which often cause a stern loss of appetite and loss in weight and physical energy. The elderly as a group seem to be at risk for nutritional deficiencies, which often become worse as a result of the use or abuse of psychotropic medication.

Nutritional status can be an important consideration in evaluating patients' strengths and limitations to be on a regimen of drug treatment. Beyond the general concerns, specific drug treatment regimens may require special attention to diet. Some of these specific considerations are adapted from Shader & Harmatz (1975) and summarized in the order of their importance and the potentials for creating hazards and adverse effects (see Shader & Harmatz, 1975, pp. 299–303 for a detailed discussion):

- MAO inhibitors. While the use of MAO inhibitors is infrequently recommended with the elderly, the foods evaluated for their tyramine contents are the most important ones that elderly patients on MAO drug agents should studiously avoid. Negligence can lead to hypertensive episodes reportedly following ingestion of the following foods: coffee, cheese, chocolate, pickles, sauerkraut, chicken livers, raisins, and yeast products such as yogurt. Several wines and beers have been evaluated for their tyramine content, and the use of most wines, beers, and alcohol should be gravely discouraged and proscribed (Verwoerdt, 1981).

- L-dopa. Elderly patients with parkinsonian symptoms or disorders treated with L-dopa may deplete their vitamin B6 store and risk neuropathy, which may be mistaken for the somatic concerns encountered in a depressive syndrome (Shader & Harmatz, 1975). It is suggested that elderly patients who are generally malnourished and have other disease states such as diabetes mellitus and chronic alcoholism will be chronically deficient in vitamin B6 and may develop peripheral neuropathy when administered L-dopa. Concurrent administration of 100 mg of vitamin B6 is a useful prophylaxis and both prevents and treats this neuropathy.

- Estrogenic steroids. Estrogenic steroids sometimes administered to postmenopausal depressed elderly women may be expected to produce functional vitamin deficiencies, although it is not clear that such deficiencies are directly linked to depression or any other adverse reaction. While routine prophylactic B6 administration is contraindicated (since evidence suggests that some women become more troubled after supplementary B6 administration), still it is important for physicians and clinicians to monitor the effects of estrogen therapy on postmenopausal depressed women's nutritional status. Women with absolute B6 deficiency may derive much benefit from supplementary B6 administration.

- Lithium carbonate. The potential for lithium to cause renal damage and thyroid dysfunction is intimately bound to that of sodium, which affects the rate of lithium reabsorption and lithium excretion. Inadequate lithium excretion is a likely consequence of restricted sodium intake in the case of many elderly with heart disease or treatment programs that require diuretics or low-salt diets.

The physician prescribing lithium is obliged to remain extremely alert to dietary changes requiring sodium loading or depletion. It is useful to monitor the elderly patient's habitual food preferences, with special focus on sodium sources, such as preserved foods, organ meats, eggs, etc. Other additives such as salts and seasoning should be evaluated and regulated. Suggestions for maintaining a daily sodium intake (just sufficient to avoid lithium toxicity) should be detailed for the elderly person on lithium administration.

Vitamin Supplements

In the elderly patient, measures of general care in eating and nutrition must be taken. Pharmacotherapy of depression will succeed to the extent that general care measures are adopted (Prange, 1973). Pharmacologic treatment without a general health care regimen is less likely to avoid side effects of medication. Suboptimal nutrition is a common problem among the elderly. Whanger and Wang's (1974) survey showed that 70 percent of the elderly studied had inadequate diets. In short, the elderly as a group seem to be at risk for nutritional deficiencies. If one deficiency persists, for example, low levels of vitamins A and C, thiamine, and riboflavin, others are frequently present. Although the direct relationship of various nutritional deficiencies and polypharmacology is still not understood, it seems safe to say that vitamin deficiencies decrease physical strength and worsen the side effects of pharmacological intervention. Although nutritional status is not often a commonly considered part of the psychological care or social work therapeutic regimen, it is important to assist the elderly in evaluating the effects of pharmacologic treatment in interaction with nutritional deficiencies and to make recommendations when appropriate.

The clinician or the family members of the elderly patient who prudently apply their general knowledge of the interaction of nutrition and pharmacology can avoid the common mistakes resulting through overuse of polypharmacy and the effects of vital vitamin deficiencies. At the same time the clinician and family members must be alert to the potentials for depressive symptoms and unspecified nervous diseases secondary to vitamin deficiencies (Chope, 1954). Several clinicians and nutritionists have documented behavioral and affective disorders attributed to vitamin deficiencies. Families and clinicians caring for elderly patients need to be aware of the following patterns of vitamin deficiencies that are nonspecifically associated with affective disorders in the elderly:

- Older persons with vitamin A deficiency have a higher incidence of general nervous diseases (Chope, 1954).
- Persons with vitamin B1 deficiencies show symptoms that mimic those of organic brain syndrome and depressive disorders, including confusion, loss of appetite, withdrawal, irritability, and inability to concentrate (Cheraskin & Ringsdorf, 1974).

Similarly Whanger (1980), based on his clinical experiences, reported that a deficiency of vitamin B2 (riboflavin) can lead to symptoms of depression, just as deficiencies in vitamin B12, niacin, pantothenic, and folic acid can lead to a host of depressive disorder symptoms such as sleeplessness, headaches, anxiety, apprehension and nervousness, apathy, physical and muscular weakness, lassitude, and depression (Dakshinamurti, 1977; Kane & Lipton, 1970; Williams, 1973).

- Attention is directed to the outcomes of vitamin C deficiency, which has been described as a neurotic triad of hysteria, depression and hypochondriasis (Kinsman & Hood, 1971).

- Attention is directed to vitamin E deficiencies in late life. Morgan, Kelleher, and Walker's (1975) data revealed that plasma levels of vitamin E were low in 67 percent of geriatric subjects admitted to hospitalization for short-term problems. In discussing the benefits of vitamin E, Whanger (1980) reports on its potentials for preventing cardiovascular disease, improving sexual functioning, and retarding the aging process.

There is little or no evidence obtained through controlled studies that vitamin E or other vitamin supplements in the diet can prevent or bring about a reversal of symptoms of aging or depression. There is no harm, however, in the clinician discussing the benefits of vitamin supplements in the diets of the elderly (Whanger, 1980). It is suggested that vitamins are generally quite safe except when taken in extreme doses; when ingested indiscriminately, toxicity may develop.

As older persons are quite susceptible to depressive symptoms secondary to vitamin deficiencies, the physician or nutritionist should be quite willing to discuss concerns about diet and the need for vitamin supplements with the elderly clients. Most elders and their families are generally quite supportive of the use of vitamin supplements. Only research will provide an answer to the potentials of vitamin therapy for stalling the aging process or reversing symptoms of depression.

We may influence not only immediate but also long-term outcomes of physical and psychological disease states in the elderly by drug treatment coordinated with a more global treatment plan of nutrition and dietary considerations. Although knowledge of what a drug can do is limited, it is a misconception that a drug affects only symptoms and not the process of health and illness (Campbell & Shapiro, 1975).

CONCLUSIONS

What is clearly indicated is a rational approach to what constitutes the legitimate role of psychoactive agents in treating a variety of recognizable behavioral and affective difficulties in an aged population. Drugs are far from safe in such a group, and the administration of both low and high doses of medication should clearly be accompanied by elaborate precautions against complications. Lennard and associates (Lennard, Epstein, Bernstein, & Ransom, 1971) report that more than 202 million prescriptions for psychotropic medication were filled by persons who saw physicians during 1970 alone. There is ever-increasing pressure on the health care specialists by drug companies to broaden the use of psychopharmacologic agents and to deal with the multiple disease entities of the elderly through the use of psychotropic drugs. The implication is that a variety of old-age affective disorders or symptoms such as depression, anxiety, and agitation should be mediated and medicated by drug management, as opposed to the more time-consuming management by physicians, staff, psychotherapists, and community caregivers.

Indeed the possibility exists of new drugs to control both the symptoms and the process of psychological and physiological changes in old age. It is conceivable that various intellectual and cognitive difficulties now a problem for many elderly may be modified by pharmacologic agents acting on the cardiovascular, autonomic, or central nervous system (Eisdorfer, 1973). Pharmacological work is exploring problems common in the elderly such as inadequate cerebral circulation and control of hypertension as well as new aspects of anticoagulation, modification of autonomic functioning, and better ANS and CNS interaction.

However, our knowledge of the biology and psychopharmacology of aging is far from sufficient. Additionally pharmaceutical progress in the development of potentially useful drugs in the elderly has not been matched by adequately controlled research to evaluate these agents. Not only must the clinician be concerned with the metabolism of drugs in elderly patients with impaired respiratory or renal function but also with understanding the complications of paradoxical drug effects on the CNS. The problems of use and abuse and the trade-off between drug effectiveness for the elderly patients' needs as opposed to long-term care by the staff become serious issues. They represent significant clinical challenges to the physician so far as effective drug use is concerned (Epstein & Simon, 1968). In the balance, however, there is no denying the fact that psychotropic drugs can be tremendously beneficial. Already drugs are proving to be valuable additions to the management of affective disorders, especially depression, in the aged. They must, however, be used with care and consideration for the special physiologic, biologic, and psychological characteristics of the patients who confront us, particularly with regard to their increased susceptibility to side effects and with attention to other available therapeutic alternatives, options, and modalities.

SUMMARY

This chapter has examined some of the major principles and issues in the psychopharmacological treatment of the elderly. The bases of altered reactions to drugs in the elderly are varied. Predominant among these are pharmacokinetic factors showing greater variability due to reduced renal and hepatic function and changing enzyme function. Numerous controlled studies have shown that the interaction of drugs increases with age and that cerebral blood flow is reduced. Furthermore, there is a loss of neurons in the brain, which often interferes with the balance and coordination of various cerebral centers, thereby producing paradoxical reactions to pharmaceutical agents.

From an overall perspective, however, it has been argued that psychopharmacologic therapy has significantly improved the prognosis of affective disorders and mental illness in older adults. Many depressive disorders are now treatable in the elderly, and drugs are a valuable addition to the management of many other biological and psychological disturbances. However, older persons are at greater risk than any other age group for problems secondary to potential toxic effects of psychotropic medication and the increased susceptibility to adverse side effects. Therefore extra caution should be used in treating the elderly with psychotropic medications. The problems of drug use and abuse, indications and contraindications, and the trade-off between drug effectiveness for the elderly person's needs as opposed to long-term care by the staff have become challenging issues for physicians and clinicians.

REFERENCES

Ayd, F.J. (1971a). Recognizing and treating depressed patients. *Modern Medicine*, Nov. 29, pp. 80–86.

Ayd, F.J. (1971b). Long term effects of doxepin (Sinequan). *Disorders of the Nervous System, 32*, 617–622.

Ayd, F.J. (1979). Trazedone: A unique broad spectrum antidepressant. *International Drug Therapy Newsletter, 14*, 33–40.

Ayd, F.J. (1980). Amoxapine: A new tricyclic antidepressant. *International Drug Therapy Newsletter, 15*, 33–40.

Baldessarini, R.J. (1977). *Chemotherapy in psychiatry*. Cambridge: Harvard University Press.

Ball, J.A.C., & Taylor, A.R. (1967). Effects of cyclandelate on mental function and cerebral blood flow in elderly patients. *British Medical Journal, iii*, 525–528.

Bazo, A.J. (1973). An ergot alkaloid preparation (Hydergine) versus papaverine in treating common complaints of the aged: Double-blind study. *Journal of American Geriatrics Society, 21*, 63–71.

Beattie, B.L., & Sellers, E.M. (1979). Psychoactive drug use in the elderly: The pharmacokinetics. *Psychosomatics, 20*(7), 474–479.

Bender, A.D. (1974). Pharmacodynamic principles of drug therapy in the aged. *Journal of American Geriatrics Society, 22*, 296–303.

Blazer, D.G. (1982). *Depression in late life*. St. Louis: C.V. Mosby Co.

Blazer, D.G., & Friedman, S.W. (1979). Depression in late life. *American Family Physician, 20*, 91–105.

Branchey, M.H., Lee, J.H., Amin, R., & Simpson, G.M. (1978). High and low potency neuroleptics in elderly psychiatric patients. *Journal of American Medical Association, 239*, 1860–1862.

Brown, G.M., & Reichlin, S. (1972). Psychologic and neural regulations of growth hormone. *Psychosomatic Medicine, 34*, 45–51.

Burgen, A.S.U., & Mitchell, J.F. (1978). *Gaddum's pharmacology*. New York: Oxford University Press.

Burrows, G.D., Vorah, J., Hunt, D., Sloman, J.G., Scoggins, B.A., & Davies, B. (1976). Cardiac effects of different tricyclic antidepressant drugs. *British Journal of Psychiatry, 129*, 335–341.

Busse, E.W., & Pfeiffer, E. (Eds.). (1973). *Mental illness in later life*. Washington: American Psychiatric Association.

Campbell, M., & Shapiro, T. (1975). Therapy of psychiatric disorders of childhood. In R.I. Shader (Ed.)., *Manual of psychiatric therapeutics*. (pp. 137–162). Boston: Little, Brown & Co.

Cheraskin, E., & Ringsdorf, W.M. (1974). *Psychodietetics*. New York: Stein & Day.

Chien, C.P. (1971). Psychiatric treatment for geriatric patients. Pub or drug? *American Journal of Psychiatry, 127*, 1070–1075.

Chope, H.D. (1954). Relation of nutrition to health in aging persons. *California Medicine, 81*, 335–339.

Cohen, S., & Ditman, K. (1974). Gerovital H3 in the treatment of the depressed aging patient. *Psychosomatics, 15*, 15–19.

Crook, T. (1979). Central nervous system stimulants: Appraisal of use in geropsychiatric patients. *Journal of American Geriatrics Society, 27*, 476–477.

Crooks, J., O'Malley, K., & Stevenson, I.H. (1976). Pharmacokinetics in the elderly. *Clinical Pharmacokinetics, 1*, 280–296.

Dakshinamurti, K. (1977). B vitamins and nervous system function. In R.J. Wurtman & J.J. Wurtman (Eds.), *Nutrition and the brain* (Vol. 1, pp. 249–318). New York: Raven Press.

Davis, J.M., Fann, W.E., & El-Yousef, M.K. (1973). Clinical problems in treating the aged with psychotropic drugs. *Advances in Behavioral Biology, 6*, 111–125.

Dilman, V.M. (1971). Age associated elevation of hypothalamic threshold to feedback control and its role in development, aging and disease. *Lancet, 1*, 1211–1221.

Domino, E.F., Dren, A.T., & Giardina, W.J. (1978). Biochemical and neurotransmitter changes in the aging brain. In M.A. Lipton, A. DiMascio, & R.F. Killam (Eds.), *Psychopharmacology: A generation of progress* (pp. 1507–1515). New York: Raven Press.

Dovenmuehle, R.H. (1965). Psychiatry: Implementation. In J.T. Friedman (Ed.), *Clinical features of the older patient* (pp. 266–272). Springfield, IL: Charles C Thomas.

Dvorim, D.V. (1977). Progressive paranoid schizophrenia in the elderly. *Zhurnal Nevropatologii i Psikhiatrii imeni S.S. Korsakova, 77*, 881–886.

Eisdorfer, C. (1973). Issues in the psychopharmacology of the aged. In C. Eisdorfer & W.E. Fann (Eds.), *Psychopharmacology and aging* (pp. 3–7). New York: Plenum Press.

Eisdorfer, C. (1980). Paranoia and schizophrenic disorders in later life. In E.W. Busse & D.G. Blazer (Eds.), *Handbook of geriatric psychiatry* (pp. 329–337). New York: Van Nostrand Reinhold Co.

Eisdorfer, C., & Fann, W.E. (Eds.). (1973). *Psychopharmacology and aging*. New York: Plenum Press.

Epstein, L.J. (1978). Anxiolytics, anti-depressants and neuroleptics in the treatment of the geriatric patients. In M.A. Lipton, A. DiMascio, & K.F. Killam (Eds.), *Psychopharmacology: A generation of progress* (pp. 1517–1523). New York: Raven Press.

Epstein, L.J., & Simon, A. (1968). Alternative to state hospitalization for the geriatric mentally ill. *American Journal of Psychiatry, 124*, 955–961.

Fann, W.E., & Lake, C.R. (1972). Drug induced movement disorders in the elderly: An appraisal of the treatment. In W.E. Fann & G.L. Maddox (Eds.), *Drug issues in geropsychiatry* (pp. 41–48). Baltimore: Williams & Wilkins Co.

Fann, W.E., & Wheless, J.C. (1975). Depression in elderly patients. *Southern Medical Journal, 68*, 468–473.

Fann, W.E., Wheless, J.C., & Richman, B.W. (1976). Treating the aged with psychotropic drugs. *Gerontologist, 16*, 322–328.

Feighner, J.P. (1980, May). *Progress in the pharmacotherapy of depression*. Symposium given at the annual meeting of the American Psychiatric Association, San Francisco.

Finch, C.E. (1973). Catecholamine metabolism in the brains of aging male mice. *Brain Research, 52*, 261–266.

Friedel, R.O. (1978). Pharmacokinetics in the geropsychiatric patient. In M.A. Lipton, A. DiMascio, & R.F. Killam (Eds.), *Psychopharmacology: A generation of progress* (pp. 1499–1505). New York: Raven Press.

Friedel, R.O. (1980). The pharmacotherapy of depression in the elderly: Pharmacokinetic considerations. In J.O. Cole & J.E. Barrett (Eds.), *Psychopathology in the aged* (pp. 157–163). New York: Raven Press.

Friedel, R.O., & Raskin, D. (1975). Relationship of blood levels of Sinequan to clinical effects in the treatment of depression in the aged patients. In J. Mendels (Ed.), *Sinequan: A monograph of recent clinical studies* (pp. 51–53). Princeton, NJ: Excerpta Medica.

Gattozzi, A.A. (1970). *Lithium in the treatment of mood disorders*. Information for Program Analysis and Evaluation Branch, National Institute of Mental Health Bulletin No. 5033. Washington: National Clearinghouse for Mental Health.

Glen, A.I.M. (1980). The pharmacology of dementia. *Hospital Update, 10*, 977–988.

Goldstein, B.J. (1977, December). Drug therapy for the depressed patient. *Hospital Formulatory*.

Goldstein, S.E. (1979). Depression in the elderly. *Journal of American Geriatrics Society, 27*, 38–42.

Greenblatt, M., Grosser, G.H., & Wechsler, H. (1964). Differential response of hospitalized depressed patients to somatic therapy. *American Journal of Psychiatry, 120*, 935–943.

Greenblatt, B., Nexhat, C., Roesel, R.A., & Natrajan, P.K. (1979). Update of the male and female climacteric. *Journal of American Geriatrics Society, 27*, 481–490.

Hale, W.E., Marks, R.G., & Stewart, R.B. (1979). Drug use in a geriatric population. *Journal of American Geriatrics Society, 27*, 374–377.

Hollister, L.E. (1972a). Psychiatric disorders. In K.L. Melmon & J.F. Morelli (Eds.), *Clinical pharmacology* (pp. 842–873). New York: Macmillan.

Hollister, L.E. (1972b). Neurologic disorders. In K.L. Melmon & J.F. Morelli (Eds.), *Clinical pharmacology* (pp. 874–912). New York: Macmillan.

Hollister, L.E. (1973). *Clinical use of psychotherapeutic drugs*. Springfield, IL: Charles C Thomas.

Hollister, L.E. (1974). Protirelin (TRH) in depression. *Archives of General Psychiatry, 31*, 468.

Hollister, L.E. (1975). Drugs for mental disorders of old age. *Journal of Medical Advancement, 234*, 195–198.

Hollister, L.E. (1979). Psychotherapeutic drugs. In A.J. Levenson (Ed.), *Neuropsychiatric side-effects of drugs in the elderly* (pp. 79–88). New York: Raven Press.

Holloway, D. (1974). Drug problems in the geriatric patient. *Drug Intelligence and Clinical Pharmacy, 8*, 632–642.

Jakobovits, T. (1970). The treatment of impotence with methyltestosterone thyroid. *Fertility and Sterility, 21*(1), 32–35.

Jeste, D.V., & Wyatt, R.J. (1981). Changing epidemiology of tardive dyskinesia. *American Journal of Psychiatry, 138*, 297–309.

Kahn, E., & Fisher, C. (1969). The sleep characteristics of the normal aged male. *Journal of Nervous and Mental Diseases, 148*, 477–494.

Kalinowsky, L.B., & Hippius, H. (1969). *Pharmacological, convulsive and other somatic treatments in psychiatry.* New York: Grune & Stratton.

Kane, F.J., & Lipton, M. (1970). Folic acid and mental illness. *Southern Medical Journal, 63*, 603–607.

Kaplan, B.H., & Herschyshen, M.D. (1971). Gas liquid chromatographic quantitation of urinary estrogens in non-pregnant women, post-menopausal women, and men. *American Journal of Obstetrics and Gynecology, 111*, 286–298.

Kaplan, H.D. (1974). Erectile dysfunction. In H.D. Kaplan (Ed.), *The new sex therapy* (pp. 255–288). New York: Brunner/Mazel.

Karasu, T.B., & Murkofsky, C.A. (1976). Psychopharmacology of the elderly. In L. Bellak & T.B. Karasu (Eds.), *Geriatric psychiatry* (pp. 225–239). New York: Grune & Stratton.

Kastenbaum, R., & Slater, P.E. (1964). Effects of wine on the interpersonal behavior of geriatric patients: An exploratory study. In R. Kastenbaum (Ed.), *New thoughts on old age* (pp. 191–204). New York: Springer.

Kay, D.W.K. (1972). Schizophrenia and schizophrenia like states in the elderly. *British Journal of Hospital Medicine, 52*, 369–372.

Kenny, A.D. (1979). Designing therapy for the elderly. *Drug Therapy, 9*, 49–64.

Kinsman, R.A., & Hood, J. (1971). Some behavioral effects of ascorbic acid deficiency. *American Journal of Clinical Nutrition, 24*, 455–461.

Klein, D.F., & Davis, J.M. (1969). *Diagnosis and drug treatment of psychiatric disorders.* Baltimore: Williams & Wilkins.

Kopell, B.S. (1977). Treating the suicide patient. *Geriatrics, 32*, 65–67.

Kral, V. (1976). Somatic therapies in older depressed patients. *Journal of Gerontology, 31*, 311–313.

Lader, M. (1982). Pharmacology of old age. In R. Levy & F. Post (Eds.), *The psychiatry of late life* (pp. 143–162). London: Blackwell Scientific Publications.

Lamy, P.P., & Kitler, M.E. (1971). Drugs and the geriatric patient. *Journal of American Geriatrics Society, 19*, 23–33.

Larson, D.B., Whanger, A.D., & Busse, E.W. (1982). Geriatrics. In B.B. Wolman (Ed.), *The therapist's handbook* (pp. 343–387). New York: Van Nostrand Reinhold Co.

Learoyd, B.M. (1972). Psychotropic drugs and the elderly patient. *Medical Journal of Australia, 1*, 1131–1133.

Lehmann, H.E. (1972). Psychopharmacological aspects of geriatric medicine. In C.M. Gaitz (Ed.), *Aging and the brain* (pp. 193–208). New York: Plenum Press.

Lennard, H.L., Epstein, L.J., Bernstein, A., & Ransom, D.C. (1971). *Mystification and drug misuse.* San Francisco: Jossey-Bass.

Linnoila, M., & Vinkari, M. (1976). Efficacy and side effects of nitrazepam and thioridazine as sleeping aids in psychogeriatric in-patients. *British Journal of Psychiatry, 128*, 566–569.

Lippincourt, R.C. (1968). Depressive illness: Identification and treatment in the elderly. *Geriatrics, 23*(11), 149–152.

Lloyd, W.H. (1967). Some clinical features of hyper- and hypothyroidism in the elderly. *Gerontologia Clinica, 9*, 337–346.

Loosen, P.T., Prange, A.J., Wilson, I.C., Lara, P.P., & Pettus, C. (1977). Thyroid stimulating hormone response after thyrotropin releasing hormone in depressed, schizophrenic, and normal women. *Psychoneuroendocrinology, 2*, 137–148.

Lowenbach, H. (1973). How well does electroshock treatment work in depression in the elderly? How safe is it, and how can it be given? In E.W. Busse & E. Pfeiffer (Eds.), *Mental illness in late life* (pp. 246–248). Washington: American Psychiatric Association.

MacFarlane, M.D. (1973). Possible rationale for procaine (Gerovital H3) therapy in geriatrics: Inhibition of monoamine oxidase. *Journal of American Geriatrics Society, 21*, 414–418.

McCrae, R.R., Bartone, P.T., & Costa, P.T. (1976). Age, anxiety and self-reported health. *International Journal of Aging and Human Development, 7*, 49–58.

Mishara, B.L., & Kastenbaum, R. (1974). Wine in the treatment of long-term geriatric patients in mental institutions. *Journal of American Geriatrics Society, 22*, 88–94.

Montgomery, S.A., Braithwaite, R.A., & Crammer, J.L. (1977). Routine nortriptyline levels in the treatment of depression. *British Medical Journal, 2*, 166.

Morgan, A.G., Kelleher, J., & Walker, B.E. (1975). A nutritional survey in the elderly: Blood and urine vitamin levels. *International Journal of Vitamin and Nutrition Research, 45*, 448–462.

Nies, A., Robinson, D.S., & Friedman, M.J. (1977). Relationship between age and tricyclic antidepressant plasma levels. *American Journal of Psychiatry, 134*, 790–793.

Obrist, W.D., Chivian, E., Cronqvist, S., & Ingvar, D.H. (1970). Regional cerebral blood flow in senile and presenile dementia. *Neurology, 20*, 315–328.

Oliver, J.E., & Restell, M. (1967). Serial testing in assessing the effects of meclofenoxate on patients with memory defects. *British Journal of Psychiatry, 113*, 219–229.

Ostfeld, A., Smith, C.M., & Stotsky, B.A. (1977). The systemic use of procaine in the treatment of the elderly: A review. *Journal of American Geriatrics Society, 25*, 1–3.

Pfeiffer, E. (1973). Multiple system interaction and high bodily concern. In C. Eisdorfer & W.E. Fann (Eds.), *Psychopharmacology and aging* (pp. 151–158). New York: Plenum Press.

Piland, B. (1979). The aging process and psychoactive drug use in clinical treatment. In *The aging process and psychoactive drug use,* Services Research Monograph Series (No. 79-813, DHEW, pp. 1–16). Washington: U.S. Department of Health, Education, and Welfare.

Prange, A.J. (1973). The use of antidepressant drugs in the elderly patient. In C. Eisdorfer & W.E. Fann (Eds.), *Psychopharmacology and aging* (pp. 225–237). New York: Plenum Press.

Prange, A.J., Wilson, I.C., Knox, A., McClane, T.K., & Lipton, M.A. (1970). Enhancement of imipramine by thyroid stimulating hormone: Clinical and theoretical implications. *American Journal of Psychiatry, 127*, 191–199.

Prentice, R. (1979). Patterns of psychoactive drug use among the elderly. In *The aging process and psychoactive drug use,* Services Research Monograph Series (No. 79-813, pp. 17–41). Washington: U.S. Department of Health, Education, and Welfare.

Prout, C.T., Allen, E.B., & Hamilton, D.M. (1956). The use of electric shock therapy in older patients. In O.J. Kaplan (Ed.), *Mental disorders in later life* (2nd ed., pp. 446–459). Stanford, CA: Stanford University Press.

Quitkin, F., Rifkin, A., & Klein, D.F. (1979). Monoamine oxidase inhibitors. *Archives of General Psychiatry, 36*, 749–760.

Ramsay, L.E., & Tucker, G.T. (1981). Drugs and the elderly. *British Medical Journal, 282*, 125–127.

Reed, K., Smith, R.C., Schoolar, J.C., Hu, R., Leelavathi, D.E., Mann, E., & Lippman, L. (1980). Cardiovascular effects of nortriptyline in geriatric patients. *American Journal of Psychiatry, 137*, 986–989.

Regli, F., Yamaguchi, T., & Waltz, A.G. (1971). Cerebral circulation. Effects of vasodilating drugs on blood flow and the microvasculature of ischemic and nonischemic cerebral cortex. *Archives of Neurology, 24*, 467–474.

Reidenberg, M.M. (1980). Drugs in the elderly. *Bulletin of the New York Academy of Medicine, 56*, 703–714.

Rhoads, F.P. (1974). Continuous cyclic hormonal therapy. *Journal of American Geriatrics Society, 22*, 443–451.

Ritschel, W.A. (1976). Pharmacokinetic approach to drug dosing in the aged. *Journal of American Geriatrics Society, 24*, 344–354.

Rosenthal, S., & Bowden, C. (1973). A double-blind comparison of thioridazine versus diazepam in patients with chronic mixed anxiety and depressive symptoms. *Current Therapeutic Research, 15*, 261–267.

Rossman, I. (1980). Bodily changes with aging. In E.W. Busse & D.G. Blazer (Eds.), *Handbook of geriatric psychiatry* (pp. 125–146). New York: Van Nostrand Reinhold Co.

Roth, G.S. (1975). Altered hormone binding and responsiveness during aging. *Proceedings of the 10th International Congress of Gerontology* (Vol. 1, pp. 44–45). New York: Excerpta Medica.

Sachar, E.J., Finkelstein, J., & Hellman, L. (1971). Growth hormone responses in depressive illness. I. Response to insulin tolerance test. *Archives of General Psychiatry, 25*, 263–271.

Salzman, C. (1975). Electroconvulsive therapy. In R. Shader (Ed.), *Manual of Psychiatric Therapeutics* (pp. 115–124). Boston: Little, Brown & Co.

Salzman, C., & Shader, R.I. (1973). Responses to psychotropic drugs in the normal elderly. In C. Eisdorfer & W.E. Fann (Eds.), *Psychopharmacology and aging* (pp. 159–168). New York: Plenum Press.

Salzman, C. & Shader, R.I. (1978). Relationship between depression in the elderly, psychologic defense mechanisms and physical illness. *Journal of American Geriatrics Society, 26*, 253–260.

Salzman, C., Van der Kolk, B., & Shader, R.I. (1975). Psychopharmacology and the geriatric patient. In R.I. Shader (Ed.), *Manual of psychiatric therapeutics* (pp. 171–184). Boston: Little, Brown & Co.

Sathananthan, G.L., Gershon, S., & Ferris, S.H. (1976). Psychological aspect of aging. Unpublished manuscript.

Shader, R.I., & Greenblatt, D.J. (1975). The psychopharmacologic treatment of anxiety states. In R.I. Shader (Ed.), *Manual of psychiatric therapeutics* (pp. 27–38). Boston: Little, Brown & Co.

Shader, R.I., & Harmatz, J.S. (1975). Practical dietary considerations. In R.I. Shader (Ed.), *Manual of psychiatric therapeutics* (pp. 299–304). Boston: Little, Brown & Co.

Smith, W.L., Lowrey, J.B., & Davis, J.A. (1968). The effects of cyclandelate on psychological test performance in patients with cerebral vascular insufficiency. *Current Therapeutic Research, 10*, 613–618.

Spiker, D.G., & Pugh, D.D. (1976). Combining tricyclic and monoamine oxidase inhibitor antidepressants. *Archives of General Psychiatry, 33*, 828–830.

Squire, L.R. (1977). E.C.T. and Memory Loss. *American Journal of Psychiatry, 134*, 997–1001.

Stotsky, B.A., & Borozne, J. (1972). Butisol sodium vs. librium among geriatric patients, younger outpatients and nursing home patients. *Diseases of the Nervous System, 33*, 254–267.

Strain, J.J. (1975). Psychopharmacological treatment of the medically ill. In J.J. Strain & S. Grossman (Eds.), *Psychological care of the medically ill: A primer in liaison psychiatry* (pp. 108–118). New York: Appleton-Century-Crofts.

Strain, J.J. (1978). *Psychological interventions in medical practice*. New York: Appleton-Century-Crofts.

Sukhovskiy, A.A. (1976). Clinical picture and dynamics of long-term remissions as an outcome of shift-like schizophrenia. *Zhurnal Nevropatologii i Psikhiatrii imeni S.S. Korsakova, 76*, 563–568.

van Scheyen, J.D., & van Kammen, D.P. (1979). Clomipramine-induced mania in unipolar depression. *Archives of General Psychiatry, 36*, 560–565.

Verwoerdt, A. (1981). *Clinical geropsychiatry*. Baltimore: Williams & Wilkins.

Verzar, F. (1961). The age of the individual as one of the parameters of pharmacological action. *Acta Physiological Academy of Science, Hungary, 19*, 313.

Vestal, R.E. (1978). A review of pharmacology and aging. *Drugs, 16*, 358–382.

Walker, J.I., & Brodie, H.K.H. (1980). Neuropharmacology of aging. In E.W. Busse & D.G. Blazer (Eds.), *Handbook of geriatric psychiatry* (pp. 102–124). New York: Van Nostrand Reinhold Co.

Weiner, R.D. (1979). The psychiatric use of electrically induced seizures. *American Journal of Psychiatry, 136*, 1507–1517.

Westreich, G., Alter, M., & Lundgren, S. (1975). Effects of cyclandelate on dementia. *Stroke, 6*, 535–538.

Whanger, A.D. (1973). Paranoid syndromes of the senium. In C. Eisdorfer & W.E. Fann (Eds.), *Psychopharmacology and aging* (pp. 203–211). New York: Plenum Press.

Whanger, A.D. (1980). Nutrition, diet, and exercise. In E.W. Busse & D.G. Blazer (Eds.), *Handbook of geriatric psychiatry* (pp. 473–497). New York: Van Nostrand Reinhold Co.

Whanger, A.D., & Busse, E.W. (1975). Care in hospital. In J.G. Howells (Ed.), *Modern perspectives in the psychiatry of old age* (pp. 450–485). New York: Brunner/Mazel.

Whanger, A.D., & Wang, H.S. (1974). Vitamin B12 deficiency in normal aged and psychiatric patients. In E. Palmore (Ed.), *Normal aging* (Vol. 2, pp. 63–73). Durham, NC: Duke University Press.

Whybrow, P.C., Prange, A.J., & Treadway, C.R. (1969). Mental changes accompanying thyroid gland dysfunction. *Archives of General Psychiatry, 20*, 48–63.

Williams, R.J. (1973). *Nutrition against disease*. New York: Bantam Books.

Wilson, R.A., & Wilson, T.A. (1972). The basic philosophy of estrogen maintenance. *Journal of American Geriatrics Society, 26*, 521–523.

Zung, W.W.K., Gianturco, D., Pfeiffer, E., Wang, H.S., Whanger, A., Bridge, T.P., & Potkin, S.G. (1974). Evaluation of Gerovital H3 as an antidepressant drug. *Psychosomatics, 15*, 127–131.

Chapter 13

Integrated Therapies
for the Aged

The emergence of numerous competing systems of treatment (medical and psycho-therapeutic) during the last three decades has been cited as one of the principal problem areas in the total range of therapeutic influence that has made its appearance in the last decade or so (Strupp, 1969). Although London (1974) described this proliferation of therapeutic influences as a necessary and vital reflection of changing times, the specific ways in which this proliferation of therapies is an answer to the elderly's problems of stress, depression, anxieties, and functional disorders are far from clear. The state of the art attests to the lack of clarity and lack of resolution of the specific versus the general elements and components of therapeutic services for the elderly. The many disparate views concerning appropriate therapeutic strategies and the increasing number of individual disciplines that are being brought to bear on diagnosis and treatment of depression, stress, and adaptation problems of the aged are indeed characteristic of the prevailing intellectual, clinical, and medical approaches to treatment of the aged. Although each approach has its own validity, such wide variation with respect to a presumed therapeutic effectiveness perpetuates concept confusion and on the clinical level engenders a system of care of the elderly that is highly inconsistent. This conflicting state of affairs is further compounded by speculations of the effectiveness of various psychotherapies (e.g., individual versus group and behav-ioral-cognitive versus psychodynamic), pharmacotherapies, and medical treatments.

In the mental health field, concern with the problems of the aged has been slow in developing. While the prevalence of psychiatric problems among the aged is high, the amount of knowledge about late-life disorders and therapies relevant to these conditions is lower than for any other age group. The amount of exploration with different combinations and integration of strategies and techniques of therapies appropriate for the elderly has been exceedingly limited. Several factors have contributed to this lack of exploration. The primary factor is that old age and the difficulties associated with growing older are perceived principally as medical problems. Important physiological changes certainly do occur in old age and must be taken into account in understanding the mental disorders of older persons and in choosing appropriate interventions. But a medical perspective with an emphasis on biological medicine and pharmacotherapy in the treatment of mental disorders has its limits. Indeed, now that the biomedical model has been so trenchantly questioned in various quarters (e.g., Engel, 1977), it is particularly important to examine an integrated model of therapies that attends not only to the more common medical and psychiatric approach but also to the social and psychological perspective and seeks to integrate the two. It is particularly important, therefore, to take an approach that is eclectic and derives from information gained from many aspects of psychological, medical, and psychopharmacological inquiry.

Until recently it was believed that the elderly could not benefit from psychotherapy. Thus even psychological disorders of older persons associated with maladaptive habits and thoughts were treated through pharmacologic therapies. However, there appears to be a growing recognition by mental health professionals of the effectiveness of one-to-one therapy and group therapy approaches and the success of behavioral and cognitive strategies. Although mental health professionals do not agree on a unitary view of psychotherapy for the elderly, there is no doubt in the minds of clinicians who have worked with older persons that they can and do respond to psychological treatment. No longer can it be maintained a priori that the aged respond only to medically oriented treatments or that they are unable to respond to cognitive or behavioral psychotherapies that go beyond the traditional supportive and psychodynamically oriented psychotherapies.

The question that needs to be answered in a more specific way is which aged, treated with which combination or integration of therapeutic elements and strategies, will respond favorably to treatment. The issues of whether the elderly benefit more from psychological treatment or pharmacotherapies or some combination are empirical questions that have not been evaluated. As in other areas of mental health there is a critical need for more and better-designed evaluation studies to assess the effects of different kinds of interventions and integrations of interventions. The lack of an integrative model of therapy for the elderly is related to the current paucity of integrative information, which in turn is a function of the poverty of interconnections between related medical and psychological fields.

This chapter argues the point that in order to provide effective mental health services to older persons, the therapeutic path must be paved in a way that allows us to consider the psychodynamic, behavioral, and cognitive dimensions of various therapeutic modalities as well as the convergence of both psychotherapy and medical treatment including pharmacotherapy. In so doing, it is hoped that some forms of integrated biopsychosocial therapies and their therapeutic processes will be more closely and critically examined. Through combining and integrating varied medical and psychological perspectives, it may be possible to document the approaches that integrate well and will lead to more refined conceptualizations and more successful approaches to the care of the depressed and stressed elderly. It may also be possible to identify those therapeutic approaches that conflict and thereby impede formulation and implementation of policies for care and treatment of the elderly.

INTEGRATION OF MEDICAL TREATMENT AND PSYCHOTHERAPY

The following rationale for an integration of medical and psychological strategies assumes that there is a natural course of psychological troubles and illness just as there is a natural history of physical and medical illness (Hodge, 1980) and that in this natural history certain identifiable factors and interactions are involved, for example, a predisposing personality, external precipitating stress and anxiety events, specific age-related changes and decline in the physiological functioning, certain developments in anxiety and stress reactions, and certain secondary gains or symptom-fixing factors commonly observed in the elderly.

It further assumes the formulation of a total treatment program (medical, pharmacologic, psychotherapeutic) in which the therapeutic goals and sites of intervention (i.e., ego personality, cognitive functions, social support networks, biological systems, genetics, and neurotransmissions) are assessed. One might consider all these sites of intervention as elements of an adaptive system. When one or more psychological, biological, or developmental capacities prove insufficient to absorb the impact of the illness, decompensation occurs and is designated as depression, stress, or maladaptation. Interventions for the elderly, whether in terms of biological medicine or psychotherapy, are selected on the basis of the individual's natural history of psychological, biological, and physical adjustments.

Assessment of Vulnerability Elements

A study of the individual's natural history often reveals vulnerable elements that increase the risk of depression and stress and weaken the person's ability to deal with the physical illness. From the perspective of biological medicine, the clinical picture presented by the elderly person tends to point to a single cause. However, in combining the medical with the psychological intervention, it is important for both the physician and psychotherapist to recognize that a given clinical picture may result from any one of several unrelated vulnerability elements. Psychological intervention will therefore have to be selected on the basis of the individual's natural history of medical illness, psychological functioning and adaptations, and predisposing personality.

The predisposing personality refers to all of the genetic, constitutional, developmental, educational, and experiential factors that constitute this basic personality of the individual (Hodge, 1980). The purpose of the intervention and the site of the intervention will have to be adapted to the predisposing personality of the elderly person. Some elderly are extremely prejudiced toward psychotherapy and will demonstrate a great deal of resistance to it. Conversely some elderly who resisted medical treatment will deny medical problems. The goals of intervention in all cases will be to promote insight into the nature of the presenting medical and psychological problem and the relationship between the past and the present and to determine how present behavior is an extension of or a repetition of past behavior, which may or may not be appropriate to the current life situation of the patient. The client's symptoms, feelings, and experience are analyzed as part of the developmental pattern so that the client may develop more of a free choice about intervention for this development.

As cognitive therapists, Gallagher and Thompson (1983) identify pathological cognition as the special vulnerability element that causes depression and stress in the elderly in response to medical illness. Adverse life situations are insufficient to produce stress and depression unless perceptions are distorted, thereby impairing the individuals' ability to appraise themselves and the event in a constructive manner (Breslau & Haug, 1983). The implications of this for the elderly are obvious. It is suggested that the most effective methods of helping the elderly deal with their medical problems and physical illness require a prophylaxis of biological medicine and psychological preparation for working through the meaning and cognitive appraisals of the disturbing illness experience.

Treatment designed to make changes in cognitions and irrational thinking need not necessarily be long-term. Information about various approaches for dealing with the client's problem (e.g., social support, caregiving services, psychotherapy, pharmacologic intervention, or combinations) may be useful in brief therapy while medical treatment is focused on other areas of the process of illness.

In choosing the sites of the intervention in accordance with this formulation, the therapist should consider the purpose of intervention at that site, the psychotherapy treatments and strategies applicable and available, and the medical facilities and pharmacologic treatment applicable. Further selection of these psychotherapeutic strategies in terms of individual, group, or family therapy always depends on the selection of the medical and pharmacological perspective or the psychological and ecological perspective. The basic psychotherapeutic goal in the integrative approach is that of promoting rational understanding, rational choice, and selection concerning the intervention.

Before and at onset of a medical illness, many elderly persons almost invariably experience a conflict in their lives. This conflict is often continuous and troublesome and disturbs the equilibrium of their lives. Physical illness, physical change, psychological upset, and environmental change usually involve the elderly persons' feelings about themselves, their activities, or their relationships with other significant persons in the family or social support networks.

The goal of integrated treatment may therefore be to relate the presenting medical and physical problems to the elderly person's problems of living and functioning. For many elderly clarification of the relationship may be all that is necessary and may lead to a positive acceptance of whatever management of physical illness is necessary to functioning. For many elderly any dominant change in thinking may not be necessary. In-depth psychotherapy intervention may not usually be necessary, though it is often helpful to relate the new insights about their medical and physical condition and the adjustments to be made in habits and styles of interaction to new patterns of thinking and behavior to be acquired. Supportive psychodynamic therapy and family therapy may be necessary to give support to the patient while the basic medical or pharmacologic therapy for the physical illness is proceeding. The following case illustrates this point.

Client 1

Mr. L. was a 76-year-old retired physician who became quite debilitated as a result of the progression of diabetes. After his wife's death, Mr. L. lost all motivation to take care of himself or to manage his diet and medication. Individual counseling with Mr. L. revealed that he had a long conflictual relationship with his son, and even in his greatly debilitated condition he resented his dependency on his son. He admitted that he often behaved recklessly and mismanaged his medication in order to spite his son.

In one-to-one counseling Mr. L. was encouraged to ventilate his feelings of resentment and to work through his conflict with his son. By means of a supportive relationship with the counselor, Mr. L. was encouraged to acquire personal mastery over his illness. Family therapy focused on promoting an effective relationship with his son and grandchildren. The use of medical and pharmacological treatment appropriate to the diabetic condition was continued. Within a matter of weeks, Mr. L. was motivated to acquire control over the progression of his illness.

INTEGRATION OF PSYCHOTHERAPY AND PHARMACOTHERAPY STRATEGIES FOR DEALING WITH PROBLEMS OF THE AGED

In discussing combined psychotherapy and psychopharmacology, a discussion of several basic assumptions is necessary to lay the framework for a discussion of the principles involved. Some of the major assumptions follow. The first assumption is that the elderly person is able to participate in psychotherapy and is able to make significant cognitive efforts to master those problems that at the moment are partially or totally unmastered. In other words a combination of psychotherapy and pharmacologic medicine is not effective in elderly who have experienced an observable degree of cognitive impairment and are therefore unable to establish a therapeutic alliance with the therapist or physician. In short the basic assumption is that the elderly person being treated with psychotherapy has some motivation and cognitive capability to deal with problems. This is true for psychotherapy for stress reactions, anxiety, and coping with drastic changes in the environment. In other words it is expected that while pharmacotherapy is in progress, the therapist will be present to relate to the patient and will help to strengthen the client's motivation to improve (Sarwer-Foner, 1980).

A second assumption is that the elderly patient recognizes that the clinical pharmacological action of this drug alone does not necessarily cure the psychological upset or disorder. The client's response to the pharmacological action of the drug will be determined by the attitudes of the doctor and of the therapist. The way in which significant others (family members, relatives, caregivers, physicians, or therapists) regard the elderly person, what they expect of that person, and the enthusiasm for or rejection of certain therapeutic agents play important roles (Sarwer-Foner, 1977, 1980). In the hands of a skilled therapist who understands both psychotherapy and pharmacotherapy, a supportive relationship with the elderly person would imply a basic therapeutic attitude that the person is potentially capable of pulling the self together and of taking responsibility at some level for the potential self-improvement.

The therapist and physician could explain the need for pharmacologic medication. After exploring this with the patient, the action of the drug may be explained, and the elderly client encouraged to use this action to collaborate with the physician, family members, nurses, etc., to improve the state. If the person sees the doctor or the therapist as someone with whom a therapeutic alliance could be formed, this sets the stage for the elderly person settling down and establishing a cooperative psychotherapeutic relationship.

A third assumption, therefore, is that the pharmacologic treatment is given with the patient implicitly and explicitly understanding that when the patient can get along without the drug, the drug will be stopped. This is perhaps the trickiest part of the psychotherapeutic and pharmacotherapeutic integration. Many elderly cohorts who grew up believing that drugs create a permanent reliance on doctors and nurses, want no part of anything, including this therapeutic relationship that reminds them of their increasing reliance on other persons and of their increasing helplessness in living, problem solving and decision making. The elderly patients especially must be helped to understand the importance of being able to deal with things themselves so as to dispel their fear that they will never be able to function without the assistance of medication.

The control of symptoms of anxiety, stress, agitation, etc., must be interpreted by the elderly person as beneficial rather than detrimental. Many elderly may resist hospitalization and institutionalization because they fear they will be doped with drugs and tranquilizers to keep them quiet and good patients. Therefore, many external factors concerned with interpersonal relations with family, friends, and authority figures are vital to effective pharmacotherapy. The average elderly who cooperates in a program of psychotherapy and pharmacotherapy does so because the person interprets the action of the drug in controlling certain symptoms as a good thing (Sarwer-Foner, 1977, 1980). For a majority of elderly much of the efficacy of the medication depends on such external variables as family support, social network support, and a supportive relationship with the physician and therapist. Their positive attitudes toward the effects of the medication and the patient's reactions to receiving it will help to give the psychopharmacological profile a good value judgment (Gottschalf, 1968). The patient's understanding of what is sociologically and therapeutically required when under the influence of drugs may play some role here.

Those elderly who do well on drugs are often those whose physicians, therapists, families, and caregivers express hope that the drug will help control symptoms of depression, anxiety, and agitation and that the person will then be better able to invest energy in more interpersonal relations and outgoing activity. Because the elderly patient's family, friends, and support networks have the expectation that the individual will feel more enthusiastic, gain self-confidence, and be more self-reliant, several elderly who previously were relatively inaccessible to psychotherapy have become potentially more accessible and are ready to use their energies to deal with problems. If this is done, many elderly respond well to a combined psychotherapeutic and pharmacotherapeutic treatment. If this situation continues for a long enough period, further ego integration takes place.

When an elderly patient is experiencing severe stress and anxiety or depression that interferes with this process of rational selection of intervention, the goal of pharmacologic treatment may be to provide just sufficient relief of anxiety, stress symptoms, and withdrawal due to depression, that this client is subsequently able to focus on what the person is doing, thinking, and feeling. Pharmacologic treatment must be particularly careful, however, of not providing too much relief of anxiety, depression, or stress symptoms through psychotropic medication, for otherwise this will increase the dependency of the elderly clients on the drugs and will interfere with the progress of the psychotherapy. When psychotherapy is combined with pharmacotherapy, it must be remembered that the goal of psychotherapy is initially to provide support, reassurance, and encouragement that there are caring individuals interested in seeing the elderly person get better or improve the medical condition. When a stable therapist-client relationship has been established, the subsequent but major goal is insight and understanding of the cognitive and attitudinal changes to be made, psychological adjustments that are necessary, and the acquisition of certain coping skills. The therapist must be prepared to help the patient in the anxiety about medical problems, social problems, and personal problems of depression, stress, or adjustment. The therapist must also be prepared to encourage the elderly person to discontinue with the pharmacologic medication as soon as the problem symptoms are under control and improvement is possible through psychotherapy alone.

Conversely many elderly show increasing paranoid tendencies during their later years. Often elderly clients with paranoid tendencies may interpret the drug effects as threatening, that is, manipulative attempts by the physicians or family members to control their assertiveness or autonomy. Such patients may resist drug therapy despite the need for characteristic pharmacological intervention to control symptoms of agitation, restlessness, suspicion, or irritability that are interfering with the process of psychotherapy. Control of these symptoms would make the person more accessible to psychotherapeutic communications, interpersonal relations, and renewed interest in externalized contacts. Conflictual relationships with family members, increased anxiety, restlessness, and suspiciousness may confirm the client's feelings of worthlessness, and the person instead of making progress in therapy may regress, relapse, or even become worse. At this point the focus of psychotherapy must be on changing the individual's attitudes toward pharmacologic treatment. If the patient initially shows symptoms of improvement through pharmacotherapy, psychotherapy may also become more meaningful. The following case illustrates this point.

Client 2

Mrs. C., who had shown paranoid symptoms for a few years, became progressively worse in her later years. She became hard of hearing and always suspected that her son and daughter-in-law were conspiring to get rid of her. She developed the notion that her daughter-in-law wanted to poison her. As a result, she stopped eating, developed severe tremors, and showed obvious signs of agitation and hyperactivity.

An integrated treatment of pharmacotherapy and supportive therapy had to be employed in order to help Mrs. C. to bring her severe agitation symptoms under control. Once a stable therapeutic alliance was established with the physician and counselor, Mrs. C. was able to communicate her fears of abandonment by the family. Psychotherapeutic intervention, even at a minimum level, was possible only after some control of symptoms was achieved through pharmacotherapy.

When an elderly person is in therapy for severe stress reactions (e.g., a spouse's death, serious financial loss) without concomitant drug therapy, there is a danger that the elderly person may experience acute signs of deterioration as a function of emotional exhaustion, intense fears and anxiety, and sleepless exhaustion mixed with fears of nightmares and bad dreams. Sometimes the first warning to the mental health professional is the emergence of severe effect and agitation. It is up to the psychotherapist to take full advantage of a knowledge of pharmacotherapy to advise the physician to medicate adequately and to generate sleep. If this is done systematically and the elderly person gets medication for several nights of good sleep, this may well counteract the fatigue and the associated symptoms of cognitive confusion, psychomotor retardation, and loss of appetite. The chances are that with the help of some concomitant drug therapy, the client may pull oneself together, the threatened psychological deterioration may disappear, and the supportive psychotherapeutic relationship may also be renewed.

The concept of time-limited interventions of a pharmacotherapy nature is suggested only when needed—and only in combination with psychotherapy efforts to strengthen the patient's ego capacity and "copabilities." All psychotropic medications including tricyclics, quadricyclics, and MAO inhibitors when given in adequate doses can be helpful, although not curative, in helping elderly subjects to acquire quick control over reactive depression and depression-induced confusional states.

Many elderly are seeking support and the recovery of significant object relatedness destroyed through losses, for example, loss of spouse through death, loss of social relationships, loss of job. Sarwer-Foner (1980) suggests that regardless of how debilitated the client looks or however helpless and abandoned the client feels, it is the responsibility of the therapist or physician to explore the possibilities of psychotherapy combined with the pharmacotherapy. The presence of unconscious hope in the patient and the potential for developing a therapeutic relationship with the physician or therapist should always be explored and assessed. The objective of antidepressant medication is mainly to help the elderly client master depression symptoms to the extent that the person can be assisted to reestablish outgoingness and object-relatedness through psychotherapy. Many elderly patients cannot talk coherently or relate even minimally while depressed. Depression may produce severe psychomotor retardation. Here the antidepressants, given in adequate doses, may improve the elderly client's capacity to reach outward and become more outgoing in approximately 70 percent of such patients after at least three weeks of treatment. Often the drugs must be maintained for the length of the depressive episode, but the patient becomes increasingly available for supportive psychotherapy as the patient's communication improves (Sarwer-Foner, 1960). The following case illustrates this point.

Client 3

Mrs. D. (age 78) lived alone in an apartment in a retirement community. Her daughter and son-in-law, who visited her regularly, were transferred to another city. Neighbors reported that shortly after her daughter's departure, Mrs. D. became sad and depressed. She refused to talk to anyone and always looked down in the mouth. When Mrs. D. was hospitalized, she had not eaten for several days. She appeared to be quite confused and incoherent in her speech. A few days immediately preceding hospitalization Mrs. D. remained in her home, refused to see anyone, and attempted an overdose of sleeping pills. Mrs. D. was put on an immediate program of antidepressant therapy. This helped her to regain appetite, and she began to communicate with the nursing staff. Mrs. D. was recommended for supportive therapy for depression and was slowly encouraged to participate in activities within the social support network. Antidepressant drugs were administered for six weeks following the depressive episode. Drug therapy was stopped after there was evidence of improvement in mood and communications. Mrs. D. was recommended for a long-term program of supportive therapy, which provided encouragement and reassurance that she would always be cared for by family and friends.

The important thing in the context of psychotherapy and supportive relationships is to withdraw the psychotropic medications as soon as the patient can control the situation. Thus as noted by Sarwer-Foner (1980), the use of drugs given in the context of endogenous or reactive depressions is a parameter that should be introduced only when needed but to be withdrawn as quickly as possible because of their complex side effects. Furthermore, drugs must be introduced and maintained only after seeking full collaboration with the elderly patients and their families.

Management of Crises through Integrated Therapy Elements

The combination of drug treatment and psychotherapy is often employed in the management of emergencies. Zinberg (1965) observed how frequently a psychiatric referral of an older person involved an emergency requiring involvement with the family members. On the one hand emergencies, whether of confusion, anxious agitation, suicidal despair, or drug interaction, call for rapid, concentrated intervention. The threat of suicide requires, of course, stringent protective measures. The immediate support of close relatives whom the elderly client trusts must be mobilized (Blazer, 1982).

There are situations in which the fundamental therapeutic injunctions to safeguard the life of the elderly client and to do no harm have certain implications for using any and all types of treatment: psychotherapy (supportive and dynamic types and individual and family approaches), pharmacotherapy, and medical treatment. The elderly clients' limited adaptability, poor tolerance of painful effects, and potential for repeated suicidal efforts dictate that we intervene in such a way that high-powered interventions are kept to a necessary minimum but that combined and well-integrated psychotherapy and pharmacotherapy procedures are used (Kahana, 1980). Medications for anxiety and mood disorders may be prescribed cautiously, in small initial doses, while carefully monitoring for any side effects to which the elderly person may be sensitive. Individual psychotherapy, depending on the person's consent and cooperation, is the best interfacing form of treatment.

The use of psychotherapy is almost indispensable in crisis situations, even when the preselection is for medical treatment, electroconvulsive therapy, or psychotropic medication. As noted by Kahana (1980), at a minimum, psychotherapy may constitute the basic support necessary to have the debilitated elderly person accept and continue with other methods of treatment. When communication with the elderly client is severely limited due to brain disorders, depression, and confusional states arising from traumatic events, then psychologically correct measures of environmental support are necessary to the management of the crisis while medical treatment or pharmacotherapy is in progress. In dealing with cases of unresolved grief reactions so frequently encountered in the elderly, rapid intervention using supportive psychotherapy and medication may relieve an incipient crisis of worsening depression.

Integration of Individual and Family Therapy

Suggestions, guidance, manipulation, and some clarification of the grief reactions are commonly utilized in the individual psychotherapy. Later, after the crisis, intervention in the form of family therapy may help to calm the elderly client and the family. Although initially medication alone may be sufficient to keep the client calm, later individual psychotherapy and family therapy may be effective in reducing the heightened resurgence of dependency conflicts that many elderly may be experiencing vis-à-vis family members. Family therapy may have to deal with the increased manifestations of ambivalence and anger toward spouse or adult children or confidants and the correlated fear of abandonment (Blau & Berezin, 1975). Given that a majority of elderly patients are dependent on the family members, family therapy is essential in both the immediate and the long-term management of the patient's crises such as suicide attempts. An effective approach calls for family therapy that is educative rather than punitive and teaches the family how to manage the elderly member's postcrises situation in the home setting. Since depressive states and suicidal tendencies in the elderly often have periodic exacerbation, it is considered essential to provide long-term maintenance therapy (Hersen & Detre, 1980), consisting of an active multifaceted treatment program of individual and group work and psychodynamic and cognitive-behavioral therapy.

Older patients frequently show increased needs for encouragement, appreciation, and even admiration following a crisis. They express depressive helplessness or demand advice, assistance, and magical help, thus placing particular strain on their therapists. During psychotherapy with elderly clients recovering from crises, substantial support from many and varied environmental sources, including family members, therapists, physicians, etc., may be necessary to maximize the older patient's ability to explore tabooed feelings and to pursue problem solutions in their own way. Therapy with members of the family and other caregivers may be necessary to facilitate their providing an appropriate form of guidance to the elderly client. Poorly structured interactions, ambiguity, or ambivalence in the interpersonal relations of the caregivers with the elderly client may elicit further anxiety and overcautiousness. Training caregivers in effective techniques of listening, respecting defenses, and conveying recognition that the patient is recovering and the reassurance that the patient will be cared for is an essential part of the therapist's or physician's function. The latter must guide caregivers in handling medication, formulating a realistic assessment of the elderly client's medical and psychological condition, and enriching the environment of the elderly client. Environmental measures, adaptive intervention, and clarification often meet with considerable success. The following case illustrates this point.

Client 4

Mr. H. (age 79) had been a jovial, happy-go-lucky person with an unsurpassed enthusiasm for life. Through a car accident Mr. H. lost his eyesight. Although his vital functions returned, Mr. H. was a changed man. He became bitter, got angry at the smallest incidents, and flew into rages, during which he yelled and screamed and threw things. This behavior frightened his wife, and she withdrew from communications with him. Anything she said to console him was always misunderstood. Mrs. H. would get very upset with her husband's behaviors and would cry and leave the home. This would aggravate Mr. H. so much that he would become quite destructive in his behaviors and needed psychotropic medication to control his violence and agitation.

Supportive therapy was recommended for Mrs. H. After she improved, she in turn was trained in effective techniques of listening and expressing empathy. She was coached in providing Mr. H. the reassurance that his condition would stabilize, that their financial status would always be sound, and that it was not her intention ever to abandon him. Both Mr. and Mrs. H. participated in individual and group therapy. One-to-one counseling with Mr. H. was helpful to him in working through his sense of loss and the bitterness associated with the loss of his sight. While Mr. H. received maintenance pharmacotherapy for several months, the wife's skills in controlling and regulating his medication, responding empathically to his condition, and giving him reassurance and encouragement that his condition would stabilize contributed greatly to his improvement.

Management of Stress Reactions through Integrated Therapy Elements

Whenever a stressful situation occurs (such as family conflict, stroke, or heart attack), the primary goal is to relieve the stress or its sequelae by whatever means possible by the use of medical, pharmacologic, or psychotherapeutic methods. Any or all of the psychotherapy and treatment strategies can be used during intervention at the level of the external precipitating stress as long as the therapist follows the basic principle that the elderly client recognizes the stressful situation and recognizes the effects on functioning and coping. Psychotherapy by promoting rational understanding is effective in helping the elderly person to understand how the stress developed, how it is related to conflicts with other people in the environment, and how other persons are contributing to the client's current conflicts.

Psychotherapy by the modification of behavior using systematic desensitization and rehearsal technique can be particularly helpful, especially in the elderly person who is taught to relax while contemplating the stressful situation. Repeated ventilation of feelings in group therapy can be especially helpful for releasing the blocked energies and emotions associated with the stress.

The direct relief or alleviation of stress symptoms through pharmacological methods, when possible, can be helpful and supportive to the patient working through the problem, but it should not allow the person to avoid working on them. Pharmacologic treatment is helpful when used to control symptoms only to the extent of allowing the elderly person to overcome intense depression states or withdrawal. Because of a variety of old persons' frailties and sensitivity to traumas, situational reactions may all too easily become major clinical psychiatric problems for the elderly (Breslau & Haug, 1983). Because of the high frequency of stressful life events in old age, elderly patients are potentially at risk for receiving a diagnosis of adjustment disorder quite commonly (Skodol & Spitzer, 1983). All this argues that the psychological reactions of the aged are a function of previous repetitive styles of coping and may quickly assume disproportionately intense clinical manifestations. This is why the most effective methods of dealing with these problems are in the prophylaxis of one-to-one counseling and family therapy, behavioral therapy, and cognitive-emotive therapy. Again, we need to call attention to the link between the developmental events of the late-life period and the resulting psychological need for emotional support and encouragement.

Supportive therapy is vitally important during stress. However, in supportive therapy it is acknowledged that no major changes are expected nor are they likely to occur. The basic goal then is to help elderly persons to accept the social or emotional losses. By modifying their support systems during periods of transitory problems such as grief, bereavement, or interpersonal conflicts, the goal is to support persons through their adjustment period.

A program of supportive therapy does not preclude the use of other psychotherapeutic strategies, which may be indicated by the specific situation. The basic tactics in this strategy are support, reassurance, encouragement, promotion of a good therapist-patient relation, and the promotion of identification with the therapist or caregiver. The use of psychological intervention appropriate to the medical condition of the client (e.g., organic brain syndrome, diabetes, or heart condition) may be essential to the medical recovery of the elderly person.

General ego-strengthening through promoting personal mastery is a valid, effective, and often undefined tactic of therapy. In the elderly many stress neuroses, especially those brought on by traumatic events, are precipitated by the elderly person feeling like a helpless victim of circumstances beyond one's control. This feeling of helplessness often occurs as a characterological state. When directive supportive therapy is used, the goal is to promote feelings of strength, competence, and "copability." Sometimes this can be accomplished by direct suggestion or through behavior therapy modeling and rehearsal (Hodge, 1980).

Another useful technique is to have the patients visualize themselves the way they were as a small helpless child (Little Johnny, Little Mary) and then to have them visualize themselves with all the assets and wisdom that they have as adults (Big John or Big Mary). Visualizing this contrast lessens the sense of helplessness and increases the elderly persons' awareness that they are not really helpless, that they handled and controlled many previous stresses, and that they will be able to cope with similar stresses. Thus, awareness of the self as an individual in the process of development is stimulated, and the elderly person often becomes aware of the differences between oneself as a helpless child and oneself as an adult feeling like a helpless child but capable of overcoming the helplessness.

Management of Anxiety through Integrated Therapy Elements

Whenever a stressful situation occurs, anxiety accompanies it or follows it. Hypochondriasis is one of the typical disturbing symptoms of older persons following stress and anxiety. It is often resistant to both medical and psychotherapy treatment and represents an unsuccessful attempt of the elderly person to control anxiety. Psychotherapy using a supportive but rational thinking approach can be used in treating the problem of anxiety. The patient is to learn that anxiety is either irrational and maladaptive or simply not currently helpful. Some elderly clients may want to learn to handle current anxiety in a healthy and productive manner.

Anxiety by its nature is future-oriented, more so in the elderly than in other age groups. If the strategy is to promote rational understanding, the current anxiety can be related to both past and future anxieties to help overcome the elderly person's fear that this could happen over and over. In this sense dynamic desensitization is particularly helpful as most elderly individuals who are anxious about one or two areas of their functioning may quickly experience anxiety generalizing to several other areas of their functioning. If the anxiety is considered maladaptive, it can be attacked directly by behavior therapy strategies of relaxation and systematic desensitization. Supportive therapy, including the use of appropriate antianxiety medication, can demonstrate that the anxiety can be relieved or modified so that it is not too intense for the debilitated and emotionally fragile elderly person to confront. This integrated approach of medication and psychotherapy is optimally suited to older adults whose illnesses are frequently characterized by marked or extreme anxiety and agitation. Indeed it may be the preferred technique for many frail and debilitated elderly persons who may need some tranquilizing medication to ameliorate the severe level of agitation accompanying the anxiety. The initial process of combined therapies usually lasts one to three weeks. It is rare for this phase to be longer.

In anxious older patients the tranquilizers may be prescribed at the time of the initial interview. The mental health practitioner would need to be working in close consultation with the physician or psychiatrist prescribing the drug in order to monitor the effects of the drug. The psychotherapeutic aspect must be strongly supportive and conducted in a face-to-face setting. It is imperative that the mental health practitioner be aware as to whether the anxiety and the symptoms are in a psychotic or self-limiting neurotic framework or are self-limiting stress reactions. Environment may exert a negative effect on the elderly person. Many older patients come expecting medication. Some older persons and their families may come with great antipathy to drug therapy or a particular type of psychotherapy. Such elderly persons, including their families, may have to be convinced of the greater effectiveness of an integrated tranquilizer-psychotherapeutic approach. Many elderly on the contrary react to the rapid relief of painful anxiety with unquestioning gratitude and indeed an eagerness to relate to the therapist. Thus the working relationship between the therapist and older person that would have taken months to establish with psychotherapy alone may be accomplished in days.

Many complications can occur, for at times an overtranquilizing may cause a panic episode in older frail persons. It is imperative that the dose of medication be optimally titrated according to intensity of manifest anxiety. This titration in elderly clients must proceed gradually, never precipitously (Lesse, 1980).

From the psychotherapeutic standpoint the level of anxiety can be affected by the relative control or encouragement of the process of catharsis. In many elderly persons a free outpouring of effect-laden material may be an effective tool leading to anxiety decompression. In family therapy other conflicts of interpersonal relations should be worked out and families must be warned of the dangers of premature termination of treatment for elderly members with severe anxiety.

If the goal is ultimately to teach the elderly person to confront the anxiety, the enduring personality characteristics of the elderly person must be carefully assessed before leading the person to take charge of the anxiety. Only those elderly individuals who had shown evidence of good internal regulatory controls in handling anxiety may be ready to confront anxiety in their later years. Elderly individuals who were poor in handling stress will continue to use the same techniques and can be expected to continue this way unless assisted through an integrated program of pharmacotherapy, supportive therapy, behavior therapy, and rational-emotive therapy. Treatment designed to make changes in anxiety management must be considered in the context of long-term supportive therapy; however, information obtained about the strategies and the processes of understanding anxiety may be usefully achieved in brief therapy. Anxiety management is also an area in which other special techniques such as environmental manipulation and family therapy may be used effectively. Direct symptom relief of anxiety or hypochondriasis may come through family members providing support, reassurance, and encouragement that they will be available to provide care and service if and when needed. Gradually through environmental manipulation and family therapy approaches elderly persons can develop a personal rational understanding of the anxiety and understand how their stresses and anxieties and concomitant behaviors affect the family environment and the other people in it.

CONCLUSIONS AND SUMMARY

The integrated therapies approach allows us to consider the dimensions of greatest departure as well as convergence in the ever-expanding field of treatment and intervention for the elderly. In clarifying treatment approaches for the elderly, each domain of individual and group therapy and psychotherapy and pharmacotherapy should be viewed as broadly congruent with the others and rarely with categorical or antithetical distinctions. Because of the multidimensional nature of the elderly's problems, traditional therapeutic boundaries must be assumed to overlap. In view of the frequent interaction of physical, psychosocial, and biomedical sites, a synthesis of various therapies will serve to strengthen the elderly person's functioning and provide controls for overwhelming anxieties, depression, or stress reactions.

The chapter has elaborated on an integration of various modes of intervention along the psychotherapeutic spectrum and the best of all therapeutic approaches. It is suggested that the stabilizing type of treatment most effective in supporting the older person's defenses and capacities to function autonomously should include components of supportive individual therapy, family therapy, and environmental manipulation of stress-inducing factors.

Karasu (1980) has noted that in attempting to supply stability to elderly clients, the therapist seeks to mobilize the client's available adaptive resources and strengths. With many elderly clients this may require an examination of stressful aspects of the environment whereby they may then be advised how to lessen these stresses in terms of conflictual relationships, financial and economic constraints, or declining physical energies. The elderly client may need ego-supportive assistance from therapist, family, and friends.

The therapist may use extrapsychotherapeutic means such as medication, pharmacotherapy, and temporary hospitalization to help the elderly person through crises or severe adjustment or to remove the elderly client from an excessively stimulating or agitating environment that may be contributing to a crisis reaction such as suicide attempt. In addition the therapist may discuss the use of temporary placements (in nursing home, hospital, or day center) for purposes of alleviating the frustration and deprivation imposed on the elderly person by a given stressful environment. Education and information about a medical problem or mental health or mental status evaluation, and how conditions can be ameliorated, can also strengthen the elderly person's defenses by enlarging their scope.

Other considerations being equal, a therapist working individually with an older adult should invariably try to include family and group approaches as adjunctive therapeutic measures. The inclusion of the family can serve to reduce the stresses on family members of the elderly client, allowing them to participate collectively in the establishment of a more therapeutic environment for the elderly member (Karasu, 1980).

With a supportive approach undertaken by therapist and family members, concrete efforts can be made to reduce disturbances in interpersonal relationships by providing information and direction with regard to everyday problems of living. The multiplicity of transference opportunities may be most beneficial for elderly clients who may have become unskilled in ways of relating to others because of their self-perceptions of helplessness and dependency. Finally, it is possible in working with elderly clients to tap intrapsychic conflicts and transference, as long as the elderly individuals' lowered capacities for tolerating frustration and stress are kept clearly in mind.

REFERENCES

Blau, D., & Berezin, M.A. (1975). Neuroses and the character disorders. In J.G. Howells (Ed.), *Modern perspectives in the psychiatry of old age* (pp. 201–233). New York: Brunner/Mazel.

Blazer, D.G. (1982). *Depression in late life.* St. Louis: C.V. Mosby Co.

Breslau, L.D., & Haug, M.R. (1983). Some elements in an integrative model of depression in the aged. In L.D. Breslau & M.R. Haug (Eds.), *Depression and aging* (pp. 269–279). New York: Springer.

Engel, G. (1977). The need for a new medical model: A challenge for biomedicine. *Science, 196,* 129–136.

Gallagher, D., & Thompson, L.W. (1983). Depression. In P.M. Lewinsohn & L. Teri (Eds.), *Clinical geropsychology: New directions in assessment and treatment* (pp. 7–37). New York: Pergamon.

Gottschalf, L.A. (1968). Some problems in the use of psychoactive drugs, with or without psychotherapy, in the treatment of nonpersonality disorders. In D.H. Efron (Ed.), *Psychopharmacology: A review of process 1957–1967* (Public Health Service Publication No. 1836, pp. 225–238). Washington: PHS.

Hersen, M., & Detre, T. (1980). The behavioral psychotherapy of anorexia nervosa. In T.B. Karasu & L. Bellak (Eds.), *Specialized techniques in individual psychotherapy* (pp. 295–303). New York: Brunner/Mazel.

Hodge, J.R. (1980). Hypnotherapy combined with psychotherapy. In T.B. Karasu & L. Bellak (Eds.), *Specialized techniques in individual psychotherapy* (pp. 400–423). New York: Brunner/Mazel.

Kahana, R.J. (1980). Psychotherapy with the elderly. In T.B. Karasu & L. Bellak (Eds.), *Specialized techniques in individual psychotherapy* (pp. 314–336). New York: Brunner/Mazel.

Karasu, T.B. (1980). General principles of psychotherapy. In T.B. Karasu & L. Bellak (Eds.), *Specialized techniques in individual psychotherapy* (pp. 33–44). New York: Brunner/Mazel.

Lesse, S. (1980). Psychotherapy of ambulatory patients with severe anxiety. In T.B. Karasu & L. Bellak (Eds.), *Specialized techniques in individual psychotherapy* (pp. 220–235). New York: Brunner/Mazel.

London, P. (1974, June). The psychotherapy boom. *Psychology Today,* pp. 63–68.

Sarwer-Foner, G.J. (1960). The role of neuroleptic medication in psychotherapeutic interaction. *Comprehensive Psychiatry, 1,* 291–300.

Sarwer-Foner, G.J. (1977). An approach to the global treatment of the borderline patient: Psychoanalytic, psychotherapeutic and psychopharmacological considerations. In P. Harticollis (Ed.), *Borderline personality disorders: The concept, the syndrome, the patient* (pp. 345–364). New York: International Universities Press.

Sarwer-Foner, G.J. (1980). Combined psychotherapy and pharmacotherapy. In T.B. Karasu & L. Bellak (Eds.), *Specialized techniques in individual psychotherapy* (pp. 479–490). New York: Brunner/Mazel.

Skodol, A.E., & Spitzer, R.L. (1983). Depression in the elderly: Clinical criteria. In L.D. Breslau & M.R. Haug (Eds.), *Depression and aging* (pp. 20–29). New York: Springer.

Strupp, H. (1969). Psychoanalytic therapy and research. In L. Eron & R. Callahan (Eds.), *The relation of theory to practice in psychotherapy* (pp. 21–62). Chicago: Aldine Publishing Co.

Zinberg, N.E. (1965). Special problems of gerontologic psychiatry. In M.A. Berezin & S.H. Cath (Eds.), *Geriatric psychiatry: Grief, loss and emotional disorders in the aging process* (pp. 147–159). New York: International Universities Press.

Chapter 14

Directions for Care
of the Elderly

A discussion of the future of the mental health needs of the elderly would not be complete without some discussion of the directions of care of the elderly and the application of therapeutic principles in the provision of mental health programs for the aged. Thus it is necessary to address special social, psychological, and environmental problems related to providing health care for the elderly.

Since clinical care of the elderly is necessarily pragmatic, efficacy is defined in terms of individual judgment. In many cases there is a considerable delay before some specific directions of psychological care or recommendations for care can be evaluated or tested rigorously. Sometimes poorly tested procedures and methods of psychological care lacking clarity are recommended in the face of preemptory need to provide care. When one considers the increasing numbers of elderly patients in need of care and the attendant rising cost factors, one can readily understand the need to provide care initially for the most preemptory needs. Those who are immediately responsible for caring for the aged in the primary care system and who make the first contact with the elderly client must play a large role in identifying the preemptory needs of each elderly client. Subsequently cooperation between primary care physicians, mental health professionals, social workers, nurses, and family members must be strengthened in the comprehensive care system as a critical element in planning treatment for the elderly. While the lack of territoriality and professional specificity in the geriatric field opens the door for conflict and uncertainty, it also has an advantage that principles of multidisciplinary care can be applied in a comprehensive approach to treatment. Accordingly the health care professional is expected to be cognizant of the client's general level of health as well as immediate health problems and to be capable of planning and coordinating health services with other types of caregiving services in a comprehensive service framework (McGivern, 1974).

One important question is the extent to which the primary caregiver provides specific service and arranges for the delayed management of an array of other problems also requiring care. The questions addressed here do not sufficiently discuss all of the major problems concerning the psychological care of the aged. However, most of the questions raised and the points discussed have a clear relevance to practitioners, professionals, paraprofessionals, and laymen who are in an everyday caregiving relationship with the elderly, whether in the home setting, community, or institution.

ALTERNATIVES TO CUSTODIAL CARE

While custodialism as a philosophy of treatment and care of the elderly is not openly advocated by physicians, psychologists, and other mental health professionals in the field of aging, it is nevertheless widely practiced in a variety of programs in health care settings such as hospitals and nursing and convalescent homes. Because custodial approaches are so deeply ingrained in our treatment of the aged, it is often overlooked that the ways we provide care allow us to treat only a small percentage of the aged population needing care and attention. Even as the number of mental health programs has increased, a smaller percentage of the aged persons has been receiving such services. Kahn (1975) notes that since 1946 there has been a considerable reduction in the use of outpatient services with a corresponding increase in the use of nursing homes, which represent an institution in which intensive care is given.

Zarit (1980) postulates that because of the lack of ameliorative community-based programs in the existing delivery of mental health services, there is an overuse of intensive, long-term institutional care, which has a deleterious impact on the independent functioning of many elderly. This philosophy of custodial care has given rise to an interesting paradox in which many elderly receive intervention that is more intensive than needed and has unfortunate negative consequences for the elderly in terms of placing them in a dependent position.

The picture in custodial care settings is bleak. The structure itself militates against the human needs of identity, connectedness, and effectualness (Blazer, 1982). Monotony, boredom, isolation, and regimentation are omnipresent (Goffman, 1961) and eventually promote more organic and affective disorders. Kahn (1975, 1977) proposes the concept of excess disabilities, which implies that through the provision of too much assistance, patients are conditioned to function at a much lower level than would be expected based on the person's physical condition alone. A number of gerontologists (e.g., Zarit & Kahn, 1974; de Vries, 1970) contend that the elderly person's cognitive and physical abilities to carry out actions or to make certain decisions and solve problems become atrophied under total care, where nursing staffs provide too much help and thereby undermine the confidence of mildly impaired or disabled elderly to care for themselves.

Excess disabilities can be prevented when an environment encourages and reinforces independent behavior. When certain functional abilities begin to deteriorate due to medical problems or illness, the functional behaviors are likely to be relearned and maintained if the environment discourages dependence and encourages and reinforces the functional capacities of the individual.

The issue of excess disabilities is an especially problematic one for facilities serving the elderly, many of whom are dementia patients, cognitively impaired, depressed, and inactive, with behavioral problems. The total care or custodial philosophy of institutions sacrifices maintenance of the individual's coping mechanisms for the needs of the institution. Elderly residents with behavioral problems are commonly given psychoactive medications, not as a part of treatment but as tranquilizers to control behaviors (Ochberg, Zarcone, & Hamburg, 1972).

The most debilitating feature of this process is that the residents become intricately tied to the institutional activities and come to rely on the institutional staff for their social identity and emotional sustenance (Glasscote et al., 1976). Holahan (1978) observed that many elderly by virtue of their long-term confinement to an institutional milieu develop a process of assimilation so subtle and complex that often they can no longer evaluate the milieu as good or bad.

One of the surprising findings, however, is that despite the demeaning quality of the institutional condition and despite substandard environments in which the elderly function, many elderly tend to evaluate their living situations more favorably than do other outpatients or objective observers (Butler, 1977). Carp (1975) and Holahan (1978) presume that the elderly are much more adaptive to unfavorable situations than is really good for them.

In view of the increasing recognition that environmental characteristics interact with human characteristics to produce passive behavior in the elderly, there is a feverish push to improve the environmental characteristics. In more traditional areas there is a tremendous emphasis on changes needed in facilities, including newer forms of treatment with wider breadth and a whole new focus on chronic illness (Burnside, 1978). There is also an emphasis on the rights and freedoms of residents and the ethical, legal and psychiatric aspects of protective services of residents (Verwoerdt, 1981). A number of alternatives to custodialism have been suggested.

Minimum Intervention

In order to be effective, a system of care that is least intrusive, maximizes the independent functioning of the residents, and attempts to improve morale through increased participation and socialization must be advocated. It is important that this increased autonomy and socialization be provided according to the principle of minimum intervention. According to Kahn (1975, p. 29) minimum intervention "is least disruptive of usual functioning in the usual setting" and provides care in mutually helpful ways in the home, day-care center, or work situation rather than in the hospital or clinic. Kahn cautions, however, that minimal intervention should not be confused with neglect and must also be differentiated from maximal-minimal intervention, in which the person is removed from the community and then placed in an institution that provides little or no psychological assistance or social compensatory measures. This would be tantamount to indifference at best and may possibly be gross abandonment. The notion of minimum intervention implies that services need to be provided by limiting professional involvement and maximizing the use of community resources to support the continued competencies of older persons.

Kahn (1975) advocates that intervention should address the client's presenting problems or the preemptory needs only as opposed to helping the elderly client deal with all of the problems, difficulties, and concerns that the individual has been experiencing. The principle of minimum intervention advocates that it is important for the caseworker to distinguish between the crisis needs of the client and other needs that the client has been able to deal with satisfactorily on one's own initiative.

Hemsi (1982) contends that the provision of basic needs constitutes reasonable and realistic care, not perfection. One of the major points in the management is to get the health care workers to do neither too little nor too much: only in this way can the families and the informal support network be helped to maintain a similar posture towards the elderly. What is required is prompt management of the client's critical problem while also supporting continued independence in the client.

The most common errors in giving service to the elderly have involved overprotection and strong intervention or neglect and indifference. The caseworker, in guiding actions according to the principle of minimum intervention, must consult with the client and get the client's opinion about the extent of intervention desired. For example, an elderly person may need help simply with transportation to the doctor's office rather than extended help to shop, cook, and do all the housework.

In the situations described, the function of the caseworker may be the formation of a trusting relationship with the family. Within that secure relationship problems, feelings, attitudes, and expectations can be expressed and ventilated. Using the principle of minimum intervention, the caseworkers' basic role is to supply practical and more general information and explanations. The process of counseling is nondirective and open-ended, and negotiation is undertaken on the most immediate needs of the client at any one time (Hemsi, 1982; Kahn, 1975).

There are times when active intervention is needed and when it will be important for the caseworker to act promptly and forcefully. For example, if the client shows symptoms or behaviors that constitute a risk to one's own life or that of others—imminent risk of suicidal behavior or aggressive tendencies toward others—then there is a clear delineation of risk to safety. The principle of minimum intervention will not be valid under these circumstances. However, even under these unusual circumstances the caseworker must accommodate the realistic needs of the elderly client to strike a balance between interventions that are constraining and those that are essential for safety.

Even when there is risk to the client's life, for instance when the client is partially blind, unsteady in walking, and in danger of falling, there must be a balancing of any risk against the potential emotional and psychological losses incurred in curtailing the client's independent functioning. In the case of clients who are cognitively alert, the client should, in consultation with the professional, ultimately decide whether to take risks with physical well-being or to seek protective services.

From an older person's perspective, minimum intervention will be perceived as consistent with individual dignity and self-esteem. The focus on maximizing the functioning of the elderly person in the setting of the home and in the familiar neighborhood surroundings will enhance the individual's sense of being important to the family and social network.

Comprehensive Services and Community Care Programs

Given the large numbers of older persons in our society and the limited resources available, professionals must have an interest in developing a comprehensive community-based approach as opposed to a custodial approach. This approach to the treatment of older persons involves attention to various types of services useful to the total population of the elderly. Based on their survey of innovative mental health programs for the aged, Glasscote, Gudeman, and Miles (1977) suggest that treatment in a comprehensive service can be categorized according to three dimensions:

1. Supportive services for the physical maintenance of the elderly including services intended to help people live in their own homes include meals on wheels, chore services, telephone links, volunteer help, and services for providing communal housing, special housing, half-way houses, intermediate-care-level nursing homes, or skilled-level nursing homes
2. Clinical services including therapeutic day programs, outpatient individual and group psychotherapy programs, and community mental health centers

3. Preventive, supportive, and life-enhancing programs including programs providing economic support, legal aid, assistance in nutrition, exercise and recreation activities, and transportation facilities

There are many reasons for a community emphasis in a comprehensive program of psychogeriatrics. As noted by Hemsi (1982), first, the nature of the mental disorders or functional disorders in the majority of the elderly is such that often no hospital investigations are necessary. Therefore, little or nothing is to be gained by the elderly patient by admission to a hospital; rather, much is to be lost in time, effort, and the energy of the frail elderly person. Second, a factor frequently overlooked by hospital professionals is that old people are integral members of community networks. Whether or not an elder has a reversible condition, the person is likely to need continuing support of the community networks. In order to provide that help, it is more important to reinforce the psychological processes already in operation within and around the elder than to create new processes. Third, except in situations of crises and medical emergencies, there are enormous problems including economic ones in caring for old persons in institutions.

If care of the elderly is to be worthwhile and comprehensive, it must be centered in the community. It must act on the premise that any assessment or management of the elder's problems outside the person's natural environment is at best incomplete and may be grossly misleading (Hemsi, 1982). For all these reasons it is realistic to expect that there will be a large shift toward community-based care.

A community-based approach to the treatment of older persons permits the geriatric medical health professional to intervene more directly in certain types of services while allowing other professionals (e.g., nurses, social workers, psychologist), paraprofessionals (e.g., nurse's aid, social work associate), and lay personnel in the community (e.g., lay counseling groups, peer counselors, pastoral counselors) to intervene more directly at certain other points in the treatment. At the core of community-oriented programs is the emphasis of the therapeutic principle that community care can be preventive, dealing as it does with problems at an early stage, before they are likely to become intransigent, requiring long-term care such as hospitalization or nursing home treatment. The second assumption is that some of the difficulties experienced by older persons that lead them to custodial care and institutionalization can be treated through a number of less intrusive ways such as home visits by practitioners and mental health assessment teams. Thus community-oriented services can have a number of major impacts. First, the elderly's impairments and problems can be treated at the primary level, through outpatient and home services. Second, institutionalization and its negative consequence can be postponed, if not prevented indefinitely. Third, the problem of scarcity and high cost of places in institutions can be avoided, and fourth, community programs can adequately meet the needs of the majority of today's elderly who can function adequately with minimal support from external agencies.

There is evidence (Blazer, 1982; Kistin & Morris, 1972) that 40 to 80 percent of the patients in long-term care do not require the extensive and intensive care provided either at the skilled nursing level or at the health-related level. It is postulated that patients, especially elderly patients, are in nursing homes or institutions because no other treatment facilities are possible.

In outlining guidelines for collaboration among the various members of the team, the Royal College of Psychiatrists and the British Geriatrics Society (1979) stress basic principles of responsibility, unity, and education, which have wide applicability for comprehensive services. The team of workers in the comprehensive care system must ensure that the intervention has been supportive and has provided the medical, psychological, or psychiatric help expected.

Responsibility is always determined by the need of the clients, rather than by quirks of referral. The clients' assessed needs should determine the services rather than these being dictated merely by what is available in that compartment of care into which a elderly client may have fallen. Criteria for division of responsibility must be clear and must be known and accepted both within and outside the services.

Underlying this notion of responsibility is the principle of coordination and integration of various services within the comprehensive services programs. Effective collaboration, coordination, and integration of services among the members of the team depend on mutual confidence, trust, and respect of each other's judgments about their own responsibility. Even within limited resources, the elderly person must be supported within the limits of feasibility.

The comprehensive service must always be a unity for consumers (i.e., patients, families, referrers). Clients should not be shuttled back and forth from one service to another merely because they fall within gray areas. Referrals and distribution of referrals should be the internal responsibility of the service. The client's right of access to specialists, particular professionals, and consultants within or outside the services, should also be respected as a part of the unity of the team.

Last, but not least, is the responsibility of comprehensive services for the elderly to contribute to education of the elderly and to the education of the public at large. Arie and Jolley (1982, p. 244) note that "ultimately, better care for the elderly depends on massive public education: education of individuals to prepare themselves for old age—and education of the public about the needs of the elderly."

Primary Care Model within Comprehensive Services

The primary care role in a comprehensive approach to the treatment of the elderly involves two overall components: (1) the initiation of care when the client first comes in contact with the health care system and (2) the responsibility for continuity of care including maintenance, evaluation and management of physical and mental health symptoms, and appropriate referral of other problems requiring management and care. One of the more comprehensive definitions of primary care is offered by Estes (1978), who relates it specifically to the elderly as follows: primary health care is accessible, comprehensive, coordinated, and continual care delivered by accountable providers of personal health services. It is usually associated with the care of the whole person rather than a particular illness and attempts to deal with major medical, psychological, and social aspects of the clients' functioning in the naturalistic setting. It is distinguished from other levels of health care by the nature of the services provided, not by the particular specialty of the provider.

What is suggested here is the development of primary care comprehensive services in which multifactorial impairments of the elderly can be treated by a multidisciplinary team of physicians, psychogeriatricians, geriatric nurses, psychotherapists, psychologists, and social workers. If an elderly client is referred for medical attention or illness, various other caregivers would be able to make input into the treatment modality.

As noted by Naegle (1983), comprehensive assessment must be followed by the assumption of responsibility for the direct provision of some care, along with coordination and collaboration in service delivery by others in light of the specific needs of the individual elderly person. It is understood that the entire team of professionals will not directly deliver many of these broad-based services, and only one or two members of the team may function as key caregivers at any given time.

It is suggested that various other factors such as economic security, education, psychological protection of families, and social and emotional support that influence or facilitate adaptation in old age should be considered in the assessment. Management goals must decidedly extend beyond the alleviation of symptoms (Futrell et al., 1980), and community-based comprehensive programs should include treatment plans addressing the social, mental, and physical problems of the elderly (Blumenthal, Davie, & Morycz, 1979).

Busse and Pfeiffer (1973), for example, note a particularly intimate relationship and interaction between the existence of significant physical illness and depressive illness in old age. In some instances depression may be obscured or may mimic organic changes when toxic states secondary to infection, cerebral trauma, psychotropic drugs, alcohol, and malnutrition produce acute brain syndrome (Blumenthal, 1980). A medical and physical assessment before mental health assessment may provide information on how old problems interface with new symptoms such as withdrawal, somatization, hypochondriasis, loss of appetite, or loss of weight (Reiff, 1980). In this context the evaluation of an aged person's physical health would receive just as high a priority as mental health.

In more pervasive symptoms of suicidal tendency, for example, the involvement of the family in both initial evaluation and ongoing contact may be important as a means of assessing the interactional patterns (both functional and dysfunctional) that characterize the family system and the extent of support the family has offered in the elderly client's previous adjustment to crises. This suggests the significance of including the family system in the treatment of the elderly client. Thus, primary care must be integrated and coordinated within the framework of comprehensive services.

Specialty Clinics in Primary Health Care Settings

As knowledge of the elderly becomes more disseminated and understood, there are few valid generalizations about this age group, especially when consideration is directed to problems of assessment, rehabilitation, and intervention (Blumenthal, 1971). Staff members working in primary care settings are often overwhelmed when confronted with current nosology of symptom classes such as cognitive and behavioral deficits, somatic symptoms, organic brain syndrome, disorientation, sleep disturbances, agitation, and death anxiety. The clinician faced with this infinite heterogeneity in symptoms, cause, and treatment possibilities feels ineffectual and untrained (Flexner, 1977) when treating elderly clients with multiple symptoms. Therefore, proponents of the coordinated comprehensive services contend that the establishment of specialty clinics to assess and recommend treatment for single-factor impairments and affective disorders should also receive a similar thrust in the primary health care model.

Newer developments in comprehensive care systems are therefore beginning to incorporate primary care principles into various specialties, including the specialty for psychotherapy for behavioral deficits and pharmacology for depression (Bellak, 1976). A more recent specialty thrust in primary health care has been seen in such programs as clinics for hypochondriasis, clinics for geriatric nutrition, and clinics for alcoholics.

Klerman (1980) suggests plans to integrate a primary care approach with specialty services for alcoholism, family services for the elderly, and practitioner programs focusing heavily on psychological needs such as support in a time of bereavement, grief, and loss

(Dono, Falbe and Kail, 1979; Rauckhorst, Stokes, & Mezey, 1980). What seems to be suggested by most of these authorities is an appropriate melding of therapeutic flexibility and creativity of specialists with the sound clinical application of primary care principles.

Integration of Social Networks and Social Support Systems

The recommendations of the President's Commission on Mental Health (1978) have stressed that "a necessary goal of community mental health should be to recognize and stengthen the natural networks to which people belong" (p. 144). Biological and psychological approaches and practices appear to have dominated the behavioral-medical scene of the elderly, but lately social network theory has indicated that social network forces are of equal importance in maintaining the elderly individual's physical and mental health status (Cassel, 1976; Cobb, 1978; Pilisuk & Froland, 1978; Syme & Berkman, 1976).

Frerichs, Aneshensel, and Clark (1980) have observed, for example, that among the elderly the rate of depression in the community was clearly related to the level of perceived network support, both in the high- and low-income level groups: the higher the perceived level of social support, the lower the depression is. When the specific concerns of the aged are considered analytically, a majority are the result of social and cultural circumstances and occur in the absence of any visibly coordinated and integrated social support network systems accessible to the elderly during crises and emergencies.

Consider, for example, some of the depressive situations that the elderly face and that suggest that much of the emotional affliction of the elderly could be helped by strengthening the social networks:

- With advancing age, mobility decreases dramatically, and so does the opportunity for social interaction. It is estimated that one of five persons, aged 65 and older, has limited mobility. At age 75 the number increases markedly (Soldo, 1980).

- Advancing age is characteristically accompanied by multiple personal losses (e.g., loss of spouse, friends, and children) and social loss of roles (e.g., work, position, and status). Soldo (1980) notes that 10 percent to 25 percent of the elderly in the sixth and seventh decade of life are widowed, and approximately 70 percent of the elderly at age 75 and older have lost their spouses.

- Advancing age is characteristically accompanied by loss of resources. With retirement, income typically drops one-half and with advancing years, income is considerably depleted, and savings and assets are rapidly used up, sometimes as a function of illness (Friedman & Sjorgren, 1981).

- Isolation is another principal social factor that causes mental health concerns in the elderly. According to Soldo (1980) approximately one of seven men and one of three women over the age of 65 lives alone. Many of these older persons experience significant psychological reactions from stress caused by social isolation. Since over 80 percent of the elderly also have loss of health problems (Raskin & Sathananthan, 1979), social isolation and chronic health problems become the two most common factors leading to nursing home placement or hospitalization.

The need for social support, therefore, is clear and obvious. In many American and Canadian cities a wide range of social networks exist, but because of lack of visibility and coordination of these natural networks, there are obstacles in the attempts to use them. Given the uncertainties of arranging for community social networks to assist in any crisis, the caseworkers invariably turn to institutional settings as the only available source of treatment following emotional affliction or other physical or emotional adjustment problems likely to be encountered by many elderly. According to a report from the U.S. Department of Health, Education, and Welfare (1979), many elderly experience an obvious impoverishment and restriction in their social contacts. What they need more than medical attention is an improvement in the emotional valence of their network interactions. Strategies to improve their opportunities for social interaction and the properties of the physical and social atmosphere are implied in the following statement of programs needed for older persons:

> Safe and affordable housing; nutritious food available through "meals on wheels," and group meal services; communication and transportation services, including telephone and escorts; recreation and education programs to promote enjoyment, challenge and stimulation; community centers to offer social opportunities; in-home services such as homemaker, visiting nurse and home health care; ready access (including by telephone) to advice from a health professional; provision of eyeglasses, hearing aids, talking books, and large-print publications; legal aid and counseling services; volunteer and employment opportunities to provide a continuing sense of purpose in life; and not least of all exercise. (p. 78)

As with all health-related studies it is necessary to determine the exact effects of specific network patterns. Some social networks are good support systems for only those elderly who are active, energetic, and self-sufficient but may have negative effects on those elderly who are philosophically accepting, timid, or mildly impaired. Social networks of some patterned nature may be invaluable to individuals before retirement, but they may lose their value for those elderly whose sphere of social influence is eroded and their morale is poor.

Social network support systems may be perceived by some elderly to be intrusive, interfering, and meddling. These are often older individuals who were self-sufficient and self-reliant in their active days and who habitually reject any offers of help and support from the community networks. Therefore, it is helpful to have demographic data about communities and their social support networks to balance the experiences of individuals and families in those communities.

Interest in social networks and in their potential as support systems has increased considerably, but much further work has to be done regarding the types of elderly individual who will be best served by a specific network pattern. As the very old and very disabled increase in number and proportion, it is essential that the formal support agencies learn from the coping strategies and procedures adopted by the families, neighbors, and friends, which form the preponderant support for the elderly (Hemsi, 1982).

Social Services and Other Support Groups

Whatever the local arrangements, it is important that regular visits are paid to residential homes so that there is a regular and dependable network of contacts between the volunteer social networks, the local authority residential homes for the elderly, and when necessary, the hospital services.

Collaboration between social networks and the social services department is at least as fruitful as collaboration with geriatric hospitals. Personal relationships here, as in all other fields, are crucial. Of special importance is liaison with residential homes, which are often administered by the social services departments in the communities. This has several important implications for staffing of the homes and for their support from psychogeriatric services.

Other informally coordinated programs include arrangement with the postmen who check on the health and welfare of older people on their route, providing human contact and supplying necessary materials in the remote areas (Outreach: Sweden, 1978). Fox (1976) describes the program in England where the Samaritans provide support, contact, comfort, and preventive services for elderly persons who are depressed, disabled, or immobile. In addition to community programs in which social workers and nurses visit the sick and infirm, many senior citizen groups and clubs offer psychological and social assistance and nurturance in the form of group therapy for widows and older women's league in Los Angeles, which provides social, recreational, and occupational diversion for elderly women.

Retirement villages in many ways create ideal environments for older citizens who have the benefit of sound health and sound incomes. In the 1980s 14 to 30 percent of older Americans and Canadians have an income below poverty level and do not qualify to be a part of the congenial neighborhood environment of the retirement villages. Nevertheless, the idea is a sound one and needs to be researched and tested for lower-income groups.

Domiciliary Assessment and Home-Care Services

Busse and Blazer (1980) advocate that greater emphasis be placed on providing services that can enable elderly individuals to remain in the home setting. It is expected that such a focus will maximize the probability that health care professionals will coordinate their activities with the home. The procedure for domiciliary assessment and home care implies that assistance to family members or other caregivers will be provided long term, will be well coordinated and integrated, and will help thereby to prevent premature institutionalization.

Kahn and Zarit (1974) stress the importance of an early intervention with the family members or other caretakers to avoid institutionalization. By seeing elderly clients in their own home, more accurate evaluations can be made of their capacities to remain in that setting and to receive treatment in a manner that conforms to their own value systems and beliefs (Macmillan, 1958; Glasscote et al., 1977).

Arie and Jolley (1983) emphasize that all geriatric patients referred for treatment should be initially assessed at home and that this assessment should be made by a mental health professional including, when necessary, other members of the team (Wattis, Wattis, & Arie, 1981). It is important, however, to make the distinction between medical geriatric patients for whom the right course is immediate admission to the hospital and psycho-geriatric patients for whom there are no emergencies and who benefit more from prior but prompt assessment in the home (Arie & Jolley, 1982).

In the reasons for home assessment, a number of important benefits are implied (Glasscote et al., 1977; Macmillan, 1958, 1967; Arie & Isaacs, 1977), principally the following:

- Psychiatric problems in old people are almost always problems of function in their normal home surroundings; old people perform quite differently in unfamiliar settings. What is at issue is not function in an outpatient clinic or hospital ward but function in that normal setting (Arie & Jolley, 1982). Thus the process of moving an old person, especially an old person who is confused and has a mild degree of disorientation, to a new institutional setting may aggravate the confusion and threaten the person's independent functioning.

- On-the-spot visit enables the psychogeriatrician to speak to other caregivers including neighbors, friends, and local shopkeepers and to obtain from them a collateral history of the client and their assessment of the elderly client's ability to remain an independent resident in the home.

- The physical environment of the home is an important factor in assessment. It may also give an important picture of the elderly's failing performance, or, by contrast, adequate adjustment despite impaired mental functioning. Other risk factors at home need to be assessed, for example, steps and stairs in the house. Brain-damaged elderly individuals often have a fragile balance or equilibrium with their surroundings. They may find it difficult to cope in a new environment such as a hospital room but may be able to function reasonably well in the limited and familiar surroundings of the home. In such cases the best setting in which the elderly person's functioning should be assessed is the home (Hemsi, 1982).

- The initial home visit may also help the specialist service establish the likely material and human resources that will be available when the geriatric patient is returned to the home and is faced with the problem of rehabilitation and eventual resettlement (Glasscote et al., 1977). "The hole in the community left by a person who is removed even temporarily from home has a way of closing rapidly and it may be very difficult to resettle that person however good the recovery" (Arie & Jolley, 1982, p. 230).

The opponents of this policy of universal home assessment, however, argue that the home is not always the best place for a proper and objective mental examination and that there are many distractions. Furthermore, investigators and practitioners contend that operating such a policy is too time-consuming. It is expensive for two or more members of a team to visit at home. Finally, such a system of domiciliary assessment is greatly hampered by the long distances of rural practice and the traffic congestion of urban life. This may well prevent the consultant from being able to make the bulk of the assessments personally. However, in a majority of cases more paraprofessional help of community nurses, social workers, and voluntary statutory workers may be quite adequate (Hemsi, 1982).

These are significant points; there is no doubt that the domiciliary assessment policy is difficult to implement. Nonetheless, based on many years of extensive practice, proponents of home services for the elderly argue that the policy represents both good practice and expediency. Such a policy, although demanding in time, actually saves time spent in trying to resettle old people whose situations have been inadequately assessed by practitioners not familiar with the normal life setting of the geriatric client.

There are countries, including the United States and Canada, where administrative or financial considerations make such a policy of home visiting by specialists difficult, if not impossible. Nevertheless, many psychogeriatricians and mental health professionals recognize the potential and the promise of success. They suggest more service and more research in this area (Glasscote et al., 1977; Kahn, 1975).

A number of programs of mental health services (e.g., Barker & Black, 1971; Plutchik, McCarthy, Hall, & Silverberg, 1973; Wallen, 1970; Zimberg, 1971) are being delivered to clients in their own homes. These programs have features of home care and assistance that are based on previous concepts of halfway houses and senior citizens' community lodges.

All these programs are based on the concept of encouraging independence in the client and implementing the principle of minimum intervention.

Promise of Future Services in the Home

Kahn (1975) suggests that the elderly who live at home with their families need the assurance that more extensive assistance will be made available to them when needed. If it is guaranteed that potential services in the form of health-related facilities, nursing care, etc., will be available, many persons will paradoxically never use them. Zarit (1978) contends that many elderly who are functioning quite independently in their homes may often make the decision to relocate to a health-related facility because they fear that it will not be available at a future date. Therefore, an important aspect of comprehensive services for the elderly lies in reassuring them and their families of the future availability of old-age assistance and special services. These services may be in the form of short-term inpatient care for the chronically ill elderly and social support and relief programs for the families of the elderly who desire some respite. Glasscote et al. (1977) have described programs in several English communities that provide temporary relief for families who provide home care for their elderly relatives. Similarly Robertson, Griffiths, and Cosin (1977) have described the considerable benefits of hospital programs that relieve the burdens of families caring for their elderly relatives at home. Such guarantees to the family that health-related agencies will assume more responsibilities for the care of the elderly have the paradoxical effect of increasing the family's willingness to provide care at home. Meeting the demands of the families in a home setting can have the same impact that short-term nursing care has on the health of the elderly.

Busse and Blazer (1980) advise that greater emphasis should be placed on organizing and coordinating a comprehensive health care program (including mental health) in which a variety of preventive and outreach services are available to support those areas of independent functioning that the elderly person can retain at home, despite some degree of physical and mental disability. The success of services for the aged needs to be measured against the goals of minimum intervention by agencies and maximum independence for the elderly clients.

Comprehensive Services and Psychological Medicine

The battle for improved health care of the elderly is being fought on many fronts—economic, political, psychological, social, and medical. Reforms in the sectors of both medicine and psychology are sorely needed if care of the elderly is to be effective. Unless psychology and medical practice are restructured to accommodate psychological as well as physiological processes, psychogeriatric care will remain unresponsive to the long-term needs of the elderly. This issue involves the identification and management of social, cultural, psychological, and medical issues in the health care of the elderly.

The point that needs to be stressed is the importance of understanding both the psychological and medical determinants of the elderly's adaptation to acute and chronic illness. Any program of comprehensive services for the elderly must include a team of professionals and semiprofessionals who are knowledgeable with respect to the four intrapsychic parameters of psychological adaptation to acute or chronic illness: (1) the elderly patient's response to the psychological stress that is universally evoked by medical illness such as coronary disease and high blood pressure; (2) the extent to which the elderly person regresses psychologically and biologically as a consequence of illness, for example, the elderly person's incontinence caused by loss of bladder or bowel control; (3) the conflicts in adult-child and elderly parent relationships; and (4) the quality of the elderly patient's relationship with the psychologist (e.g., questions of transference and emotional dependence) and the relationship with the medical doctor (e.g., questions of the omnipotence of the physician or surgeon).

Both the medical personnel and mental health personnel in the comprehensive health care team need to recognize a number of changes in the course of the elderly's development. Both sets of professionals (psychologists and physicians) in the health care team must agree to treatments that are based on principles of minimum intervention, prevention of institutionalization, prevention of excess disabilities, and reinforcement of functional capacities of the elderly.

The mental health professionals and medical professionals both need to advance their knowledge and skills in the other's areas of expertise. The implementation of reciprocal training programs and basic education programs in each other's disciplines is urgently necessary. In addition to good will and good sense, physicians, psychologists, therapists, clinicians, and mental health professionals need to develop mutual confidence, skills, and knowledge about various sectors of geriatric functioning. In short the efficacy of their efforts to provide optimal care for the chronically ill elderly patients depends first on their acquiring sufficient knowledge of the biological and psychological determinants of adaptation to medical illness and the effects of medical illness on the psychological adaptation of the chronically ill elderly. Second, both must be able to elicit significant psychosocial and medical data from the elderly patient. Third, the coordination of comprehensive services for the elderly must be such that treatment plans reflect both the psychosocial and biological-medical data (cf. Strain, 1978) that have been elicited in the primary care setting.

PROTECTIVE SERVICES: PSYCHOLOGICAL AND ETHICAL TRENDS

In North American cities protective services have developed as part of a broad range of social services for older persons (Blenckner, Bloom, & Nielson, 1971). These services pertain to those aspects of medical, psychiatric, or social treatment modality required to protect an individual from abuse, neglect, safety hazards, mistreatment, or exploitation. "These are undertaken with or on behalf of persons who are unable or unwilling to secure such protection for themselves or who are without able or responsible persons acting on their behalf" (Verwoerdt, 1981, p. 299). Protective services can range from a casework or legal relationship established through a local agency to the establishment of a guardianship or conservatorship.

The elderly compared to other age groups are still the main adult population in need of protective services because of a wide range of physical as well as mental conditions that cause them to become unable to act competently on their own behalf. Protective services for the elderly are also defined in terms of measures necessary to protect them against neglect or abuse.

In Britain, Canada, and the United States the law gives the elderly persons the right to decide whether they will consent to protective services from the department of social services. If an elderly person is abused or neglected and refuses to accept protective services or lacks the capacity to consent, statutes allow protection for the elderly and flexibility to permit a guardian in assisting or in making only necessary decisions.

The central issue in protective services may not be whether they are necessary, but rather the manner in which these services are provided (Verwoerdt, 1981). Concern about the ethics of protective intervention should be foremost in the mind of the providers of these services for each elderly individual they see. The history of social services contains numerous examples of the social workers, caseworkers, or mental health professional imposing their own values and preferences on clients. The aged as a group are likely to have some values different from those of a younger social worker because of generational and educational differences. Moreover, old age carries with it certain firm notions and beliefs about self-reliance, self-esteem, and financial independence that are inconsistent with the concept of protective service, which suggests in part the recipients' inability to care for themselves. For those reasons it is critical for the caseworkers, social workers, or social services administrators to develop protective services plans that reflect the objectives and values of the elderly client. The elderly individual is more likely to give consent to some form of protective service if the necessary consultation has taken place.

By contrast a therapist, caseworker, or other professional may have to intervene directly or even forcefully with other family members or the elderly client if aware that a vigorous treatment is available for a reversible condition. Salzman and Shader (1979), for example, have noted that many cases of depression, delirium, and disorientation in the elderly may in fact be toxic reactions to medication, acute infections, and other reversible organic brain syndromes. By treating these reversible problems the extent of physical and mental disabilities in an elderly patient can be markedly reduced. However, many health care professionals may be reluctant for political reasons to intervene in the private decisions of the elderly and to recommend vigorous protective intervention.

In a caseworker's evaluation elderly clients may need protective services because they are a danger to themselves or a danger to others. When elderly clients are viewed as a danger to themselves, this suggests that they show a number of patterns of passive and active self-destructiveness, principally the following:

- inability to care for themselves in basic living activities such as eating, personal hygiene, and mobility
- inability to make use of available mental health and medical facilities because of physical isolation and lack of transportation facilities
- denial of illness, disability, or need for protective services as often seen in the responses of many elderly with chronic illness and elderly with organic brain syndrome who may be unaware of the hazards surrounding them
- poor judgment in decision making, problem solving, or function, which may be a reflection of psychiatric disturbance or mild to moderate degree of cognitive impairment in many elderly
- deterioration in personal hygiene and poor eating habits, alcoholism and other addictions, and many other obsessive-compulsive behaviors, perhaps posing a serious threat to the safety of the elderly person
- deterioration in vision, hearing acuity, and physical coordination, perhaps predisposing many elderly to accidents

Active self-destructive patterns, although less frequent, may take the form of extreme withdrawal and social and physical isolation. Refusal of medical care and nursing attention in the case of many paranoid and depressed elderly patients with suicidal tendencies may clearly warrant protective services.

An even more complex set of obstacles to the provision of protective services is presented by the elderly who are judged a danger to others. In the case of such elderly the goal of protective services is to alleviate the distress, anguish, and burden that these elderly may be causing other individuals by virtue of specific age-related impairments. Many of these stresses that the elderly involuntarily cause to others around them may take the form of encroachments on the family members' time and physical and emotional energies. A cognitively impaired elderly or one with mental disturbance may be a source of social nuisance and embarrassment to family members and neighbors.

Other forms of geriatric delinquency (Wolk, Rustin, & Scotti, 1963) may take the form of behaviors of combativeness and aggressiveness and sexual deviancy such as exhibitionism or assault. Several factors are included in deciding how much risk of endangerment to take with an elderly client. First, there should be some assessment of the probability of a particular danger to self (such as slipping in the bathtub or leaving the burners on) or danger to others, which is rare but possible (such as when an elderly person is disoriented and confused but insists on driving a car).

If the danger is minimal (i.e., it is feared but has not occurred), then the therapist or caseworker working in consultation with the family may decide to take a risk in order that the elderly client may function as independently as possible. The worker should have a frank discussion with the elderly client (unless the person has moderate or severe cognitive impairment that affects understanding of the situation) and with the family members about the advantages or limitations of the risk. The mental health worker should not presume to know what is best for the elderly client (Zarit, 1980) or that the client is unable to undertake the risk.

Legal considerations are important in the decision to provide protective services to the elderly who are neglected by families, who are unable to care for themselves, or who are a risk to the emotional health and mental well-being of the families with whom they live. However, other equally important considerations are the legal rights of the elderly to be functionally independent as long as the social system will permit. Regardless of the views of the professional, the opinion of the elderly person or the opinion of the family must be given more weight in matters that affect the functioning of the elderly client.

In some cases of severe depression, cognitive impairment, or paranoid condition, there is increasing loss of rational control on the part of the elderly client and increasing resistance to accept protective intervention. In such situations there may be an increasing need for substitute authority to step in and take over. When transfer of authority for protective intervention is sought, all auxiliary individuals such as members of the family, physicians, consultants, clergy, and the family lawyer may have to be consulted before implementation of mandatory protective intervention.

As to the question of how much pressure, force, or persuasion is necessary in enforcing intervention, the client's active self-destructiveness and active deliberate danger to others call for forceful application of external controls and intervention. Verwoerdt (1981) cautions practitioners to use the authority inherent in their professional role with discrimination and discretion and to implement protective intervention for elderly clients in a manner that is rational and well thought through. As far as possible, mandatory protective intervention should be discussed and advised only as a last resort (Muir Gray, 1980; Norman, 1980).

Whenever an old person has a disability that is persistent and impairs independence, alternatives to remaining at home may have to be considered, especially if the elder lives alone (Akhtar, Broe, Crombie, McLean, & Caird, 1973). Hemsi (1982) cautions practitioners that when the elder can make an informed decision and has the means to make the arrangements, the professional worker has the ethical obligation not to become involved. From an ethical standpoint it is imperative that protective services act in the best interests of the elderly. First, it must be ascertained that everything possible has been done to support the elder in the home setting, using all the available services and not simply those informal services that happen to be available or on the scene. Second, as far as possible some assessment must be made about how the change of environment will affect the old person. As there can be no certainty about the effects of the change, the elderly's admission to a shelter, home, or institution must be viewed as a trial or experiment.

Institutionalization is often the only feasible alternative for elders who are a danger to themselves and exploited by caretakers. Even when danger to the self is evident and the need for protective intervention is clearly established among the elderly client, the family, and the health care professional, the choice of the institution should still be given to the elderly person. The institution's ability to offer a psychotherapeutic and rehabilitative approach much be balanced against those services that the older persons cannot receive living in their own homes, and against the personality needs of the elderly clients.

When the elderly does not, or cannot, make the decision about an institution, Norman (1980) suggests that protective social services may be called on to make the difficult judgment. Such a judgment must take into account whether the elder can cognitively tell the difference between one environment and another; the balance of risks and the availability of support in the previous and new alternative accommodation; the ethical aspects raised by conflicts of interest between the elder and others; and whether medical treatment for disease and any reversible conditions will always be promptly available in the shelter or home (*British Medical Journal,* 1981).

CARE OF THE MENTALLY ILL ELDERLY

Mentally ill elderly are usually, although not always, supported in the home. Nonmedical techniques may be expected to assume increasing importance in the case of elderly patients who have few prospects of recovery, or are medically and mentally impaired. In this connection, any preventive or rehabilitation program for aged persons must take account of the extent of social disintegration or deterioration that can be avoided. It would appear that these aged persons are still capable of learning, provided the level of teaching is adapted to them and developed step by step; provided also that this happens in a therapeutic milieu that encourages them to create their own humane environment and considers their preferences within the course of treatment (Kahana, 1973). Paul (1969) proposes a number of preventive measures that would enable the mentally ill elderly to move toward some degree of independent action within the framework of the "communal life of the home":

- It is advisable to stimulate social interactions and skills by the availability of a range of social activities, by bringing into the home volunteers from the neighborhood.
- It is advisable to stress clarity in communication, with concrete instructions for appropriate conduct that are imposed on the elderly person consistently and firmly, but with compassion and empathy.
- It is advisable to provide practical opportunities for practicing domestic skills, with feedback and specific training for those skills that are useful in client self-care.

- It is advisable to use in the home a system in which the expectations for the elderly person (in terms of the degree of independence and level of responsibility) are realistic, and explained in concrete terms.

Much potential functional incapacity can be avoided or prevented in mentally ill elderly if they can be encouraged to remain involved in instrumental roles in the home. For such aged persons, the objective of preventive care is to maintain functional capacity and some degree of independent action in the home.

PREVENTIVE APPROACH TO HEALTH CARE OF THE ELDERLY

If we are to develop rational and effective strategies for a preventive approach to the psychological, psychiatric, and physical problems in the aged, it is essential that we be able to describe systematically and with some insight important psychosocial, medical, and ecological aspects of prevention. Methods of prevention, in terms of both primary prevention and secondary prevention, and the implementation and coordination of both forms need to be delineated with much greater clarity than has been achieved.

Ascertainment, Prevention, and Supervision

The dictum that old people are ill not because they are old but because there is some progressive disease process at work is true often enough to make some clear form of identification of risk factors, predisposing factors, morbidity factors, and vulnerability factors essential. The first significant thesis that has evolved, therefore, is that old people require some form of ascertainment so that their problems of physical illness, psychological anxieties, social isolation, and functional disabilities may be detected at an early stage. Simple and timely measures and continued surveillance in the form of diagnostic assessment and follow-up will prevent or at least slow physical or cognitive deterioration. This ascertainment applies not only to description but to the potential etiology of the concerns and problems anticipated in old age.

Primary health caregivers, including physicians, psychiatrists, geropsychologists, and other mental health practitioners find that old patients have come to them at a late stage in their illness. Williamson (1966) showed clearly that old people tend not to report physical illness or other mental health concerns to their doctors or other caregivers in community health services. It is probably accurate to attribute some of the underutilization of mental health and medical resources to lack of public education (Waxman, Carver, & Klein, 1984) and to the sensitivity of the elderly to negative attitudes of caregivers toward them (Levin & Levin, 1980). For a significant proportion of the elderly population, however, feelings of pessimism with regard to the inevitability of deterioration in old age are severe enough to keep them from seeking early causal factors of disease. It is fairly typical for elders or families of elders to seek medical or psychological intervention only when the elderly patient is very ill or when the social environment of the elderly patient has collapsed. It is important, therefore, from both the perspective of the patient and the community in which the normal older person resides, that the prevalence of behavioral, emotional, or physical disorders or potential disorders be ascertained within the framework of community health services. This requires an extensive program of community health services responsible for ascertainment, prevention, and supervision functions toward the older population.

The iceberg phenomenon of undetected disease and medical, psychological, and social problems of the aged living in the communities was first emphasized in Britain. The impetus for early detection was provided by Williamson et al. (1964) with respect to physical illness, and similar impetus was provided with regard to the merits of preventing mental illness and social problems (Kay, Beamish, & Roth, 1964; Brockington & Lempert, 1966).

A practical endeavor in the early diagnosis of physical, mental, and social illness has been since undertaken by Berezin and Stotsky (1977) and Bloom and Blenkner (1970), stressing the need for a preventive mobilization of community health resources for the early detection of high-risk groups in the elderly. From the experience of earlier preventive medical and mental health experimental projects (see Anderson & Cowan, 1965; Miller, 1963; Richardson, 1964) it is obvious that high-risk individuals in the older population require special and continual observation in terms of assessment, diagnosis, therapeutic intervention, and follow-up of their problems (Blenckner, Bloom, and Nielson, 1971)

High-risk groups, suggested by Williamson (1966) as needing special observation, are those living alone, those recently bereaved, those with locomotor difficulties from whatever cause, and those showing signs of mental impairment. Furthermore, Williamson emphasizes the need for a special observation of the physical, mental health, and social status of elderly recently discharged from hospitals—especially if these individuals were admitted with any evidence of self-neglect, self-injury, or a potential for suicide. The latter group may need special rehabilitation with the objective of restoring the patient to the maximum level of psychological, physical, and functional self-sufficiency. Rehabilitation, however, overlaps with prevention and intervention in so many ways that any distinction between them must be artificial. However, specific mention must be made of the fact that in preventive care, as opposed to rehabilitative care, old age should be anticipated and that prophylactic care should be given in middle life. Problems of unreported illness and methods needed for early detection are also stressed in preventive care (Currie, 1975).

Once an older person has been found to be a risk, such a person must be followed up for a long time by a member of the primary health care unit, working always in unison with the patient, the patient's family, and other medical or mental health specialists who were involved in the early ascertainment of the elderly person's problems, concerns, or disease. In any form of early ascertainment one member of the primary health care team should be kept informed of any results or implications with regard to physical factors—the use of medication and other physical agents; psychological factors—anxieties and fears, family conflict, predisposition to self-injurious behaviors, psychological interventions, or counseling being sought; and social factors—social, institutional, and environmental facilities or the lack thereof.

Methods of Prevention

In describing a preventive approach to health care, a number of modes of conceptualizing health care have emerged.

Medical Model

The medical model—probably the most frequently used by health care teams—is based on the assumption of a dichotomy between health and disease. Medical indexes of disease and health are formulated and patients' complaints and other indexes of disorders are explicated. This approach, probably more appropriately called the *medical-pathology model,* focuses on secondary as opposed to primary prevention.

Recently, several surveys and investigations of elderly samples were done within the secondary prevention framework, that is, that the goal of prevention is to prevent the progress of acute illness. For example, Andrews, Cowan, and Anderson (1971) observed a marked increase in physical illness around the age of 70 years and they identified common medical problems (i.e., cardiac insufficiency, diminishment in metabolic activity, urinary symptoms, and loss in visual and auditory acuity). Within a preventive approach this investigation suggested that there is a critical period in old age when people are more subjected to physical illness. Similar studies done within a secondary prevention model implicated nutritional deficiencies as critically contributing to ill health at age 70 (Stanton & Exton-Smith, 1970) and steady increase in disability around age 70. This assemblage of studies suggests that the potential for various physical and neurological disabilities and illness increases from 12 percent around age 65 to 80 percent at the age of 85 and over (Akhtar et al., 1973).

From a medical-preventive perspective it has been identified that a combination of obesity, hypertension, and advancing age is hazardous to health in late life and makes older men and women more prone to diseases of cerebral or coronary artery. Thus clinical judgment is important in deciding whether hypotensive agents should be used with elderly persons. Clinical judgment is needed also in deciding how much medication and supervision are necessary to the prompt forestalling of the acute progress of the illness. Acute physical and psychotic reactions demand a different mode of medical and drug management in the elderly than in middle adulthood, and the presence of concomitant factors such as bereavement, time before retirement, social isolation, and lack of social support complicates the management of physical disorders by medical or pharmacological means.

In deciding on secondary prevention methods, therefore, the health specialist must consider other factors commonly affecting older people's health such as chronic bronchitis, coronary artery disease, anemia, and diabetes. Patients with complaints can be kept active and out of the hospital by careful preventive supervision. An important aspect of the secondary prevention of physical illness in the elderly is information directed toward the prevention of accidents. A complete physical examination on a regular basis is advised, and it normally should include a rectal examination, urine test for albumin and sugar, a chest x-ray, and a routine ECG. An oral hygiene test is also recommended for preventive care of the teeth.

In older age groups the medical model puts less emphasis on primary prevention. *Primary prevention* means the use of health education starting in youth, progressing through middle age, and advancing to old age. Through proper dissemination of information the elderly can be helped to keep in good health, be self-sufficient in daily functional activities, and avoid custodial care as long as possible. As medical knowledge about the psychobiological changes of late life is improving and there appears to be a clearer identification of normal aging and disordered aging, it is possible to anticipate some of the changes of old age that will require prophylactic care in middle life. Primary prevention can be stimulated by health education programs designed for elderly persons. Broadcasts by radio and television and home visits by health workers can generate interest and give information on health care facilities available for the elderly and how to keep fit by nutrition, exercise, and recreation.

Adaptational Models

These models are not related to disease, and prevention is designed not merely to overcome barriers to effectiveness but to promote maximal integration of mental and physical health through early identification of factors promoting positive attitudes toward old age. Included in the adaptational models is a social welfare model of care, which posits that all individuals in a culture should be supplied minimal resources for maintaining sound physical and mental health. This model, contrary to the medical model of health versus disease or pathology, assumes that lack of effectiveness or pathology may be offset by increasing one's resource capacity (Eisdorfer & Stotsky, 1977) in regard to physical, psychological, or social adaptation. The criteria for effectiveness in preventive health care may be personal or social and, in the case of the aged, may relate to cohort differences and socially mitigated expectancies.

With respect to preventive mental health the adaptational model endeavors to assess the common causes of emotional disturbance in the elderly (defined as anxiety and depression) as related to physical illness. For example, a preventive adaptational model may anticipate that emotional disturbance is much commoner in those who have a physical disease. It may be concluded that the incidence of emotional disturbance does not necessarily increase with age but is more commonly associated with other factors such as bereavement, personal ill-health, neglectful family members, enforced retirement, and financial difficulties (Sheldon, 1948).

Identification of important causes and secondary factors leading to emotional upset in old age is a key component of the prevention of mental health problems in late life. Similarly social isolation increases the risk to mental ill-health as does social rejection or lack of social support, which emphasizes the need for an early ascertainment of the kinds of social activities, recreational activities, and interpersonal interactions that can stimulate and encourage health care of older people. Women are more liable to be emotionally upset in late life than are men, but this greater susceptibility to emotional upset may be attributed to the fact that more women than men live till the seventh and eighth decade of life, when chronic illness is more preponderant and contributes to anxiety and depression. Since the commonest primary causes of emotional upset in elderly women are physical disease and the adverse environment of widowhood and financial stress, preventive mental health care should emphasize the greater need for preparing women in middle life for the adverse effects of widowhood, falling income, and bereavement. Information directed toward elderly helping themselves and being encouraged to live independently, building a network of social supports and relationships, is essential to good mental health.

While the incidence of need for social support in the two sexes is comparable, older women are at greatest risk if they experience psychological or social illness in late life. Figures of 50 percent are given for the frequency of confusional states in elderly women over the age of 70; figures of 3 percent to 27 percent are given for the frequency of dementia in a community population of the elderly. This greatly increases the chances that many elderly with mild to moderate degrees of cognitive deterioration resulting from brain syndromes will be taken care of by family members and adult children. Few relatives do not play some part in caring for their older people.

Therefore, in any program of preventive health care for older persons the idea of reciprocity and mutuality in family relations must be stressed. The focus must be on healthy family relationships and the resolution of conflicts between adult children and their elderly parents. Programs of preventive family life education would be essential in an endeavor to overcome friction or potential hostility between parent and daughter or son. A supervised conference between elders and their children to formulate a proper course of action may also be required. The objective of such a conference would be to conduct a functional assessment of the various members of the family and what each member is capable of offering to the elderly relative in terms of caregiving, nurturance, and emotional support (Blazer, 1982). The early detection of suicidal impulses in the elderly person and the lack of personal and emotional resources on the part of the other family members to handle the potential crisis need to be ascertained long before a crisis. Numerous studies have revealed the high incidence of depression and suicide of 10 percent to 30 percent in older people in the community and the close association between suicidal tendencies in the elderly and lack of family support and encouragement.

Trends in Preventive Care

In recent years much emphasis has been placed on encouraging the elderly to adopt more positive and constructive attitudes toward aging and to overcome their stereotypic expectancies of the impact of old age. The emphasis more recently is on the elderly helping themselves, being assertive, and living independently.

Elliott and Stevenson (1973) have insisted that the preventive care of the elderly is the responsibility of entire communities and no one in the community should be absolved from the responsibility of looking after the aged. Custodial care of the elderly should be avoided as long as possible, and excess disability of the elderly generally fostered through custodial care should also be discouraged. The amount of unknown medical, psychological, and social need among the elderly indicates that some structured form of ascertainment of the needs of elderly persons in the community is required. Physicians, health visitors, mental health practitioners, and families are the ideal community to undertake this work.

Anderson (1978) recommends the implementation of a series of preventive health care policies and procedures, principally the policy for a biannual physical and mental health examination for older persons, including an assessment of stress, anxiety, and depression factors. Home visits by the physician and social worker are encouraged. Preventive care would call for a greater degree of coordination and better liaison between community health services, hospital staff, mental health practitioners, and social welfare agencies but would be a great advantage to the elderly (Arie & Jolley, 1982).

Preparation for retirement is stressed as a part of preventive health care of aging persons. Most mental health practitioners agree that although retirement may not represent a crisis to some elderly, preretirement assistance programs have been helpful to many elderly in anticipating problematic changes and in marshaling resources to compensate for potential financial and emotional losses following retirement (Slover, 1982; Palmore, 1982). Verwoerdt (1981) proposes a program of structured education for leisure time activity, which would be an essential part of retirement counseling both at the pre- and postretirement phase.

It will take many years to prove that the type of preventive policies and procedures suggested are of any value, but according to Anderson (1976), who reviewed the effect of early diagnostic measures procedures on the quality of life after 70, when such preventive services have been provided there has been a considerable improvement in the morale of older persons.

SUMMARY

This chapter has brought into focus a broad range of services and interventions that can be enlisted on behalf of the elderly into a model of community care and comprehensive services. Our present system of care for the psychological and physical disabilities of the elderly has been sustained by a philosophy of custodialism and long-term care in institutional facilities. Preventive community-oriented services and home-care services designed to restore and maintain the functioning of the elderly have not been readily available or accessible. The lack of viable alternatives to custodial care has caused mental health professionals to refer many elderly to long-term care facilities. Research shows that the decision to institutionalize may also be necessitated by the lack of coordinated and unified services. Such coordination requires the development of a comprehensive and community-oriented system of care with interdisciplinary professional planning and collaboration. Leaders in various disciplines related to gerontology are beginning to advocate a system of consultation between specialists and primary care practitioners. Options for including primary care components in comprehensive services are being explored.

The thesis has evolved, therefore, that a system of preventive health care (in terms of both primary and secondary prevention) is essential to the successful aging and the well-being of increasing numbers of elderly. The elderly require some special form of ascertainment so that their physical and mental health problems are detected at an early age, when preventive measures can slow deterioration. This requires the identification of high-risk groups among the elderly, but it also requires a system of primary prevention using health education, leisure education, and retirement education starting in youth through middle age and on to old age. Coordination of efforts at the community level is of prime importance.

Comprehensive services should be implemented according to the principle of maximizing the older person's functional capacities by minimum intervention and maximum reinforcement of the remaining competencies of the elderly. The development of social networks and their potential as support systems for the elderly are also stressed. Although many forms of natural and community support systems have been tried for the elderly— some with great success—more integration of these services into a program of comprehensive services is recommended. With the increasing trend toward deinstitutionalization and treatment of the elderly in the community, greater emphasis should be placed on providing services that can enable elderly individuals to remain in the home setting. Therefore, a policy of home assessment and home care that will maximize the probability of health care professionals coordinating their activities with the home is advocated.

Along with our role as clinicians, practitioners, researchers, and educators, our primary role is as social advocates of the elderly. Our obligation is to press for a change in the quality of service for older persons that leaves in the clients' own hands as much control as possible over their decisions, options, and preferences. Rather than sponsoring the traditional long-term care facilities, the emphasis must be on building up alternative services in which the elderly can be supported in the communites in which they have lived, worked, and endured.

REFERENCES

Akhtar, A.J., Broe, A., Crombie, A., McLean, W.M.R., & Caird, F.I. (1973). Disability and dependence in the elderly at home. *Age and Ageing, 2,* 102–110.

Anderson, W.F. (1976). *Practical management of the elderly.* Oxford: Blackwell Scientific Publications.

Anderson, W.F. (1978). Preventive medicine in old age. In J.C. Brocklehurst (Ed.), *Textbook of geriatric medicine and gerontology* (pp. 783–790). Edinburgh: Churchill Livingstone.

Anderson, W.F., & Cowan, N.R. (1955). A consultative health centre for older people. *Lancet, ii,* 239–240.

Andrews, G.R., Cowan, N.R., & Anderson, W.F. (1971). The practice of geriatric medicine in the community. In G. McLachlan (Ed.), *Problems and progress in medical care* (5th series) (pp. 57–86). London: Oxford University Press.

Arie, T., & Isaacs, A.D. (1977). The development of psychiatric services for the elderly in Britain. In F. Post & A.D. Isaacs (Eds.), *Studies in geriatric psychiatry* (pp. 241–261). New York: John Wiley & Sons, Inc.

Arie, T., & Jolley, D. (1982). Making services work: Organization and style of psychogeriatric services. In R. Levy & F. Post (Eds.), *The psychiatry of late life* (pp. 222–251). London: Blackwell Scientific Publications.

Barker, A., & Black, S. (1971). An experiment in integrated psychogeriatric care. *Nursing Times, 67,* 1395–1399.

Bellak, L. (1976). Geriatric psychiatry as comprehensive health care. In L. Bellak & T.B. Karasu (Eds.), *Geriatric psychiatry. A handbook for psychiatrists and primary care physicians* (pp. 3–12). New York: Grune & Stratton.

Berezin, M.A., & Stotsky, B.A. (1970). The geriatric patient. In H. Grunebaum (Ed.), *The practice of community mental health* (pp. 219–244). Boston: Little, Brown & Co.

Blazer, D.G. (1982). *Depression in late life.* St. Louis: C.V. Mosby Co.

Blenkner, M., Bloom, M., & Nielson, M. (1971). Protective services for older people: Findings for the Benjamin Rose Institute study. *Social Casework, 52,* 483–499.

Bloom, M., & Blenkner, M. (1970). Assessing functioning of older persons living in the community. *Gerontologist, 10,* 31–37.

Blumenthal, M.D. (1971). Measuring depressive symptomatology in a general population. *Archives of General Psychiatry, 32,* 971–991.

Blumenthal, M.D. (1980). Depressive illness in old age: Getting behind the mask. *Geriatrics, 35*(4), 34–43.

Blumenthal, M.D., Davie, J.W., & Morycz, R.K. (1979). Developing a curriculum in psychogeriatrics. *American Journal of Psychiatry 136*(19), 1157–1161.

British Medical Journal (1981). Leading article. *British Medical Journal, 282,* 1817–1818.

Brockington, F., & Lempert, S.M. (1966). *The social needs of the over-80's.* Manchester, England: University Press.

Burnside, I.M. (1978). *Working with the elderly: Group processes and techniques.* North Scituate, MA: Duxbury Press.

Busse, E.W., & Pfeiffer, E. (Eds.). (1973). *Mental illness in late life.* Washington: American Psychiatric Association.

Busse, E.W., & Blazer, D.G. (1980). The future of geriatric psychiatry. In E.W. Busse & D.G. Blazer (Eds.), *Handbook of geriatric psychiatry* (pp. 521–532). New York: Van Nostrand Reinhold Co.

Butler, R.N. (1977). *Alternatives to retirement.* Washington: U.S. Department of Health, Education, and Welfare.

Butler, R.N. (1977). Myths and realities of clinical geriatrics. In S.S. Steury & M. Blank (Eds.), *Readings in psychotherapy with older people.* Rockville, MD: National Institute of Mental Health.

Carp, F. (1975). Ego defense or cognitive consistency effects as environmental evaluations. *Journal of Gerontology, 30,* 707–717.

Cassel, J. (1976). The contribution of the social environment to host resistance: The fourth Wade Hampton Frost lecture. *American Journal of Epidemiology, 104,* 107–123.

Cobb, S. (1978). Social support as a moderator of life stress. *Psychosomatic Medicine, 38,* 300–314.

Currie, G. (1975). The care of the elderly. In J.H. Barber & F.A. Boddy (Eds.), *General practice medicine* (pp. 280–287). Edinburgh: Churchill Livingstone.

de Vries, H.A. (1970). Physiological effects of exercise training regimen upon men aged 52–88. *Journal of Gerontology, 25,* 325–336.

Dono, J.E., Falbe, C.M., & Kail, B.L. (1979). Primary groups in old age structure and function. *Research on Aging, 1,* 403–433.

Eisdorfer, C., & Stotsky, B.A. (1977). Intervention, treatment and rehabilitation of psychiatric disorders. In J.E. Birren & K.W. Schaie (Eds.), *Handbook of the psychology of aging* (pp. 724–748). New York: Van Nostrand Reinhold Co.

Elliott, A.E., & Stevenson, J.S.K. (1973). Geriatric care in general practice. *Journal of the Royal College of General Practitioners, 23,* 615–625.

Estes, E.H. (1978). A manpower policy of primary care. *Tar Heel Practitioner,* Summer, pp. 13–15.

Flexner, J. (1977). Dying, death, and front line physician. In D. Barton (Ed.), *Dying and death: A clinical guide for caregivers* (pp. 170–182). Baltimore: Williams & Wilkins.

Fox, R. (1976). The recent decline of suicide in Britain: The role of the Samaritan Suicide Prevention movement. In E.S. Shneidman (Ed.), *Suicidology: Contemporary development* (pp. 499–524). New York: Grune & Stratton.

Frerichs, R.R., Aneshensel, C.A., & Clark, V.A. (1980, June). *Prevalance of depression in Los Angeles County.* Paper presented at the Society of Epidemiological Research, Minneapolis.

Friedman, J., & Sjorgren, J. (1981). Assets of the elderly as they retire. *Social Security Bulletin, 44*(1), 16–31.

Futrell, M., Brovender, S., McKinnon, E., Mullett, H., & Brower, T. (1980). *Primary health care for the older adult.* North Scituate, MA: Duxbury Press.

Glasscote, R., Biegel, A., Butterfield, A., Clark, E., Cox, B., Elpers, K., Gudeman, J.E., Gurel, L., Lewis, R., Miles, D., Raybin, J., Reifler, C., & Vito, E. (1976). *Old folks at home: A field study of nursing and board and care homes.* Washington: American Psychiatric Association.

Glasscote, R., Gudeman, J.E., & Miles, C.D. (1977). *Creative mental health services for the elderly.* Washington: American Psychiatric Association.

Goffman, E. (1961). *Asylums: Essay on the social situation of mental patients and other inmates.* Garden City, NJ: Doubleday.

Hemsi, L. (1982). Psychogeriatric care in the community. In R. Levy & F. Post (Eds.), *The psychiatry of late life* (pp. 252–287). London: Blackwell Scientific Publications.

Holahan, C. (1978). *Environment and behavior.* New York: Plenum Press.

Kahana, E. (1973). The humane treatment of old people in institutions. *Gerontologist, 13,* 282–289.

Kahn, R.L. (1975). The mental health system and the future aged. *Gerontologist, 15*(1, pt. 2), 24–31.

Kahn, R.L. (1977). Excess disabilities. In S.H. Zarit (Ed.), *Readings in aging and death: Contemporary perspectives* (pp. 228–229). New York: Harper & Row.

Kahn, R.L., & Zarit, S.H. (1974). Evaluation of mental health programs for the aged. In P.O. Davidson, F.W. Clark, & L.A. Hamerlynck (Eds.), *Evaluation of behavioral programs: In community, residential and school settings* (pp. 223–251). Champaign, IL: Research Press.

Kay, D.W.K., Beamish, P., & Roth, M. (1964). Old age mental disorders in Newcastle-upon-Tyne. *British Journal of Psychiatry, 110,* 146–158.

Kistin, H., & Morris, R. (1972). Alternatives to institutional care for the elderly and disabled. *Gerontologist, 12,* 139–142.

Klerman, G.L. (1980). Klerman outlines goals of ADAMHA programs. *Psychiatric News, 40,* 23.

Levin, J., & Levin, W.C. (1980). Blaming the elderly. In J. Levin & W.C. Levin (Eds.), *Ageism: Prejudice and discrimination against the elderly* (pp. 132–147). Belmont, CA: Wadsworth.

Macmillan, D. (1967). Problems of a geriatric mental health service. *British Journal of Psychiatry, 113,* 175–181.

Macmillan, D. (1958). Hospital community relationships. In *An approach to the prevention of disability from chronic psychoses: The open mental hospital within the community.* New York: Millbank Memorial Fund.

McGivern, D. (1974). Baccalaureate preparation of the nurse practitioner. *Nursing Outlook, 22,* 94–98.

Miller, H.C. (1963). *The ageing countryman: A sociomedical report on old age in a country practice.* London: National Corporation for the Care of Old People.

Muir Gray, J.A. (1980). Section 47. *Age and Ageing, 9,* 205–209.

Naegle, M.A. (1983). The role of the psychotherapist within the primary health care model. In L.D. Breslau & M.R. Haug (Eds.), *Depression and aging: Causes, care and consequences* (pp. 156–167). New York: Springer.

Norman, A.J. (1980). *Rights and risk: A discussion document on civil liberty in old age.* London: National Corporation of the Care of Old People.

Ochberg, F.M., Zarcone, V., & Hamburg, D.A. (1972). Symposium on institutionalism. *Comprehensive Psychiatry, 13,* 91–104.

Outreach: Sweden (1978). *Ageing International, 5*(1), 8.

Palmore, E.B. (1982). Preparation for retirement: The impact of preretirement programs on retirement and leisure. In N.J. Osgood (Ed.), *Life after work* (pp. 330–341). New York: Praeger Publications.

Paul, G.L. (1969). Chronic mental patient: Current status future directions. *Psychological Bulletin, 71,* 81–94.

Pilisuk, M., & Froland, C. (1978). Kinship, social networks, social su   rt and health. *Social Science and Medicine, 12,* 273–280.

Plutchik, R., McCarthy, M., Hall, R.H., & Silverberg, S. (1973). Evaluation of a comprehensive psychiatric and health care program for elderly welfare tenants in a single-room occupancy hotel. *Journal of American Geriatrics Society, 21,* 451–459.

President's Commission on Mental Health, Special Populations Subpanel of Mental Health of Hispanic Americans. (1978). *Report to the President's Commission on Mental Health.* Washington: Government Printing Office.

Raskin, A., & Sathananthan, G. (1979). Depression in the elderly. *Psychopharmacology Bulletin, 15*(2), 14–16.

Rauckhorst, L.M., Stokes, S.A., & Mezey, M.D. (1980). Community and home assessment. *Journal of Gerontological Nursing, 6,* 319–327.

Reiff, T.R. (1980). The essentials of geriatric evaluation. *Geriatrics, 35,* 59–68.

Richardson, I.M. (1964). *Age and need: A study of older people in North East Scotland.* Edinburgh: Churchill Livingstone.

Robertson, D., Griffiths, A., & Cosin, L.Z. (1977). A community-based continuing care program for the elderly disabled: An evaluation of planned intermittent hospital admission. *Gerontologist, 32,* 334–339.

Royal College of Psychiatrists. (1979, November). Guidelines for collaboration between geriatric physicians and psychiatrists in the care of the elderly. *Bulletin, 168.*

Salzman, C., & Shader, R.I. (1979). Clinical evaluation of depression in the elderly. In A. Raskin & L.F. Jarvik (Eds.), *Psychiatric symptoms and cognitive loss in the elderly* (pp. 39–72). Washington: Hemisphere.

Sheldon, J.H. (1948). *The social medicine of old age.* London: Oxford University Press.

Slover, D. (1982). Preparation for retirement. In N.J. Osgood (Ed.), *Life after work* (pp. 342–350). New York: Praeger Publications.

Soldo, B.J. (1980). *America's elderly in the 1980s: Population Bulletin* (Vol. 35, No. 4). Washington: Population Reference Bureau, Inc.

Stanton, B.R., & Exton-Smith, A.N. (1970). *A longitudinal study of the dietary of elderly women.* London: King Edward's Hospital Fund.

Strain, J.J. (1978). *Psychological interventions in medical practice.* New York: Appleton-Century-Crofts.

Syme, S.L., & Berkman, L.F. (1976). Social class, susceptibility and sickness. *American Journal of Epidemiology. 104*(1), 1–8.

U.S. Department of Health, Education and Welfare (1979). *Healthy people: The surgeon general's report on health promotion and disease prevention.* Washington: Government Printing Office.

Verwoerdt, A. (1981). *Clinical geropsychiatry* (2nd ed.). Baltimore: Williams & Wilkins.

Wallen, V. (1970). Motivation therapy with the aging geriatric veteran patient. *Military Medicine, 135,* 1007–1010.

Wattis, J., Wattis, L., & Arie, T. (1981). Psychogeriatrics: A national survey of a new branch of psychiatry. *British Medical Journal, 282,* 1529–1533.

Waxman, H.M., Carver, E.A., & Klein, M. (1984). Underutilization of mental health professionals by community elderly. *Gerontologist, 24,* 23–30.

Williamson, J. (1966, 9 November). *Ageing in modern society.* Paper presented to the Royal Society of Health, Edinburgh.

Williamson, J., Stokoe, I.H., Gray, S., Fisher, M., Smith, A., McGhee, A., & Stephenson, E. (1964). Old people at home: Their unreported needs. *Lancet, i,* 1117–1120.

Wolk, R.L., Rustin, S.L., & Scotti, J. (1963). The geriatric delinquent. *Journal of American Geriatrics Society, 11,* 653–659.

Zarit, S.H. (1978). Predictors of outcome among day care participants. *Long Term Care and Health Services Administration Quarterly, 1,* 150–162.

Zarit, S.H. (1980). *Aging and mental disorders: Psychological approaches to assessment and treatment.* New York: Free Press.

Zarit, S.H., & Kahn, R.L. (1974). Impairment and adaptation in chronic disabilities. *Journal of Nervous and Mental Diseases, 159,* 63–72.

Zimberg, S. (1971). The psychiatrist and medical home care: Geriatric psychiatry in the Harlem community. *American Journal of Psychiatry, 127,* 1062–1066.

Index

About the Author

P.S. FRY is a counseling psychologist trained at the Pennsylvania State University and the University of Michigan. She is professor of educational psychology and chairman of the general studies program at the University of Calgary, Alberta, Canada. A former Fulbright Fellow, Woodrow Wilson Fellow, and Killam Scholar, she has published widely in mental health, clinical-developmental and gerontology journals. She serves on the editorial boards of several psychology journals. Her current longitudinal psychotherapy research on depression in the aged is supported by grants from the Department of Health and Welfare, Canada, and the Social Sciences and Humanities Research Council of Canada. She is editor of *Changing Conceptions of Intelligence and Intellectual Functioning* and author of a book (soon to be published), *Stress and Coping in the Aged: Psychological Assessment and Intervention*.